Handbook of
Veterinary Pharmacology

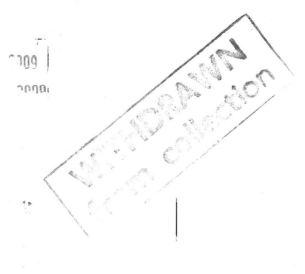

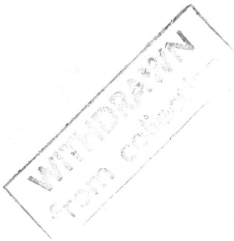

Handbook of
Veterinary Pharmacology

Walter H. Hsu

Professor of Pharmacology
Department of Biomedical Sciences
College of Veterinary Medicine
Iowa State University
Ames, Iowa

(W)WILEY-BLACKWELL

A John Wiley & Sons, Ltd., Publication

Edition first published 2008
© 2008 Wiley-Blackwell

Blackwell Publishing was acquired by John Wiley & Sons in February 2007. Blackwell's publishing program has been merged with Wiley's global Scientific, Technical, and Medical business to form Wiley-Blackwell.

Editorial Office
2121 State Avenue, Ames, Iowa 50014-8300, USA

For details of our global editorial offices, for customer services, and for information about how to apply for permission to reuse the copyright material in this book, please see our website at www.wiley.com/wiley-blackwell.

Library of Congress Cataloguing-in-Publication Data
Hsu, Walter H.
  Handbook of veterinary pharmacology / Walter H. Hsu. – 1st ed.
     p. ; cm.
  Includes bibliographical references and index.
  ISBN-13: 978-0-8138-2837-4 (alk. paper)
  ISBN-10: 0-8138-2837-6 (alk. paper)
  1. Veterinary drugs–Handbooks, manuals, etc. I. Title.
  [DNLM: 1. Veterinary Drugs–Handbooks.   2. Drug Therapy–veterinary–Handbooks.
  3. Pharmacology–Handbooks. SF 917 H873h 2008]

SF917.H78 2008
636.089'51–dc22

                            2008007204

A catalogue record for this book is available from the U.S. Library of Congress.

Set in Optima by Aptara
Printed in Singapore by Markono Print Media Pte Ltd

Disclaimer

1 2008

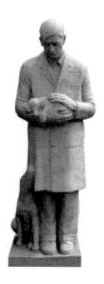

To the memory of my parents, Han-Po Hsu and Hua-Eng Yuan Hsu, for their discipline and endless love. They are the ones who taught me: "Never give up, no matter what is going on."

To my wife, Rou-Jean, for her love and putting up with me all these years with my long working hours.

To my children, Susan, Karen and her husband, Bob, for their love and patience.

To my lovely grandson, Nathan Wei-Ming.

To my brothers, Hong and Tsao, my sisters, Yun and Hui (Michelle) for their love and support since childhood.

To my old friend, Charles Cheng-Chau Wang, for sharing many thoughts and interests for more than forty years.

To my mentors, Dr. Cary W. Cooper, Dr. Gordon L. Coppoc, Dr. Franklin A. Ahrens, and Dr. Donald C. Dyer, who guided me to do research and teaching in pharmacology.

To my teachers, friends, colleagues, and students for their teaching so I can keep improving myself and treat people and animals with care and fairness.

Contents

Contributors

Franklin A. Ahrens, D.V.M., Ph.D.
Professor Emeritus of Pharmacology
Department of Biomedical Sciences
College of Veterinary Medicine
Iowa State University
Ames, Iowa

Daniel M. Betts, D.V.M., Diplomate A.C.V.O.
Professor
Department of Veterinary Clinical Sciences
College of Veterinary Medicine
Iowa State University
Ames, Iowa

Leslie E. Fox, D.V.M., M.S., Diplomate A.C.V.I.M. (Internal Medicine)
Associate Professor
Department of Veterinary Clinical Sciences
College of Veterinary Medicine
Iowa State University
Ames, Iowa

Walter H. Hsu, D.V.M., Ph.D.
Professor of Pharmacology
Department of Biomedical Sciences
College of Veterinary Medicine
Iowa State University
Ames, Iowa

Albert E. Jergens, D.V.M., Ph.D., Diplomate A.C.V.I.M. (Internal Medicine)
Professor
Department of Veterinary Clinical Sciences
College of Veterinary Medicine
Iowa State University
Ames, Iowa

Anumantha G. Kanthasamy, M.S., M.Phil., Ph.D.
Professor and Lloyd Chair in Neurotoxicology
Department of Biomedical Sciences
College of Veterinary Medicine
Iowa State University
Ames, Iowa

Arthi Kanthasamy, Ph.D.
Assistant Professor
Department of Biomedical Sciences
College of Veterinary Medicine
Iowa State University
Ames, Iowa

Richard J. Martin, B.V.Sc., Ph.D., D.Sc., M.R.C.V.S., Diplomate E.C.V.P.T.
Professor of Pharmacology
Department of Biomedical Sciences
College of Veterinary Medicine
Iowa State University
Ames, Iowa

Stephen D. Martin, Pharm.D., M.B.A.
Chief Staff Pharmacist
Veterinary Teaching Hospital
College of Veterinary Medicine
Iowa State University
Ames, Iowa

James O. Noxon, D.V.M., Diplomate A.C.V.I.M. (Internal Medicine)
Professor
Department of Veterinary Clinical Sciences
College of Veterinary Medicine
Iowa State University
Ames, Iowa

Dean H. Riedesel, D.V.M., Ph.D., Diplomate A.C.V.A.
Professor
Department of Veterinary Clinical Sciences
College of Veterinary Medicine
Iowa State University
Ames, Iowa

Wendy A. Ware, D.V.M., M.S., Diplomate A.C.V.I.M. (Cardiology)
Professor
Departments of Veterinary Clinical Sciences and Department of Biomedical Sciences
Staff Cardiologist
Veterinary Teaching Hospital
College of Veterinary Medicine
Iowa State University
Ames, Iowa

Preface

The *Handbook of Veterinary Pharmacology* is written in a concise format, which is the extension of the *National Veterinary Medical Series Pharmacology Book* (Editor: F. A. Ahrens) published in 1996. This book is not intended to provide a lengthy discussion of veterinary drugs; instead, it is designed as a handbook that contains concise descriptions of pharmacological concepts and information for the commonly used veterinary drugs available in the United States. Every effort has been made to keep the information on basic and clinical veterinary pharmacology up-to-date and concise. Whenever possible, each class of drugs is explored under the heading of "general considerations" or "introduction" to convey the basic concept and information, which is followed by a description of the pharmacology of each drug with the headings of (1) chemistry/preparations, (2) pharmacological effects/mechanism of action, (3) therapeutic uses, (4) administration, (5) pharmacokinetics, and (6) adverse effects/contraindications.

The ultimate goal of this book is to provide to both the veterinary students and practitioners the information on pharmacology that is applicable and easily retrievable. A list of suggested reading at the end of each chapter is provided for further reading of the subject. In addition, 10–20 study questions and explanations are presented at the end of each chapter.

There are two appendices at the end of the book; one on the withdrawal times for drugs used in production animals and the other on the drug dosages in various domestic species. The drug dosages in both generic name and selected trade names are listed according to chapter, drug class, route of administration, and species. I hope these two appendices will be useful to veterinary practitioners, particularly when a quick decision is needed on drug therapy.

To complete the task of writing such a book requires strong commitment of many of my colleagues. I am most grateful to the 11 contributors who put a great deal of effort in writing chapters amid their busy schedules and to their acceptance and tolerance of my editing. A special thanks to Mr. Nasser Syed, one of my graduate students, for providing many of the illustrations and helping create the index. I would also like to thank Dr. Dai Tan Vo, another graduate student of mine, for his meticulous efforts in compiling the appendices and some of the tables for this book. I am grateful to Dr. Kim D. Lanholz and Dr. Alison E. Barnhill for reviewing some of the chapters. I am indebted to Dr. Donald C. Dyer for his generosity in allowing us to utilize the information and illustrations in the chapters that he wrote for the *National Veterinary Medical Series Pharmacology Book*. The secretarial assistance of Ms. Hilary Renaud and Ms. Marilee Eischeid in preparing the manuscripts is greatly appreciated.

It is our hope that the *Handbook of Veterinary Pharmacology* will become a valuable tool for both veterinary students and practitioners.

Please send me an e-mail (whsu@iastate.edu) if you detect errors and/or have comments/suggestions for improvement of the book in the next edition. Your input will be deeply appreciated.

Walter Haw Hsu

Chapter 1

Principles of Drug Absorption, Drug Disposition, and Drug Action

Richard J. Martin and Walter H. Hsu

I. **INTRODUCTION. Pharmacology** is the study of the properties of chemicals used as drugs for therapeutic purposes. It is divided into the study of pharmacokinetics and pharmacodynamics. Veterinary pharmacology focuses on drugs that are used in domestic animals. Pharmacokinetics is the study of drug absorption, distribution, biotransformation (metabolism), and excretion. Pharmacokinetic processes affect the route of administration, doses, dose intervals, and toxicities of drugs given to animals. Pharmacodynamics is the study of cell/tissue responses and selective receptor effects. In this chapter, we introduce standard concepts of pharmacokinetics and pharmacodynamics and comment on the need to be aware of species variation when considering principles of veterinary pharmacology.

II. **DRUG ABSORPTION AND DISPOSITION**

 A. **General principles.** An overview of the principles involved in a drug's journey in the body beginning from its administration to the pharmacologic response.

 How do drugs reach their site of action? It is apparent from Figure 1-1 that a drug usually crosses several biological membranes from its locus of administration to reach its site of action and thereby produce the drug response. The manner by which drugs cross membranes are fundamental processes, which govern their absorption, distribution, and excretion from the animal.

 1. **Passive diffusion**. Cell membranes have a bimolecular lipoprotein layer, which may act as a barrier to drug transfer across the membrane. Cell membranes also contain pores. Thus, drugs cross membranes based on their ability to dissolve in the lipid portion of the membrane and on their molecular size, which regulates their filtration through the pores.

 a. **Weak acids and weak bases**. The majority of drugs are either weak acids or weak bases. The degree to which these drugs are fat soluble (nonionized, the form which is able to cross membranes) is regulated by their pK_a and the pH of the medium containing the drug. $pK_a =$ pH at which 50% of the drug is ionized and 50% is nonionized.

 b. To calculate the percent ionized of a drug or to determine the concentration of a drug across a biological membrane using the **Henderson–Hasselbalch** equation one needs to know whether a drug is an acid or a base.

 If the drug is a weak acid use:

$$pK_a = pH + \log \frac{\text{Concentration of nonionized acid}}{\text{Concentration of ionized acid}}$$

 If the drug is a weak base use:

$$pK_a = pH + \log \frac{\text{Concentration of ionized base}}{\text{Concentration of nonionized base}}$$

 c. In monogastric animals with a low stomach pH, weak acids such as aspirin ($pK_a = 3.5$) tend to be better absorbed from the stomach than weak bases because of the acidic conditions. In ruminants, the pH varies with feeds and the pH is often not low.

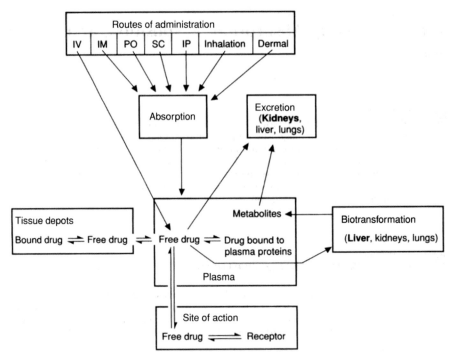

FIGURE 1-1. This diagram relates what may be expected to occur to a drug in the animal following its administration (IV, intravenous; IM, intramuscular; PO, per os or oral; IP, intraperitoneal; SC, subcutaneous; inhalation, dermal). (From Figure 1-1, *NVMS Pharmacology.*)

    d. Weak bases are poorly absorbed from the stomach since they exist mostly in the ionized state (low lipid solubility) because of the acidic conditions. Weak bases are better absorbed from the small intestine due to the higher environmental pH.

2. Filtration

    a. Some low molecular weight chemicals, water, urea, and so forth, cross membranes better than predicted on the basis of their lipid solubility, suggesting that membranes possess pores/channels.

    b. The glomerular filtration process in the kidney provides evidence for large pores, which permit the passage of large molecular weight substances but small enough to retain albumin (mw ~60,000).

3. Facilitated diffusion

    a. No cellular energy is required and it does not operate against a concentration gradient.

    b. Transfer of drug across the membrane involves attachment to a carrier (a macro-molecular molecule).

    c. Examples: Reabsorption of glucose by the kidney and absorption from the intestine of vitamin B_{12} with intrinsic factor.

    d. This is not a major mechanism for drug transport.

4. Active transport

    a. Requires cellular energy and operates against a concentration gradient.

    b. Chemical structure is important in attaching to the carrier molecule.

    c. Examples: Penicillins, cephalosporins, furosemide, thiazide diuretics, glucuronide conjugates, and sulfate conjugates are examples of acidic drugs that are actively secreted by the proximal renal tubule. Amiloride, procainamide, quaternary ammonium compounds, and cimetidine are examples of basic drugs that are actively secreted by the proximal renal tubule cells. Intestinal absorption of 5-fluorouracil, an anticancer drug, which is transported by the same system used to transport uracil.

5. Pinocytosis. This is a minor method for drug absorption, but it may be important in the absorption process for some polypeptides, bacterial toxins, antigens, and food proteins by the gut.

B. **Routes of administration**. All routes of administration except intravascular (see Figure 1-1) involve an absorption process in which the drug must cross one or more membranes before getting into the blood.

1. Alimentary routes
  a. Oral (per os, PO)
    (1) Advantages
      (a) Usually safest, convenient, economical, but some animals are difficult to administer this way.
      (b) May require the drug to be mixed in the food to facilitate administration.
      (c) Food may stimulate bile secretion, which will help dissolve lipophilic drugs to increase absorption.
    (2) Disadvantages
      (a) Acidic environment of stomach and digestive enzymes may destroy the drug.
      (b) In ruminants the bacterial enzymes may inactivate the drug.
      (c) Some drugs may irritate the GI mucosa.
      (d) The presence of food may adversely alter absorption.
      (e) Some drugs are extensively metabolized by the GI mucosa and the liver before they reach the systemic circulation (e.g., propranolol) and this is referred to as the **first-pass effect**.
      (f) Antimicrobials may alter the digestive process in ruminants and other herbivores.
  b. Rectal
    (1) Advantages
      (a) Can be used in the unconscious animal and in those vomiting.
      (b) Absorption is slower compared to the intramuscular route.
      (c) There are some drugs like diazepam and phenytoin that have an erratic oral absorption and are better given rectally.
      (d) In dogs, influence of the first-pass effect is reduced because the rectal veins bypass the portal circulation and go to the caudal vena cava.

2. Parenteral routes (circumvents the GI tract)
  a. Examples
    (1) Intravenous (IV)
    (2) Intramuscular (IM)
    (3) Subcutaneous (SC)
    (4) Intraperitoneal (IP)
    (5) Spinal and subdural. Used for regional anesthesia.
  b. Advantages
    (1) Rapid onset (IV > IM > SC), may be useful in an unconscious or vomiting patient, absorption is more uniform and predictable.
    (2) Absorption from IM and SC injection sites is mostly determined by the amount of blood flow to that site. The absorption of local anesthetics is often purposely slowed by coadministration with epinephrine, which decreases the blood flow to the injection site.
  c. Disadvantages
    (1) Asepsis is necessary.
    (2) Cause pain.
    (3) May penetrate a blood vessel during IM injection.
    (4) The speed of onset is so rapid as with IV administration that cardiovascular responses may occur to drugs, which normally have minimal effects on this system.
    (5) In food animals, discoloration of the meat or abscess formation may occur to IM injection and these may be expected to devalue the carcass.

3. Other routes

a. Dermal or topical

(1) Degree of absorption is dependent on the drug's lipid solubility.

(2) Abraded or damaged skin may be expected to absorb more drug than intact skin.

(3) Animals with thin skin, like cats, may absorb drugs like corticosteroids readily if they are applied topically than animals with thicker skin.

(4) It is convenient and allows nonskilled operators to administer the drugs by pour-on methods. For example, topical application of anthelmintics that are lipophilic, like levamisole and macrocyclic lactones, is frequently performed in this manner.

b. Inhalation

(1) It is used for volatile or gas anesthetics. Example: isoflurane.

(2) Response is rapid because of the large surface area of the lungs and large blood flow to the lungs.

(3) It is reversible if the anesthetic is turned off and the animal ventilated.

C. Drug distribution

1. Distribution refers to the reversible transfer of drug from one site in the body to another site.

2. In much of the body, the junctions between the capillary endothelial cells are not tight thereby permitting free (unbound to plasma proteins) drug to rapidly reach equilibrium on both sides of the vessel wall.

3. Distribution of drugs into the central nervous system (CNS) and cerebrospinal fluid (CSF) is restricted due to the **blood–brain barrier** (BBB).

a. There are three processes that contribute to keeping drug concentration in the CNS low:

(1) In much of the CNS (except: area postrema, pineal body, posterior lobe of hypothalamus), the capillary endothelial junctions are tight and glial cells surround the precapillaries. This reduces the filtration process and requires that drugs diffuse across cell membranes to leave the vascular compartment and thereby enter the extracellular fluid or CSF. This ability to cross cell membranes is dependent upon the drug's lipid solubility.

(2) Cerebrospinal fluid production within the ventricles circulates through the ventricles and over the surface of the brain and spinal cord to flow directly into the venous drainage system of the brain. This process continues to dilute out the drug's concentration in the CSF.

(3) Active transport mechanisms are found for organic acids and bases in the choroid plexus, which transports drug from the CSF into the blood. P-glycoprotein is one transporter protein that is present in the endothelial cells of the choroid plexus (blood–brain barrier) that contributes to drug entry into and exit from the brain.

Examples: The macrocyclic lactones, ivermectin, and selamectin but less so with moxidectin, are excluded from the brain via P-glycoprotein. In some breeds of dog, particularly the Collies, P-glycoprotein is defective and ivermectin accumulates in the CNS, leading to toxicity.

Penicillin (a weak acid) concentrations in the CNS are kept low due to an active organic ion transporter system.

4. Plasma protein binding of drug can affect drug distribution since only the free (unbound) drug is able to freely cross cell membranes (see Figure 1-1, II A).

$$\text{drug} + \text{protein (free)} \leftrightharpoons \text{Drug} - \text{protein (bound)}$$

Acidic drugs are bound primary to **albumin** and basic drugs are bound primarily to α_1-**acid glycoprotein**. Steroid hormones and thyroid hormones are bound by specific **globulins**, respectively, with high affinity.

a. Drug–protein binding reaction is **reversible** and obeys the laws of mass action.

b. Binding does not prevent a drug from reaching its site of action but retards/slows the rate at which it reaches a concentration sufficient to produce a pharmacologic effect.

c. Drug–protein binding limits glomerular filtration as an elimination process since bound drugs cannot be filtered. Example: sulfa drugs with a high degree of binding to protein are eliminated more slowly in urine than those sulfa drugs with a lower binding affinity for plasma proteins.

d. Binding to albumin does not totally prevent the elimination of drugs that are actively secreted by the kidney or metabolized by the liver, rather it slows the rates of metabolism and/or secretion. Binding lowers the free drug concentration but there is still release from the drug–protein complex for the metabolism or secretion.

e. Drug interactions may occur when two drugs are used that bind at the same site on the plasma proteins. Competition for the same site will increase the percent of drug in the free form, thereby increasing the pharmacologic/toxicological response by the displaced drug.

5. Drug redistribution can terminate the drug response.

a. The biologic response to a drug is usually terminated by metabolism/biotransformation and excretion.

b. Redistribution of a drug from its site of action to other tissues will lower its concentration at its site of action, thereby terminating the drug response.

c. Drugs exhibiting the redistribution phenomenon are highly lipid soluble. Thiopental is the classic example in dogs where redistribution from the brain to less vascular area of the body, including the muscle and fat, allows recovery. In sheep and goats, however, liver biotransformation takes place at such a high rate so that in these species it is metabolism, not redistribution that dominates the duration of anesthesia. Propofol is very lipophilic and is rapidly redistributed following IV injection so that in goats and dogs anesthesia is ultrashort. Interestingly, the redistribution process varies between breeds of dogs due to the different leanness of the different breed. Very lean breeds like Greyhounds with less fat for the lipophilic anesthetics to redistribute to, take longer to recover.

6. Drug distribution from dam to fetus.

a. Drug transfer across the placenta occurs primarily by simple diffusion.

b. Drugs cross the placenta best if they are lipid soluble (nonionized weak base or acid).

c. The fetus is exposed to some extent even to drugs with low lipid solubility when given to the dam.

d. General rule: Drugs with an effect on the maternal CNS have the physical–chemical characteristics to freely cross the placenta and affect the fetus. Examples: anesthetics, analgesics, sedatives, tranquilizers, and so forth.

D. **Drug metabolism/biotransformation** is the term used to describe the chemical alteration of drugs (xenobiotics) as well as normally found substances in the body.

1. Principles

a. Following filtration at the renal glomerulus most lipophilic drugs are reabsorbed from the filtrate.

b. Biotransformation of drugs to more water-soluble (polar) chemicals reduces their ability to be reabsorbed once filtered by the kidney. This enhances their excretion and reduces their volume of distribution.

c. The **liver** is the most important organ for biotransformation but the lung, kidney, and GI epithelium also play a role.

d. Drug biotransformation frequently reduces the biological activity of the drug/chemical/toxicant.

e. Drug metabolism/biotransformation is not synonymous with drug inactivation as the parent chemical may be transformed to a chemical with greater or significant biologic activity.

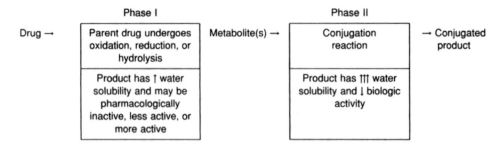

FIGURE 1-2. Phases of biotransformation. (From Figure 1-2, *NVMS Pharmacology.*)

Example:

Acetylsalicylic acid	→	salicylate
Inactive (aspirin)		active anti-inflammatory
febantel	→	fenbendazole/oxfendazole
Inactive		active anthelmintic
Primidone	→	phenobarbital
Inactive		active anticonvulsant
codeine	→	morphine
active analgesic		more active analgesic

2. Enzymatic reactions in biotransformation usually occur in two phases (Figure 1-2):
    a. **Phase I** biotransformation enzymes are found in the **smooth endoplasmic reticulum** of the hepatic cells (also referred to as the **microsomal enzymes** since they are found in the microsomal fraction following high-speed centrifugation).
       (1) **Oxidation** is carried out by a family of isozymes termed cytochrome P450s.
       (2) The enzyme system is also called a **mixed function oxidase** since one atom of oxygen is incorporated in the drug molecule and the other atom of oxygen combines with hydrogen to form water. Nicotinamide adenine dinucleotide phosphate (NADPH) provides the reducing equivalents. Examples of microsomal oxidation:
          (a) **Side chain and aromatic hydroxylation**: pentobarbital, phenytoin, phenylbutazone, propranolol
          (b) **O-dealkylation**: morphine, codeine, diazepam
          (c) **N-oxidation**: acetaminophen, nicotine, phenylbutazone, pentobarbital
          (d) **S-oxidation**: phenothiazines (acepromazine, chlorpromazine), cimetidine
          (e) **Deamination or N-dealkylation**: lidocaine
          (f) **Desulfuration**: thiopental
       (3) **Nonmicrosomal oxidation**
          A few chemicals are oxidized by cytosol or mitochondrial enzymes.
          (a) **Alcohol dehydrogenase** and **aldehyde dehydrogenase. Example:** ethanol, acetaldehyde, ethylene glycol
          (b) **Monoamine oxidase. Example:** epinephrine, norepinephrine, dopamine, serotonin
          (c) **Xanthine oxidase. Example:** theophylline
       (4) **Oxidative metabolism.** There are considerable differences among the species in the activity of the oxidative enzymes. Generally, the difference has been attributed to differences between the kinetic parameters (Michaelis constants and Max velocity) of the species enzymes. Oxidation is higher in horses than cattle, which in turn are higher than dogs. Oxidation is lowest in cats among domestic animals. The level of oxidative enzymes is lower in very young animals. The duration of pentobarbital anesthesia in horses is much shorter than in dogs. Young calves are much more sensitive to pentobarbital and lindane than adult cattle.

TABLE 1-1. Drug Conjugation Reactions

Conjugation Reaction	Drug Conjugated
Glucuronidation	Aspirin, morphine, sulfadimethoxine, digitoxin, steroids, thyroxine, phenobarbital, phenytoin, chloramphenicol, phenylbutazone
Acetylation	Sulfonamides, clonazepam, procainamide
Glutathione formation	Ethacrynic acid
Glycine formation	Salicylic acid, nicotinic acid
Sulfate formation	Catecholamines, acetaminophen
Methylation	Catecholamines, histamine

(5) **Reduction** biotransformation reactions are **less frequent** than oxidation-type reactions. Enzymes are located in both microsomal and nonmicrosomal fractions. **Examples:** chloramphenicol and naloxone.

(6) **Hydrolysis** reactions occur with either ester (esterases) or amide linked chemicals (amidases).

(a) **Esterases** occur primarily in nonmicrosomal systems and are found in the plasma, liver, and other tissues. Examples of drugs hydrolyzed: acetylcholine, succinylcholine, and procaine.

(b) **Amidases** are nonmicrosomal enzymes found primarily in the liver. Examples of drugs hydrolyzed: acetazolamide, lidocaine, procainamide, sulfacetamide, and sulfadimethoxine.

b. **Phase II** biotransformation (conjugation) may occur to a phase I metabolite or to a parent drug/chemical. This involves the coupling of an endogenous chemical (glucuronic acid, acetate, glutathione, glycine, sulfate, or methyl group to the drug). Enzyme systems are present in the microsomes, cytosol, and in the mitochondria.

(1) Products of phase II biotransformation have greater water solubility and are more readily excreted via the kidney.

(2) Examples of drugs undergoing phase II biotransformation (Table 1-1).

(3) **Species variation in phase II metabolism.** There are considerable species defects in certain conjugation reactions:

(a) In the cat, glucuronide synthesis where the target is $-OH$, $-COOH$, $-NH_2$, $=NH$, $-SH$ is only present at a low rate. Thus, cats often have longer plasma $t_{1/2}$ for many drugs than other species.

(b) In the dog acetylation of aromatic-NH_2 groups is absent and this affects the metabolism of sulfonamides and other drugs.

(c) In the pig sulfate conjugation of aromatic-OH, aromatic-NH_2 groups are only present at a low extent.

(4) Enterohepatic recirculation

(a) Drugs biotransformed via the formation of a glucuronic acid metabolite may be eliminated via the bile.

(b) Glucuronide metabolites can be hydrolyzed by intestinal or bacterial β-glucuronidases, thereby releasing free drug, which can then be reabsorbed. This process can greatly increase a drug's residence in the body. This is recognized for etorphine in horses and may give rise to relapse despite initial reversal with the antagonist diprenorphine.

(5) Biotransformation by GI microflora. In addition to the liver, metabolism of drugs can also take place in the rumen and GI tract by the microflora where hydrolytic activity and reductive activity may occur. Gut-active sulfonamides (phthalylsulfathiazole) require hydrolysis for the release of sulfathiazole for antimicrobial action. Cardiac glycosides are hydrolyzed in the rumen and become inactive, the chloramphenicol $-NO_2$ group is reduced and the drug is inactivated.

FIGURE 1-3. Proximal renal tubule. Only drugs (D) which are free in the plasma are filtered. Once in the tubular lumen the drug may be passively re-absorbed. In the proximal renal tubule active transport mechanisms exist for se-creting acid and base drugs (D) from the extracellular fluid into the renal tubule.

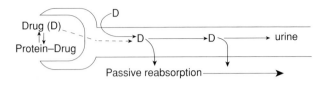

E. **Drug excretion** refers to the processes by which a drug/drug metabolite is eliminated from the body. The **kidney** is the primary organ for drug excretion.

1. **Renal excretion.** Primary mechanisms.
   a. **Glomerular filtration.** All drugs (**D**, Figure 1-3) not bound to plasma proteins are filtered.
   b. **Active tubular secretion.** In the **proximal** portion of the renal tubule **active transport** mechanisms exist for both **acidic** and **basic drugs**. Examples of drugs actively secreted into the tubule lumen are presented above. **Competition** among the acidic drugs or basic drugs can be expected to occur for the secretion pro-cess (Table 1-2).
   c. **Passive tubular reabsorption.** The lipid nature of the cellular membrane lining the tubule dictates that only **lipophilic drugs will be reabsorbed**.
      (1) Since most drugs are weak acids or bases the degree of ionized (water sol-uble, non-reabsorbable) or nonionized (lipid soluble, reabsorbable) form of the drug will vary with the pK_a of the drug and the pH of the lumen urine.
      (2) Urinary pH of carnivore animals is acidic (pH 5.5–7.0).
      (3) Urinary pH range of herbivore animals is 7.0–8.0.
      (4) Food will influence the urinary pH for both carnivores and herbivores.
      (5) **Excretion** can be **enhanced** for drugs eliminated primarily by the kidney through altering the pH of the urine. For practical purposes this is limited to weak acidic or weak basic drugs with a pK_a of 5–8.
      (6) Quaternary drugs (R_4-N^+) are polar at all urine pH and can be expected to be eliminated rapidly, since they cannot be reabsorbed.
2. **Other routes of excretion**
   a. **Biliary secretion.** Both the parent drug and glucuronide form of the drug may be eliminated via the bile.
      (1) **Glucuronide-drug** conjugates eliminated via the bile may be hydrolyzed by β-glucuronidases from gut bacteria. The free drug then may be reabsorbed giving rise to "enterohepatic recycling."
      (2) Transport processes exist in the liver for actively transporting acidic, basic, and neutral drugs into the bile. Since these drugs may eventually be re-absorbed from the gut lumen, biliary elimination processes tend to be less important than are renal excretion processes.

TABLE 1-2. Examples of Drugs Actively Secreted

Acid Drugs	Basic Drugs
Penicillin	Histamine
Ampicillin	Amiloride
Cephalosporins	Cimetidine
Thiazine duretics	Procainamide
Furosemide	Neostigmine
Probenecid	Trimethoprim
Salicylate	Atropine
Ethacrynic acid	
Phenylbutazone	

(3) **Role of P-glycoprotein in drug excretion.** P-glycoprotein is a transmembrane efflux pump that has a role in the "first-pass clearance" of some oral drugs. P-glycoprotein is also found in the biliary and renal tubular epithelia and thus plays a role in the "secretion" of some but not all drugs into the gut and renal tubules. As stated earlier, this protein is also found in the BBB and its effect there is to "expel" the drug from the CNS. Substrates of P-glycoprotein include azole antifungal agents, corticosteroids, cyclosporine, digoxin, diltiazem, doxorubicin, opioids, macrocyclic lactones, macrolide antibiotics, quinidine, and vincristine/vinblastine.

b. **Milk.** While this is not a major route for drug excretion for the dam, it is important since the drugs given to the dam appear in the milk and produce residues requiring a withdrawal period if the milk is to be used for human consumption. Antimicrobial drugs given to the dam appear in concentrations sufficient to treat mastitis. **Milk is acidic relative to plasma.** Therefore, weak organic bases will diffuse from the plasma into the milk where they will become more ionized, thereby preventing passage back to the plasma. This is an example of **ion trapping.** Drugs which are basic (tylosin, erythromycin, and lincomycin) can be expected to be found in milk in higher concentrations than in the plasma.

c. **Saliva.** This is not a major route for excretion but is important in herbivores receiving parenteral antimicrobial drugs. Drugs enter the saliva by passive diffusion from the blood. Copious salivation by cattle and sheep and the swallowing of antimicrobial-drug-laden saliva may upset the digestive process in the rumen.

d. **Expired air.** This route of elimination is primarily important for volatile drugs such as gas anesthetic drugs.

e. **Minor routes of excretion: tears and sweat.**

F. **Pharmacokinetics** is the mathematical description of drug concentrations in the body. Frequently in pharmacokinetics, the distribution of drugs is depicted as being in a compartment, that is, a one-compartment model or in a two- or three-compartment model. Since many drugs used in veterinary medicine can be described by a two-compartment open model this will be the only model described but the reader should refer to standard textbooks for information on other pharmacokinetic models.

1. **Two-compartment model (Figure 1-4)**
    a. Mathematically, the log-concentration–time graph can be depicted as composed of two straight lines.
        (1) The line representing the distribution phase has an intercept "A" and a slope $-\alpha$.
        (2) The line representing the elimination phase has an intercept "B" and a slope $-\beta$; β is used to calculate the elimination half-life, see below.
    b. The theoretical plasma concentration at time zero (C_p^0) is: $C_p^0 = A + B$. Units are usually µg/mL or µg/L.
    c. The apparent volume of distribution (V_d) is a proportionality constant relating the plasma drug concentration to the total amount of drug in the body.

$$V_d = \frac{\text{Dose}}{\left(\dfrac{A}{\alpha} + \dfrac{B}{\beta}\right)\beta}.$$

The apparent volume of distribution gives a measure of how well distributed the drug is within the body. A high volume of distribution like 1 L/kg for a drug implies that the drug is widely distributed throughout the body water.

    d. **Half-life** $(t_{1/2})$ of a drug is the time needed for the drug concentration to be reduced by half. This value is determined during the elimination phase of the drug.

$$t_{1/2} = \frac{\ln 2}{\beta} = \frac{0.693}{\beta}$$

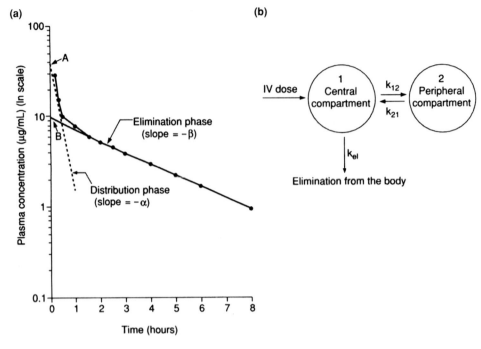

(a)

(b)

FIGURE 1-4. (a) The plasma-concentration–time graph following IV injection of a drug exhibiting two-compartment pharmacokinetics. The distribution phase is represented by the line with intercept A and slope $-\alpha$. The elimination phase is represented by the line with intercept B and slope $-\beta$. **(b)** A model of a two-compartment open model. The central compartment represents rapid equilibration and represents fluids such as the blood, interstitial fluid, and highly perfused organs (e.g., the lungs). The peripheral compartment reaches equilibrium more slowly and represents organs such as bone and fat. K_{12} and k_{21} = the rate constants of distribution between the central and peripheral compartments. (From Figure 1-3, *NVMS Pharmacology*.)

    (1) $t_{1/2}$ is usually limited by the processes of biotransformation and renal excretion; sometimes it is governed by slow release from tissue sites like bone or fat.

    (2) Indicates the time required to attain 50% of the steady state or to lose 50% of the steady state concentration.

    (3) Has limited value as an indicator of drug residues or distribution.

  e. Total body clearance (Cl_B) is the volume of blood that is effectively cleared of a drug in a specified period of time.

$$Cl_B = \beta \cdot V_d = \frac{0.693\, V_d}{t_{1/2}}$$

Clearance expresses the rate of drug removal from the body that is independent of $t_{1/2}$. Disease and infection may alter drug distribution and clearance, but not necessarily the $t_{1/2}$ value. Therefore, the volume of distribution and clearance can be altered and thus the $t_{1/2}$ will be altered. We can rewrite the equation as:

$$t_{1/2} = \beta \cdot V_d = \frac{0.693 \cdot V_d}{Cl_B}$$

  f. Bioavailability (F) is a term that describes the fraction of drug entering the systemic circulation intact from the site of administration; it is the fraction absorbed or taken up.

    By definition the bioavailability of an IV dose = 100% or 1. All other routes of administration will have a bioavailability of less than one. Knowledge of F for oral dosage is particularly important. The presence of **food** may alter the bioavailability of some drugs.

$$F = \frac{(AUC)^{nIV} \cdot dose^{IV} \cdot \beta^{n.IV}}{(AUC)^{IV} \cdot dose^{nIV} \cdot \beta^{IV}},$$

where AUC is the area under the plasma concentration curve; nIV is the non-intravenous route of administration; IV is the intravenous route of administration; and β is the slope of the elimination phase.

g. Determination of dosage

Knowledge of a drug's bioavailability (F), clearance (Cl_B), and the average steady state concentration ($\overline{C}_P\infty$) of a drug needed to produce the pharmacologic response permits dosage calculation.

$$\frac{F \cdot dose}{\text{Dosing interval}} = \overline{C}_{P\infty} \cdot Cl_B.$$

G. **Species variation.** Veterinarians must be aware of differences between species and also of differences that can occur among breeds.

1. Examples of species variation

a. It is recognized that xylazine (an α_2-adrenergic agonist) is a much more potent sedative in cattle than other species; the reason that ruminants are more sensitive to α_2-agonists such as xylazine is because the difference is at the pharmacodynamics level; ruminants have α_{2D}-receptors and nonruminants have α_{2A}-receptors.

b. It is recognized that morphine (a μ-opioid agonist) is more potent in cats than dogs. In dogs, the dose is 1 mg/kg where it consistently produces sedation. In cats, the dose for analgesia is 0.1 mg/kg. Higher doses in cats may produce excitement. The excitement in cats appears to be mediated by central dopamine receptors and is inhibited by sedatives with dopamine antagonist actions like droperidol. The detailed explanation for this species difference between dogs and cats is not known.

c. Certain breeds of dog: Great Dane and Irish Setters are more sensitive to bloat following xylazine administration due to aerophagia.

d. Ivermectin can cause CNS depression in collies at normal doses due to a defect in the P-glycoprotein transporter which excludes ivermectin from the brain.

e. Ivermectin should not be used in tortoises or crocodiles because of potential toxic effects; it is possible that the BBB in these species against ivermectin maintained by the P-glycoprotein is not secure.

f. Succinlycholine, a depolarizing muscle relaxant, can be used in horses where it is broken down rapidly by the plasma esterases, but in ruminants where the esterase levels are much lower require only 0.02 mg/kg, but horses require 0.1 mg/kg.

g. Cats have a low level of glucuronyl transferase so that the $t_{1/2}$ of many drugs that are conjugated to glucuronide by the liver is much longer. The classic example is aspirin where the $t_{1/2}$ in cats is 25–35 hours compared to 8 hours in dogs and 1 hour in horses.

h. GI absorption will differ between nonherbivores animals and ruminant herbivores. The GI transit time in monogastrics animals means that oral suspensions are swept out of the intestine within 24 hours. The benzimidazoles are examples of drugs where the GI transit time in herbivores is longer than in nonherbivores. In most cases, benzimidazoles are administered once to herbivores, but to nonherbivores, in daily doses over a period of 3–5 days.

i. Most lipophilic organic bases, like ivermectin, lincosamide, tulathromycin, erythromycin, tylosin, ketamine, metronidazole, enrofloxacin, theophylline, and trimethoprim have larger volumes of distribution in ruminants than in monogastrics animals.

2. **Drug metabolism.** The differences in the rate of elimination for drugs that are metabolized by the liver usually accounts for most of the differences in the $t_{1/2}$ values between species. There is a wide variation in the $t_{1/2}$ of most drugs that are eliminated mainly by hepatic metabolism.

  a. The general trend is that cattle and horses have shorter $t_{1/2}$ values than the dog and cats which often have longer $t_{1/2}$ values. Cattle and horses oxidize drugs more efficiently than dogs and cats.

  b. Because pharmacokinetic parameters including $t_{1/2}$ values are more available for humans, it is important to appreciate that human values are usually longer than those of domestic animals (except cats), because the oxidation of drugs by liver P450 oxidative enzymes in domestic animals is usually faster than in humans.

  c. The exceptions include the methylxanthines (e.g., theophylline) in horses and phenylbutazone in cattle, which have longer $t_{1/2}$ values in these animals than in humans.

  d. There are also differences between more closely related species. Cefitofur, trimethoprim, and sulfamethazine have a shorter $t_{1/2}$ value in goats than sheep, while $t_{1/2}$ of phenylbutazone is shorter in donkeys than horses.

  e. The $t_{1/2}$ of extensively metabolized drugs is shorter in mice, rats, rabbits, and guinea pigs (lab animals) than in domestic animals.

  f. It is also important to be careful about comparing duration of action between different species of birds. There is significant variation between $t_{1/2}$ values of chickens, turkeys, and different wild birds which is again related to differences in metabolism.

  g. Although there are different types of cholinesterase in the tissues and blood, the overall levels in ruminants are lower than in horses and humans. This means that sheep, goats, calves, and cattle, are more sensitive to organophosphorous compounds than horses and humans. Sheep have been suggested as possible "sentinel" animals for the detection of toxic anticholinesterase (organophosphate nerve gases) because of their sensitivity.

3. **Ionized drugs.** There is much less variation in the $t_{1/2}$ values between the species for drugs that are more ionized, and have a lower volume of distribution: renal excretion is the main route of elimination. For example, the $t_{1/2}$ of gentamicin for cats is 82 minutes, for dogs it is very similar, 75 minutes. Penicillins and cephalosporins also have short $t_{1/2}$ values of 30–90 minutes in different species. Thus, highly "ionized drugs" are less likely to show species variation.

4. **Cold-blooded animals.** Fish and reptiles have longer $t_{1/2}$ values compared to mammalian species due to the much lower metabolic rates. However, the temperature of the ambient environment affects the metabolic rate of the animals and this, in turn, affects the $t_{1/2}$ values of the drug. The $t_{1/2}$ value of trimethoprim given IV to carp is 41 hours at 10°C but 20 hours at 24°C. Fish also have a lower renal function and more enterohepatic recycling than warm-blooded animals.

5. **Distribution and species variation.** Distribution does vary with species, but less so than $t_{1/2}$ values. There is a significant difference between nonruminant and ruminants in the distribution of lipid-soluble organic base drugs. The rumen has a pH of 5.5–6.5 and is a large volume relative to the whole body water; because of the large capacity of the rumen, which is up to 25 liters in sheep and up to 220 liters in cattle, the phenomenon of "ion-trapping" leads to the accumulation of weak bases in the rumen fluids. This means that xylazine, furosemide, and phenylbutazone have larger volumes of distribution in ruminants so that these compounds have a greater clearance in ruminants than nonruminants.

H. **Effect of disease states on pharmacokinetic parameters.** We have seen above that the distribution of drugs (V_d) and $t_{1/2}$ values are key factors that affect access, concentration, and duration of action of drugs. These parameters are usually determined in healthy animals. However, veterinarians need to treat sick animals with these drugs, so **how do the pharmacokinetics change in diseased animals?**

  1. **Effects of fever.** Endotoxin-induced fever can increase the extravascular distribution of ionized drugs like penicillins, cephalosphorins, and aminoglycosides,

although without much effect on $t_{1/2}$ values and renal clearance. Bacterial infections induced experimentally in pigs can increase the volume of distribution of penicillin G, ampicillin, and decrease that of oxytetracyline. The volume of distribution of the penicillins probably increases because the permeability of the inflamed tissue barriers to penicillins increases. The distribution of oxytetracyline may decrease because of binding to inflammatory exudates.

2. **Liver disease.** Drugs whose $t_{1/2}$ values are determined by liver metabolism, that is, lipophilic drugs in general, and which undergo conjugation to convert them to more polar drugs can be affected by liver disease. Liver microsomal activity can be reduced in the presence of moderate or severe liver damage and so the effect and duration of drugs metabolized by the liver can be increased.

3. **Kidney disease.** The rates of elimination of drugs that are eliminated mostly via the kidney are decreased with renal disease. Renal blood flow affects all three renal excretion mechanisms of glomerular filtration, carrier-mediated secretion, and pH-dependent passive reabsorption.

I. **Effect of stereoisomers.** Many of the drugs that are used for therapeutic purposes have a chiral carbon so that a number of stereoisomers are possible; they are produced during the chemical synthesis of the compounds. Many of the commonly used therapeutic drugs are produced as a mixture of racemates. Because of the stereoselective nature of drug receptors, the mixture of racemates will contain the active moiety and the isomeric ballast (reduced activity racemates).

1. Tetramisole was originally produced by Jansen Pharmaceutical and subsequently the l-isomer, levamisole, was produced as the active compound and the d-isomer, dexamisole, found to be less active but contributed to toxicity of the racemic mixture.

2. Medetomidine is a racemate mixture, whereas dexmedetomidine, the d-isomer, has much more potent α_2-agonistic activity than the l-isomer of medetomidine.

3. The metabolism of the stereoisomers may also be selective, favoring one isomer over others. The more potent isomer is referred to as the **eutomer** and the less potent enantiomer as the **distomer**. The stereoselective processes involved in the pharmacokinetic processes can be species-dependent and so concentration–time plots may vary between enantiomers and between the different species of animal.

III. PHARMACODYNAMICS: MECHANISMS OF DRUG–RECEPTOR INTERACTIONS

A. Drugs and drug receptors

1. Many drug receptors are protein macromolecules present in cell membranes, which when activated initiate a biochemical change within the cell/tissue that in turn produces a pharmacologic response.
   a. **Receptors bind ligands (drugs) and transduce signals (a process referred to as signal transduction)**
   b. Drug binding to receptors uses similar **chemical bonds** as that used for enzyme–substrate interaction: hydrogen bonds coordinate covalent bonding and Vander Waals forces. Examples of covalent bonding involved in drug–receptor interactions are few in number.
   c. Drugs have two identifiable properties: **affinity** for the receptor and **intrinsic activity**.
      (1) **Intrinsic activity** is the property of the drug that permits it to initiate post-receptor processes, which lead to a response.
         (a) **Agonists** are drugs that have both **affinity** and **intrinsic activity**. Examples: epinephrine, acetylcholine, angiotensin, and prostaglandin $F_{2\alpha}$.
            i. **Full agonists versus partial agonists.** A *full agonist* is a drug that appears able to produce the full cell/tissue response. A *partial agonist* is a drug that provokes a response, but the maximum response is less than the maximum response to a full agonist; this is because a partial

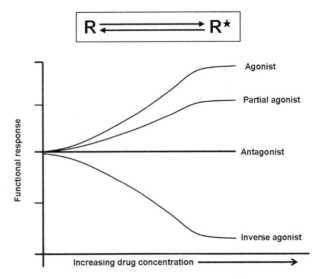

FIGURE 1-5. Ligands may be classified as agonists (full, partial, and inverse) and antagonists. Both full and partial agonists stabilize the active state (R*) and thus increase receptor signaling, whereas inverse agonists stabilize the inactive state and thus decrease basal receptor signaling. Antagonists, which have equal affinity for both R* and R and thus do not affect the equilibrium between the two states, but will reduce the ability of full, partial, and inverse agonists to bind to the receptor. (Modified from Leurs R. et al., *Clin. Exp. Allergy*, 32:4989–498, 2002.)

agonist has much higher affinity for the receptor, but less intrinsic activity than a full agonist. Concurrent administration of a partial agonist can reduce/antagonize the effect of a full agonist (Figure 1-5).

ii. **Inverse agonists.** In the context of receptors which exert constitutive signaling activity, even in the absence of an agonist, *inverse agonists* are drugs that bind to the receptor, suppressing the constitutive signaling activity. Recent evidence suggests that propranolol and antihistamines are inverse agonists (Figures 1-5 and 1-6).

(b) **Receptor antagonists** are drugs which have an **affinity** for the receptor site but which lack intrinsic activity. Antagonists block or reduce the effects of agonists (Figure 1-5).

Examples:

Antagonists	Agonists
atropine (M_1–M_5)	cholinergic agonists
yohimbine (α_2)	α_2-adrenergic agonists
phenoxybenzamine (α_1)	epinephrine
diphenhydramine (H_1)	histamine
cimetidine (H_2)	histamine
naloxone	opioids
naltrexone	carfentanil
flumazenil	benzodiazepines
spironolactone	aldosterone

i. Antagonists may act in a **competitive (these are reversible on removal, washout)** manner. Example: phentolamine-norepinephrine.

ii. **Noncompetitive (these may be reversible or irreversible on removal, washout)** manner. The noncompetitive antagonism may be due to the antagonist binding to separate site to the agonist or due to covalent bonding. Examples: phenoxybenzamine blockade of α_1-adrenergic receptors are irreversible due to covalent bonding with the receptor protein; picrotoxin antagonism of GABA receptors is reversible but noncompetitive because picrotoxin blocks the open Cl^- channel pore not the GABA binding site.

2. **Antagonism**

a. Antagonism is the interaction between two drugs such that the response of one drug (the agonist) is reduced in the presence of the second drug (the antagonist).

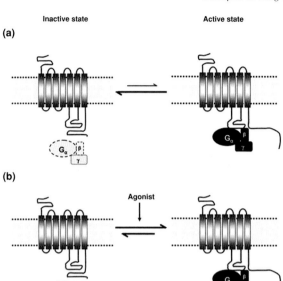

(a)

Inactive state   Active state

(b)

FIGURE 1-6. Two-state model of the G protein-coupled receptor. **(a)** At rest, the inactive state isomerizes with the active state, but favors the latter. **(b)** A full agonist converts the inactive state to active state. **(c)** An inverse agonist converts more active state to inactive state than during the resting state.

(c)

There are three types of antagonism in pharmacology: **receptor, physiologic**, and **chemical**.

(1) **Receptor antagonism** occurs on the same receptor protein such that two drugs, an agonist and an antagonist, compete and bind to the same receptor protein. See above for examples.

(2) **Physiologic antagonism** occurs as the result of activating receptors with opposite physiological effects.

Examples:

acetylcholine   →↓ heart rate
epinephrine   →↑ heart rate
histamine   → bronchoconstriction
epinephrine   → bronchodilation
histamine   →↓ blood pressure
epinephrine   →↑ blood pressure

(3) **Chemical antagonism** occurs as the result of a drug combining with two or more molecules via the formation of chemical bonds. This type of antagonism often does not require animal tissue to be demonstrated, and has been used to treat heavy metal intoxication.

Examples:

Drug	Metal chelated
Dimercaprol (BAL)	Hg, As
Penicillamine	Cu, Pb, Hg

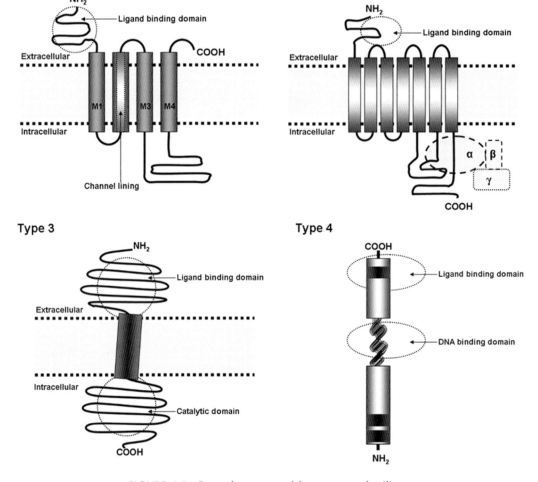

FIGURE 1-7. General structure of four receptor families.

3. **Signal transduction**. Four general types of receptor **mechanism can be described** (Figure 1-7):
   a. **Ligand-gated ion channels (Type 1 receptor mechanisms)** regulate the flow of ions through the cellular plasma membrane channels.
      (1) Response time is very rapid, for example, milliseconds, once the drug/ligand binds to the receptor.
      (2) Examples of synaptic transmitters which act via ion channels: acetylcholine (at nicotinic receptors), gamma-aminobutyric acid ($GABA_A$ receptors), glycine, and glutamate (ionotropic receptors).
   b. **GTP-binding proteins (G proteins, Type 2)** couple the binding of the ligand on the cell surface receptor to intracellular second messengers. These receptors are 7-transmembrane (serpentine) receptors, which cross the plasma membrane seven times. More than 80% of receptors in animals are G protein-coupled receptors (Figure 1-8).
      (1) Agonists (acetylcholine—on muscarinic receptor, catecholamines—on α- and β-adrenergic receptors, and many others) acting on receptors cause the displacement of guanosine diphosphate (GDP) from the G protein and its replacement by guanosine triphosphate (GTP).
      (2) The G protein–GTP complex in turn regulates the activity of enzymes (e.g., adenylyl cyclase, phospholipase C-β) or ion channels (e.g., Na^+, K^+, Ca^{2+}).

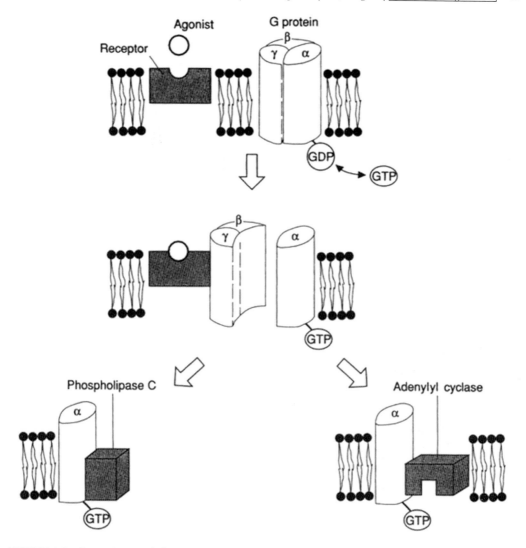

FIGURE 1-8. G protein-coupled receptor and its effectors. When an agonist binds to a receptor that is linked to a G protein-mediated second messenger system, the conformation of the receptor in the membrane is changed, enabling it to encounter a G protein complex. When the activated receptor encounters the G protein, it induces the G protein to exchange GDP for GTP. The presence of GTP causes the α-subunit to separate from the G protein and diffuse within the membrane until it encounters the effector (e.g., adenylyl cyclase, phospholipase C) that initiates the second messenger response. This response may involve regulation of enzymatic activity or opening/closure of ion channels. Hydrolysis of the GTP to GDP on α-subunit returns the G protein to inactive state. (From Figure 1-4, *NVMS Pharmacology.*)

        Hydrolysis of the GTP to GDP stops the activation of enzyme or ion channels.

(3) The G protein–GTP complex may last 10 seconds whereas the initial agonist/ligand–receptor complex formation may have lasted for a few milliseconds. This leads to an **amplification** of the original agonist–receptor signal.

(4) G proteins may **couple stimulatory responses** as well as **inhibitory responses**. Each cell may have more than one G protein type. In general, there are three G proteins: G_s, $G_{i/o}$, and G_q (Figure 1-9).

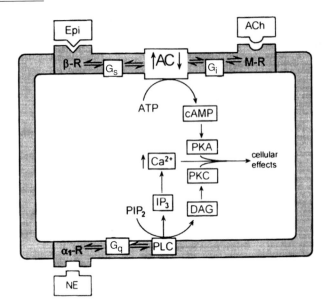

FIGURE 1-9. Signal transduction pathways for G protein-coupled receptors (R). Activation of β-adrenergic receptor (β-R) by epinephrine (Epi) involves a stimulatory G (G_s), which activates adenylyl cyclase (AC) to synthesize cyclic AMP (cAMP); cAMP activates protein kinase A (PKA). Acetylcholine (ACh) binds a muscarinic-2 receptor ((M-R) linked to an inhibitory G (G_i), which inhibits AC and hence PKA. Activation of α_1-R by norepinephrine (NE) activates another G (G_q), which in turn activates phospholipase C-β (PLC). PLC hydrolyzes PIP_2, a membrane phospholipid to form IP_3 and diacylglycerol (DAG). IP_3 releases Ca^{2+} from the endoplasmic reticulum, whereas DAG activates protein kinase C. PKA and PKC phosphorylate various cellular constituents that, in concert with elevated cystosolic Ca^{2+} levels, elicit characteristic changes in the cellular functions. (From Fig. 5.9 of Adams' *Veterinary Pharmacology and Therapeutics*, 8th ed.)

    (a) G_s protein couples to adenylyl cyclase, which increases the formation of cyclic AMP. Cyclic AMP activates protein kinase A, which phosphorylates cellular constituents. **Examples:** glucagon, glucagons-like peptide 1, β-adrenergic agonists, D_1- and D_5-dopaminergic agonists, 5-HT_4 agonists, gonadotropins, thyrotropin, vasopressin V_2-agonists, ACTH, and many other hormones/drugs use this mechanism.

    (b) $G_{i/o}$ protein couples negatively to adenylyl cyclase, thereby decreasing the formation of cyclic AMP. In addition, $G_{i/o}$ protein can close Ca^{2+} and open K^+ channels. **Examples:** α_2-adrenergic agonists, M_2- and M_4-muscarinic agonists, D_2-, D_3-, D_4-dopaminergic agonists, $5HT_1$-agonists, opioids, $GABA_B$-agonists, somatostatin, neuropeptide Y, and many other hormones/drugs use this mechanism.

    (c) G_q protein couples to phospholipase C-β, which increases the formation of inositol 1,4,5-triphosphate (IP_3) and diacylglycerol (DAG). IP_3 elevates intracellular Ca^{2+} concentrations by increasing Ca^{2+} release from the endoplasmic reticulum and Ca^{2+} influx through store-operated calcium (SOC) channels. DAG activates protein kinase C, which phosphorylates cellular constituents. Vasopressin V_1-agonists, oxytocin, muscarinic M_1- and M_3-agonists, α_1-adrenergic agonists, bradykinin, and many other hormones/drugs use this mechanism.

  c. Kinase-linked receptors (Type 3 receptor mechanism)

    (1) Receptors with tyrosine kinase activity. Some hormones (e.g., **insulin, certain growth factors**) have tyrosine kinase as a part of the plasma membrane receptor. The insulin receptor is used as an example to explain how the tyrosine kinase receptor works (see Figure 12-5).

(a) The activated insulin receptor (tyrosine kinase) phosphorylates its substrates [e.g., insulin receptor substrate (IRS) 1-4].

(b) Activated IRS is thought to phosphorylate a number of cellular constituents including phosphoinositol-3 kinase (PI3-kinase), which can activate other cellular proteins including glucose transporter 4 (GLUT4) in the skeletal muscle cells and adipocytes, leading to increased glucose transport into these cells.

(2) Cystosolic tyrosine kinase (also see Figure 12-1). Growth hormone, prolactin, leptin, and cytokines also have the plasma membrane receptors. Activation of these receptors will lead to the phosphorylation of Janus kinase (JAK), a form of tyrosine kinase present in the cytosol. Activation of JAK, in turn, phosphorylates the signal transduction and activation of transcription (STAT) proteins. The phosphorylated STATs form dimers, and move into the nucleus where they act as transcription factors.

(3) Guanylyl cyclase–protein kinase G. Guanylyl cyclase catalyzes cyclic GMP formation from GTP. The plasma membrane receptors of atrial natriuretic peptide (ANP) and guanylin have guanylyl cyclase activity. In addition, nitric oxide (NO) can activate cytosolic quanylyl cyclase. Cyclic GMP activates protein kinase G, which mediates many effects, including closure of Na^+ and Ca^{2+} channels, and opening of K^+ channels.

d. Intracellular receptors (Type 4 receptor mechanisms) Steroid hormones (including vitamin D) and thyroid hormone (T_3) bind to these receptor proteins. Corticostereoid receptors are in cytosol and the receptors of other steroid hormones and T_3 are in nucleus. Activated receptor proteins form dimer and move to the promoter region of the DNA, altering transcription processes (and thereby changing protein synthesis; see Figure 12-3).

B. Dose–response relationships

1. Graded dose–response relationships

a. The response is measured in an individual animal or tissue. Increases in the dose produce increases in the response. Example: progressive increases in epinephrine dose produce increases in cardiac output and vasoconstriction, which lead to increases in blood pressure (Figure 1-10).

b. Drug concentration–effect relationships have four important characteristics: **potency, slope, maximum efficacy,** and **individual variation**.

(1) Potency refers to the dose (concentration) of a drug needed to produce the effect. Potency is not an important property of a drug, provided the formulated form of the drug can be conveniently administered. The smaller the dose to produce the effect, the greater the potency. Assume drug [A] and drug [B] have similar pharmacological activity. The fact that drug [A] is five times more potent than drug [B] does not automatically make drug [A] the drug of choice. Strong consideration must also be given to side effects,

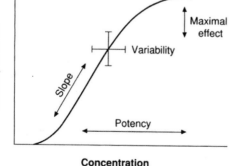

FIGURE 1-10. The log dose–effect relationship, showing the four characteristic variables. (From Figure 1-5, *NVMS Pharmacology.*)

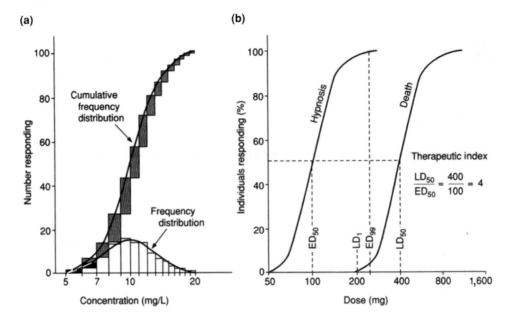

FIGURE 1-11. (a) The effective concentration to produce a quantal response was determined in each of 100 subjects. The number of subjects who required each dose is plotted, giving a log normal frequency distribution (bars with diagonal lines). The stippled bars demonstrate that the normal frequency distribution, when summated, yields the cumulative frequency distribution—a sigmoid curve that is a quantal concentration–effect curve. **(b)** Quantal dose–response curves for the useful action and death action of a drug. ED_{50} is the dose needed to treat 50% of the population. LD_{50} is the dose which will kill 50% of the population. (From Figure 1-6, *NVMS Pharmacology.*)

toxicities, cost, duration of action, and so forth, in deciding which of the two drugs to use.

(2) Slope is of both practical and theoretical importance. Drugs that act on a common receptor (e.g., norepinephrine and phenylephrine acting on the α_1-adrenoceptor) have dose–response curves with parallel slopes. Drugs that have steep slopes for their concentration–response relationship curves are potentially more difficult to use, since small increases in the dose may produce toxicity.

(3) Variability in the response can be expected from a specific dose and variation in dosage may be required to produce a given response.

(4) Maximum effect is the maximum response possible for that effector.

2. Quantal dose–response relationships

a. A **quantal** response is based on an **all or none response** (death, pregnant, vomit, and convulsion). The assumption is made that individual animals respond to the maximum possible or not at all. Thus, dose is not expressed as to the intensity of the effect but to the **frequency** with which any dose produced the all-or-none response. The **frequency distribution curve** is shown in Figure 1-11.

b. Quantal dose–response relationships are used to establish the useful drug effect and the toxic (death) drug effect curves.

(1) Therapeutic index is a ratio used to evaluate the safety of the drug. Using information available from Figure 1-11 the therapeutic index (TI) can be calculated:

$$TI = \frac{LD_{50}}{ED_{50}}$$

Theoretically, the larger the TI the safer the drug. However, if the effectiveness and lethality curves are not parallel, the TI may be misleading.

(2) **Standard safety margin** is a more conservative measure of a drug's safety than is TI and is used to relate the therapeutic effect in all animals without the risk of producing a hazardous effect. The standard safety margin is the percent by which the ED_{99} must be increased before an LD_1 is reached.

$$\text{Standard safety margin} = \frac{LD_1 - ED_{99}}{ED_{99}} \cdot 100$$

(a) Assume 10 mg/kg of a drug is effective in 99% of the animal population and that a dose of 100 mg/kg will cause toxicity in 1% of the same population.

$$\text{Standard safety margin} = \frac{100 - 10}{10} \cdot 100$$

The dose which is effective in 99% of the population must be increased by 900% to produce a toxic effect in 1% of the population.

SUGGESTED READING

Foreman JC, Johansen G. 1996. *Textbook of Receptor Pharmacology*. Boca Raton, FL: CRC Press.

Halpert JR. 1995. Structural basis of selective cytochrome P450 inhibition. *Annu Rev Pharmacol Toxicol* 35:29–53.

Koch-Weser J, Sellers EM. 1976. Binding of drugs to serum albumin. *N Engl J Med* 294:311–316.

Leurs R, Church MK, Talialatea M. 2002. H_1-antihistamines: Inverse agonism, anti-inflammatory actions and cardiac effects. *Clin Exp Allergy* 32:489–498.

Milligan G, Bond RA, Lee M. 1995. Inverse agonism: Pharmacological curiosity or potential therapeutic strategy? *Trends Pharmacol Sci* 16:10–13.

Riviere J. 2004. *Comparative Pharmacokinetics: Principles, Techniques and Application*. Ames, IA: Blackwell Publishing.

Simonds QF. 1999. G-protein regulation of adenylate cyclase. *Trends Pharmacol Sci* 20:66–72.

STUDY QUESTIONS

DIRECTIONS: Each of the numbered items or incomplete statements in this section is followed by answers or by completion of the statement. Select the **one** lettered answer or completion that is **best** in each case.

1. The same dose of a drug is given by two different routes of administration (A, B) and the plasma concentration is followed over time as shown in the drawing.

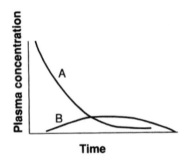

(A) Curve A results from intramuscular administration
(B) Curve B results from intravenous administration
(C) Curve A results from oral administration
(D) Curve A results from intravenous administration
(E) The bioavailability of the drug in curve B is the greatest

2. The first-pass effect is most apt to occur after which route of drug administration?

(A) Intravenous
(B) Intramuscular
(C) Subcutaneous
(D) Oral
(E) Inhalation

3. All of the following statements about the therapeutic index (TI) are true EXCEPT

(A) a high TI suggests that the drug is safe to use.
(B) a low TI suggests that the drug is dangerous to use therapeutically.

(C) a high TI indicates that the ED_{50} far exceeds the LD_{50}.
(D) the standard safety margin is a better measure of the drug's safety than is TI.
(E) quantal dose–response curves are used in the calculation of the TI.

4. Which of the following statements concerning drug receptors is true?

(A) Drug receptors play an important role in the bioavailability of a drug.
(B) Drugs cannot act unless they are first released from a drug receptor.
(C) A drug can act as an antagonist even if it is bound to a drug receptor.
(D) Drugs cannot act unless they are first bound to a receptor.
(E) Most drugs combine with their receptor by forming covalent bonds.

5. The maximum effect (E_{max}) achieved by a drug is a measure of

(A) the drug's potency.
(B) the drug's efficacy (intrinsic activity).
(C) the drug's antagonistic magnitude.
(D) the drug's therapeutic index.
(E) the drug's lipid solubility.

6. A drug is eliminated by first-order processes. Assume 50 mg of the drug is administered intravenously and at 6 hours, 25 mg remain in the body. How much drug will remain in the body at 24 hours.

(A) 18 mg
(B) 15 mg
(C) 10 mg
(D) 6 mg
(E) 3 mg

7. A 20-kg dog is dosed with 5 mg of drug X. If the half-life of drug X is 30 minutes, how long will it take for the animal to have less than 1 mg of the drug remaining in the body?

(A) 90 minutes
(B) 120 minutes
(C) 150 minutes
(D) 180 minutes
(E) 210 minutes

8. You are presented with a severely dehydrated dog in renal failure. Its glomerular filtration rate is one fourth normal. The antibiotic you want to administer is cleared solely by glomerular filtration. Assume the drug's volume of distribution is only in the extracellular fluid and that V_d is one half normal. In a normal animal the antibiotics half-life is 60 minutes, what would it be in this animal?

(A) 30 minutes
(B) 60 minutes
(C) 90 minutes
(D) 120 minutes
(E) 240 minutes

9. The plasma concentration of drug X in a dairy cow is 5 µg/mL. Assume drug X is a weak base with a pK_a of 8.4, and the milk pH is 6.4 and the pH of plasma is 7.4. What is the concentration of drug X in the milk?

(A) 5 µg/mL
(B) 30 µg/mL
(C) 45 µg/mL
(D) 55 µg/mL
(E) 500 µg/mL

10. The mechanism by which most drugs are absorbed following an intramuscular injection is

(A) simple diffusion.
(B) active transport.
(C) pinocytosis.
(D) facilitated diffusion.

11. Drug X is a weak acid with a pK_a of 4. Approximately, what percent of the drug is ionized in a pH 2 environment?

(A) 10%
(B) 5%
(C) 1%
(D) 0.1%
(E) 0.5%

12. The mechanism by which pretreatment with phenobarbital for several days decreases the duration of action of pentobarbital involves

(A) stimulation by phenobarbital of the synthesis of microsomal enzymes in the liver.
(B) neutralization by phenobarbital of naturally occurring inhibitors.
(C) acceleration of the excretion of pentobarbital.
(D) competition for receptor sites in the CNS.
(E) increased binding of pentobarbital to plasma proteins.

13. The renal clearance of a drug (weak organic base) is favored if the drug

(A) has low solubility in water.
(B) reduces renal blood flow.
(C) has a high degree of binding to plasma protein.
(D) is put in the ionized form by acidifying the urine.
(E) is put in the nonionized form by alkalinizing the urine.

14. The major organ for drug excretion is the

(A) brain.
(B) liver.
(C) kidney.
(D) spleen.
(E) gastrointestinal tract.

15. Biotransformation of drugs usually results in the

(A) formation of metabolites which are usually more polar.
(B) formation of metabolites which are less polar.
(C) formation of substances which are more active than the drug itself.
(D) liver toxicity.
(E) formation of a carcinogen.

16. Which of the following drug characteristics will tend to favor a low apparent volume of distribution?

(A) Extensive plasma protein binding
(B) A large molecular weight
(C) High water solubility
(D) All of the above are correct
(E) None of the above (A, B, C)

17. The two curves below were obtained for drug A and drug B. The ordinate represents the percent of animals responding to the beneficial effect of the drug. Which of the following statements is **most** correct?

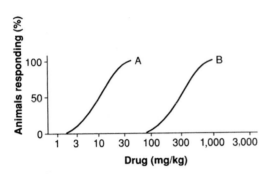

(A) Drug A is more potent than Drug B.
(B) Drug B is more potent than Drug A.
(C) Drug A is 30 times more potent than Drug B.
(D) Drug A is 300 times more potent than Drug B.
(E) Drug B is 30 times more potent than Drug A.

18. Which of the following is a correct statement regarding a partial agonist?

(A) It is a drug that is able to produce the full cell/tissue response.
(B) It is a drug that induces a response, but the maximum response is less than the maximum response to a full agonist.
(C) It is a drug that binds to the receptor, suppressing the receptor's basal intrinsic activity.

(D) It is the drug that has high affinity for the receptor, but has no intrinsic activity.

19. Activation of which of the following G protein-coupled receptors will mostly likely cause an increase in Ca^{2+} release from the endoplasmic reticulum?

(A) G_s
(B) $G_{i/o}$
(C) G_q

20. Which of the following is a correct statement regarding species variation in pharmacokinetics/pharmacodynamics?

(A) In the dog, glucuronidation of drugs is only present at a low rate.
(B) Xylazine is a much more potent sedative in horses than cattle.
(C) Horses have higher levels of plasma esterases than cattle to break down succinylcholine.
(D) Nonherbivores have a more complete GI absorption of a benzimidazole anthelmintic than herbivores.
(E) Most of lipophilic organic bases have smaller volumes of distribution in ruminants than monogastric animals.

21. Acidifying the urine would be expected to increase the rate of elimination for

(A) a weak acid with a pK_a of 7.
(B) a weak base with a pK_a of 6.
(C) both (A) and (B) are correct.
(D) neither (A) nor (B) is correct.

ANSWERS AND EXPLANATIONS

1. The answer is D.
There is no absorption phase for IV administration. Curve B shows an ascending (absorption phase) plasma concentration phase followed by a descending (elimination phase) plasma concentration phase.

2. The answer is D.
The first-pass effect indicates that a significant amount of drug is lost during the absorption process and a large quantity of drug is then not available for distribution. Usually, the first-pass effect is evident for drugs which are metabolized significantly by the gut epithelium and liver prior to distribution via the systemic circulation.

3. The answer is C.
The formula for determining the therapeutic index is:

$$LD_{50}/ED_{50}$$

If the ED_{50} was larger than the LD_{50} the TI would be small.

4. The answer is C.
Antagonists have a high affinity for the receptor and therefore occupy the receptor sites. The degree of binding and occupancy of the receptor site is a measure of the drug's affinity. Answer D is not correct since some drugs can exert an effect without acting on a receptor system, for example, neutralization of acid as with antacids and drugs acting through chelation.

5. The answer is B.
Drug efficacy or intrinsic activity is a measure of the drug to produce an effect.

6. The answer is E.
Since the drug is eliminated by a first-order process, this indicates that a constant fraction of drug is eliminated per unit of

time. Since 25 mg remains at 6 hours, this indicates that the $t_{1/2}$ is 6 hours. Using this reasoning we can determine the following:
50 mg in body at time 0
25 mg in body at time 6 hours
12.5 mg in body at time 12 hours
6.25 mg in body at time 18 hours
3.12 mg in body at time 24 hours (correct answer)

7. The answer is A.
The dog's body will contain the following amounts of drug at the time indicated: 30 minutes = 2.5 mg; 60 minutes = 1.25 mg; 90 minutes = 0.62 mg (the correct answer).

8. The answer is D.
The drug's half-life ($t_{1/2}$) is influenced by the volume of distribution (V_d) and body clearance (Cl_B) according to the following formula:

$$t_{1/2} = \beta \cdot V_d = \frac{0.693 \cdot V_d}{Cl_B}$$

Since clearance is reduced to 0.25 of normal and volume of distribution is 0.5 of normal, the $t_{1/2}$ is doubled. Thus, in this dog the expected $t_{1/2}$ would be 120 minutes.

9. The answer is C.
Knowledge of the Henderson–Hasselbalch equation is necessary to solve this problem. Since the drug is a weak base the proper formula to use is:

$$pK_a = pH + \log$$
$$\times \frac{\text{ionized base (I)}}{\text{nonionized base (U)}}$$

It is the U form of the drug which is lipid soluble and able to cross the biologic membrane. At equilibrium the concentration of U will be the same on both sides of the biologic membrane. The drug will dissociate on both sides of the membrane based on the pH of the environment.

Membrane

Milk (pH 6.4)

$$8.4 = 6.4 + \log \frac{I}{U}$$

$$2 = \log \frac{I}{U}$$

take the antilog of both sides

$$100 = \frac{I}{U}$$

If $U = 1$ drug unit, then $I = 100$

Total drug: $U + I = 100 + 1 = 101$ drug units

Plasma (pH 7.4)

$$8.4 = 7.4 + \log \frac{I}{U}$$

$$1 = \log \frac{I}{U}$$

take the antilog of both sides

$$10 = \frac{I}{U}$$

If $U = 1$ drug unit, then $I = 10$

Total drug: $U + I = 10 + 1 = 11$ drug units

$$\frac{\text{milk}}{\text{plasma ratio}} = \frac{101}{11} = 9.18$$

If the plasma concentration is 5 µg/mL then the milk concentration (X) can be determined as follows:

$$\frac{\text{milk}}{\text{plasma}} = \frac{101 \text{ drug units}}{11 \text{ drug units}} = \frac{X \, \text{µg/mL}}{5 \, \text{µg/mL}}$$

thus, $505 = 11\,X$
and $X = 45.9 \, \text{µg/mL}$ in milk.

10. The answer is A.
Absorption from an injection site into the vascular compartment permits the drug to be distributed systematically. Diffusion of the drug through the capillary membrane or capillary channels (pores) permits its absorption.

11. The answer is C.
Use the Henderson–Hasselbalch equation for an acid:

$$pK_a = pH + \log$$

$$\times \frac{\text{nonionized acid (U)}}{\text{ionized acid (I)}}$$

$$4 = 2 + \log \frac{U}{I}$$

$$2 = \log \frac{U}{I}$$

take the antilog of both sides:

$$100 = \frac{U}{I}$$

If $U = 1$ unit of drug then $I = 0.01$ unit of drug; $U + I = 1.01$ units of drug. By

definition, $U + I = 100\%$. Thus 1.01 units of drug $= 100\%$. Thus:

$$\frac{0.01 \text{ ionized drug}}{1.01 \text{ total drug}} = \frac{X\%}{100\%}$$

$$X = 0.99\% \text{ or approx. } 1\%$$

12. The answer is A.
Pentobarbital is oxidized by the cytochrome P450 enzyme system present in the endoplasmic reticulum (microsomes) of the liver. Pretreatment with phenobarbital induces the liver cells to synthesize more cytochrome P450 enzymes. Thus, animals pretreated with phenobarbital for several days have a greater capacity to metabolize pentobarbital.

13. The answer is D.
Acidification of the urine increases the percent of the weak base in the ionized form. The ionized form of the drug crosses biologic membranes poorly and thus is not able to be passively reabsorbed from the tubule once filtered. This enhances its elimination. Answer E is incorrect since in the nonionized form it is reabsorbed to the greatest extent thus decreasing excretion.

14. The answer is C.
Drugs in the urine are voided along with the urine thereby eliminating the drug from the body. However, some drugs are excreted into the feces, particularly the ones that are not absorbed when administered orally.

15. The answer is A.
Following phase I and phase II biotransformation the chemical is usually more polar (more water soluble) and has less biological activity.

16. The answer is D.
A high percent of drug bound to plasma proteins will keep the majority of the drug in the vascular compartment as will a drug with high molecular weight. Drugs with a high degree of water solubility generally have low solubility in lipids and therefore would be expected to cross biologic membranes less well, thereby limiting their distribution.

17. The answer is C.
Potency refers to the amount of drug required to produce a specified effect or response. Drug A is more potent than drug B. The ED_{50} for drug A is 10 mg/kg, while that for drug B is 300 mg/kg. Drug A is 30 times more potent than drug B.

18. The answer is B.
A partial agonist is a drug that induces a response, but the maximum response is less than the maximum response to a full agonist. A full agonist is a drug that is able to produce the full cell/tissue response. An inverse agonist is a drug that binds to the receptor, suppressing the receptor's basal intrinsic activity. A receptor antagonist is a drug that has high affinity for the receptor, but has no intrinsic activity.

19. The answer is C.
Activation of G_q-coupled receptors will stimulate phospholipase C-β to synthesize IP_3 from PIP_2. IP_3 will bind to its receptors on the endoplasmic reticulum to release Ca^{2+} from this organelle. G_s activates adenylyl cyclase, which increases the synthesis of cyclic AMP. $G_{i/o}$ inhibits adenylyl cyclase.

20. The answer is C.
Horses have higher levels of plasma esterases than cattle to break down succinylcholine, this is the reason the dosage of succinylcholine is higher than cattle. In the cat, glucuronidation of drugs is only present at a low rate; this is one reason that acetaminophen is contraindicated in the cat because metabolism of this drug depends on glucuronidation. Xylazine is a much more potent sedative in cattle than horses, since their receptors (α_{2D}) are very sensitive to xylazine. Herbivores have a more complete GI absorption of benzimidazoles than nonherbivores, since they have a larger GI tract to perform this function. Most of lipophilic organic bases have larger volumes of distribution in ruminants than monogastric animals.

21. The answer is B.
Use the Henderson–Hasselbalch equations to ascertain the percent of drug in ionized form. It is the ionized form which is not subject to passive reabsorption following the filtration process. Assume acidification of urine to pH 5.

Weak acid	Weak base
$pK_a = pH + \log \dfrac{U}{I}$	$pK_a = pH + \log \dfrac{I}{U}$
$7 = 5 + \log \dfrac{U}{I}$	$6 = 5 + \log \dfrac{I}{U}$
$2 = \log \dfrac{U}{I}$	$1 = \log \dfrac{I}{U}$
take the antilog of both sides	take the antilog of both sides
$100 = \dfrac{U}{I}$	$10 = \dfrac{I}{U}$
If $U = 1$ drug unit, then $I = 0.01$	If $U = 1$ drug unit, then $I = 10$
1.01 drug units $= 100\%$	11 drug units $= 100\%$
$\dfrac{0.01}{1.01} = \dfrac{X\%}{100\%}$	$\dfrac{10}{11} = \dfrac{X\%}{100\%}$
$X = 0.99\%$ ionized (approx. 1%)	$X = 90.9\%$ of drug is ionized

Since the base will be ionized the greatest at pH 5 it will be eliminated the fastest.

Chapter 2

Drugs Affecting Peripheral Nervous System

Walter H. Hsu

I. INTRODUCTION TO THE PERIPHERAL EFFERENT NERVOUS SYSTEM

A. **The somatic nervous system innervates skeletal muscle** and controls motor functions of the body. Axons originate from the spinal cord and release the neurotransmitter acetylcholine (ACh) at the neuromuscular junction. Some drugs can affect both the somatic and the autonomic nervous systems because ACh is a transmitter in both systems.

B. **The autonomic nervous system** regulates the activity of the **heart, secretory cells, and smooth muscle.** Two neurons are involved in the transmission process. The first neuron originates in the central nervous system (CNS) and synapses in a ganglion outside the CNS. A second neuron then innervates the target (effector) tissue.

1. **Organization** (Figure 2-1)
   a. **Sympathetic nervous system**
      (1) **Preganglionic neurons** originate from the thoracic and lumbar portions of the spinal cord and terminate in the para- or post-vertebral ganglia, or they directly innervate the adrenal medulla. Functionally, the adrenal medulla responds as if it were a ganglion.
      (2) **Postganglionic neurons** originate from the ganglia and innervate the effector cell.
   b. **Parasympathetic nervous system**
      (1) **Preganglionic neurons** originate from either the midbrain, the medulla oblongata, or the sacral portion of the spinal cord. They terminate on postganglionic neurons. The terminals of the preganglionic neurons and ganglia are located in or close to the effector cell.
      (2) **Postganglionic neurons** innervate the tissue.
2. **Neurotransmitters** are chemical substances that transmit impulses across junctions such as synapses (e.g., nerve-to-nerve, nerve-to-effector cell).
   a. **Sympathetic nervous system**
      (1) **Preganglionic neurons** release **ACh** onto **nicotinic receptors** of postganglionic neurons or the adrenal medulla.
      (2) **Postganglionic neurons** release **norepinephrine (NE) onto adrenergic receptors (adrenoceptors)** in the effector tissue.
   b. **Parasympathetic nervous system**
      (1) **Preganglionic neurons** release **ACh** onto **nicotinic receptors** of postganglionic neurons.
      (2) **Postganglionic neurons** release **ACh** onto **muscarinic receptors** in the effector cell.
3. **Receptors** (Table 2-1)
   a. **Cholinergic receptors** mediate the effects of **ACh.** They are muscarinic or nicotinic, named after plant alkaloids responsible for the physiologic effects of poisonous mushrooms and tobacco, respectively.
      (1) **Muscarinic receptors** have five subtypes, M_1–M_5. M_1 receptors are found in neurons to mediate excitatory postsynaptic potential (EPSP); M_2 receptors are found in the heart (to decrease excitability); M_3 receptors are found in smooth muscles, sphincters, and secretory glands; M_4 receptors are found in the CNS; and M_5 receptors are found in the midbrain dopaminergic neurons [to increase dopamine (DA) release], cerebral arteries and arterioles, possibly peripheral blood vessels, and lymphocytes. M_1, M_3, and M_5 receptors

TABLE 2-1. Tissue Receptors and Response to Stimulation

Effector Organ	Adrenergic		Cholinergic	
	Receptor Type	Response to Stimulation	Receptor Type	Response to Stimulation
Heart				
S-A node	$\beta_1 > \beta_2$	↑Heart rate	M_2	↓Heart rate
Atria	$\beta_1 > \beta_2$	↑Contractility ↑Conduction velocity	M_2	↓Contractility
A-V node	$\beta_1 > \beta_2$	↑Automaticity ↑Conduction velocity	M_2	↓Conduction velocity A-V block
Ventricles	$\beta_1 > \beta_2$	↑Contractility ↑Conduction velocity ↑Automaticity	M_2	↓Contractility
His-Purkinje system	$\beta_1 > \beta_2$	↑Conduction velocity ↑Automaticity	—	—
Arteries				
Coronary	α_1, α_2 β_2	Constriction Dilation	M_3^*	Dilation
Renal	α_1, α_2 β_1, β_2	Constriction Dilation	M_3^*	Dilation
Skin and mucosa	α_1, α_2	Constriction	M_3^*	Dilation
Skeletal muscle	α_1 β_2	Constriction Dilation	M_3^*	Dilation
Pulmonary	α_1 β_2	Constriction Dilation	M_3^*	Dilation
Abdominal viscera	α_1 β_2	Constriction Dilation	M_3^*	Dilation
Veins	α_1, α_2 β_2	Constriction Dilation	—	—
Endothelium	—.	—	M_3	↑ NO synthesis
Eye				
Iris				
Radial muscle	α_1	Contraction (mydriasis)	—	—
Sphincter muscle	—	—	M_3	Contraction (miosis)
Ciliary muscle	β_2	Relaxation (far vision)	M_3	Contraction (near vision)
Salivary glands	α_1	↑ Secretion	M_3	↑ Secretion
Lung				
Tracheal and bronchial smooth muscle	β_2	Relaxation	M_3	Contraction
Bronchial glands	α_2 β_2	↓Secretion ↑Secretion	M_3	↑Secretion
Stomach				
Motility and tone	$\alpha_2, \beta_1, \beta_2$	Decrease	M_3	Increase
Sphincters	α_1	Contraction	M_3	Relaxation
Secretion	α_2	Inhibition	M_3	Stimulation
Intestine				
Motility and tone	$\alpha_2, \beta_1, \beta_2$	Decrease	M_3	Increase
Sphincters	α_1	Contraction	M_3	Relaxation
Secretion	α_2	Inhibition	M_3	Stimulation
Gallbladder and ducts	β_2	Relaxation	M_3	Contraction

TABLE 2-1. (*continued*)

Effector Organ	Adrenergic		Cholinergic	
	Receptor Type	Response to Stimulation	Receptor Type	Response to Stimulation
Kidney				
Renin secretion	α_2	Decrease	—	—
	β_1	Increase		
Urinary bladder				
Detrusor	β_2	Relaxation	M_3	Contraction
Trigone and sphincter	α_1	Contraction	M_3	Relaxation
Ureter				
Motility and tone	α_1	Increase	M_3	Increase (?)
Uterus	α_1, α_2	Pregnant, contraction	M_3	Contraction
	β_2	Nonpregnant, relaxation		
Sex organs, male	α_1	Ejaculation	M_3	Erection
Skin				
Pilomotor muscles	α_1	Contraction		
Sweat glands	α_1	↑ Localized secretion (Adrenergic sweating)	M_3	↑Generalized secretion
Spleen capsule	α_1	Contraction	—	
	β_2	Relaxation	—	
Adrenal medulla	—		Nicotinic (N_N)	↑Epi, NE secretion
Skeletal muscle	β_2	↑Contractility, Glycogenolysis, K^+ uptake	—	
Liver	α_1, β_2	↑Glycogenolysis	—	—
Pancreas				—
Acini	α_2	↓Secretion	M_3	Secretion
Islets (β cells)	α_2	↓Secretion	M_3	Secretion
	β_2	↑Secretion		
Fat cells	α_1, β_{1-3}	↑Lipolysis (thermogenesis)	—	—
	α_2	↓lipolysis		
Salivary glands	α_1	↑K^+ and H_2O secretion	M_3	↑K^+ and H_2O secretion
Nasopharyngeal glands	—	—	M_3	↑Secretion
Pineal glands	β	↑Melatonin secretion	—	—
Posterior pituitary	α_2	↓AVP secretion	—	—
Autonomic nerve endings				
Sympathetic				
Autoreceptor	α_2	↓NE release		
Heteroreceptor		—	M_2	↓NE release from sympathetic nerve terminal
Parasympathetic				
Autoreceptor		—	M_2	↓ACh release
Heteroreceptor	α_2	↓ACh release from myenteric plexus		

*These receptors are in endothelium, which respond to ACh by increasing NO synthesis. NO diffuses into muscle and causes vasodilation.

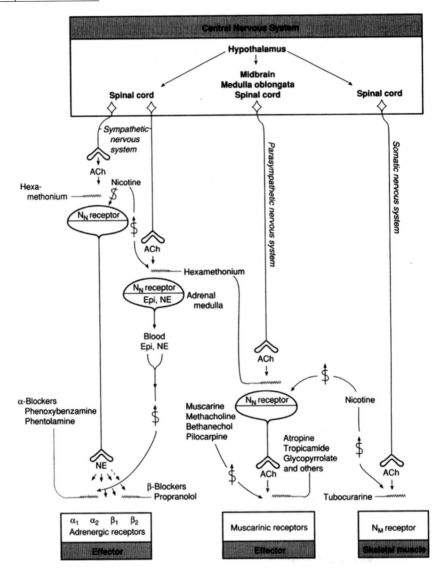

FIGURE 2-1. Effector neurons of the peripheral nervous system. Drugs that stimulate ($) and block (〰〰) receptors are also shown. N_N, ganglionic nicotinic receptor; N_M, skeletal muscle nicotinic receptor; NE, norepinephrine; Epi, epinephrine; ACh, acetylcholine. (From Figure 2-1, *NVMS Pharmacology.*)

are coupled to G_q, whereas M_2 and M_4 receptors are coupled to $G_{i/o}$ (Table 2-2).

(2) Nicotinic receptors have two subtypes, N_M and N_N. N_M receptors are found in the muscle of neuromuscular junctions, whereas N_N receptors are found in the neurons of the CNS and autonomic ganglia. Nicotinic receptors are part of the nonselective cation channels; activation of these receptors will open the channels to permit the passage of Na^+, K^+, and Ca^{2+}, predominantly Na^+. As a result, membrane is depolarized, which triggers the opening of voltage-dependent Ca^{2+} channels to further increase Ca^{2+} influx.

b. Adrenergic receptors mediate the effects of **NE** and **epinephrine (Epi)**.

(1) α-Receptors: α_1, α_2

These receptors are found in many tissues (Table 2-1). α_2-Receptors are also found in presynaptic site of the adrenergic neuron. α_1-Receptors are coupled to G_q, whereas α_2-receptors are coupled to $G_{i/o}$.

TABLE 2-2. Cholinergic Receptor Pharmacology—An Overview

	Cholinergic Receptors						
	Nicotinic Receptors		Muscarinic Receptors				
	N_M	N_N	M_1	M_2	M_3	M_4	M_5
Agonists	◄·· Acetylcholine ···►						
	◄·················· Nicotine ····················►						
	◄ Succinylcholine ►		◄·····························Bethanechol·····························►				
Antagonists	◄·· Tubocurarine ··►	◄·Hexamethonium··►	◄··································· Atropine ····································►				

(2) β-Receptors: $\beta_1, \beta_2, \beta_3$

Both β_1- and β_2-receptors are found in many tissues and elicit many different effects (Table 2-1). β_3-Receptors are found mainly in adipocytes and some in myocardium. All three β-receptor subtypes are coupled to G_s.

II. ADRENERGIC AGONISTS (SYMPATHOMIMETIC AMINES). An overview is presented in Table 2-3.

A. Catecholamines

1. **Epi, NE, and DA** are endogenous substances that serve as hormones and neurotransmitters. They are also used therapeutically as drugs.
   a. **Chemistry and biosynthesis** are illustrated in Figure 2-2.
   b. **Mechanism of action** (Figure 2-3)
      (1) **Epi** is a potent agonist of all adrenergic receptors (i.e., α_1, α_2, β_1, β_2, and β_3).
      (2) **NE** is a potent agonist of α_1-α_2-, and β_1-receptors. It has little effect on β_2-receptors.
      (3) **Dopamine**
         (a) DA causes the release of NE from adrenergic neurons, which activates α_1-and β_1-receptors.
         (b) DA activates specific DA receptors.
            i. **D_1-receptors** are present in the **renal, mesenteric, and coronary** circulation and are activated by low concentrations of DA. Activation

TABLE 2-3. Adrenergic Receptor Pharmacology—An Overview

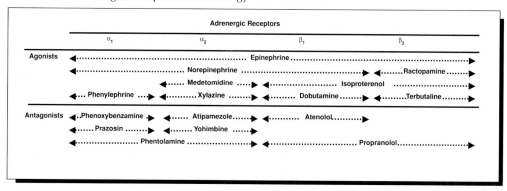

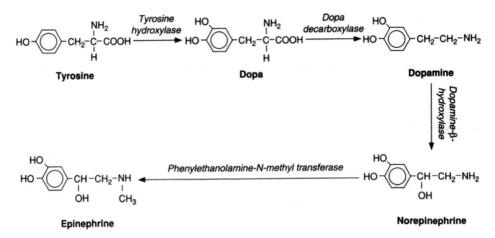

FIGURE 2-2. Biosynthesis of dopamine, norepinephrine, and epinephrine. (From Figure 2-2, *NVMS Pharmacology.*)

of these receptors evokes **vasodilatation**, which is blocked by DA receptor antagonists (e.g., **haloperidol**), but not by β-adrenergic receptor antagonists. **D_1-receptors are coupled to G_s, thereby stimulating cyclic AMP synthesis** (more cyclic AMP, more relaxation of smooth muscle).

    ii. **D_2-receptors** are present in **ganglia, adrenal cortex, and certain areas of the CNS**, including the **substantia nigra and pituitary gland**. Activation of these receptors **inhibits neuroendocrine release**. **D_2-receptors are coupled to $G_{i/o}$, thereby inhibiting cyclic AMP synthesis** (less cyclic AMP, less neurosecretion).

    iii. **D_3-receptors** are present in the nucleus accumbens located at the base of the striatum. D_3-receptors are coupled to $G_{i/o}$.

    iv. **D_4-receptors** are present in the heart and CNS. D_4-receptors are coupled to $G_{i/o}$.

    v. **D_5-receptors** are present in lymphocytes, hippocampus, and nucleus accumbens. D_5-receptors are coupled to G_s.

c. Pharmacokinetics

    (1) Absorption

      (a) Catecholamines are poorly absorbed following oral administration, partly because the drugs are rapidly oxidized and conjugated.

      (b) They are absorbed from the respiratory tract when nebulized and inhaled.

      (c) SC absorption is slow because of vasoconstriction.

    (2) Fate

      (a) Distribution. Catecholamines do not cross the blood–brain barrier readily.

      (b) Deactivation (see Figure 2-3)

        i. Tissue uptake mechanisms remove the drug from the receptor site, thereby decreasing the number of receptors being occupied and decreasing the response.

        Uptake$_1$ is the active uptake of the drug into the **presynaptic** sympathetic nerve terminal. **Cocaine** produces a sympathomimetic effect by **blocking uptake$_1$**.

        Uptake$_2$ is the uptake of catecholamines into the **effector** cell. Effector cell contains monoamine oxidase (**MAO**) and catechol-*O*-methyltransferase (**COMT**), which metabolize catecholamines to inactive products.

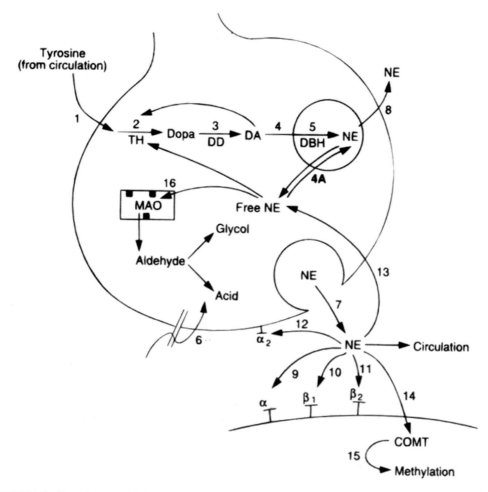

FIGURE 2-3. Site of action of drugs affecting the sympathetic nervous system. The figure depicts the events taking place at the junction of a sympathetic nerve terminal and an end-organ cell.

Tyrosine from the circulation enters the nerve terminal **(1)** and is converted first **(2)** via tyrosine hydroxylase (TH) into dopa and then **(3)** via dopa decarboxylase (DD) into dopamine (DA). DA enters the vesicle of the nerve terminal **(4)**, where it is converted **(5)**, via DA β-hydroxylase (DBH), into norepinephrine (NE), which is stored in the vesicles. Free NE in the axoplasm also enters and leaves the vesicles **(4A)**.

In the process of nerve impulse transmission across the neuroeffector junction, the nerve terminal is depolarized **(6)** by action potential. The storage vesicle fuses with the plasma membrane, and NE is released into the junction **(7)** by exocytosis. Indirect-acting sympathomimetics can also cause NE to leave the vesicles and enter the junction **(8)**.

Once released from the neuron, NE activates the postsynaptic $\alpha(\alpha_1, \alpha_2)$, β_1, and β_2 receptors **(9, 10, 11)** on the effector cell, thereby producing the response. NE also activates presynpatic α_2-receptors to inhibit further NE release **(12)**.

Several mechanisms terminate the action of NE. Most important is the reentry of NE into the nerve terminal (a process known as uptake-1) **(13)**. Some of the NE enters the effector cell (uptake-2) **(14)**, and some enters the circulation.

Two enzymes play a role in the metabolism of NE. The NE that enters the effector cell is methylated **(15)** by catechol-*O*-methyltransferase (COMT) to normetanephrine. The NE in the axoplasm of the nerve terminal is converted **(16)** by monoamine oxidase (MAO) in the neuron's mitochondria, first to the aldehyde, and then to the glycol or to vanillylmandelic acid (VMA). The glycol and the acid are the major metabolites excreted in the urine. (From Figure 2-3, *NVMS Pharmacology*.)

       ii. The liver and kidneys, which are rich in **MAO** and **COMT**, inactivate circulating catecholamines.

    (c) Excretion. The metabolites are excreted in the urine.

  d. Pharmacologic effects. The pharmacologic response to an agonist is a function of the affinity of the agonist for the receptor, the number of receptors, and the efficacy of the agonist (see Table 2-1).

    (1) Epinephrine

      (a) Blood pressure effects

        i. Low doses may cause little change in blood pressure. They increase skeletal muscle **blood flow** via activation of β_2-**receptors** and increase **heart rate and force of contraction via activation of β_1-receptors**. β_2-Receptors have a higher affinity than do α-receptors for Epi, producing a preferential activation at low doses.

        ii. Higher doses. Increasing the dose of Epi leads to the activation of α receptors, which causes **vasoconstriction** and reduces the blood flow to the skeletal musculature. **Because α-receptors predominate in the cutaneous, mesenteric, and renal vascular beds**, the net result is an increase in blood pressure.

        Activation of the α-receptors increases total peripheral resistance and counters the β_2-receptor-mediated vasodilatation. In addition, the larger dose of Epi activates more β_1-receptors in the heart, which increases cardiac output and contributes to the increase in blood pressure.

        As the blood pressure increases, **baroreceptors in the aorta arch and carotid sinus** are activated. They, in turn, activate the vagus nerve and **increase vagal tone** on the heart to reduce the cardiac output, lowering the systemic blood pressure.

      (b) Vascular effects

        i. Skin. Activation of α-**receptors causes vasoconstriction**, decreasing blood flow.

        ii. Skeletal muscle. At low concentrations, β_2-**receptors** are activated, **increasing blood flow** to skeletal muscle. At higher concentrations, activation of α-adrenergic receptors reduces blood flow.

        iii. Mesentery and kidneys. Activation of α-**receptors** leads to a decreased blood flow.

        iv. Lungs. Decreased blood flow results from **vasoconstriction** of arteries and veins.

        v. Heart. Blood flow increases, largely because of the metabolic products created by the increase in cardiac work.

      (c) Cardiac effects. β_1-**Receptors** predominate in the heart, but α_1, β_2, and β_3-receptors are also present. Epi causes

        i. Increased force of contraction (positive inotropic effect).

        ii. Increased rate of contraction (positive chronotropic effect).

        iii. Increased output.

        iv. Increased excitability.

        v. Increased automaticity.

        vi. Increased potential for arrhythmias.

        vii. Decreased efficiency (greater oxygen consumption).

      (d) Smooth muscle effects

        i. Gastrointestinal (GI) tract. Epi and NE **relax GI smooth muscle via activation of α_2- and β-receptors**, and increase the **contraction of the sphincters by activating α_1-receptors**. Activation of α_2-**receptors** in the presynaptic nerve of the parasympathetic ganglia **inhibits ACh release**, thereby decreasing parasympathetic tone.

        ii. Uterus. Contraction (mediated by α-receptors) or relaxation (mediated by β_2-receptors) may occur, depending on the state of estrous cycle, pregnancy, and species.

        iii. Urinary bladder. Urinary retention occurs when the fundus relaxes (as a result of β-receptor stimulation) and the trigone and sphincter contract (as a result of α_1-receptor stimulation).

    iv. Bronchioles. Relaxation occurs via activation of β_2-receptors.

    v. Eye. Mydriasis (pupillary dilation) results when α_1- receptors in the radial muscles of the iris are stimulated, intraocular pressure may be reduced by a local vasoconstriction that decreases the production of aqueous humor.

    vi. Spleen. Contraction (mediated by α_1-receptors) increases blood erythrocyte levels, particularly in dogs.

    vii. Pilomotor muscles. Contraction (mediated by α_1-receptors) erects the hairs on the skin, particularly in carnivores during fear or rage reactions.

  (e) Metabolic effects

    i. Blood concentrations of glucose, free fatty acids, and lactic acid increase when β-receptors in the liver, skeletal muscle, and adipose tissue are stimulated.

    ii. Some of the effects of Epi on plasma glucose concentrations are secondary (e.g., inhibition of insulin secretion via activation of α_2-receptors and stimulation of glucagon secretion via activation of β_2-adrenergic receptors).

(2) NE elicits most of the effects produced by Epi that are mediated via α_1-, α_2-, and β_1-receptors, with the following exceptions:

  (a) At similar doses, NE will increase the mean blood pressure more than Epi because it is not able to relax the skeletal blood vessels via β_2-adrenergic receptors.

  (b) Baroreceptor activation and vagal reflex will occur at lower doses for NE than Epi. This reflex can be strong enough to decrease cardiac output despite the direct activation of cardiac β_1-receptors.

(3) DA has unique pharmacologic actions. The release of NE from the sympathetic postganglionic nerve terminal by DA contributes to its pharmacologic effects.

  (a) Activation of D_1-receptors causes vasodilatation of the renal, mesenteric, and coronary vasculature at low rates of infusion. Natriuresis and diuresis result from the increased glomerular filtration rate and renal blood flow.

  (b) Activation of D_2-receptors in the CNS decreases blood pressure and heart rate in the same manner as activation of α_2-adrenergic receptors in the CNS. It is unlikely that CNS D_2-receptors are activated when DA is infused, because DA does not cross the blood–brain barrier.

  (c) Activation of β_1-receptors, which occurs at somewhat greater concentrations, produces a positive inotropic effect on the heart.

  (d) Activation of α_1-receptors causes vasoconstriction; however, very high concentrations are necessary to produce this effect.

e. Therapeutic uses. Epi, NE, and DA are used parenterally or topically.

  (1) Epinephrine

    (a) Epi will reduce **bronchospasm.**

    (b) Epi is used to **treat hypersensitivity** reactions and **anaphylactic shock** that is characterized by bronchospasm and hypotension.

    (c) Epi reduces cutaneous blood flow, which makes it useful for **prolonging local anesthetic effects.**

    (d) Applied topically, it can be used to **control localized hemorrhage**.

    (e) Epi promotes the outflow of aqueous humor, making it useful for the **treatment of open-angle glaucoma.**

    (f) Epi is used to **restore cardiac activity** following cardiac arrest.

  (2) NE may be used to **correct the hypotension** induced by spinal anesthesia. It is not useful for correcting hypotension in most types of shock, because sympathetic activity is already high and further vasoconstriction may compromise the renal and mesenteric circulations.

  (3) DA may be used to treat

    (a) Cardiogenic shock

    (b) Septic shock

    (c) Acute heart failure (usually as supportive therapy)

    f. Adverse effects
        (1) Epinephrine
            (a) Anxiety, fear, and restlessness
            (b) Palpitations
            (c) Cerebral hemorrhage
            (d) Cardiac arrhythmias (especially in hyperthyroid patients)
        (2) Norepinephrine. Adverse effects are similar to those of Epi. In addition, extravasations following IV injection may cause necrosis and sloughing at the site because of intense vasoconstriction.
        (3) Dopamine. Adverse effects include those of Epi and NE, but they are short-lived because DA is rapidly metabolized.
  2. Isoproterenol (Isuprel®)
    a. Mechanism of action. Isoproterenol, a potent **nonselective β-receptor agonist**, increases **cyclic AMP** levels as β_1- and β_2-receptors activate adenylyl cyclase through **coupling to G_s.**
    b. Pharmacologic effects
        (1) IV infusion decreases mean blood pressure by reducing peripheral resistance, primarily in skeletal muscle.
        (2) Cardiac output increases, owing to increases in cardiac contractility and heart rate.
        (3) Smooth muscle tissues possessing β-receptors (e.g., bronchiolar and GI smooth muscle) are relaxed.
    c. c. Therapeutic uses
        (1) Acute bronchial constriction
        (2) Complete atrioventricular (A-V) block.
    d. d. Pharmacokinetics
        (1) Absorption. Isoproterenol is readily absorbed parenterally or as an aerosol.
        (2) Fate. It is principally metabolized by COMT and MAO, but MAO is less effective than with Epi and NE.
        (3) Excretion. Metabolites are excreted in urine.
    e. Adverse effects
        (1) Tachycardia
        (2) Arrhythmias (as a result of general stimulation of cardiac tissues).

B. | **Noncatecholamines**

  1. Phenylephrine (Neo-synephrine®)
    a. Mechanism of action. Phenylephrine is an **α_1-receptor agonist** (Figure 2-4). It also has **some β-adrenergic** stimulatory properties at high doses.
    b. Pharmacologic effects. Phenylephrine **increases blood pressure** (primarily by vasoconstriction).
    c. Therapeutic uses. It is administered parenterally, orally, or topically.
        (1) Phenylephrine has an advantage over Epi as a **vasopressor** in situations where cardiac stimulation is undesirable, such as during gas anesthesia.
        (2) Phenylephrine is used as a topical nasal decongestant.
        (3) It is used in ophthalmology as a **mydriatic** agent (during examinations), to reduce posterior synechiae formation, and to relieve the pain associated with uveitis.
    d. Pharmacokinetics
        (1) Following IV administration, vasopressor effects begin immediately and persist for ≤20 minutes.
        (2) It is **metabolized** by the liver (to phenolic conjugates mainly after oral ingestion, and to m-hydroxymandelic acid after IV administration), and the effects of the drug are also terminated by uptake into tissues. The biological $t_{1/2}$ is 2–3 hours.
    e. Adverse effects
        (1) Phenylephrine may elicit a **reflex bradycardia** when administered IV.
        (2) Hypertension, especially in geriatric, hyperthyroid, or hypertensive patients, may occur.

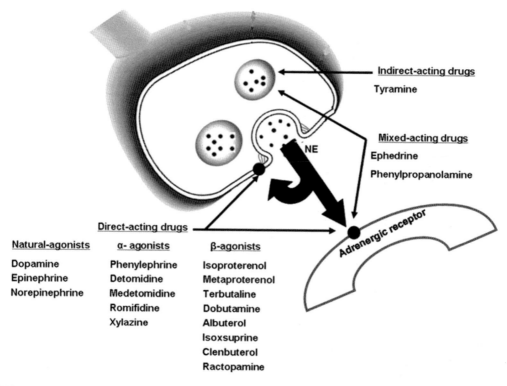

FIGURE 2-4. Comparison of direct-, mixed-, and indirect-acting sympathomimetic drugs. Direct-acting drugs are able to elicit a pharmacologic response independently of the sympathetic neuron. Indirect-acting drugs produce a response by releasing norepinephrine (NE) from the neuron after they are transported into the neuron. Mixed-acting drugs stimulate the adrenergic receptor directly and by inducing the release of NE from the neuron.

    (3) Nasal irritation and rebound congestion may occur following long-term nasal use.

2. Dobutamine (Dobutrex®, see also Chapter 8)

    a. Chemistry. The clinically used formulation of dobutamine is the racemic mixture of two enantiomeric forms, the negative and positive isomers.

    b. Mechanism of action. Dobutamine activates β_1-**receptors**, and activates weakly β_2- and α_1-receptors as well.

    c. Pharmacologic effects

        (1) Dobutamine produces an **inotropic effect**, which is greater than its chronotropic effect.

        (2) It increases cardiac output by increasing cardiac contractility and stroke volume.

        (3) Increased myocardial contractility may **increase myocardial oxygen demand** and coronary blood flow.

    d. Therapeutic uses. Dobutamine is used for the short-term treatment of **heart failure.**

    e. Pharmacokinetics

        (1) Dobutamine is administered by IV infusion. Upon IV infusion, the onset of action generally occurs within 2 minutes and peaks after 10 minutes.

        (2) Dobutamine is metabolized rapidly in the liver and other tissues and has a plasma $t_{1/2}$ of 2 minutes in humans. The drug's effects diminish rapidly after cessation of therapy.

    f. Adverse effects

        (1) Dobutamine may increase oxygen use; therefore, it should be used with care after **myocardial infarction** to avoid increasing infarct size.

        (2) It may induce **cardiac arrhythmias.**

(3) Other adverse effects may include those described for Epi [see II A 1 f (1)].

3. Ephedrine (Ephedra®)

    a. Mechanism of action. Ephedrine is a mixed-acting agent (i.e., it has direct and indirect actions); however, its primary action is indirect. Thus, a significant portion of its action is indirectly from the **NE release. Its direct effect is activation of α_1-adrenergic receptors and β-receptors.**

    b. Pharmacologic effects

        (1) Ephedrine **increases blood pressure** by causing peripheral vasoconstriction and cardiac stimulation.

        (2) It causes **bronchodilation** by activating β_2-adrenergic receptors.

        (3) It causes the **urinary bladder sphincter constriction** by activating α_1-adrenergic receptors.

    c. Therapeutic uses. Ephedrine is a scheduled drug (i.e., additional regulations for its use are imposed by FDA).

        (1) It is used to treat **asthma-like** conditions.

        (2) It is used as a **mydriatic.**

        (3) It can be used to treat primary **urinary bladder sphincter incompetence. However, phenylpropanolamine has been used more commonly than ephedrine for urinary incontinence.**

    d. Pharmacokinetics

        (1) Absorption. Ephedrine is absorbed from the GI tract and can be administered orally.

        (2) Metabolism. It is resistant to metabolism by MAO and is not a substrate for COMT, so it has a prolonged action. It is metabolized very slowly in the liver and excreted mostly unchanged in the urine. Urine pH may alter excretion characteristics. In humans: at urine pH of 5, $t_{1/2}$ is ~3 hours; at urine pH of 6.3, $t_{1/2}$ is ~6 hours.

    e. Adverse effects are similar to those of Epi.

        (1) Hypertension and cardiac arrhythmias may occur with systemic use.

        (2) CNS stimulation may cause nervousness, nausea, and agitation.

        (3) Tachyphylaxis (i.e., diminished response following repeated administration) may occur. It is thought to be caused by a depletion of NE in the adrenergic nerve terminals susceptible to ephedrine.

4. Phenylpropanolamine (PPA®)

    a. Chemistry and mechanism of action. PPA is a mixed-acting agent (i.e., it has direct and indirect actions); however, its primary action is indirect. Thus, part of its action is indirectly from the **NE release. Its direct effect is activation of α_1-adrenergic receptors.**

    b. Pharmacologic effects. The effects of PPA are similar to those of ephedrine, except **PPA has little CNS stimulatory activity**.

    c. Therapeutic uses. PPA is used **primarily for urinary incontinence.** Tachyphylaxis has not been seen when it is used for this purpose.

    d. Pharmacokinetics

        (1) Absorption. PPA is absorbed from the GI tract and can be administered orally.

        (2) PPA is resistant to metabolism by MAO and is not a substrate for COMT.

        (3) The drug is partially metabolized to an active metabolite by the liver, but 80–90% is excreted unchanged in the urine within 24 hours of dosing.

        (4) The plasma $t_{1/2}$ is 3–4 hours.

    e. Adverse effects are similar to those of ephedrine. In addition, anorexia may occur.

5. Terbutaline (Brethine®) is an orally effective **β_2-receptor agonist** used as a bronchodilator. It can be administered SC as well. It is the **bronchodilator of choice for animals with heart disease, hyperthyroidism, or hypertension**; however, it should be administered with caution because **high doses may stimulate β_1-receptors.** Terbutaline can be administered parenterally or orally.

    a. Pharmacokinetics

        (1) No information is available for dogs and cats. Terbutaline has **a high pKa (10.1)**; as a result, **most of terbutaline is in ionized form at physiological**

pH. In humans, <50% of oral dose is absorbed because of the high pKa value for this drug; peak bronchodilation occurs within 3 hours and lasts for ≤8 hours. It is well absorbed following SC administration, peak bronchodilation occur within 1 hour, and lasts for ≤4 hours.

(2) **In horses, terbutaline should not be administered orally, since <1% is being absorbed via this route.** When administered IV, bronchodilation lasts for ~30 minutes. Thus, terbutaline should be administered as constant infusion when given IV.

(3) Terbutaline is excreted mainly as the parent drug in the urine (60%), the rest as metabolites (sulfate conjugate).

b. Adverse effects. Tachycardia, tremors, and excitation may be seen, particularly at high doses. Sweating may be seen in horses.

6. **Albuterol** (Torpex®)

a. **Mechanism of action.** Albuterol is a selective β_2- **agonist**, which causes bronchodilation.

b. **Therapeutic uses.** Albuterol is used as an aerosol and oral tablets, mainly in dogs, cats, and horses as a bronchodilator and for its effects on bronchial smooth muscle to alleviate bronchospasm or cough.

c. **Pharmacokinetics**

(1) **Albuterol has a high pKa (9.3)**, thus most of the compound is in ionized form in the blood and other tissues at physiological pH. The absorption following oral administration is limited because of the high pKa value for this drug. The absorption following inhalation is rapid and complete; bronchodilation occurs within 5 minutes of inhalation.

(2) **Duration of bronchodilation** generally persists for 1–7 hours after inhalation and ≤12 hours after oral administration.

(3) **Albuterol is extensively metabolized** in the liver, principally to the inactive metabolite, albuterol $4' - O$-sulfate, which is excreted into urine. Plasma $t_{1/2}$ is 3–5 hours after oral administration.

7. **Isoxsuprine** (Vasodilan®)

a. **Pharmacologic effects and mechanism of action. Isoxsuprine is a selective β_2-adrenergic agonist**, which causes vasodilatation in skeletal muscle. In horses with navicular disease, isoxsuprine raises distal limb temperatures. Isoxsuprine also relaxes uterine smooth muscle and may increase heart rate and contractility. At high doses, isoxsuprine can decrease blood viscosity and reduce platelet aggregation.

b. **Therapeutic uses. Isoxsuprine is used to treat navicular disease in horses**, and should be administered IV; the efficacy is disappointing when used orally.

c. **Pharmacokinetics.** Very limited information is available for horses. After oral administration of isoxsuprine, the plasma concentrations of the drug are highly variable. The elimination $t_{1/2}$ is ~3 hours in horses.

d. **Adverse effects.** Horses may show signs of **CNS stimulation** (uneasiness, hyperexcitability, nose-rubbing) or **sweating, hypotension, and tachycardia**.

8. **Clenbuterol** (Ventipulmin® Syrup)

a. **Mechanism of action.** Clenbuterol is a selective β_2-**adrenergic agonist**.

b. **Therapeutic uses.** Clenbuterol is used in horses as a **bronchodilator** for airway obstruction, such as chronic obstructive pulmonary disease. It had been **misused as a repartitioning agent** before ractopamine became available. It is administered orally.

c. **Pharmacokinetics**

(1) After oral administration to horses, plasma levels of clenbuterol peak at 2 hours and $t_{1/2}$ is ~12 hours.

(2) Urinary concentrations of clenbuterol are 100 times of those found in the plasma and can persist for 12 days in urine after the last oral dosing.

d. **Adverse effects**

(1) Muscle tremors, sweating, restlessness, urticaria, and tachycardia may be noted, particularly early in the course of therapy. Increase in serum creatine kinase concentrations (an indicator for muscle damage) has been noted in some horses and ataxia can occur.

(2) Clenbuterol can induce tachycardia at high doses. Thus, it **should not be used in horses suspected of having cardiovascular impairment.**

(3) Clenbuterol can induce **uterine relaxation**, which may offset the effects of oxytocics, for example, oxytocin and prostaglandin $F_{2\alpha}$.

9. Ractopamine (Optaflexx®, Paylean®). This is **one of the two approved repartitioning agents for animals.** It is used in cattle and swine.

   a. Mechanism of action. Ractopamine is a selective **β_2-adrenergic agonist.**

   b. Therapeutic uses. Ractopamine is used as a feed additive to improved rate of weight gain, feed efficiency, and increase carcass Leanness. Ractopamine increases lipolysis.

   c. Pharmacokinetics

     (1) The **pKa** of ractopamine is **9.4**, thus it is mostly **in ionized form when present in the blood or tissues at the physiological pH of 7.4.** As a result, the **GI absorption of ractopamine is low**, and the tissue concentrations of the drug are also low following oral administration. **No preslaughter withdrawal period is needed when animals are on ractopamine.**

     (2) Ractopamine is metabolized in the liver into glucuronide form, and the latter is excreted mostly into urine. Thus, both liver and kidney have the highest levels of residues. The residues in liver and kidney decline rapidly, that is, after a 24-hour withdrawal period, only 45% and 10% of the total residues present after a zero-day withdrawal period remained in liver and kidney, respectively.

   d. Adverse effects. Anorexia, bloat, and locomotion disorder have been seen. Personnel protection is needed when handling ractopamine. **Persons with cardiovascular disease should exercise special caution to avoid exposure.**

10. Zilpaterol (Zilmax®). It is a new and selective β_2-agonist that is used as a repartitioning agent in beef cattle. The pharmacokinetics of zilpaterol are largely unknown. The preslaughter withdrawal period is 48 hours.

III. ADRENERGIC ANTAGONISTS

A. α-**Adrenergic antagonists**

   1. Phenoxybenzamine (Dibenzyline®)

     a. Mechanism of action. Phenoxybenzamine differs from most α_1-receptor antagonists in that it **binds covalently to the α_1-receptor.** This is a stable chemical bond that **produces a long-lasting and irreversible block of the receptor.**

     b. Pharmacologic effects

       (1) Phenoxybenzamine **decreases total peripheral resistance,** causing hypotension.

       (2) Heart rate may be increased via de-activation of the baroreceptor reflex.

       (3) Phenoxybenzamine can block pupillary dilation, lid retraction, and contraction of the nictitating membrane.

     c. Therapeutic uses. It is administered orally.

       (1) In dogs and cats, phenoxybenzamine **reduces hypertonus at the urethral sphincter.**

       (2) In horses, phenoxybenzamine has been used to **treat laminitis and secretory diarrhea.**

     d. Pharmacokinetics. No information is available for animals. In humans, it is poorly absorbed from the GI tract with a bioavailability of 20–30%. Onset of action of the drug is slow (several hours) and increases over several days after regular dosing. Effects persist for 3–4 days after discontinuation of the drug.

       Phenoxybenzamine is highly lipid soluble and may store in adipose tissue. It is metabolized (dealkylated) and excreted in both the urine and bile. The plasma $t_{1/2}$ is ~24 hours in humans.

  e. **Adverse effects**
    (1) **Hypotension** may be enhanced in hypovolemic animals.
    (2) **It should not be used in horses with colic.**
2. **Prazosin** (Minipress®)
  a. **Mechanism of action.** Prazosin is a competitive and selective α_1-**receptor antagonist.**
  b. **Pharmacologic effects**
    (1) **Prazosin relaxes arterial and venous smooth muscle.**
    (2) There is a decrease in total peripheral resistance. High doses may cause **hypotension.**
  c. **Therapeutic uses. It is administered orally.**
    (1) Prazosin is used in the treatment of **congestive heart failure.** It decreases arterial pressure, which **improves cardiac output.**
    (2) Prazosin is also used in the treatment of **hypertension.**
  d. **Pharmacokinetics.** No information is available for animals. In humans, it is variably absorbed after oral administration. Peak levels occur in 2–3 hours. It is widely distributed throughout the body and is ~97% bound to plasma proteins. It is metabolized in the liver and some metabolites are active. Metabolites and ≤10% of unchanged drug are eliminated in feces.
  e. **Adverse effects include diarrhea, tachycardia, hypotension, and fluid retention.**
3. **Phentolamine** (Regitine®)
  a. **Mechanism of action.** Phentolamine is a **competitive** α_1- **and** α_2-**receptor antagonist.**
  b. **Pharmacologic effects**
    (1) Heart rate may be increased by de-activation of the baroreceptor reflex or by blocking the presynaptic α_2-receptors of the heart.
    (2) Blood pressure is lowered by inhibition of α_1- and α_2-receptors in vascular smooth muscle.
  c. **Therapeutic uses.** Phentolamine is administered IV or IM to treat hypertension and to **control high blood pressure resulting from sympathomimetic amine overdose.**
  d. **Pharmacokinetics.** No information is available for animals. In humans, it is metabolized in the liver and is excreted into the urine mostly as metabolites. The elimination $t_{1/2}$ is ~20 minutes.
  e. **Adverse effects.** Tachycardia is frequently observed.
4. **Yohimbine** (Yobin®, see also Chapter 4).
  a. **Mechanism of action.** Yohimbine is a competitive α_2-**receptor antagonist** that promotes the formation of cyclic AMP by blocking α_2-receptor activation.
  b. **Pharmacologic effects**
    (1) **Yohimbine can cause CNS stimulation, increased heart rate, and increased blood pressure by increasing NE release from the adrenergic nerve endings.**
    (2) **Yohimbine can increase GI motility by increasing parasympathetic tone.**
    (3) Yohimbine may increase plasma insulin levels, because α_2-receptors inhibit insulin release.
  c. **Therapeutic uses.** Yohimbine is used IV and IM in **monogastric animals to reverse the effects of** α_2-**receptor agonists** (i.e., xylazine, detomidine, medetomidine, and romifedine) and amitraz, a miticide that has α_2-agonistic activities. Yohimbine is marginally effective in ruminants.
  d. **Pharmacokinetics**
    (1) Yohimbine is distributed evenly after IV administration. The total body clearance is 35 mL/min/kg in horses and 30 mL/min/kg in dogs.
    (2) The $t_{1/2}$ of the drug is 0.5–1.5 hours in horses and 1.5–2 hours in dogs.
  e. **Adverse effects** are primarily **CNS stimulation, tachycardia, hypertension, and increase in GI motility.**
5. **Tolazoline.** It is a competitive antagonist for α_1- and α_2-receptors. The pharmacologic effects are similar to phentolamine.

   a. Therapeutic uses. It is administered IV (slowly) to reverse the pharmacologic effects of α_2-agonists, for example, xylazine, **particularly in ruminants.**
   b. Pharmcokinetics. After IV administration in horses, it is widely distributed. It is concentrated in the liver and kidneys. The plasma $t_{1/2}$ in horses is ~60 minutes. In cattle after an IV dose of 4 mg/kg, the concentration of tolazoline was <10 µg/kg by 96 hours in tissues and by 48 hours in milk. On the basis of these data, it is recommended the preslaughter withdrawal period of 8 days and milk withdrawal time of 48 hours in cattle.
   c. Adverse effects. Tolazoline can cause tachycardia, hypotension, and increased GI motility. Because of hypotension, it should not be administered to animals exhibiting signs of stress, debilitation, cardiac disease, sympathetic blockage, hypovolemia, or shock.
6. **Atipamezole**. It is an α_2-antagonist, which is labeled for use as a reversal agent for medetomidine. It can reverse the effects of other α_2-agonists as well (e.g., amitraz, xylazine). It is effective in all species, including ruminants. However, it is too expensive to be used in food animals.
   a. Pharmacokinetics. It is administered IM, IV, or SC, but IM route is preferred. After IM administration in the dog, peak plasma levels occur in 10 minutes. It is metabolized in the liver to compounds that are eliminated in the urine. The elimination $t_{1/2}$ is 2–3 hours.

B. **β-Adrenergic antagonists**

1. **Propranolol** (Inderal®, see also Chapter 8).
   a. Mechanism of action. Propranolol is a **nonselective β-receptor antagonist** that competitively blocks both β_1- and β_2-receptors. Recent evidence indicates propranolol is an inverse agonist of β-receptors.
   b. Pharmacologic effects
      (1) Propranolol decreases the sinus heart rate and depresses A-V conduction.
      (2) It decreases cardiac output.
      (3) It decreases myocardial oxygen demand.
      (4) It decreases the automaticity of cardiac tissue.
      (5) It increases airway resistance.
   c. Therapeutic uses. It is administered IV, IM, SC, or orally for following conditions:
      (1) Propranolol is used to treat **cardiac arrhythmia and hypertension associated with thyrotoxicosis and pheochromocytoma**, respectively.
      (2) It is used to treat **arrhythmias** (e.g., atrial and ventricular premature complexes and supraventricular and ventricular tachycardia).
   d. Pharmacokinetics
      (1) Absorption. Propranolol is well absorbed following oral administration.
      (2) Propranolol is highly lipid soluble and readily crosses the blood–brain barrier.
      (3) The $t_{1/2}$ in dogs is 1–2 hours and <2 hours in horses.
      (4) There is a significant first-pass effect, which reduces the systemic bioavailability. In dogs, only 2–27% of an oral dose reaches the blood. Rapid metabolism occurs in the liver to form 4-hydroxypropranolol, which is followed by conjugation. More than 99% of propranolol is excreted as metabolites.
   e. Adverse effects
      (1) Up-regulation of β-receptors (i.e., an increased number of receptors) occurs with long-term therapy.
      (2) Abrupt cessation of therapy may lead to excessive stimulation of β-receptors, thereby exacerbating the symptoms.
   f. Contraindications
      (1) Propranolol may cause **bronchospasm** and is contraindicated in asthmatic animals.

(2) Propranolol is contraindicated in animals with **heart failure or sinus brady-cardia**.

(3) It is contraindicated in animals with **hepatic disease.**

2. **Atenolol** (Tenormin®)

a. **Mechanism of action.** Atenolol is a competitive β_1-**receptor antagonist.**

b. **Pharmacologic effects.** Atenolol decreases heart rate, cardiac output, and systolic and diastolic pressures.

c. **Therapeutic uses.** Atenolol is administered orally to treat **supraventricular arrhythmias, hypertrophic cardiomyopathy** in cats, and hypertension.

d. **Pharmacokinetics**

(1) Atenolol has low lipid solubility and unlike propranolol, only small amounts of atenolol are distributed into the CNS.

(2) Atenolol is minimally biotransformed in the liver; 40–50% is excreted unchanged in the urine and the bulk of the remainder is excreted in feces as the parent compound.

(3) The plasma $t_{1/2}$ in dogs is 3.2 hours and in cats, it is 3.7 hours. Duration of β-adrenergic blockade in cats is ~12 hours.

e. **Adverse effects**

(1) Although atenolol is selective for β_1-receptors, it should be used cautiously in animals with asthma or a history of bronchospasm, because at high doses it can block β_2-receptors as well.

(2) Excessive β_1-blockade can greatly reduce cardiac output.

(3) It is a negative inotrope, so it must be used with caution in patients with congestive heart failure, in renal failure patients, and in patients with sinus node dysfunction.

(4) Atenolol can cause lethargy, hypotension, or diarrhea.

3. **Metoprolol** (Lopressor®)

a. **Mechanism of action.** Metoprolol is a selective β_1-**receptor antagonist.** However, at high doses it blocks β_2-receptors as well.

b. **Pharmacologic effects**

(1) Cardiovascular effects secondary to metoprolol's negative inotropic and chronotropic actions include decreased sinus heart rate, slowed AV conduction, diminished cardiac output, decreased myocardial oxygen demand, reduced blood pressure, and inhibition of the β-agonist-induced tachycardia.

(2) Metoprolol does not possess membrane-stabilizing activity like propranolol.

c. **Therapeutic uses.** Metoprolol can be used to treat **supraventricular tachyarrhythmias, premature ventricular contractions, systemic hypertension, hypertrophic cardiomyopathy, and thyrotoxicosis** in cats. It is administered orally at every 12 hours. Because metoprolol is relatively safe to use in animals with bronchospastic disease, it is often chosen over propranolol.

d. **Pharmacokinetics**

(1) Metoprolol tartrate/succinate is rapidly and nearly completely absorbed from the GI tract, but it has a relatively high first-pass effect (50%) so systemic bioavailability is reduced.

(2) Metoprolol has very low protein binding characteristics (5–15%) and is distributed well into most tissues.

(3) Metoprolol crosses the blood–brain barrier, and CSF levels are ~80% of those found in the plasma.

(4) Metoprolol is metabolized in the liver; unchanged drug and metabolites are then principally excreted in the urine. The reported $t_{1/2}$ in dogs is 1.6 hours and in cats it is 1.3 hours.

e. **Adverse effects.** They are similar to the adverse effects of propranolol.

4. **Esmolol** (Brevibloc®)

a. **Mechanism of action.** Esmolol is a selective β_1-**receptor antagonist. Not like propranolol, it has little membrane-stabilizing activity.**

b. **Therapeutic uses. Esmolol and propranolol are the first choices for IV use for tachyarrhythmias** and occasionally for acute management of dynamic left

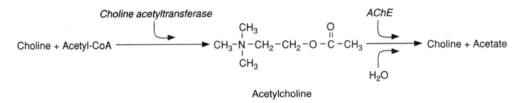

FIGURE 2-5. Synthesis and hydrolysis of acetylcholine (ACh). CoA, coenzyme A; AChE, acetylcholinesterase.

     ventricular outflow obstruction in cats. **Esmolol, very short-acting (~20 minutes), is still used in selected cases and can "test" whether a β-adrenergic antagonist would be helpful, while not lasting long if it is not.**

    c. Pharmacokinetics. Esmolol has a plasma $t_{1/2}$ of ~10 minutes. The short duration of action of esmolol is attributable to **rapid enzymatic hydrolysis by red blood cell esterases.**

    d. Adverse effects. Excessive β₁-blockade can greatly reduce cardiac output.

  2. Sotalol (Betapace®)

    a. Mechanism of action. Sotalol is **a nonselective β-receptor antagonist**, which can selectively prolong the duration of action potential and refractory period (see Chapter 8).

    b. Therapeutic uses. Sotalol is **a class III antiarrhythmic drug**, which can be used orally to treat **ventricular tachycardias** in dogs.

    c. Pharmacokinetics. Unlike propranolol, **sotalol does not have any appreciable first-pass effect after oral administration**. Food may reduce the bioavailability of sotalol by 20% (human data). The drug has relatively low lipid solubility and virtually no protein binding. Elimination is almost all via the kidney and most of the drug is excreted unchanged. In dogs, sotalol's elimination $t_{1/2}$ is 5 hours.

    d. Adverse effects. At high doses, sotalol may show negative inotropic effects and proarrhythmic effects. Sotalol may cause dyspnea/bronchospasm, fatigue/dizziness, and nausea/vomiting.

IV. CHOLINERGIC AGONISTS (Table 2-2)

A. Acetylcholine (ACh)

  1. Chemistry and biosynthesis (Figure 2-5). ACh is a quaternary chemical, synthesized by the enzyme choline acetyltransferase from choline and acetyl coenzyme A (acetyl-CoA).

  2. Mechanism of action. ACh stimulates muscarinic and nicotinic receptors.

  3. Pharmacologic effects (see Tables 2-1 and 2-2)

    a. Cardiovascular. The actions of ACh on the heart are similar to the effects produced by vagal stimulation. ACh decreases systemic blood pressure following IV injection. Possible mechanisms include negative inotropic or chronotropic action and vasodilatation.

      (1) Vasodilatation in response to nerve-released ACh is of little physiologic importance in the maintenance of blood pressure, because most peripheral blood vessels are not cholinergically innervated. However, drugs that are analogs of ACh are capable of producing vasodilatation via activation of muscarinic receptors in the blood vessels.

      (2) Vasodilatation is thought to be caused by two processes as follows:

        (a) Inhibition of the release of NE from the sympathetic nerve terminal by activating M₂-receptors.

(b) **Interaction with M$_3$-receptors on the endothelial cells to release nitric oxide, which initiates the relaxation of vascular smooth muscle.**
  b. **Smooth muscle and glands**
    (1) Stimulation of muscarinic M$_3$-receptors increases GI motility and secretion.
    (2) ACh causes smooth muscle contraction in the uterus, ureters, bladder, bronchi, and sphincter muscles of the iris via activation of M$_3$-receptors.
    (3) Activation of M$_3$-receptors increases salivary and lacrimal gland secretions.
  4. **Therapeutic uses.** ACh has little or no use as a therapeutic drug, but it is used topically to **constrict pupil** in intraocular surgery.
  5. **Antagonists. Atropine** is a specific antagonist at muscarinic receptors.

B. **Carbachol (Carbamylcholine, Carbastat$^\circledR$, etc.)**

  1. **Chemistry.** Carbachol has a carbamic acid-ester bond that is not hydrolyzable by cholinesterase. Like ACh, carbachol is a quaternary nitrogen compound.
  2. **Mechanism of action.** Carbachol activates both muscarinic and nicotinic receptors.
  3. **Therapeutic use.** Carbachol is used topically to produce **miosis** in ophthalmology. It could be administered SC to treat GI and uterine atony, but its use in such cases should be performed with extreme caution to prevent rupture of the tracts.
  4. **Pharmacokinetics.** No information is available for animals.

C. **Bethanechol**

  1. **Chemistry.** Bethanechol chemically resembles carbachol and is a **quaternary** compound. It is resistant to hydrolysis by cholinesterase.
  2. **Pharmacologic effect.** Bethanechol is an **agonist of muscarinic receptors**.
  3. **Therapeutic uses.** Bethanechol is administered SC to treat the **distention of the urinary bladder** by increasing contractility. It could be administered SC to treat **GI and uterine atony**, but its use in such cases should be performed with extreme caution to prevent rupture of the tracts.
  4. **Pharmacokinetics.** No information is available for animals. Because bethanechol is a quaternary ammonium compound, the **GI absorption is nil** after oral administration.

D. **Pilocarpine**

  1. **Chemistry.** Pilocarpine is a **tertiary amine** alkaloid.
  2. **Pharmacologic effects.** Pilocarpine resembles carbachol in actions; however, because it does not contain a quaternary ammonium, it can cross the biologic membranes.
  3. **Therapeutic uses.** Pilocarpine is primarily used topically to produce **miosis** and to lower **intraocular pressure** in glaucoma.
  4. **Pharmacokinetics.** No information is available for animals.
  5. **Adverse effects**
    (1) Pilocarpine can cause local irritation and inflammation of the uveal tract.
    (2) With repeated use, pilocarpine may cause systemic effects (**vomiting, diarrhea, and increased salivation**).

V. **ANTICHOLINESTERASE AGENTS (INDIRECT CHOLINERGIC AGONISTS)**

A. **Mechanism of action.** These agents act indirectly by **preventing the hydrolysis of ACh by acetylcholinesterase** (AChE). Therefore, at synaptic junctions, more cholinergic receptors are occupied by ACh, causing increased muscarinic and nicotinic responses. Anticholinesterase (anti-ChE) agents prevent the hydrolysis of ACh via three following **primary mechanisms:**

    1. Reversible AChE inhibition. The quaternary nitrogen of the drug reversibly binds to the active center of the enzyme at the anionic site.

    2. Carbamylation of AChE. The carbamates are substrates for AChE and occupy the active site for an extended period of time, thereby increasing the ACh concentration at synapses.

    3. Phosphorylation of AChE. The organophosphates form a stable covalent bond with the enzyme, and their effects are long-lasting (Figure 2-5).

B. **Preparations**

    1. Carbamates
      a. Physostigmine (Antilirium®)
        (1) Chemistry. Physostigmine is a tertiary amine.
        (2) Pharmacologic effects. The pharmacologic effects mimic those of ACh.
          (a) Physostigmine produces miosis, salivation, and increased GI motility.
          (b) In large doses, it causes fasciculation followed by paralysis of skeletal muscle (caused by the accumulation of ACh at the neuromuscular junction).
        (3) Therapeutic uses. Physostigmine can be used topically to treat simple and secondary **glaucoma**, and can be used IM, SC, or orally to counteract intoxication by atropine and other antimuscarinic drugs.
        (4) Pharmacokinetics. Physostigmine is well absorbed from the GI tract, SC tissues, and mucous membranes. It crosses the blood–brain barrier. It is largely hydrolyzed at the ester linkage by plasma esterases. Duration of action is 3–6 hours.
      b. Neostigmine (Prostigmin®)
        (1) Chemistry. Neostigmine contains a quaternary ammonium.
        (2) Pharmacologic effects
          (a) The pharmacologic effects of neostigmine mimic those of ACh, causing effects similar to those of physostigmine.
          (b) Neostigmine reverses the neuromuscular block produced by tubocurarine-like drugs by
            i. Inhibition of AChE
            ii. Increasing the release of ACh from nerve endings
            iii. Acting directly on the skeletal neuromuscular junction
        (3) Therapeutic uses. It is administered SC, IM, or IV to treat the following conditions:
          (a) Reversal of tubocurarine-like blockade at the skeletal neuromuscular junction
          (b) Paralytic ileus
          (c) Atony of the urinary bladder
          (d) Myasthenia gravis-like conditions
        (4) Pharmacokinetics
          (a) Absorption. Typical of quaternary ammoniums, neostigmine is not well absorbed orally nor does it cross the blood–brain barrier.
          (b) Metabolism. Neostigmine is hydrolyzed by plasma esterases.
          (c) Excretion. It is excreted in the urine as parent compound. Duration of action is 0.5–2 hours.
        (5) Adverse effects and contraindications. Adverse effects of neostigmine are **cholinergic** in nature. It is contraindicated in the presence of **GI or urinary obstruction**.
      c. Edrophonium (Tensilon®, etc.)
        (1) Pharmacologic effects. Like neostigmine, edrophonium is a quaternary ammonium compound. Its actions are similar to those of neostigmine.
        (2) Therapeutic uses. Edrophonium is used to diagnose myasthenia gravis-like disease and antagonize tubocurarine-like drugs.
        (3) Pharmacokinetics. Edrophonium is administered parenterally and has a short duration of action (10–15 minutes). Other aspects of pharmacokinetics have not been well-described.

   (4) Adverse effects are generally dose-related and cholinergic in nature. Severe
   adverse effects are possible with large overdoses.
   d. **Pyridostigmine** (Mestinon®) and **demecarium** are similar to neostigmine (quaternary compounds); however, they have a longer duration of action of 4–6 hours.
   Pyridostigmine is used orally to treat myasthenia gravis, but should be given parenterally to increase effectiveness of the treatment. Demecarium is used topically
   to treat glaucoma. Adverse effects are similar to those of neostigmine.
   e. Carbaryl and propoxur are carbamate ectoparasiticides. See Chapter 16 for further information. The effects of overdose are similar to organophosphate poisoning and are treatable with atropine.
2. **Organophosphates**
   a. **Preparations**
      (1) **Echothiophate.** It is a quaternary organophosphate (OP), and has a long du-
      ration of action (>12 hours). It is used topically in the treatment of open
      angle glaucoma.
      (2) **OPs used as ectoparasiticides are discussed in Chapter 16.**
   b. **Adverse effect (see also Chapter 16)**
      (1) **Clinical signs**
         (a) SLUDD (i.e., salivation, lacrimation, urination, defecation, and dyspnea)
         refers to a constellation of signs that are related to muscarinic stimula-
         tion. In addition, miosis and bradycardia may be seen.
         (b) Anorexia and vomiting may occur.
         (c) Neurologic signs include convulsions and fasciculation of skeletal
         muscle. Respiratory failure caused by inhibition of respiratory center,
         bronchial spasm and excessive secretions, and weakness of the respira-
         tory muscles ultimately leads to death.
      (2) **Treatment**
         (a) Detoxification
            i. Dermal exposure. The skin should be washed with soap and water
            to remove unabsorbed toxin. These chemicals are highly lipid-soluble
            and are readily absorbed via the skin; therefore, personnel should
            wear protective gear to prevent contact with the toxin.
            ii. Oral exposure. Gastric lavage should be considered if the organo-
            phosphates have been ingested.
         (b) Stabilization
            i. Respiratory assistance may be required.
            ii. Anticonvulsants may be administered.
         (c) Antidotal therapy
            i. Atropine will reduce the muscarinic effects.
            ii. Pyridine-2-aldoxime methiodide (2-PAM, pralidoxime) reactivates
            AChE (Figure 2-6).

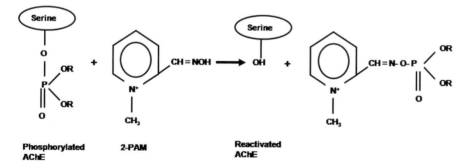

FIGURE 2-6. Pralidoxime (2-PAM) reactivates acetylcholinesterase (AChE). An organophosphate phosphorylates AChE by binding to the serine residue of the enzyme. 2-PAM works by binding to the
organophosphate, which then pulls the compound from ACh, regenerating the enzyme.

VI. PARASYMPATHETIC ANTAGONISTS (ANTIMUSCARINIC DRUGS)

A. Atropine sulfate

1. **Chemistry.** Atropine, a tertiary amine, is the prototype for all antimuscarinic drugs. It is an alkaloid obtained from the plant *Atropa belladonna* (deadly nightshade).
2. **Mechanism of action. Atropine is a competitive and nonselective antagonist of ACh at muscarinic receptors.**
3. **Pharmacologic effects**
   a. **Heart**
      (1) **Heart rate.** The effect of atropine on the heart rate is variable.
         (a) The rate may be slow initially or following a low dose, possibly as a result of central vagal stimulation.
         (b) As the muscarinic receptors on the sinoatrial (SA) node are blocked by higher concentrations of atropine, tachycardia results.
      (2) The PR interval is shortened.
   b. **Vasculature.** Because blood vessels are regulated primarily by the sympathetic nervous system, atropine at therapeutic doses has a small to modest effect on the systemic blood pressure.
   c. **CNS.** Toxic doses of atropine produce excitation, possibly followed by depression as the toxicity progresses.
   d. **Smooth muscle**
      (1) **GI contractions are reduced in amplitude and frequency.** Muscle tone is also reduced.
      (2) Biliary tract smooth muscle is relaxed.
      (3) **Urinary bladder and ureter tone is reduced.**
      (4) **Bronchodilation** occurs in the large bronchi.
   e. **Eye**
      (1) **Mydriasis.** Atropine blocks the muscarinic receptors for ACh on the sphincter smooth muscle of the iris.
      (2) **Cycloplegia** is the inability to accommodate for near vision. Atropine inhibits cholinergic control of the ciliary muscle of the lens.
      (3) Sweat gland secretions are reduced.
      (4) Gastric secretions are reduced at high doses.
4. **Therapeutic uses.** It is administered IV, IM, SC, or orally.
   a. **Atropine** is used as a **preanesthetic agent to reduce salivary and respiratory Secretions.**
   b. Antimuscarinic agents are used in ophthalmology to produce **cycloplegia and mydriasis**; however, because atropine has a **long duration of action**, its usefulness in this capacity is limited.
   c. It may be used to treat **renal and biliary colic** when combined with opioids.
   d. **It is used to counter anti-ChE overdose or toxicity.**
   e. It may be useful in treating mushroom toxicity if **muscarine** is the toxic agent.
5. **Pharmacokinetics**
   a. Atropine is rapidly and well absorbed when given orally or parenterally. After IV administration, peak effects in heart rates occur within 3 minutes.
   b. Atropine is well distributed throughout the body and crosses into the CNS.
   c. Atropine is metabolized into noratropine, atropin-*n*-oxide, and tropic acid by the liver and excreted into the urine. Thirty to fifty percent of a dose is excreted unchanged into the urine. The $t_{1/2}$ of atropine is ~2.5 hours, and most of the drug is excreted in the urine within the first 12 hours.
6. **Adverse effects include tachycardia, photophobia (from mydriasis), xerostomia, increased body temperature in horses (caused by a decrease in sweating), restlessness, disorientation, and CNS stimulation.**
7. **Treatment of toxicity.** An anti-ChE agent (e.g., neostigmine, physostigmine) should be administered to increase the concentration of ACh at muscarinic receptor sites. **CNS stimulation may be controlled by benzodiazepines.**

B. **Scopolamine (hyoscine) and *N*-butylscopolammonium (Bucospan®), alkaloids resemble atropine** in chemical structure and pharmacologic properties. Scopolamine can be used orally to control motion sickness. *N*-butylscopolammonium is administered IV in horses as an antispasmodic and antimuscarinic drug to treat colic and intestinal impaction. These two drugs may produce excitement or sedation.

C. **Propantheline** (Pro-Banthine®)

1. **Chemistry.** Propantheline is a synthetic quaternary ammonium antimuscarinic agent.
2. **Therapeutic uses**
   a. In small animals, propantheline is used orally as an **antispasmodic/antisecretory** agent in the treatment of diarrhea, colitis, and acute irritable bowel syndrome. It is also used orally in the treatment of hyperreflexic detrusor or urge **urinary incontinence** and as oral treatment in anticholinergic responsive **bradycardias**. However, doubts have been raised with the effectiveness, since GI absorption of the drug is rather poor.
   b. In horses, propantheline has been administered IV to reduce **colonic peristalsis** and to relax the rectum to allow easier **rectal examination and perform surgical procedures** to the rectum.
3. **Pharmacokinetics.** It is poorly absorbed after oral administration, only <25% of oral dose is absorbed. After being absorbed, it cannot penetrate the blood–brain barrier. After oral administration, it is believed to be prevalently metabolized (hydrolyzed) in the GI and/or liver; <5% of an oral dose is excreted unchanged in the urine. The plasma $t_{1/2}$ in humans is 1.6 hours and duration of action is 6 hours; no information is available for animals.
4. **Adverse effects** are similar to those of atropine, except propantheline does not effectively enter the CNS, since it is a quaternary ammonium compound.

D. **Glycopyrrolate** (Robinul®-V)

1. **Chemistry.** Glycopyrrolate is a synthetic quaternary ammonium.
2. **Therapeutic uses**
   a. It is used as a preanesthetic drug by parenteral administration (IV, IM, or SC).
   b. It can be administered IV or IM to treat sinus bradycardia, S-A arrest, and incomplete A-V block.
   c. It can be administered SC to control hyersalivation in cats.
3. **Pharmacokinetics**
   a. After parenteral administration, it does not effectively enter the CNS or eye.
   b. After IM administration, plasma levels reach at peak in 30–45 minutes. Vagal blocking actions persist for 2–3 hours and antisalivation effect persists up to 7 hours.
   c. It is eliminated primarily via the kidney; metabolism plays a small role in its elimination. The plasma $t_{1/2}$ is ~1 hour after IM or IV administration..

E. **Tropicamide**, a synthetic tertiary amine antimuscarinic drug, is used topically in ophthalmology to induce mydriasis and cycloplegia. It has an advantage over atropine in that its duration of action is shorter (4–8 hours) (see also Chapter 14).

F. **Aminopentamide** (Centrine®)

1. **Therapeutic uses.** It is used orally, IM, or SC in dogs and cats for the treatment of **acute abdominal visceral spasm, pylorospasm or hypertrophic gastritis** and associated nausea, vomiting, and/or diarrhea. When compared with atropine as an anticholinergic drug, it has a greater effect on **reducing colonic contractions** and **less mydriatic and salivary effects**. Aminopentamide may **reduce gastric acid secretion** as well.
2. **Pharmacokinetics.** No information is available.

VII. GANGLIONIC NICOTINIC AGONISTS AND ANTAGONISTS. Ganglionic nicotinic agonists and antagonists are of limited use in veterinary medicine. Skeletal neuromuscular junction nicotinic antagonists (see VIII) have more therapeutic uses.

A. **Nicotine and nicotine-like antinematodal drugs**, for example, levamisole, pyrantel, and morantel (see also Chapter 16).

1. **Mechanism of action (see Figure 2-1; Table 2-2)**
   a. These compounds activate nicotinic receptors in both the sympathetic and parasympathetic ganglia, where they stimulate the postganglionic neuron. They mimic the actions of ACh in this aspect.
   b. These compounds stimulate the adrenal medulla to release Epi and NE into the blood stream.
   c. In the somatic nervous system, they stimulate the skeletal neuromuscular junction at nicotinic receptors.
2. **Pharmacologic effects**
   a. **CNS.** Stimulation of the motor cortex by nicotine produces tremors.
   b. **Respiratory.** Respiration may be initially stimulated and then depressed.
   c. **Cardiovascular.** Increases in blood pressure, heart rate, and peripheral resistance result from stimulation of sympathetic ganglia and the adrenal medulla.
   d. **Smooth muscle and glands.** Stimulation of parasympathetic ganglia may increase GI motility and salivary secretion.
3. **Therapeutic uses.** Nicotine has no therapeutic use, but **nicotine-like compounds are available as antiparasitic drugs.**
4. **Pharmacokinetics**
   a. **Absorption.** Nicotine and nicotine-like compounds are well absorbed by all routes, including the dermal route.
   b. **Metabolism.** They are metabolized by the liver via phase I and II metabolism.
   c. **Excretion.** They are eliminated by the kidney both as metabolites and parent compound. The plasma $t_{1/2}$ of levamisole is 4–6 hours and of pyrantel tartrate is ~6 hours.
5. **Adverse effects**
   a. Convulsions may occur with high doses.
   b. Vomiting and muscle fasciculation may occur.
   c. Depolarizing neuromuscular blockade paralyzes skeletal muscle, particularly respiratory muscle, which can be fatal.

B. **Hexamethonium, trimethaphan, and mecamylamine are antagonists of post-ganglionic nicotinic receptors.** These drugs have been used as pharmacological tools to characterize nicotinic receptors in the ganglia, but have not been used in veterinary medicine. The primary disadvantage to their use is that they are **not selective** (i.e., they block transmission in both sympathetic and parasympathetic ganglia).

VIII. NEUROMUSCULAR BLOCKING DRUGS

A. **Mechanism of action.** These drugs act on nicotinic receptors at neuromuscular junction (N_M receptors) via two different mechanisms to relax skeletal muscle.

1. **Depolarizing drugs** [e.g., succinyicholine (SuCh, Anectine®)]. SuCh acts like ACh to depolarize the neuromuscular junction, but it is hydrolyzed by AChE less rapidly. Solutions of SuCh should always be kept cold in the field, since it undergoes spontaneous hydrolysis.
   a. **Phase I.** The nonselective cation channel associated with the N_M receptor is opened and the receptor is depolarized. Persistent binding of succinylcholine to the N_M receptor transforms the receptor so that it is incapable of transmitting further impulses. This phase is associated with **muscle fasciculation.**

TABLE 2-4. Duration of Action of Competitive N_M Blockers When Administered IV

Animal	Tuborcurarine Dose (mg/kg)	Tuborcurarine Duration (min)	Pancuronium Dose (mg/kg)	Pancuronium Duration (min)	Atracurium Dose (mg/kg)	Atracurium Duration (min)	Vecuronium Dose (mg/kg)	Vecuronium Duration (min)
Horse	0.3	60	0.06	40	0.15	30	0.1	30
Cow	0.06	30	0.04	40	—	—	—	—
Sheep	0.04	30	0.025	45	0.5	30	0.04	15
Pig	0.4	30	0.1	30	—	—	—	—
Dog	—	—	0.06	30	0.5	40	0.1	25
Cat	—	—	—	—	0.5	40	0.1	25

Modified from Table 2-4, *NVMS Pharmacology.*

      b. Phase II. Over time, the nonselective cation channel closes and repolarization occurs, rendering the neuromuscular junction resistant to depolarization. Flaccid paralysis ensues.

  2. Competitive blocking drugs (e.g., tubocurarine, pancuronium, atracurium, vecuronium)—nondepolarizing drugs. These drugs occupy the N_M receptor but do not activate it. By reducing the number of N_M receptors available for ACh, the end-plate potential is reduced, the threshold required to excite the muscle is not reached, and the muscle relaxes.

B. **Pharmacokinetics**

  1. Depolarizing drugs
    a. Following IV or IM administration (IV is preferred), SuCh has a rapid onset of action. Since there is a species difference in the level of pseudocholinesterase, the duration of action varies according to species and dosages. Ruminants have lower levels of this enzyme than other species, that is, horses. For unknown reasons, dogs may show prolonged paralysis after SuCh administration.
    b. SuCh is hydrolyzed by pseudocholinesterase of liver and plasma. Animals that have been exposed to an organophosphate cholinesterase inhibitor (e.g., in ectoparasiticides or eyedrops) up to 30 days before SuCh administration may experience a prolonged duration of action caused by a reduced rate of hydrolysis.
  2. Competitive blocking drugs. Each drug has a specific duration of action that varies according to species following IV administration (Table 2-4).
    a. Tubocurarine is not significantly metabolized in animals. Approximately 50% is excreted unchanged in the urine and 50% in the bile. Caution should be taken not to administer tubocurarine to animals with liver or kidney disease.
    b. Pancuronium is metabolized by the liver, but the kidney is the major route for elimination.
    c. Atracurium has a unique mechanism for metabolism. It undergoes spontaneous degradation in the plasma called Hoffman elimination and ester hydrolysis, which do not involve the liver or kidneys. Thus, in patients with renal or liver disease, atracurium may be the drug of choice for relaxing skeletal muscle.
    d. Vecuronium is eliminated by the kidney (~15%) and by metabolism and biliary excretion.

C. **Therapeutic uses**. Neuromuscular blockers are used to

  1. Promote and enhance skeletal muscle relaxation during surgery. This permits less general anesthetic to be used and enhances safety of the surgery.
  2. Facilitates endotracheal intubation.

D. Adverse effects

1. General aspects
   a. These drugs do not affect sensory mechanisms. Though paralyzed, conscious animals still feel pain.
   b. Prolonged apnea may occur.
   c. These drugs should not be used unless facilities are available for administering artificial respiration.

2. Succinylcholine
   a. Succinylcholine elicits uncoordinated muscle contraction that may last for ~30 seconds and be painful. ACh receptors in autonomic ganglia and muscarinic receptors may be stimulated by SuCh. This may result in bradycardia and increases in bronchiolar and salivary secretion.
   b. SuCh may serve as a trigger for malignant hyperthemia in the pig and horse.

3. Tubocurarine
may reduce blood pressure by causing histamine release and by blocking transmission in autonomic ganglia. Dogs and cats are prone to histamine release by tubocurarine, which precludes its use in these species. Histamine release may also cause bronchospasm, bronchial secretion, and salivation.

4. Pancuronium
causes a small increase in heart rate.

5. Atracurium
does induce histamine release but the extent of release is less than that of tubocurarine.

6. Vecuronium
does not have other adverse effects.

E. Factors influencing the action of neuromuscular blocking drugs

1. Genetic or ChE inhibitor-induced decreases in plasma. ChE activity will prolong the duration of action of SuCh.
2. Hepatic disease may prolong the duration of action of SuCh, since the liver synthesizes plasma ChE.
3. Aminoglycoside antibiotics have neuromuscular blocking activities since they inhibit ACh release.
4. Inhalant anesthetics, for example, isoflurane, enhance nondepolarizing neuromuscular blockade since they stabilize the postjunctional membrane.
5. Concomitant administration of SuCh with inhalation anesthetics may induce increased incidences of bradycardia, arrhythmias, sinus arrest, and apnea (owing to ganglionic blockade).

F. Reversal of neuromuscular blockade

1. Competitive neuromuscular blockers can be antagonized by ChE inhibitors such as edrophonium and neostigmine.
2. No good antagonists exist for SuCh. The patient should be ventilated until recovery occurs.

SUGGESTED READING

Adams HR. 2001. "Introduction to neurohumoral transmission and the autonomic nervous system." In *Veterinary Pharmacology and Therapeutics*. Edited by Adams HR. 8th ed., pp. 69–90. Ames, IA: Iowa State University Press.

Adams HR. 2001. "Neuromuscular blocking agents." In *Veterinary Pharmacology and Therapeutics*. Edited by Adams HR. 8th ed., pp. 137–152. Ames, IA: Iowa State University Press.

Atri A, Chang MS, Strichatz GR. 2006. "Cholinergic pharmacology." In *Principles of Pharmacology:The Pathophysiologic Basis of Drug Therapy*. Edited by Golan DE, Tashjian AH, Jr, Armstrong EJ, Armstrong AW. 2nd ed., pp. 109–128. Baltimore, MD: Lippincott Williams & Wilkins.

http://www.drugs.com

Plumb DC. 2005. *Veterinary Drug Handbook*. 5th ed. Ames, IA: Blackwell Publishing.

Westfall TC, Westfall DP. 2006. "Neurotransmission: The autonomic and somatic motor nervous system." In *Goodman & Gilman's The Pharmacological Basis of Therapeutics*. Edited by Brunton LL, Lazo JS, Parker KL. 11th ed., pp. 237–295. New York: McGraw-Hill.

STUDY QUESTIONS

DIRECTIONS: Each of the numbered items or incomplete statements in this section is followed by answers or by completion of the statement. Select the **one** lettered answer or completion that is **best** in each case.

1. α_1-Receptors are associated with which one of the following effects?

(A) Cardioacceleration
(B) Vasodilation
(C) Pupillary dilation
(D) Bronchodilation
(E) Pupillary constriction

2. What is the most likely cause of death in organophosphate poisoning?

(A) GI bleeding
(B) Hypertension
(C) Respiratory failure
(D) Congestive heart failure
(E) Cardiac arrhythmia

3. Which of the following adrenergic agonists at clinical doses produces dilation of vessels in muscle, constriction of cutaneous vessels, and positive inotropic and chronotropic effects on the heart?

(A) Phenylpropanolamine
(B) Isoproterenol
(C) Isoxsuprine
(D) Epinephrine
(E) Dobutamine

4. Which of the following drugs produces pupillary dilation (mydriasis) without causing cycloplegia?

(A) Scopolamine
(B) Pilocarpine
(C) Isoproterenol
(D) Tropicamide
(E) Phenylephrine

5. Which of the following bronchodilators is considered the safest for use in an animal with cardiac disease?

(A) Isoproterenol
(B) Terbutaline
(C) Ephedrine
(D) Epinephrine

6. Nicotinic receptor sites are found in all of the following locations, *except*

(A) parasympathetic ganglia.
(B) sympathetic ganglia.
(C) skeletal muscle.
(D) bronchial smooth muscle.

7. When placed in the eye, echothiophate can cause all of the following, *except*

(A) mydriasis.
(B) ciliary spasm.
(C) reversal of cycloplegia.
(D) reduction in intraocular pressure.

8. Which of the following autonomic drugs would be most likely to increase myometrial contractility?

(A) Atropine
(B) Phenoxybenzamine
(C) Ractopamine
(D) Xylazine

9. Which of the following is the sign of bethanechol stimulation of muscarinic receptors?

(A) Skeletal muscle twitching
(B) Urination
(C) Constipation
(D) Dry mucous membranes

10. Which of the following muscarinic receptor subtype mediates the bethanechol-induced decrease in heart rate and contractility?

(A) M_1
(B) M_2
(C) M_3
(D) M_4
(E) M_5

11. Which of the following adrenergic receptors subtype mediates the phenylpropanolamine-induced contraction of the trigone and sphincter muscle of the urinary bladder? This effect is useful to treat urinary incontinence.

(A) α_1
(B) α_2
(C) β_1
(D) β_2
(E) β_3

12. Metoprolol is used in a cat with hyperthyroidism showing cardiac arrhythmia. The use of metoprolol in this cat will most likely cause

(A) hypersalivation.
(B) mydriasis.
(C) bronchoconstriction.
(D) hyperglycemia.
(E) decreased renin secretion.

13. Which of the following would be most likely to increase airway resistance in a dog with pulmonary obstruction?

(A) Albuterol
(B) Atenolol
(C) Isoproterenol
(D) Phenoxybenzamine
(E) Propranolol

14. In patients with liver or renal disease, which of the following neuromuscular blockers would be the choice for these patients?

(A) Atracurium
(B) Pancuronium
(C) Succinylcholine
(D) Tubocurarine
(E) Vecuronium

15. Administration of which of the following neuromuscular blockers will cause transient and painful skeletal muscle contractions and an increase in bronchial and salivary secretions?

(A) Atracurium
(B) Pancuronium
(C) Succinylcholine
(D) Tubocurarine
(E) Vecuronium

16. Which of the following β_2-adrenergic agonists can be used legally as a repartitioning agent in cattle and swine and use of it does not require preslaughter withdrawal?

(A) Albuterol
(B) Clenbuterol
(C) Ractopamine
(D) Terbutaline

17. Which of the following β-blockers has the shortest duration of action of 20 minutes? Such a drug can be used to test if the treatment is beneficial to animals.

(A) Atenolol
(B) Esmolol
(C) Metoprolol
(D) Propranolol
(E) Sotalol

18. Which of the following is not a pharmacological effect of yohimbine?

(A) CNS excitation.
(B) Hyperglycemia.
(C) Hypertension.
(D) Increased GI motility.
(E) Tachycardia.

19. Which receptor subtype mediates DA-induced vasodilatation in renal, mesenteric, and coronary arteries?

(A) D_1
(B) D_2
(C) D_3
(D) D_4
(E) D_5

ANSWERS AND EXPLANATIONS

1. The answer is C.
Sympathetic stimulation causes the α_1-receptors in the iris to contract, causing pupillary dilation (mydriasis). An increased heart rate is associated with β_1-receptors. Vasodilation and bronchodilation are associated with β_2-receptors. Miosis (i.e., constriction of the pupils) is associated with stimulation of muscarinic cholinergic receptors.

2. The answer is C.
Organophosphate cholinesterase inhibitors prevent the hydrolysis of acetylcholine (ACh). ACh accumulates at cholinergic synapses. All autonomically innervated tissues may be affected by the excess ACh; one of the important effects is to evoke bronchoconstriction and bronchial secretion. In addition, excess ACh at the skeletal muscle neuroeffector junction ultimately leads to paralysis of the respiratory muscles, and inhibition of the respiratory center in the medulla. The primary cause of death is respiratory failure.

3. The answer is D.
Activation of β_2-receptors, α_1-receptors, and β_1-receptors produces vasodilation in muscle, constriction of skin vasculature, and positive inotropic and chronotropic effects on the heart, respectively. The only drug listed that activates α_1-, β_1-, and β_2-receptors at clinical doses is epinephrine. Phenylpropanolamine activates predominantly α_1-receptors. Isoproterenol activates both β_1- and β_2-receptors but not α_1-receptors. Isoxsuprine is a selective β_2-agonist, whereas dobutamine is a selective β_1-agonist.

4. The answer is E.
Phenylephrine, an α_1-agonist, constricts the radial muscles of the iris to induce mydriasis. Scopolamine and tropicamide are muscarinic antagonists that produce mydriasis and cycloplegia. Pilocarpine is a muscarinic agonist that produces miosis when placed in the eye. Activation of β-receptors in the eye, such as that caused by isoproterenol, does not change pupil size.

5. The answer is B.
Terbutaline would be the drug of choice when it is necessary to induce bronchodilation in an animal with heart disease. A drug with β_2-agonistic activity is necessary to produce bronchodilation. Although isoproterenol and epinephrine are β_2-agonists, they are also strong β_1-agonists and thus would be expected to excite the heart. Ephedrine increases the release of norepinephrine from the sympathetic nerve terminal, and also activates both α- and β-adrenergic receptors. Although terbutaline is the drug of choice in this situation, caution is warranted because at high doses, terbutaline may stimulate β_1-receptors as well.

6. The answer is D.
Bronchial smooth muscle contains muscarinic receptors, not nicotinic receptors. Both the parasympathetic and sympathetic ganglia contain N_N-nicotinic cholinergic receptors, and the skeletal neuromuscular junction contains N_M-nicotinic cholinergic receptors.

7. The answer is A.
Echothiophate, a cholinesterase inhibitor that increases the buildup of acetylcholine (ACh) causes miosis, ciliary spasm, reversal of cycloplegia, and reduced intraocular pressure. Mydriasis can be induced by blocking M_3-muscarinic receptors in the sphincter smooth muscles of the iris or by contracting the radial muscles of the iris via α_1-receptors.

8. The answer is D.
Myometrial contractility is increased by activation of α_1-, α_2-, and M_3-receptors and is decreased by activation of β_2-receptors. Xylazine is an α_2-agonist, and it can facilitate parturition and cause abortion. Atropine is a muscarinic receptor antagonist, ractopamine is a β_2-agonist, and phenoxybenzamine is an α-blocker. These latter drugs evoke uterine relaxation.

9. The answer is B.
Stimulation of M_3-muscarinic receptors causes urination by increasing contractions

of the urinary bladder. Bethanechol does not stimulate nicotinic receptors, and thus it does not cause skeletal muscle twitching. Constipation and dry mucous membranes are due to antagonism of M_3-receptors.

10. The answer is B.
M_2-receptors mediate the decrease in all aspects of cardiac activities and this effect is due to inhibition of norepinephrine release from the sympathetic nerve endings of the heart. M_2-receptors are found in these nerve endings and they are inhibitory receptors, coupling to $G_{i/o}$. Activation of M_2-receptors inhibits norepenephrine release and thus decreases cardiac activities.

11. The answer is A.
The α_1-receptors are found in sphincter muscles (except iris sphincter muscle). Activation of α_1-receptors evokes contractions of the trigone and sphincter muscle of the urinary bladder, and thus α_1-agonists can be used to control urinary incontinence.

12. The answer is E.
β_1-Receptors mediate renin secretion, and thus blockade of these receptors will decrease the secretion. Hypersalivation, mydriasis, bronchoconstriction, and hyperglycemia cannot be induced by β_1-blockade.

13. The answer is E.
Since β_2-receptors mediate bronchodilation, the blockade of these receptors will increase airway resistance, which is detrimental to the animals with pulmonary obstruction. Propranolol can block β_2-receptors, and thus should not be used in these animals. Albuterol and isoproterenol can activate β_2-receptors to induce bronchodilation. Atenolol is a selective β_1-blocker and should not block β_2-receptors at the clinical doses. Phenoxybenzamine is an α-blocker, and it does not cause bronchoconstriction.

14. The answer is A.
Atracurium is spontaneously degraded in the plasma by a process called Hoffman elimination and ester hydrolysis. Thus, the degradation of atracurium does not require the participation of the liver and kidneys. Atracurium is the choice for the patients with liver or renal disease. Other neuromuscular blockers required the participation of liver and/or kidney to eliminate the drug.

15. The answer is C.
Succinylcholine (SuCh) is a depolarizing neuromuscular blocking agent, which causes transient but strong muscle contractions before paralyzing them, which can be painful. SuCh can stimulate muscarinic receptors to increase bronchial and salivary secretions.

16. The answer is C.
Ractopamine is the only FDA-approved repartitioning agent used in cattle and swine. The pKa of ractopamine is 9.4, thus it is mostly in ionized form when present in the blood or tissues at the physiological pH of 7.4. As a result, the GI absorption of ractopamine is low, and the tissue concentrations of the drug are also low following oral administration. Thus, no preslaughter withdrawal period is needed after ractopamine administration.

17. The answer is B.
Esmolol is a β_1-blocker and has a plasma $t_{1/2}$ of ~10 minutes. The short duration of action of esmolol is attributable to rapid enzymatic hydrolysis by red blood cell esterases. Other β_1-blockers have longer $t_{1/2}$ and thus do not have the advantages of esmolol.

18. The answer is B.
Yohimbine is an α_2-antagonist that exerts many effects opposite to the ones exerted by α_2-agonists. α_2-Agonists induce CNS depression, long-lasting hypotension, hyperglycemia, decreased GI motility, and bradycardia. Yohimbine does not cause hyperglycemia.

19. The answer is A.
Dopamine activates D_1-receptors in renal, mesenteric, and coronary arteries to induce vasodilatation. D_1-receptors are coupled to G_s, just like β-receptors.

Chapter 3

Autacoids and Their Pharmacological Modulators

Anumantha G. Kanthasamy and Walter H. Hsu

I. INTRODUCTION

A. Definitions

1. **Autacoids** are chemical mediators that are synthesized and function in a localized tissue or area and participate in physiologic or pathophysiologic responses to injury. They act only locally and therefore also termed "local hormone." Autacoids normally do not function as the classical blood-borne hormones. Typically, autacoids are short-lived and rapidly degraded.
2. **Autacoid modulators** interfere with the synthesis, inhibit the release or the receptors upon which they act.

B. Physiologic function

1. Autacoids modulate blood flow in specific tissues.
2. Some autacoids modulate secretory processes, for example, histamine on gastric acid formation.
3. Autacoids modulate smooth muscle function.
4. Autacoids play a key role in allergy, inflammation, smooth muscle function, pain, and certain types of drug reactions (Anaphylaxis).

C. Major classes. The autacoids to be discussed in this chapter can be divided into three categories based on their chemical structure. Not all known autacoids will be discussed and the reader should consult a standard pharmacology text for information on vasoactive intestinal polypeptide, substance P, and the cytokines.

1. **Biogenic amines**: Histamine, serotonin (5-hydroxytryptamine)
2. **Polypeptides**: Bradykinin, angiotensin
3. **Lipid-derived autacoids**
   a. **Eicosanoids**. Prostaglandins, leukotrienes, thromboxane
   b. **Platelet activating factor**

II. BIOGENIC AMINES

A. Histamine

1. **Biosynthesis**. Dietary **histidine** is decarboxylated by l-histidine decarboxylase to form **histamine** (Figure 3-1).
2. **Metabolism**. Two pathways are involved in the degradation of histamine. The major degradation pathway (>50% histamine degradation) involves conversion of histamine to an inactive metabolite 1-methylhistamine by imidazole-*N*-methyltransferase. The minor pathway (25% histamine degradation) involves breakdown of histamine by diamine oxidase (histaminase) to form imidazoleacetic acid.
3. **Distribution and storage sites**. Histamine is widely distributed in tissues and its concentration and rate of synthesis varies greatly from tissue to tissue.
   a. The primary tissue sites storing histamine are the **lungs**, **skin**, mucosal layer of the **stomach** and **basophils**.
      (1) Food and vagal stimulation can release histamine from the stomach mucosal enterochromaffin-like (ECL) cells. The released histamine then initiates gastric acid secretion (see Chapter 11, Figure 11-2).

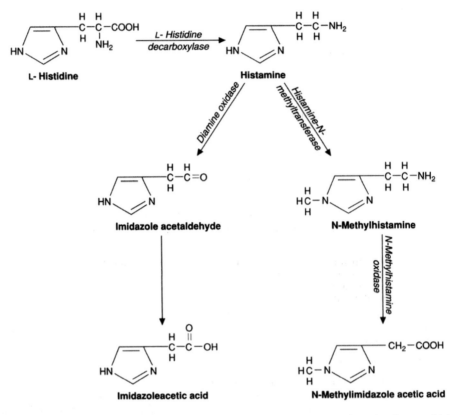

FIGURE 3-1. Synthesis and catabolism of histamine. Note: The conversion of imidazole acetaldehyde to imidazoleacetic acid is catalyzed by acetaldehyde dehydrogenase.

  (2) Allergic responses in the skin and lungs are due in part to histamine release from mast cells.
  b. **Mast cells** are the primary cells that store histamine where it exists in a complex with heparin sulfate and chondroitin sulfate E in storage granules. The rate of histamine synthesis and turnover in mast cells is low.
  c. Histamine is also found in CNS where it may act as a neurotransmitter.
  d. Many **venoms** and **insect stings** contain histamine, as well as other biologically active substances.
  e. Histamine is found in the digesta where it is formed in large part by bacterial action. This histamine normally does not reach the systemic circulation since it is metabolized by enzymes in the gut wall and liver.
4. **Release**
  a. **Immune release.** When sensitized mast cells or basophils are coupled to IgE antibodies and then exposed to the proper antigen; the mast cell degranulates, thereby releasing histamine and other autacoids. This is also referred to type I IgE-mediated hypersensitivity reaction.
  b. **Drug-induced release.** Drugs, usually strong bases (morphine, polymyxin, tubocurarine, codeine, lidocaine, penicillin), and/or their vehicles are capable of releasing histamine but this release does not involve degranulation or mast cell injury. These drugs displace or compete with histamine for the binding sites with heparin.
  c. **Plant and animal stings** are capable of releasing histamine, which is an important component of the physiologic reaction (erythema, pain, itch) to these stings.
  d. **Physical injury** such as heat, cold, or trauma can disrupt the mast cells thereby releasing histamine.

TABLE 3-1. Histamine Pharmacology—An Overview

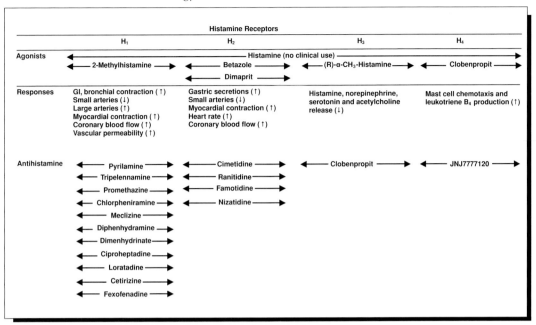

	Histamine Receptors			
	H_1	H_2	H_3	H_4
Agonists	◄———————————————— Histamine (no clinical use) ————————————————►			
	◄——— 2-Methylhistamine ———►	◄——— Betazole ———►	◄——— (R)-α-CH₃-Histamine ———►	◄——— Clobenpropit ———►
		◄——— Dimaprit ———►		
Responses	GI, bronchial contraction (↑) Small arteries (↓) Large arteries (↑) Myocardial contraction (↑) Coronary blood flow (↑) Vascular permeability (↑)	Gastric secretions (↑) Small arteries (↓) Myocardial contraction (↑) Heart rate (↑) Coronary blood flow (↑)	Histamine, norepinephrine, serotonin and acetylcholine release (↓)	Mast cell chemotaxis and leukotriene B₄ production (↑)
Antihistamine	◄——— Pyrilamine ———► ◄——— Tripelennamine ———► ◄——— Promethazine ———► ◄——— Chlorpheniramine ———► ◄——— Meclizine ———► ◄——— Diphenhydramine ———► ◄——— Dimenhydrinate ———► ◄——— Ciproheptadine ———► ◄——— Loratadine ———► ◄——— Cetirizine ———► ◄——— Fexofenadine ———►	◄——— Cimetidine ———► ◄——— Ranitidine ———► ◄——— Famotidine ———► ◄——— Nizatidine ———►	◄——— Clobenpropit ———►	◄——— JNJ7777120 ———►

5. **Receptor pharmacology (see Table 3-1 for overview of histamine receptor pharmacology).**

Four classes of receptors (H_1, H_2, H_3, and H_4) mediate the action of histamine.

a. **H_1-receptors are coupled to G_q protein–phospholipase C and mediate the following effects:**

(1) Contraction of smooth muscle and neuronal actions are due to increases in $[Ca^{2+}]_i$ and activation of protein kinase C (see Chapter 1 for detailed information).

(2) Relaxation of vascular smooth muscle involves Ca^{2+}-induced formation of nitric oxide (NO).

(3) H_1-receptors mediate contraction of bronchiolar and intestinal smooth muscle, vasodilation of small arteries and veins, increased capillary permeability and pruritus. There are considerable species variations in their sensitivity of bronchial smooth muscle to contraction by histamine. The guinea pig bronchi are the most sensitive but the bronchi of rabbit, dog, goat, calf, pig, horse, and human also contract. In contrast, histamine relaxes respiratory smooth muscle in cats (via H_1 and H_2) and sheep (via H_2). The mechanisms by which H_1-receptors mediate brochodilation in cats are not known. H_2-receptors mediate bronchodilation via an increase in cAMP levels (see below). H_1-agonists and H_1-antihistamines are listed in Table 3-1.

b. **H_2-receptors are coupled to G_s protein-adenylyl cyclase**

Stimulation of G_s-coupled H_2 receptors activate adenylyl cyclase and increase tissue cAMP levels. This is the mechanism by which vascular smooth muscle relaxes, and gastric acid secretion is stimulated.

H_2-receptor primarily mediates gastric acid secretion and vasodilatation.

(1) Agonists include 4-methylhistamine and dimaprit.

(2) H_2-Antihistaminec include: cimetidine, ranitidine, famotidine, and nizatidine. Recent evidence suggests, just like H_1-antihistamines, these drugs are inverse agonists. (Table 3-1).

c. **H_3-receptors are coupled to $G_{i/o}$ protein.** Inhibition of the release of histamine and other neurotransmitters involves inhibition of cAMP synthesis, opening of K^+ channels to increase K^+ efflux, and closure of Ca^{2+} channels to block Ca^{2+} entry into the nerve.

H_3-receptors are located presynaptically on neurons and inhibit neurotransmitter release. There are no drugs used in veterinary medicine that specifically activate or block these receptors.

   d. H_4-receptors are coupled to $G_{i/o}$ protein and activate phospholipase C-β by Gβγ (see Chapter 1 for detailed information). These receptors are selectively expressed in mast cells, basophils, and eosinophils. Activation of H_4-receptors mediates histamine-induced mast cell chemotaxis and leukotriene B_4 production via activation of phospholipase C-β. Thus, H_4-receptors may play a role in early events of inflammation, edema, and thermal hyperalgesia.

      H_4-receptor antagonists are being developed as anti-inflammatory drugs that involve mast cells and eosinophils.

6. Physiologic and pathologic roles

  a. Gastric acid secretion. Histamine is the most important regulator of gastric acid secretion and it stimulates secretion via H_2 receptors (see below under pharmacological effects).

  b. Allergic reactions and anaphylactic shock. The binding of antigenic substances to IgE molecules on mast cells causes the release of histamine. Other biologically active substances such as prostaglandin D_2 and leukotrines (LTC_4 and LTD_4) are also released.

  c. Inflammation. Histamine may be involved in the vasodilation observed in the inflammatory process.

  d. Neurotransmission. Histamine is a neurotransmitter in various brain areas and is involved in activating sensory nerves resulting in pain and itch sensations.

  e. Microcirculation. Histamine relaxes arterioles and increases capillary permeability.

7. Pharmacologic effects (summarized in Table 3-1).

  a. Cardiovascular system

    (1) Histamine dilates arterioles, capillaries, and venules, increases cardiac contractility and heart rate by activating both H_1- and H_2-receptors. The cardiovascular effects are complex. There is a decrease in peripheral resistance (vasodilatation), resulting in **hypotension**. The stimulation of cardiac activity involves a direct action and reflex activation of the sympathetic nervous system, which is activated by the low blood pressure.

    (2) There is an increase in capillary permeability brought about by contracting the endothelial cells, which exposes the basement membrane. Fluid and protein pass across the basement membrane to produce edema.

  b. Respiratory system. Respiratory smooth muscle is contracted in most species via H_1-receptors (see II A 5 a). There is also stimulation of glandular secretion and prostaglandin formation. Asthmatics are generally more sensitive to histamine than normal animals.

  c. Glandular tissue. Histamine can stimulate glandular tissues to increase secretion. A most important action of histamine is its ability to increase gastric acid and pepsin secretion from the gastric mucosa via H_2-receptors (see Chapter 11, Figure 11-2).

    (1) Regulation of gastric acid production is quite complex. Acid secretion by parietal cells is regulated by histamine, acetylcholine (ACh), gastrin, and prostaglandin E_2 (PGE_2).

    (2) Sight and smell of food activate the vagus via the CNS to release ACh on parietal cells (M_3-muscarinic receptor) and on enterochromaffin-like (ECL) paracrine cells (M_1-muscarinic receptor).

    (3) The presence of food and an increase in antral pH initiate the release of gastrin. Gastrin acts on CCK_2 receptors of the parietal and ECL cells. Histamine is released from ECL cells that are close by, and activate parietal H_2-receptors.

    (4) ACh has both a direct and indirect action on gastric acid production. Activation of M_3-receptors directly activates the parietal cell, whereas activation of the M_1-receptor on the ECL cells releases histamine which in turn activates H_2-receptors on the parietal cell.

(5) Gastrin has both a direct and indirect action. Gastrin directly activates CCK_2-receptors on parietal cells to increase gastric acid secretion and in-directly increases gastric acid secretion by activating the release of histamine from ECL cells, which again in turn activates H_2-receptors on the parietal cells. Thus, **histamine release is a major factor in the stimulation of acid production by both ACh and gastrin**.

(6) Activation of H_2-receptors enhances the gastric acid secretion by ACh and gastrin on parietal cells. Upon H_2-receptor stimulation, intracellular cAMP is increased. Activation of PKA by cAMP translocates H^+, K^+-ATPase in tuberovesicles to canalicular membrane, which subsequently releases H^+ into the lumen. Upon stimulation of M_3-receptors and gastrin (CCK_2) re-ceptors, calmodulin kinase is activated to translocate the H^+, K^+-ATPase to canalicular membrane as well. Chloride is released into lumen by K^+ and Cl^- carrier, evoking next increase in HCl level in the lumen (see Figure 11-2).

(7) H_2-antihistamines inhibit not only HCl secretion by histamine but secre-tion stimulated by gastrin, ACh (vagus), and food. This explains why H_2-antihistamines are effective therapy for peptic ulcers. Proton pump inhibitors (e.g., omeprazole) block the H^+, K^+-ATPase in canalicular membrane. PGE_2 act as a negative regulator of gastric acid secretion as PGE_2 activates $G_{i/o}$-coupled EP_3 receptors on parietal cells.

(8) Histamine can increase the release of catecholamines from the adrenal medulla and stimulate salivary secretion.

d. Intradermal tissue. Intradermal injection of histamine produces a **triple response (of Lewis)**. Insect and plant stings mimic many of these responses.

(1) A **reddening** at the site of injection is due to dilation of the small arterioles.

(2) Dilation of arterioles extends beyond injection site (**Flare**). The flare involves an axon reflex since cutting the cholinergic nerves abolishes the reflex.

(3) Swelling (**Wheal**) occurs at the injection site due to separation of the en-dothelial cells and edema caused by the increased capillary permeability, which is due to H_1-receptor-mediated contraction of endothelial cells.

(4) The intradermal injection of histamine causes pain and itching by stimula-tion of H_1-receptors on sensory nerve endings.

8. Therapeutic uses of histamine agonists

a. Histamine phosphate can be used for diagnostic purposes for testing of gastric acid secretion and pheochromocytoma. However, its profound side effects limit its use.

b. Betazole is an analog of histamine, which is an H_2-receptor agonist. Betazole has a 10-fold selectivity for stimulation of gastric acid production over vasodila-tion. Pentagastrin is also used for this purpose.

B. **Antihistamines**. Therapeutically useful antihistamine drugs are H_1-antihistamines and H_2-antihistamines. At present there are no clinically useful H_3 or H_4-antihistamines.

1. H_1-antihistamines were the first type of antihistaminic drugs discovered and are sometimes referred to as the classical antihistaminics. See Table 3-1 for examples of drugs in this class.

a. Mechanism of action. Traditionally, it was thought that H_1-antihistamines act as competitive antagonists of histamine receptors. However, recently it has been demonstrated that most, if not all, of H_1-antihistamines act as **inverse agonists** rather than the receptor antagonists. (See Chapter 1 for detailed information on inverse agonists.)

b. Classification of H_1-antihistamines. Histamine can be broadly classified into two groups based on usage: (1) first-generation H_1-antihistamines and (2) second-generation H_1-antihistamines.

Most frequently used first-generation H_1-antihistamines are **diphenhydramine, dimenhydrinate, hydroxyzline, chlorpheniramine, meclizine, promethazine,** and **cyproheptadine**. These drugs are unionized drugs at physiological pH and

TABLE 3-2. H_1-Receptor Antagonists

Class	Side Effects	Elimination $t_{1/2}$ (Humans) (hours)
First-generation H_1 antihistamines		
Ethanolamines		
Diphenhydramine	$+++, \mu$	3–9
Dimenhydrinate	$+++, \mu$	3–9
Ethylenediamines		
Pyrilamine	$++$	?
Tripelennamine	$++$	?
Alkylamines		
Chlorpheniramine	$+$	20
Piperazines		
Hydroxyzine	$+$	20–25
Meclizine	$+$	6
Phenothiazines		
Promethazine	$+++, \mu$	16–19
Trimeprazine	$+++, \mu$	16–19
Piperidines		
Cyproheptadine	$+$	1–4
Second-generation H_1 antihistamines		
Piperazines		
Cetirizine	$-$	8
Piperidines		
Loratadine	$-$	8
Fexofenadine	$-$	14

$-$ Low incidence of sedation; $+$, Slight sedation; $++$, Moderate sedation; $+++$, Strong sedation; μ, Antimuscarinic.

easily cross the blood–brain barrier (BBB). Therefore, they produce CNS side effects, in particular, sedation.

Commonly used second-generation drugs are **loratadine (Claritin®), cetirizine (Zyrtec®), and fexofenadine (Allegra®).** This class of drugs is ionized at physiological pH and is difficult to cross BBB. See Table 3-2 for chemical classification of H_1-antihistamines (Table 3-2).

  c. Pharmacologic effects of H_1-antihistamines

    (1) Relaxation of contracted bronchiolar smooth muscle.

    (2) Relaxation of contracted intestinal smooth muscle.

    (3) Inhibition of histamine-induced vasodilation and increased capillary permeability and thereby blocking formation of edema and wheals.

    (4) Inhibition of itch sensation by prevention of stimulation of sensory nerves. Many H_1-antihistamines have a potent **local anesthetic action** that may contribute to their inhibition of itching and pain.

       Note: **H_1-antihistamines alone are not effective for treatment of systemic anaphylaxis because large amount of other autacoids are released during anaphylaxis.**

  d. Other pharmacologic effects of H_1-antihistamines (Table 3-2).

    (1) Sedation is a common effect of first-generation H_1-antihistamines but sedation does not correlate with their potency for inhibiting H_1-receptors. Sedation may be a desirable/undesirable effect and can be expected to be additive to other CNS depressants.

    (2) Antimuscarinic effects are prominent for some H_1-antihistamines, for example, **diphenhydramine** and **promethazine**, which decrease secretions and relax smooth muscles.

    (3) Antimotion sickness (antiemetic) effects. This effect is due to the inhibition of histaminergic signals from the vestibular nucleus to the vomiting center in the medulla. All H_1-antihistamine have this effect, but some of them (diphenhydramine, dimenhydrinate, and meclizine) have more potent antimotion sickness effect than others in the group.

e. **Therapeutic uses.** H_1-antihistamines are administered orally, parenterally, or topically for the following conditions.

(1) Treatment of patients with allergic conditions and to reduce or ameliorate the effects due to histamine. Conditions benefited from H_1-antihistamines include:

(a) Urticaria and pruritus

(b) Allergic reactions to drugs

(c) Anaphylaxis

(2) Prevention of motion sickness. Diphenhydramine, dimenhydrinate, and meclizine are more effective in preventing motion sickness than other H_1-antihistamines.

(3) Sedation induction. Promethazine and diphenhydramine are the most potent for inducing sedation.

f. **Pharmacokinetics**

(1) The pharmacokinetics of vast majority of H_1-antihistamines have not been studied in domestic animals. Most information is derived from humans.

(2) All H_1-antihistamines are effectively absorbed following oral administration and T_{max} = 1–3 hours.

(3) All H_1-antihistamines that have been studied for pharmacokinetics are well distributed and are bound by plasma proteins ($\geq 60\%$).

(4) All H_1-antihistamines are metabolized by cytochrome P450 enzymes, and these metabolites further undergo conjugation.

(5) The first-generation antihistamines are excreted primarily by the kidneys as metabolites.

(6) The second-generation antihistamines that cause least or no sedation are excreted more into feces when compared with the first-generation drugs: cetirizine (70% in urine, 30% in feces); loratadine (40% in urine, 40% in feces as metabolites); fexofenadine (11% in urine, 80% in feces).

(7) **Elimination** $t_{1/2}$: See Table 3-2 for information in humans. The $t_{1/2}$ information for animals is mostly not available.

g. **Adverse effects** (see also Table 3-2)

(1) CNS depression (lethargy, somnolence, ataxia) are the most common but they may diminish with time. The performance of working dogs may be adversely affected.

(2) Antimuscarinic effects (dry mouth, urinary retention) occur with many H_1-antihistaqmines. They should be used with caution in patients with angle closure glaucoma.

(3) In high doses CNS stimulation is possible, for example, pyrilamine in the horse.

(4) Some individuals could develop allergy to the use of H_1-antihsitamines.

(5) Drug tolerance. The decrease in efficacy and sedation (also called subsensitivity) can develop during the use of H_1-antihistamines for days or weeks. The mechanisms underlying this phenomenon are not understood.

2. **H_2-antihistamines**. These drugs are inhibitors of gastric acid secretion. They have little action on H_1-receptors.

a. **Chemistry.** H_2-antihistamines contain imidazole ring with uncharged side chains and are smaller than H_1-antihistamines. See Figure 3-2 for an example of drugs in this class.

b. **Pharmacologic effects.** H_2-antihistamines competitively inhibits histamine (H_2-receptors) in parietal cell and thereby decreases gastric acid production during basal conditions and when stimulated by food, vagal activity, pentagastrin, gastrin, or histamine. H_2-antihistamines have been reported to act as inverse agonists, but further validation of this observation is needed.

c. **Therapeutic uses.** H_2-antihistamines are administered orally to treat gastric, abomasal and duodenal ulcers, drug-induced erosive gastritis, duodenal

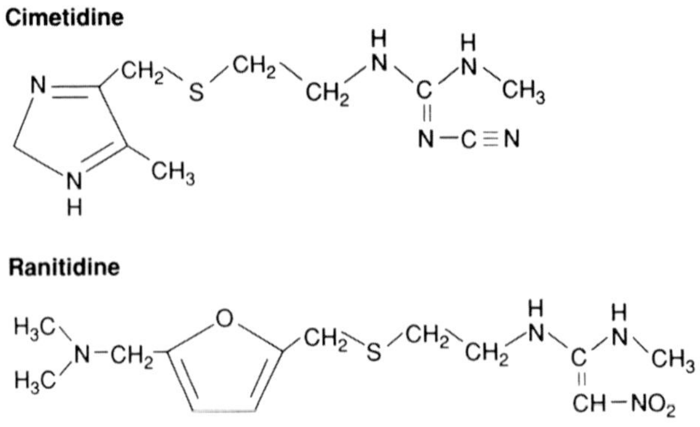

Cimetidine

Ranitidine

FIGURE 3-2. Chemical structure of two H_2-antihistamines, cimetidine and ranitidine.

gastric reflux, and esophageal reflux. Cimetidine is least potent among the four H_2-antihistamines. Lack of therapeutic effect of cimetidine has been reported in dogs.

d. Pharmacokinetics

(1) All four drugs are well absorbed when administered orally. T_{max} is 2–3 hours for all four drugs. The bioavailability for cimetidine, ranitidine, nizatidine, and famotidine is 95%, 81%, >70%, and 40–50%, respectively.

(2) All four drugs are well distributed in the body, with 10–20% bound by plasma proteins.

(3) Cimetidine, ranitidine, and famotidine are metabolized by cytochrome P450 enzymes. Only <10% of nizatidine is metabolized by CYP450 enzymes.

(4) All four drugs are excreted by the kidneys as the primary route. The majority of cimetidine, ranitidine, and famotidine is excreted as metabolites and 30–50% is excreted as the unchanged drug. A total of ≥60% of nizatidine is excreted as the unchanged drug.

(5) Plasma $t_{1/2}$ of cimetidine, ranitidine, and famotidine are 2–3 hours for all three drugs. The $t_{1/2}$ for cimetidine and ranitidine in dogs are 1.3 hours and 2.2 hours, respectively. Plasma $t_{1/2}$ of nizatidine is 1–2 hours in humans; no information is available for animals.

e. Adverse effects are uncommon when recommended dosages are used. Cimetidine possesses weak antiandrogenic activity and can cause gynecomastia and decreased libido in humans. The antiandrogenic effect is, in part, due to decreased testosterone synthesis.

Ranitidine, famotidine, and nizatidine seem to be very well tolerated. Rarely, agranocytosis has been seen with the use of ranitidine and famotidine.

f. Drug interactions. Cimetidine can inhibit the hepatic cytochrome P450 enzymes. It may reduce the metabolism of other drugs, which undergo hepatic metabolism, thereby elevating and prolonging their concentration in the plasma.

3. Inhibitors of histamine release. The one drug in this category, cromolyn sodium, differs in mechanism of action from the H_1- and H_2-antihistamines discussed above.

a. Cromolyn sodium inhibits the release of histamine and other autacoids from mast cells. It **does not** inhibit H_1- and H_2-receptors, but opens chloride channel to hyperpolarize the cells.

(1) It is primarily used to treat pulmonary and nasal allergic reactions.

(2) It is not well absorbed from the gut and has no clinical use when given orally.

(3) It is used in a prophylactic manner.

(4) It has been used in the horse where it is nebulized and delivered via a face mask.

(5) **The 4% eye drop is used to control allergic conjunctivitis.**

4. Physiologic antagonists to histamine. The sympathomimetic drugs, for example, epinephrine, phenylephrine, phenylpropanolmaine, and ephedrine (see Chapter 2) antagonize the actions of histamine by antagonizing histamine's physiological

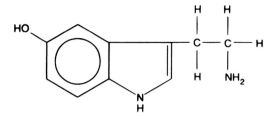

FIGURE 3-3. Chemical structure of serotonin.

function. These drugs either directly or indirectly activate α- and β-adrenoceptors to elevate blood pressure and relax the bronchi. This counters the blood pressure lowering and bronchoconstrictive actions of histamine.

Epinephrine is the preferred drug to treat the immediate effects of anaphylaxis.

C. **Serotonin** (5-hydroxytryptamine, 5-HT)

1. **Biosynthesis**. 5-HT is present in high concentration in platelets, the enterochromaffin cells and myenteric plexus of the GI tract and CNS. Its synthesis starts from dietary tryptophan, which is acted upon by the enzyme tryptophan hydroxylase to form 5-hydroxytryptophan, which in turn is acted upon by the enzyme L-aromatic acid decarboxylase to form 5-hydroxytryptamine (serotonin; Figure 3-3).

2. **Metabolism, distribution, and function**

   a. Serotonin is deaminated by monoamine oxidase (MAO) to form 5-hydroxyindoleacetaldehyde, which is then oxidized to 5-hydroxyindole acetic acid.

   b. Approximately 90% of the body's serotonin is found in the GI tract in enterochromaffin cells. It is involved in regulating motility.

   c. Platelets actively transport serotonin and store it. This keeps the concentration of free 5-HT low in the blood flow.

   d. Serotonin is synthesized and stored in the CNS where it acts as a neurotransmitter.

   e. Serotonin is also found in venoms and stings. Sensory nerve ends are stimulated by serotonin and this action may be responsible in part for the pain and itch of stings.

3. **Serotonin receptors**. There are more receptors for serotonin than any other biogenic amine. At the present time there are >14 receptor subtypes. Some of these have recently been discovered and their function is uncertain. The major categories of serotonin receptors include: 5-HT$_1$(G$_{i/o}$-coupled), 5-HT$_2$(G$_q$-coupled), 5-HT$_3$(a ligand-gated ion channel), 5-HT$_{4-7}$(G$_s$-coupled) with some categories having more than two receptor subtypes.

4. **Functions of serotonin**. While none of the following proposed functions are known for certain, the current evidence suggests that serotonin is involved in regulating gut motility, body temperature, sleep, aggression, pain, mood, and endocrine function.

5. **Pharmacologic effects**. Serotonin may produce vasoconstriction or vasodilatation, which is dependent upon the vascular bed, 5-HT receptor subtypes, and the species. Many smooth muscles (bronchi, uterus, GI) contract in response to serotonin.

6. **Therapeutic uses**. Serotonin has no therapeutic use.

D. **Serotonin agonists in nature**

1. **Ergot alkaloids** (ergotamine, ergonovine, ergocryptine, ergocornine, ergocristine, ergosine) occur in various combinations and are found in the fungi of the genus *Claviceps*. *Claviceps purpurea* is the common mold that attacks the seed of rye, oats, wheat, and barley. Another ergot, **ergovaline** is produced by the endophytic fungus *Acremonium coenophialum* and is the major toxicant associated with tall fescue grass toxicosis.

   a. **Pharmacologic effects**. Ergot alkaloids exhibit a complex pharmacology. They have the ability to act on both adrenergic and serotonergic receptors either as partial agonists or antagonists. They stimulate the smooth muscle of the gut, uterus, bronchi, and blood vessels.

b. Therapeutic uses. Because of complicated pharmacologic effects, ergot alkaloids with serotonin agonistic activity are in general not clinically useful. Ergonovine is used in obstetrics to stop postpartum hemorrhage and induce uterine involution (see Chapter 12 for more information).

c. Ergot alkaloid poisoning in cattle. Chronic ingestion of plant materials infected with the fungus produces a syndrome referred to as ergotism. In the acute form, the animal may exhibit nervousness or convulsions and in the chronic form, gangrene (due to severe vasoconstriction). When consumed in small amounts over days or weeks animals may develop gangrene of the extremities (ear, tail, legs). Agalactia, small litter size, decreased birth weight, decreased rate of gain and abortion may occur.

(1) Fescue grass toxicity
This is prominent in the southeast quarter of the United States where ~35 million acres of tall fescue grass are infected with endophytic fungus (*Neotyphodium coenophialum*). Loss of weight, agalactia, rough hair coat, retained placenta, and dystocia are common symptoms of fescue toxicosis. It is estimated that the cattle industry loses $700 million annually to this infection.

(2) Ergovaline is a major toxicant. It is a potent constrictor of bovine and ovine uterine, umbilical, placental, and tail arteries. The vasoconstriction is mediated by G_q-coupled 5-HT$_2$ receptors and can be blocked by ketanserin, a 5-HT$_2$ antagonist.

E. **Serotonin-receptor modifying drugs.** Some serotonin agonists/antagonists in veterinary medicine are listed below:

1. GI prokinetic agents: These drugs increase GI motility by increasing ACh release from the vagus nerve.
a. Cisapride
(1) Therapeutic uses. It is an agonist for G_s-coupled 5-HT$_4$ receptor, and is used for gastric/intestinal stasis, reflux esophagitis, and constipation/megacolon in cats.
(2) Pharmacokinetics. Only information in humans is available: Cisapride is rapidly absorbed following oral administration with an absolute bioavailability of 35–40%. The drug is highly bound to plasma proteins and is extensively distributed throughout the body. Its elimination $t_{1/2}$ is 8–10 hours.
(3) Adverse effects. The primary adverse effects are GI in origin, including diarrhea and colic.
b. Metoclopramide (Reglan®)
(1) Therapeutic uses. It is a $G_{i/o}$-coupled D_2-receptor antagonist/5-HT$_4$ agonist, and is used for treating vomiting disorders, reflux esophagitis, and gastric stasis, or hypomotility.
(2) Pharmacokinetics. Metoclopramide is administered PO, SC, and IM.
(a) It is absorbed well after oral administration. Bioavailability after IM administration is 74–96%. After oral dosing, T_{max} is ≤2 hours.
(b) It is well distributed in the body and enters the CNS. A total of 13–22% of metoclopramide is bound by plasma proteins.
(c) It is primarily excreted in the urine in humans. The majority of the drug is metabolized to glucuronidated or sulfated conjugate forms and then excreted in the urine. Only ~20% of the drug is excreted unchanged in the urine.
(d) The $t_{1/2}$ of metoclopramide in the dog is ~90 minutes.
(3) Adverse effects
(a) In dogs, changes in mental state and behavior (restlessness and hyperactivity to drowsiness/depression). Cats may exhibit signs of frenzied behavior or disorientation. Both dogs and cats can develop constipation while taking this medication.

    (b) In adult horses, IV metoclopramide administration has caused alternating periods of sedation and excitement, behavioral changes, and abdominal pain.

    (c) Other side effects include nausea, diarrhea, transient hypertension, and increased prolactin secretion.

2. Cyproheptadine (5-HT_2 antagonist and H_1-antihistamine)

  a. Therapeutic uses. It is useful in cats as an appetite stimulant. It is useful in the treatment of feline asthma or pruritus in cats. It also has H_1-antihistamine activity, and thus is useful in managing hives. In horses, it is for treating photic head shaking.

  b. Pharmacokinetics. Orally administered cyproheptadine is well absorbed from the gut and is metabolized and excreted in both feces and urine, with <20% of the total dose is eliminated in feces, with 5.7% of the total dose remaining as the unchanged parent compound. Over 40% of the dose is eliminated in urine, predominantly as a quaternary ammonium glucuronide conjugate.

  c. Adverse effects include sedation, anticholinergic activity, anorexia, and lethargy. Higher doses of cyproheptadine can produce polyphagia.

3. Ketanserin (G_q-coupled $5HT_2$ receptor antagonist)

  a. Therapeutic uses. The potential use of ketanserin is to treat ergovaline-induced severe vasoconstriction. It also has significant α-adrenergic blocking activity and thus reduces blood pressure. It can be used to reduce intraocular pressure in glaucoma.

4. Other serotonin modifying drugs used are antidepressants (see Chapter 5 for information).

III. PHOSPHOLIPID-DERIVED MEDIATORS

A. Eicosanoids

1. Chemistry and biosynthesis (Figure 3-4)

  a. The eicosanoids include the **prostaglandins (PGs)**, **thromboxanes (TXs)**, and **leukotrienes (LT)**. They are derived from polyunsaturated acids and arachidonic acid, a 20 carbon essential fatty acid with 4 double bonds (20:4) as the primary substrate. The eicosanoids play key role in inflammatory, cardiovascular, and reproductive functions.

  b. Arachidonic acid is released from membrane phospholipids primarily by phospholipase A_2 in response to physical, chemical, hormonal, and neurotransmitter stimuli. Another source of arachidonic acid results from the action of phospholipase C on membrane phosphoinositides to yield a diglyceride plus inositol phosphate. The resulting diglyceride is acted upon by diglyceride lipase to yield arachidonic acid.

  c. Arachidonic acid can be metabolized by three pathways.

    (1) The **cyclooxygenase** pathway leads to prostaglandin, thromboxane, and prostacyclin production.

    (2) The **5-lipoxygenase pathway** leads to the synthesis of leukotrienes.

    (3) The **15-lipoxygenase pathway** leads to the synthesis of hydroperoxyeicosatetraenoic acid (15-HPETE) and 15(S)-hydroxyeicosatetraenoic acid (15-HETE) as intermediates for many eicosanoids. The function of these eicosanoids is still under investigation.

2. Nomenclature and structure

  a. The Greek work *eikosi*, meaning "20," serves as the stem word for eicosanoid. Arachidonic acid is 5,8,11,14-eicosatetraenoic acid.

  b. The name prostaglandin is a misnomer. It was originally thought that the origin of the smooth muscle stimulating and blood pressure lowering substance in human seminal fluid was the prostate, hence the name prostaglandin for this substance. Many years later, the substance was shown to originate from the seminal vesicles but the name prostaglandin remained.

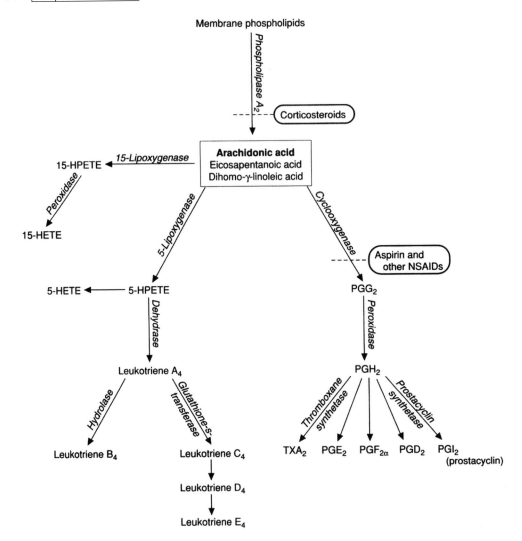

FIGURE 3-4. Eicosanoid synthesis pathway. Various stimuli, including certain hormones, activate phospholipase A_2 to release arachidonic acid from membrane phospholipids. There are three pathways that arachidonic acid metabolism can follow, which lead to biologically active products. What determines which pathway is followed appears to depend on the enzyme concentration in each tissue and the local environmental conditions in each tissue. (1) The cyclooxygenase pathway ultimately leads to the synthesis of thromboxane (TXA_2), prostacyclin (PGI_2), and three prostaglandins (PGE_2, $PGF_{2\alpha}$, and PGD_2). (2) The 5-lipoxygenase pathway leads to the formation of the leukotrienes (LTA_4, LTB_4, LTC_4, LTD_4, and LTE_4). (3) The 15-lipoxygenase pathway produces hydroperoxyeicosatetraenoic acid (15-HPETE) and 15(S)-hydroxyeicosatetraenoic acid (15-HETE) as intermediates for many eicosanoids.

    c. Prostaglandin nomenclature identifies 10 specific molecular groups which are designated by the letters A through J. Each group is characterized by the substituent attached to position 9 and 11 of the cyclopentane ring.

    d. Prostaglandin can be synthesized from three fatty acids: dihomo-γ-linolenic acid (20:3), arachidonic acid (20:4), and eicosapentaenoic acid (20:5) with 3, 4, and 5 double bonds can lead to the synthesis of prostaglandin E_1 (PGE_1), PGE_2, and PGE_3, respectively. The subscript numbers 1, 2, and 3 denote the number of double bonds in the aliphatic side chains attached to the cyclopentane ring. For the PGF series of prostaglandins the subscript α or β refers to the configuration of the hydroxyl group at carbon 9. See Figure 3-5 for nomenclature and structural characteristics.

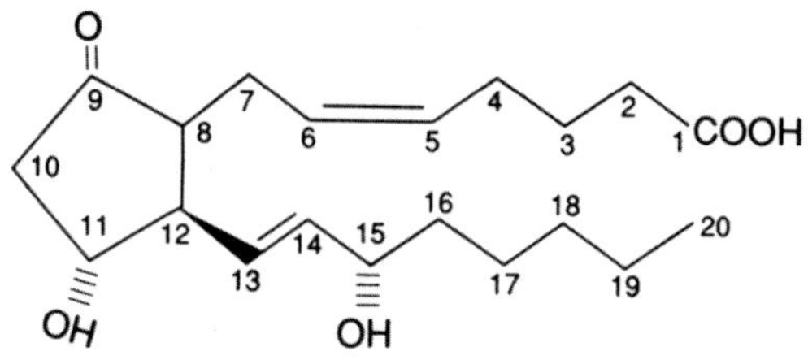

FIGURE 3-5. Chemical structure of two prostaglandins, PGE_2 and $PGF_{2\alpha}$.

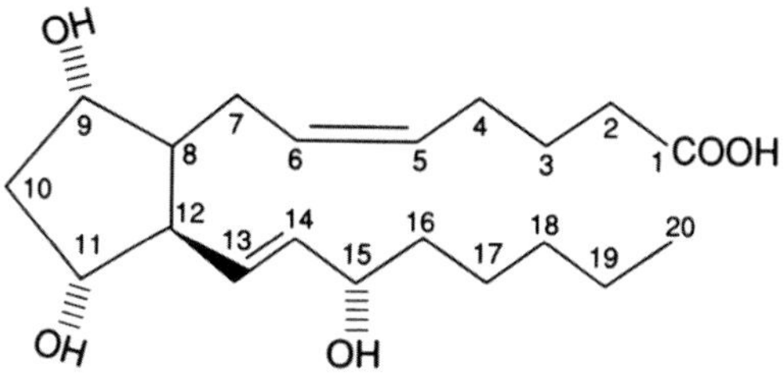

3. Prostaglandins (PGs) and thromboxanes (TXs)

a. Synthesis, release, and fate. They are not stored but are synthesized de novo in response to appropriate stimuli and enter the extracellular space. The PGs are short-lived molecules and exert their actions in the region where they are synthesized. Circulating PGs are rapidly catabolized by degrading enzymes in the lung, kidney, spleen, adipose tissue, and intestine. Lung tissue is particularly effective and can remove about 90% of PGE_2 or $PGF_{2\alpha}$ from blood in one passage through the lungs. Thromboxane A_2 (TXA_2) spontaneously hydrolyzes ($t_{1/2} = 30$ seconds) in blood fluids to the biologically inactive thromboxane B_2 (TXB_2). Prostacyclin (PGI_2) is spontaneously hydrolyzed ($t_{1/2} = 3$ minutes) in body fluids to the biologically inactive 6-keto-$PGF_{1\alpha}$.

b. Pharmacologic effects

(1) Table 3-3 summarizes the receptor pharmacology of various prostaglandins, which serves as the basis for the pharmacologic effects of prostaglandins.

(2) Smooth muscle

(a) Blood vessels. PGE_2 and PGI_2 relax arteriolar smooth muscle and promote vasodilatation. TXA_2 and $PGF_{2\alpha}$ are vasoconstrictors with TXA_2 being the most potent. TXA_2 also promotes platelet adhesion and aggregation. TXA_2 receptor signals through G_q-coupled receptor. The $t_{1/2}$ of TXA_2 is extremely short (10–20 seconds). PGI_2 (commonly referred as prostacylin) is synthesized by vascular endothelial cells and acts as physiological antagonist of TXA_2. PGI_2 functions as vasodilator and inhibits platelet aggregation. PGI_2 receptor signals through G_s-coupled receptor. Endothelial cell damage may result in a hemostatic plug as a result of a decrease in PGI_2 synthesis and an increase in TXA_2 synthesis.

(b) Gut. PGE_2 and $PGF_{2\alpha}$ contract longitudinal muscle, whereas PGI_2 and $PGF_{2\alpha}$ contract circular muscle, but PGE_2 relaxes it.

(c) Bronchioles. PGE_1, PGE_2, and PGI_2 relax respiratory smooth muscle, whereas TXA_2 and $PGF_{2\alpha}$ cause contraction. PGE_2 is an important PG, produced in many tissues including macrophages and mast cells. Depending on the type receptor activation, PGE_2 mediates various biological functions including vasodilatation, bronchoconstriction, pyrexia, and mucus production.

TABLE 3-3. The Eicosanoid Receptor Signaling

Ligand	Receptor	Receptor Signaling
PGE$_2$	EP$_1$	↑PLC (G$_q$)
	EP$_2$	↑cAMP (G$_s$)
	EP$_{3A-D}$	A, D: ↓ cAMP (G$_i$) B, C: ↑ cAMP (G$_s$) D: ↑ PLC (G$_q$)
	EP$_4$	↑cAMP (G$_s$)
PGF$_{2\alpha}$	FP$_{A,B}$	↑PLC (G$_q$)
PGI$_2$	IP	↑cAMP (G$_s$)
TXA$_2$	TP$_{\alpha,\beta}$	↑PLC (G$_q$), ↓cAMP (G$_i$), G$^*_{12/13}$
LTB$_4$	BLT$_1$	G$_i$
	BLT$_2$	↑PLC (G$_q$), ↓cAMP (G$_i$)
LTD$_4$	CysLT$_1$	↑PLC (G$_q$)
LTC$_4$/LTD4	CysLT$_2$	↑PLC (G$_q$)

*Effectors of G$_{12/13}$ include NO synthase, Rho, phospholipase D, and Na$^+$/H$^+$ exchanger.
PLC, phospholipase C-β.

    (3) Platelets. As discussed above, PGI$_2$ inhibits aggregation, whereas TXA$_2$ is synthesized by the platelets and strongly promotes aggregation. In human medicine, small daily doses of aspirin are used to permanently inhibit platelet cyclooxygenase and thereby prevent thromboxane A$_2$ formation in cardiovascular disease.

    (4) Reproductive system (also see Chapter 12)

        (a) Female. PGF$_{2\alpha}$ is the luteolytic hormone produced by the ovaries and endometrium, which causes ovulation and regression of corpus luteum (luteolysis) in cycling animals. In the prepartum period, PGF$_{2\alpha}$ initiates luteolysis, which decrease plasma progesterone levels. PGF$_{2\alpha}$ is a stimulant of myometrium and is involved in parturition. PGF$_{2\alpha}$ receptor is coupled to G$_q$. PGF$_{2\alpha}$-induced luteolysis and myometrial contractions are use therapeutically to control reproduction.

        (b) Male. The role of PGs in the male is uncertain.

    (5) Central and peripheral nervous systems

        (a) Fever. Administration of PGE$_1$ or PGE$_2$ into the cerebral ventricles increases body temperature. Pyrogen initiates the release of interleukin-1, which promotes PGE$_2$ formation. The inhibition by aspirin and other NSAID drugs of PGE$_2$ synthesis explains their antipyretic activity (see also Chapter 7).

        (b) Sleep. Infusion of PGD$_2$ into the cerebral ventricles induces sleep. PGD$_2$ receptor is coupled to G$_s$.

        (c) Neurotransmission. PGEs inhibit the release of norepinephrine from sympathetic neurons via activation of EP$_3$ receptors.

    (6) Neuroendocrine. PGEs can enhance the secretion of the anterior pituitary hormones, growth hormone, prolactin, thyroid-stimulating hormone, corticotropin, follicle-stimulating hormone, and luteinizing hormone by activating EP$_1$ and EP$_4$ receptors. This effect may be a direct one and may be an indirect one by stimulating the release of the hypothalamic releasing hormones.

  c. Therapeutic uses. Only PGE and PGF$_{2\alpha}$ analogs are used therapeutically in veterinary medicine.

    (1) Misoprostol. It is a PGE$_1$ analog that has two functions which make it a useful protective agent for the GI tract. It directly inhibits gastric acid secretion by parietal cells and it facilitates PGE-mediated mucosal defenses and healing in response to GI injuries. Misoprostol is used to treat gastric ulceration when caused or aggravated by NSAIDs. Misoprostol can cause diawhea, bloat, colic, and abortion.

 (2) Dinoprost and cloprostenol. Dinoprost is the drug name for $PGF_{2\alpha}$ and cloprostenol is a synthetic $PGF_{2\alpha}$ analog. They are used to induce luteolysis for the control of estrous cycle, to terminate pregnancy, and to induce parturition. See Chapter 12 for more information.

 (3) Precautions to the use of $PGF_{2\alpha}$ drugs:

  (a) Animals with respiratory or GI disorders may be compromised by the bronchoconstriction and stimulation of the GI motility by the $PGF_{2\alpha}$ compounds. Older animals may exhibit exacerbated vasoconstriction-associated complications.

  (b) Women of child-bearing age or who are pregnant, persons with asthma, or respiratory disease should use extreme caution in handling these drugs as they are readily absorbed via the skin. If contact with the skin is made, the skin must be washed immediately with soap and water.

4. Leukotrienes (LTs)

 a. Chemistry (see Figure 3-4)

  (1) LTs are synthesized by the 5-lipoxygenase (5-LOX) in neutrophils, monocytes, macrophages, mast cells, and keratinocytes.

  (2) LTs are also synthesized in the lungs, spleen, brain, and heart.

  (3) Stimuli for LT production include:

   (a) Phagocytosis and immune complexes in macrophages.

   (b) Mast cell anti-IgE antibody.

   (c) Release of platelet-activating factor (PAF) by basophils and mast cells.

  (4) The enzyme 5-LOX reacts with arachidonic acid to form 5-HPETE (an intermediate), which is reduced by a dehydrase to LTA_4 (the subscript indicates the number of double bonds present). In human leukocytes a single enzyme is responsible for the synthesis of 5-HPETE and LTA_4. LTA_4 is either hydrolyzed to LTB_4 or converted to LTC_4 in the presence of glutathione and glutathione s-transferase. Removal of the glutamic acid moiety by γ-glutamyltranspeptidase yields LTD_4. Removal of the glycine by a dipeptidase forms LTE_4. **The slow-reacting substance of anaphylaxis (SRS-A)** is now known to be a mixture of LTC_4, LTD_4, and LTE_4.

 b. Pharmacologic effects. The LTs (e.g., LTD_4) contract most smooth muscle. LTC_4, LTD_4, and LTE_4 are also known as cysteinyl leukotrienes and mediate their effect by binding to the CysLT type 1 receptor (see Table 3-3 for details). The cysteinyl leukotrienes are responsible for airway and smooth muscle contractions during asthma. They also play various other inflammatory processes in vascular and skin diseases.

  (1) LTC_4, LTD_4, and LTE_4

   (a) These LTs are potent vasoconstrictors.

   (b) They are potent bronchoconstrictors and cause brochospasm. They are 1,000 times more potent than histamine.

   (c) They increase capillary permeability.

   (d) They increase mucous secretion and impair mucus clearance by inhibiting the movements of cilia on airway epithelium.

  (2) LTB_4 is a potent chemotactic chemical for leukocytes, eosinophils, and monocytes. Other LTs do not possess this action. It promotes adhesion of neutrophils to the vascular endothelium and their transendothelial migration.

 c. LT antagonists. The production of LTs can be blocked by LOX inhibitors (e.g., zileuton), which inhibits 5-LOX enzyme by chelating the enzyme's nonheme iron. The clinical use of zileuton is limited in veterinary medicine due to the cost and adverse effects (e.g., liver toxicity).

  The LT receptor antagonists are emerging as effective treatment for asthma symptoms. **Montelukast (Singulair®)** and **zafirukast (Accolate®)** are now used in small animals. These drugs reduce bronchial spasm and improve pulmonary function.

(1) Therapeutic uses. They are used as adjunctive treatment for atopic dermatitis in dogs and asthma in cats. However, they are not effective for acute asthma attacks.

(2) Pharmacokinetics. The information is available for humans only. The pharmacokinetics of LT antagonists has not been studied in domestic animals.

    (a) Zafirukast is rapidly absorbed following oral administration, though the absolute bioavailability is unknown; zafirukast administered with food shows a reduced bioavailability of 40%. Montelukast is similarly administered, and its bioavailability in humans is 63–73%. T_{max} for both drugs is 2–4 hours.

    (b) Both drugs show strong binding to plasma proteins (99%).

    (c) Both drugs are extensively metabolized by cytochrome P450 enzymes to hydroxylated metabolites.

    (d) The metabolites of these two LT antagonists are eliminated in feces (>80% of dose). Less than 10% is eliminated in the urine.

    (e) Plasma $t_{1/2}$ of montelukast and zafirukast are 2.7–5.5 hours and 8–16 hours, respectively.

(3) Adverse effects: No adverse effects have been reported in animals because of limited experience with these two drugs. In humans, common adverse effects include GI distress, hallucinations, and agitation. More serious, but rare adverse effects include hepatitis, agranulocytosis, and allergic granulomatous vasculitis.

5. Platelet-activating factor (PAF)

  a. Chemistry

    (1) PAF is 1-O-alkyl-2-acetyl-sn-glycerol-3phosphocholine. It is derived from 1-O-alkyl-2-acyl-glycerophosphocholine found in the membrane of many cells.

    (2) PAF synthesis involves the action of phospholipase A_2 on 1-O-alkyl-2-acyl-glycerophosphocholine to yield 1-O-alkyl-2-lyso-glycerophosphocholine (lyso-PAF). Lyso-PAF is acetylated by acetyl coenzyme A in the presence of lyso-PAF acetyltransferase. It is released from many different cells including neutrophils, activated macrophages, eosinophils, mast cells, and of course from platelets. The action of PAF is not only limited to platelets but also acts on many different cells. Even very low concentration (10^{-10} M, 100 pM).

  b. Pharmacologic effects

  PAF mediates its effect by binding to PAF receptor, which couples with at least two different types of G proteins, $G_{i/o}$ and G_q. The downstream effect of the receptor signaling is mediated nitric oxide synthesis in the endothelium.

    (1) PAF is a potent vasodilator and it lowers blood pressure and total vascular resistance.

    (2) PAF increases vascular permeability and the movement of fluid out of the vascular compartment. PAF is ~1000× more potent than histamine or bradykinin.

    (3) PAF is a potent promoter of platelet aggregation.

    (4) PAF stimulates polymorphonuclear leukocytes and monocytes to aggregate.

    (5) PAF commonly contracts GI, uterine, and small bronchiolar smooth muscle.

  c. Pathophysiological roles for PAF include:

    (1) Stimulation of platelet aggregation.

    (2) Involvement in ovulation, implantation, and parturition.

    (3) Promotion of inflammation and allergic responses.

    (4) Implication in the toxicological action of beestings and snakebites.

    (5) Delineation of the pathophysiologic function of PAF is complicated, since the activation of phospholipase A_2 in the synthesis of PAF also releases arachidonic acid, which in turn can be synthesized to the PGs, TXA_2, or LTs, all with significant biological activity.

  d. Therapeutic uses. There are no clinical uses of PAF, its synthesis inhibitors or receptor antagonists. This remains an active research area. PAF receptor antagonist lexipafant has recently been used for management of acute pancreatitis. The anti-inflammatory property of glucocorticoids is, in part, attributed to inhibition of PAF synthesis.

IV. POLYPEPTIDES (see also Chapter 8)

A. **Angiotensins** are polypeptides that elevate blood pressure by inducing vasoconstriction.

1. **Chemistry (see Figure 8-1).**
   a. **Angiotensinogen** is an α_2-globulin synthesized in the liver and is present in the circulation. It is the precursor for all angiotensins.
   b. **Renin** is an enzyme secreted by juxtaglomerular cells in the renal arterioles, which metabolizes angiotensinogen to form the decapeptide angiotensin I.
   c. **Angiotensin-converting enzyme (ACE)**, an enzyme found in large amounts in lung capillary endothelial cells as well as in other vascular beds, metabolizes angiotensin I to the biologically active octapeptide **angiotensin II**.
   d. Angiotensin II is metabolized by an aminopeptidase to **angiotensin III** that has less biologic activity than angiotensin II. Other peptidases metabolize angiotensin II to inactive products.

2. **Mechanism of action**
   a. Two receptor subtypes for angiotensin II have been identified: AT_1 and AT_2. AT_1 receptors are stimulatory, whereas AT_2 receptors are inhibitory, which mediate effects usually are opposite to those of AT_1.
   b. AT_1 receptors mediate most of the actions of angiotensin II.
      (1) AT_1 receptors utilize G_q-coupled signaling (IP_3, Ca^{2+}) and thereby mediate the contraction of smooth muscle.
   c. AT_2 receptors are G protein-coupled receptors. It is still not known which G protein is coupled to these receptors. However, NO synthesis is increased after activation of AT_2 receptors, which stimulates guanylyl cyclase to increase cGMP formation. In addition, PKC synthesis, particularly PKCα synthesis is inhibited by activation of AT_2 receptors.

3. **Pharmacologic effects. Angiotensin II regulates blood pressure and fluid and electrolyte balance.**
   a. Hypertensin, edema, and electrolyte imbalances can occur from overactivity of the renin–angiotensin system.
   b. Angiotensin II is 40-times more potent as a vasoconstrictor than norepinephrine.
   c. Angiotensin II promotes the synthesis and secretion of aldosterone by zona glomerulosa of the adrenal cortex. Aldosterone promotes sodium and water retention and potassium loss (see also Chapter 12).
   d. Angiotensin II stimulates the thirst center in the hypothalamus and increases vasopressin (antidiuretic hormone) secretion.
   e. AT_1 receptors mediate the above stimulatory effects.
   f. AT_2 receptors, in general, mediate the inhibition of the above effects mediated by AT_1 receptors.

4. **Therapeutic uses of angiotensin II.** Angiotensin II has not been used clinically.

5. **Antagonists of the renin–angiotensin system.**
   a. **ACE Inhibitors.** These drugs effectively inhibit ACE, resulting in inhibition of angiotensin II production and accumulation of angiotensin I and bradykinin. **(See Chapter 8 for detailed information.)**
      (1) Captopril, enalapril, lisinopril, benazepril, and others inhibit the enzymatic conversion of angiotensin I to angiotensin II.
          Drugs in this class do not block angiotensin II receptors nor do they have agonist activity.
      (2) ACE inhibitors produce the following pharmacologic/therapeutic effects:
          (a) Decreased retention of sodium and water by reducing the secretion of aldosterone.
          (b) An increase in the levels of bradykinin (a vasodilating polypeptide) since bradykinin is inactivated by ACE.
          (c) A decrease in blood pressure and fluid retention in patients with elevated angiotensin I blood levels. (See Chapter 8 for detailed information regarding therapeutic uses of ACE inhibitors.)

    b. **β₁-Adrenergic antagonists.** The sympathetic nervous system promotes the release of renin from juxtaglomerular cells via β_1-receptors. Drugs such as propranolol inhibit activation of β_1-receptors and thereby reduce renin release (see Chapter 2 for information on β-receptors and antagonists).

    c. **Angiotensin I (AT₁) receptor antagonists.** Several AT_1 receptor antagonists, including losartan, candesartan, and valsartan are now added to antihypertensive treatment in human medicine. These drugs do not have the adverse effects associated with chronic use of ACE inhibitors and appear to have a number of ancillary beneficial effects such as anticancer activity and neuroprotective effects in experiment model systems. The veterinary use of AT_1 blockers is limited due to the high cost of this class of drugs.

    d. **Renin receptor inhibitor—aliskiren.** The renin receptor inhibitor aliskiren inhibits the conversion of angiotensinogen to angiotensin I. It is for controlling hypertension in humans. The use of aliskiren in veterinary medicine is yet to be established.

B. **The kinins: bradykinin and kallidin** are polypeptides that dilate blood vessels.

1. **Chemistry**
   a. Two distinct enzymes (one from plasma and the other from tissue) called **kallikreins** catalyze the formation of two polypeptides: **bradykinin**, a nonapeptide and **kallidin** (lysyl-bradykinin), a decapeptide.
   b. α_2-Globulins serve as the precursor for the synthesis of the two peptides.
   c. Proteases inactivate both bradykinin and kallidin. The major peptidase is ACE. ACE inhibitors prolong the duration of action of both peptides and this contributes to their blood pressure lowering activity as well as bronchoconstriction.

2. **Mechanism of action.** Bradykinin acts on bradykinin-1 (BK_1) and bradykinin-2 (BK_2) receptors. Both BK_1 and BK_2 receptors are coupled to G_q. No antagonists are available for therapeutic uses.

    In addition to their own activity, bradykinin may stimulate the formation of prostaglandins by activating PLA_2, which in turn have pronounced biologic effects.

3. **Pharmacologic effects:**
   a. Kinins are potent **vasodilators** of resistance arteries. The vasodilating effect is due to production of NO and prostaglandins that stimulate NO and cAMP synthesis, respectively.
   b. Kinins contract nonvascular smooth muscle such as the bronchial and intestinal smooth muscles.
   c. They cause veins to contract by stimulating BK receptors in the venous smooth muscle.
   d. Kinins increase vascular permeability and edema by contracting endothelial cells to increase leakage of plasma into interstitial space.
   e. Kinins increase secretion of fluids in the lungs and GI tract.
   f. Both kinins are potent pain-inducing chemicals.
   g. Various venoms and stings from snakes and insects owe their toxic effects to the formation of kinins.

4. **Therapeutic uses of bradykinin and its antagonists.** They are not available yet for clinical use.

SUGGESTED READING

Armstrong AW, Kvedar JC. 2008. "Histamine pharmacology." In *Principles of Pharmacology: The Pathophysiologic Basis of Drug Therapy.* Edited by Golan DE, Tashjian AH, Jr, Armstrong EJ, Armstrong AW. 2nd ed., pp. 769–779. Baltimore, MD: Lippincott Williams & Wilkins.

http://www.drugs.com

Leurs R, Church MK, Talialatea M. 2002. H₁-antihistamines: Inverse agonism, anti-inflammatory actions and cardiac effects. *Clin Exp Allergy* 32:489–498.

Plumb DC. 2005. *Veterinary Drug Handbook.* 5th ed. Ames: Blackwell Publishing.

Smyth EM, Burke A, FitzGerald GA. 2006. "Lipid-derived autacoids: Eicosanoids and platelet-activating factors." In *Goodman & Gilman's The Pharmacological Basis of Therapeutics.* Edited by Brunton LL, Lazo JS, Parker KL. 11th ed., pp. 653–670. New York: McGraw-Hill.

STUDY QUESTIONS

DIRECTIONS: Each of the numbered items or incomplete statements in this section is followed by answers or by completions of the statement. Select the **one** lettered answer or completion that is **best** in each case.

---

1. Which of the following is a major effect of angiotensin II?

(A) Stimulation of thirst and vasopressin secretion.
(B) Vasodilation.
(C) Inhibition of aldosterone secretion.
(D) Tachycardia.

2. Which of the following is a function of angiotensin converting enzyme (ACE)?

(A) Converts angiotensinogen to angiotensin I.
(B) Converts bradykinin to inactive metabolites.
(C) Directly promotes aldosterone secretion.
(D) Converts angiotensin II to angiotensin III.

3. Which one of the following is the most frequently associated side effect of H_1-antihistamines?

(A) Anti-androgenic activity in males.
(B) Sedation.
(C) Inhibition of cytochrome P450 enzymes.
(D) Constipation.

4. How does diphenhydramine work to relieve the symptoms of hypersensitivity?

(A) It competitively antagonizes the effect of histamine at H_1-receptors.
(B) It stabilizes mast cells to inhibit histamine release.
(C) It inhibits the binding of allergens to IgE.
(D) It promotes the endocytosis of H_1-receptors.
(E) It promotes the shift of active H_1-receptors to the inactive state.

5. Which of the following statements is incorrectly associated with prostacyclin (PGI_2)?

(A) PGI_2 is a vasoconstrictor.
(B) PGI_2 is formed from platelet endoperoxides.

(C) PGI_2 inhibits platelet aggregation.
(D) PGI_2 is spontaneously hydrolyzed into inactive 6-keto-$PGF_{1\alpha}$.

6. Which of the following statements regarding histamine H_2-antihistamines is correct?

(A) Nizatidine may cause drug interactions because of its inhibition of the cytochrome P450 enzyme system.
(B) Ranitidine is more potent than cimetidine.
(C) Ranitidine is a potent CNS depressant.
(D) Famotidine has a plasma half-life much longer than that of cimetidine.

7. Which of the drugs listed below inhibits the release of histamine?

(A) Betazole
(B) Cimetidine
(C) Dimenhydrinate
(D) Cromolyn sodium

8. Which of the following statements regarding serotonergic receptors is incorrect?

(A) All serotonergic receptors are G protein-coupled receptors, except 5-HT_3 receptors.
(B) There are more classes of serotonergic receptors than any other receptors of biogenic amines.
(C) Stimulation of 5-HT_1 receptors increases GI motility.
(D) Stimulation of 5-HT2 receptors evokes severe vasoconstriction, which accounts for fescue grass toxicity.

9. Which one of the following statements is incorrect?

(A) Arachidonic acid is the precursor for the synthesis of the leukotrienes.
(B) Aspirin inhibits the formation of $PGF_{2\alpha}$.

(C) PGE_2 increases body temperature.

(D) Leukotrienes are potent relaxants of bronchiolar smooth muscle.

10. Which of the following autacoid inhibitors/antagonists is a leukotriene (LT) receptor antagonist that blocks LT-induced bronchoconstriction?

(A) Cetirizine

(B) Lisinopril

(C) Montelukast

(D) Zileuton

11. Why doesn't fexofenadine cause sedation?

(A) It is a drug that blocks H_2 receptors in the CNS.

(B) It is not effective blocking cerebral H_1 receptors.

(C) It is an excellent substrate for P-glycoprotein, which pumps drugs including fexofenadine out of the CNS efficiently.

(D) It is ionized at pH 7.4 and does not cross the blood–brain barrier.

ANSWERS AND EXPLANATIONS

1. The answer is A.
Angiotensin II stimulates the thirst center in the hypothalamus, and increases vasopressin (antidiuretic hormone) secretion from the posterior pituitary gland. Angiotensin II does not cause vasodilation, but is a potent vasoconstrictor. Angiotensin II increases, but not decreases, aldosterone secretion. It could cause bradycardia, but not tachycardia, which is attributable to baroreceptor reflex in response to hypertension.

2. The answer is B.
ACE converts bradykinin to biologically inactive products. This is the reason that the feline patients on an ACE inhibitor may have bronchoconstriction as a side effect. ACE converts angiotensin I to angiotension II, but does not affect the conversion of other angiotensin-related proteins, nor does ACE directly affect aldosterone secretion.

3. The answer is B.
Most of the older (first generations) H_1-antihistamines possess some sedative properties. The newer (second generations) H_1-antihistamines tend to have minimal or no sedative properties. Cimetidine, an H_2-antihistamine, is a potent inhibitor of cytochrome P450 enzymes, which also inhibits testosterone synthesis. Many H_1-antihistamines have antimuscarinic properties, which will decrease GI motility, and they cause constipation occasionally.

4. The answer is E.
In the past, the general concept was that H_1-antihistamines competitively antagonized H1-receptors. However, recent evidence indicates that H_1-antihistamines shift the active H_1-receptors to the inactive state. These drugs do not stabilize mast cells to inhibit histamine release, nor do they evoke H_1-receptor endocytosis.

5. The answer is A.
PGI_2 is a vasodilator, but not a vasoconstrictor. PGI2 receptors are coupled to G_s, thereby increasing cAMP synthesis and leading to relaxation of vascular smooth muscle and a decrease in platelet aggregation. PGI_2 is synthesized in endothelial cells utilizing platelet endoperoxides, which can be inhibited by NSAIDs, aspirin in particular.

6. The answer is B.
Ranitidine is more potent than cimetidine as an H2-antihistamine. Cimetidine, but not nizatidine, may cause drug interactions, because of its inhibition of the cytochrome P450 system. Ranitidine at very high doses may cause CNS disturbances including depression. Famotidine, cimetidine, ranitidine, and nizatidine have similar plasma half-lives of 2–3 hours.

7. The answer is D.
Cromolyn sodium inhibits histamine release. This is due to cell membrane hyperpolarization induced by opening of chloride channels. Dimenhydrinate, betazole, and cimetidine are H_1-antihistamine, H_2-agonist, and H_2-antihistamine, respectively.

8. The answer is C.
Stimulation of 5-HT$_4$ receptors by agonists such as cisapride, but not stimulation of 5-HT$_1$ receptors, increases GI motility. Because 5HT$_4$-receptors are coupled to G_s, which results in an increase in cAMP synthesis and acetylcholine release from the vagus nerve.

9. The answer is D.
Leukotrienes are potent stimulators of the contraction of bronchiolar smooth muscle. The other statements are all true.

10. The answer is C.
Montelukast is a leukotriene (LT) receptor antagonist that blocks LT-induced bronchoconstriction. Because asthma in cats may be attributable to increased autacoid release including histamine and LT, LT receptor antagonists can be used as adjunctive therapy. Cetirizine is a second-generation H_1-antihistamine; lisinopril is an ACE inhibitor; zileuton is a 5-lioxygenase inhibitor, which inhibits LT synthesis.

11. The answer is D.

The second-generation H_1-antihistamines including fexofenadine are ionized at physiological pH and the ionized form of the drug does not cross the blood–brain barrier to cause sedation. Fexofenadine can block cerebral H_1-receptors in vitro, but it cannot reach the target site in the CNS in vivo. P-glycoprotein is not the reason that fexofenadine does not cause sedation.

Chapter 4

Drugs Acting on the Central Nervous System

Walter H. Hsu and Dean H. Riedesel

I. INTRODUCTION

A. Function. Drugs can alter the function of the central nervous system (CNS) to provide

1. Anticonvulsant effects
2. Tranquilization (sedation)
3. Analgesia

B. Neurotransmitter–receptor relationship. Neurotransmitters released by a presynaptic neuron combine with receptors on the plasma membrane of a postsynaptic neuron, altering its membrane potential.

1. Neurotransmitters in the CNS include dopamine, γ-aminobutyric acid (GABA), acetylcholine (ACh), norepinephrine, dopamine, serotonin, histamine, glutamate, glycine, substance P, and many neuropeptides.
2. Receptors for neurotransmitters are the site of action for exogenous drugs.
   a. The neurotransmitter–receptor complex may directly alter the permeability of the cell membrane by opening or closing specific ion channels.
   b. Second messengers. The neurotransmitter-receptor complex may initiate a sequence of chemical reactions that alter ion transport across the membrane, thereby altering the membrane potential. Specific intracellular signal molecules, or second messengers, may be generated. The second messenger system sustains and amplifies the cellular response to drug–receptor binding (see Chapter 1). The vast majority of these neurotransmitters have G protein-coupled receptors (GPCRs).

C. Blood–brain barrier (BBB). Circulating drugs must cross BBB in order to gain access to the neurons of the brain.

1. Drugs that are lipid soluble, small in molecular size, poorly bound to protein, and nonionized at the pH of cerebrospinal fluid (CSF) will cross BBB most readily.
2. The BBB tends to increase in permeability in the presence of inflammation or at the site of tumors.
3. The BBB is poorly developed in neonates; hence, chemicals can easily gain access to the neonatal brain.

II. ANTICONVULSANT DRUGS

A. General features

1. **Preparations.** Only a few of the anticonvulsant drugs available for human use have been proven to be clinically useful in dogs and cats.
   a. Some of the drugs are too rapidly metabolized in dogs to be effective, even at high dosages.
   b. Clinical experience and pharmacokinetic data are unavailable for many of these compounds in cats. Cats are generally assumed to metabolize drugs more slowly and poorly than dogs.
2. **Mechanism of action.** Anticonvulsant drugs stabilize neuronal membranes.

   a. They may act directly on ion channels, resulting in hyperpolarization of the neuronal membrane.

   b. They activate GABA-gated Cl⁻ channels increasing the frequency of Cl⁻ channel opening produced by GABA, thereby evoking hyperpolarization of the neurons.

3. Therapeutic uses. Anticonvulsant drugs reduce the incidence, severity, or duration of seizures.

4. Administration

   a. Plasma concentrations of anticonvulsant drugs should be adequate to ensure an effective concentration in the brain. Treatment for at least five half-lives must occur before stable plasma levels of these drugs are achieved; thus, serum analyses for drug concentrations are beneficial.

     (1) Trough concentrations should be within the therapeutic range.

     (2) Peak concentrations should be below toxic levels.

   b. Drugs with long-elimination $t_{1/2}$ are more convenient to use in veterinary medicine because owners are usually only able to administer the drug 2–3 times daily.

5. Adverse effects

   a. Withdrawal symptoms, seizures, or status epilepticus may follow rapid cessation of administration of these drugs.

   b. A lowered seizure threshold, precipitating seizures in an otherwise well-controlled patient, may follow the administration of other drugs, such as

     (1) Phenothiazine tranquilizers (e.g., acepromazine)

     (2) Some antiparasitic drugs (e.g., pyrantel, levamisole, pyrethroids, methoxychlor, lindane, and anticholinesterases).

     (3) Metoclopramide, a dopamine receptor antagonist, is used to increase gastrointestinal (GI) motility.

   c. Enzyme induction

     (1) Phenobarbital, primidone, and phenytoin increase the cytochrome P450 enzymes of the liver. This enzyme induction may increase the biotransformation of other endogenous and exogenous chemicals.

     (2) Membrane-bound enzymes (e.g., alkaline phosphatase) can also be induced, leading to increases in serum concentrations that could be mistaken as an indication of liver injury.

   d. Hepatotoxicity is the most common adverse effect of anticonvulsant therapy in dogs. It develops in 6–15% of dogs treated with primidone alone or in combination with phenytoin.

     (1) The liver should be evaluated every 6–12 months for signs of toxicity, including

       (a) Elevated serum enzyme concentrations, particularly alanine transaminase (ALT) and glutamyl transferase activity.

       (b) Rising serum phenobarbital concentrations in dogs receiving a constant dosage.

       (c) Decreasing serum albumin concentrations.

       (d) Elevated postprandial serum concentration of bile acids.

     (2) If hepatotoxicity is detected, the dosage of primidone or phenobarbital should be decreased and KBr therapy implemented.

B. Barbiturates

1. Phenobarbital

   a. Chemistry. Phenobarbital is an oxybarbiturate.

   b. Mechanism of action. Barbiturates activate GABA-gated Cl⁻ channels, thereby evoking hyperpolarization of the neurons.

   c. Pharmacologic effects

     (1) Phenobarbital limits the spread of action potentials and thus elevates the seizure threshold.

     (2) Most barbiturates have anticonvulsant effects, but phenobarbital is unique in that it usually produces this effect at lower doses than those necessary to cause pronounced CNS depression (sedation).

d. **Therapeutic uses.** Phenobarbital is used for the long-term control of seizures. **It is not useful for terminating an ongoing seizure because the time span from administration until the onset of effect is too long (~20 minutes).**

e. **Pharmacokinetics**

   (1) When given orally, its GI absorption is practically complete in all animals. Peak levels occur in 4–8 hours after oral dosing in dogs.

   (2) It is widely distributed throughout the body, but because of its lower lipid solubility, it does not distribute as rapidly as most other barbiturates into the CNS. The amount of phenobarbital bound to albumin is 40–50%.

   (3) The oxybarbiturates are primarily metabolized in the liver. The major metabolite of phenobarbital is a parahydroxyphenyl derivative that is inactive and excreted in the urine.

   (4) Hepatic cytochrome P450 enzyme activity is increased by chronic administration of barbiturates, producing increased rates of barbiturate metabolism as well as increased metabolism of other drugs.

   (5) Hepatic cytochrome P450 enzyme activity is inhibited by certain drugs (e.g., chloramphenicol; see Chapters 1 and 19), thereby decreasing the elimination rate of barbiturates.

   (6) The elimination $t_{1/2}$: dogs, 32–90 hours; cats, 34–43 hours; horses, 13–18 hours.

f. **Administration**

   (1) Phenobarbital is usually administered orally, but can be injected IV or IM.

   (2) A serum drug concentration of 15–45 µg/mL is usually effective in controlling seizures; however, because of phenobarbital's long $t_{1/2}$, 14 days of therapy are required to develop a steady serum concentration.

g. **Adverse effects**

   (1) Sedation, polydipsia, polyuria, and polyphagia are common side effects. Dogs develop a tolerance to the sedative effects after 1–2 weeks, but cats may experience more pronounced sedation with longer duration.

   (2) **Hepatotoxicity.** Chronic administration to dogs may result in elevated serum concentrations of hepatic enzymes, for example, alkaline phosphatase and alanine tranaminase (ALT) and, in a small percentage of cases, liver damage.

   (3) Patients on phenobarbital may show a small decrease in serum thyroid hormone levels and an increase in plasma thyroid-stimulating hormone (TSH) levels. The decrease in thyroid hormone levels is attributed to the increase in liver enzymes that metabolize these hormones.

2. **Primidone.** It was a commonly used antiepileptic drug in dogs, but it is rarely used to control seizures.

   a. **Chemistry.** Primidone is a deoxybarbiturate (an analog of phenobarbital).

   b. **Pharmacokinetics**

      (1) Primidone is slowly absorbed after oral administration in dogs, with peak levels occurring 2–4 hours after dosing.

      (2) In dogs, primidone is rapidly metabolized by the liver to phenylethylmalonamide (PEMA) and phenobarbital. Primidone, PEMA, and phenobarbital are all anticonvulsants, but the $t_{1/2}$ of the first two are too short for them to be effective. The potency of primidone and PEMA is only 1/30 that of phenobarbital. Thus, ~85% of the anticonvulsant activity of primidone is attributable to phenobarbital.

      (3) **In cats, the metabolism to phenobarbital is slower and the $t_{1/2}$ is very long; thus, primidone should not be used in this species.**

   c. **Administration.** In dogs, an oral dose of 4–5 mg of primidone will produce a serum phenobarbital concentration that is equivalent to an oral dose of 1 mg of phenobarbital.

   d. **Adverse effects.** Prolonged use of primidone in dogs may lead to decreased serum albumin and elevated serum concentrations of liver enzymes. Occasionally, serious liver damage occurs.

3. **Pentobarbital**

   a. **Chemistry.** Pentobarbital is an oxybarbiturate.

b. Therapeutic uses. Pentobarbital will terminate seizures at a dose that produces anesthesia. This dose usually results in significant cardiopulmonary depression but may be the only way to control status epilepticus, if a benzodiazepine fails to work. However, there are two following problems associated with pentobarbital in the treatment of status epilepticus:

   (1) IV pentobarbital (2–6 mg/kg) requires 15–20 minutes to take effect; ≥ 6 mg/kg can cause cardiopulmonary depression.

   (2) IV pentobarbital induces paddling reflex activity during recovery; such activity may be confused with continued seizure activity.

c. Pharmacokinetics. It has a rapid onset (<1 minute) after IV injection and short duration of action.

   (1) It is distributed rapidly to all body tissues with highest concentrations found in the liver and brain. It is ~40% bound to albumin.

   (2) It is metabolized in the liver mainly by oxidation via cytochrome P450 enzymes. The $t_{1/2}$ in dogs is ~8 hours.

d. Administration. Pentobarbital is administered IV.

e. Adverse effects

Pentobarbital is a CNS depressant; close monitoring and respiratory assistance must be readily available. It may cause excitement during recovery from anesthesia. Hypothermia may develop in animals receiving pentobarbital, if exposed to temperatures <27°C. The barbiturates can be very irritating when administered perivascularly.

C. **Phenytoin**

1. **Chemistry.** Phenytoin is a hydantoin derivative.

2. **Mechanism of action.** Phenytoin stabilizes neuronal membranes and limits the development and spread of seizure activity.

   a. It reduces Na^+ influx during the action potential, reduces Ca^{2+} influx during depolarization, and promotes Na^+ efflux. The resultant effect is an inhibition of the spread of seizure activity.

   b. K^+ movement out of the cell during the action potential may be delayed, producing an increased refractory period and a decrease in repetitive depolarization.

3. **Therapeutic uses**

   a. Phenytoin is an anticonvulsant drug; however, because of its short $t_{1/2}$ in dogs, use of phenytoin may be impractical.

   b. Because of its lidocaine-like effects, phenytoin has been recommended for the treatment of digitalis-induced ventricular arrhythmias in dogs (see Chapter 8).

4. **Pharmacokinetics**

   a. After oral administration, phenytoin is 40% absorbed in dogs. Phenytoin is well distributed throughout the body and is ~80% bound to albumin in dogs.

   b. It is metabolized in the liver and with much of the drug conjugated to a glucuronide form and then excreted by the kidneys. Phenytoin induces hepatic cytochrome P450 enzymes, which may enhance the metabolism of itself and other drugs.

   c. The plasma $t_{1/2}$ are 3–7 hours in dogs, 8 hours in horses, and 42–108 hours in cats. Because of the pronounced hepatic enzyme induction in dogs, phenytoin metabolism is increased with shorter $t_{1/2}$ within 7–9 days after the beginning dose.

D. **Benzodiazepines** (see also IV C)

1. **General consideration**

   a. Diazepam, midazepam, clonazepam, and lorazepam are used as anticonvulsants.

   b. They are the preferred drugs for the treatment of status epilepticus (continuous seizure activity lasting >5 minutes or recurrent seizures between which the patient does not fully recover) and cluster seizures (≥ 2 discrete seizure events within a 24-hour period).

    c. They can be used as a maintenance anticonvulsant in cats. However, they have a very limited use as a maintenance anticonvulsant in dogs, because the development of tolerance occurs rapidly in this species due to drug metabolism into inactive metabolites. In contrast, cats metabolize benzodiazepines poorly and thus do not have problems with these drugs as dogs do.

2. Diazepam

    a. Mechanism of action. Benzodiazepines activate GABA-gated Cl^- channels to potentiate the channel opening activity of GABA, thereby evoking hyperpolarization of the neurons.

    b. Therapeutic uses and administration. Diazepam is used as an anticonvulsant, muscle relaxant, tranquilizer, and appetite stimulant.

        (1) In cats, it is administered orally for seizure control. The longer $t_{1/2}$ and lower incidence of developing tolerance make diazepam clinically useful for long-term seizure control in cats.

        (2) In dogs, it is administered IV for the control of status epilepticus and cluster seizures.

        (3) Diazepam is well absorbed after intrarectal administration, and thus can be used as an at-home treatment of animals with cluster seizures. Other benzodiazepines are not well absorbed after this route.

        (4) It is not used orally in dogs as a maintenance anticonvulsant because it has a short $t_{1/2}$ of 2–4 hours and its tendency to develop tolerance in this species due to drug metabolism.

    c. Pharmacokinetics

        (1) Absorption. Diazepam is dissolved in propylene glycol and Na benzoate for injection.

            (a) Because of its poor water solubility, diazepam solution (in propylene glycol) via the IM route is slowly absorbed.

            (b) Diazepam is very lipid soluble and rapidly crosses BBB.

        (2) Distribution. It is highly (>85%) albumin bound.

        (3) Metabolism and excretion. Diazepam is metabolized in the liver to several metabolites, including desmethyldiazepam (nordiazepam), temazepam, and oxazepam, all of which are pharmacologically active. These metabolites are conjugated to glucuronide and excreted by the kidneys.

        (4) The plasma $t_{1/2}$ of diazepam: dogs, 2–4 hours; cats, 5.5 hours; horses, 7–22 hours. The plasma $t_{1/2}$ of nordiazepam: dogs, ~3 hours; cats, ~24 hours.

    d. Adverse effects

        (1) Changes in behavior (irritability, depression, and aberrant demeanor) may occur after receiving diazepam.

        (2) Cats may develop acute fatal hepatic necrosis after receiving oral diazepam for several days. As a result, some neurologists do not recommend the use of diazepam as a maintenance anticonvulsant in cats.

        (3) Complications related to the propylene glycol carrier include venous thrombosis, transient cardiovascular depression, and arrhythmias following rapid IV injection.

3. Midazolam. It is more potent than diazepam for its anticonvulsant/sedative effects, but its duration of action is shorter than diazepam.

    a. Therapeutic uses. Midazolam is used as an anticonvulsant for status epilepticus, muscle relaxant, tranquilizer, and appetite stimulant the same way as diazepam.

    b. Pharmacokinetics. Midazolam has a shorter elimination $t_{1/2}$ of 77 minutes in dogs, which is shorter than diazepam (~3 hours).

        (1) Distribution. At low pH values (<4.0), midazolam is water soluble, but at higher pH values, it is lipid soluble. Thus, in the bottle (pH = 3.5), it is an aqueous solution, but in the body (pH = 7.4), it is lipid soluble and readily crosses BBB and cell membranes. A total of 95% of midazolam is bound by albumin.

        (2) Metabolism and excretion. Midazolam is metabolized by cytochrome P450 enzymes. An active metabolite α-hydroxymidazolam has less pharmacologic effect than the parent drug. The metabolites are conjugated to glucuronide and excreted by the kidneys.

c. **Administration.** It is administered IM or IV.
d. **Adverse effects.** Midazolam may cause mild respiratory depression, vomiting, restless behavior, agitation, and local irritation.

4. **Clonazepam**
   a. **Therapeutic uses.** The uses are the same as diazepam without distinct advantages over diazepam. It is administered orally or IV. IV administration is for the treatment of status epilepticus. However, clonazepam injectable is not available in the United States. It can be used as an adjunctive therapy to be in combination with phenobarbital in order to reduce the dosage of the latter. Clonazepam alone has very limited value as a maintenance anticonvulsant because of the rapid development of drug tolerance.
   b. **Pharmacokinetics.** It is well absorbed from the GI tract; crosses BBB and placenta. A total of 85% of clonazepam is bound by albumin. It is metabolized in the liver by cytochrome P450 enzymes to several metabolites that are excreted in the urine. Peak plasma levels occur ~3 hours after oral administration. The $t_{1/2}$ ranges from 20 to 40 hours in humans. No information is available for animals.
   c. **Adverse effects.** Tolerance to the anticonvulsant effects of clonazepam has been reported in dogs, which is usually noted after weeks of therapy. GI disturbances, including vomiting, hypersalivation, and diarrhea/constipation may occur.

5. **Lorazepam**
   a. **Therapeutic uses**
      (1) It can be administered orally for a short-term at-home treatment of dogs having cluster seizures.
      (2) It is also useful in cats as a maintenance anticonvulsant, and the chances of developing idiopathic hepatic necrosis are minimal.
      (3) It may be safely used in individuals with compromised liver function and in geriatric dogs because it does not produce active metabolites.
   b. **Pharmacokinetics**
      (1) After oral administration, it is rapidly absorbed from the GI tract in dogs, although, to a lesser degree in cats. The time to peak plasma concentrations is ~2 hours.
      (2) Approximately 85% of lorazepam is bound by albumin.
      (3) It is primarily metabolized to its glucuronide conjugation in dogs and cats. The formation of the conjugate is much faster in dogs as compared to humans and cats.
      (4) It is excreted primarily in the urine and to a lesser extent in the feces of dogs. In cats, the drug is excreted in equal parts in both feces and urine.
      (5) In humans, the mean $t_{1/2}$ is ~12 hours, whereas $t_{1/2}$ of lorazepam glucuronide is ~18 hours. No information is available for animals.
   c. **Adverse effects.** Increased appetite, paradoxical excitation, and anxiety have been reported to occur early in therapy, although they resolve with continued use or by decreasing the dose.

E. **Potassium bromide (KBr)**

1. **Mechanism of action**
   a. It is hypothesized that Br^- enters neurons via Cl^- channels, resulting in hyperpolarization of the neuronal membrane.
   b. Barbiturates and benzodiazepines, which enhance Cl^- conductance, may act in synergy with KBr to hyperpolarize neurons, thus raising the seizure threshold.
2. **Therapeutic uses**
   a. KBr is administered orally to **treat refractory seizures** in dogs. The use in cats is not recommended, since it evokes **severe asthma in this species**.
   b. It is used in combination with phenobarbital to terminate refractory generalized tonic-clonic convulsions in dogs.
3. **Pharmacokinetics**
   a. **Absorption.** Br^- is quickly absorbed from the GI tract following oral administration.

    b. Metabolism. Br$^-$ is neither metabolized nor bound to plasma proteins. It has a long $t_{1/2}$ (25 days in dogs and 10 days in cats), and it may take up to 6 months to achieve stable plasma Br$^-$ concentrations.

    c. Elimination. Br$^-$ is eliminated exclusively by the kidneys.

4. Adverse effects

    a. Transient sedation at the beginning of therapy may occur.

    b. GI effects. Stomach irritation can produce nausea and vomiting. Vomiting, anorexia, and constipation are indications of toxicity.

    c. Polydipsia, polyuria, polyphagia, lethargy, irritability, and aimless walking are additional adverse effects of Br$^-$.

    d. Pancreatitis may be precipitated by Br$^-$.

    e. Severe asthma can be seen in Br$^-$-treated cats.

F. Valproic acid and sodium valproate

1. Chemistry. Valproic acid is a derivative of carboxylic acid. It is structurally unrelated to other anticonvulsant drugs.

2. Therapeutic uses

    a. In dogs, valproic acid is effective in controlling seizures when given orally, but its short $t_{1/2}$ makes it impractical for long-term use. It is a second to fourth-line anticonvulsant that may be useful as an adjunctive treatment in some dogs.

    b. Its clinical usefulness in cats has not been evaluated.

3. Pharmacokinetics

    a. Sodium valproate is rapidly converted to valproic acid in the acidic environment of the stomach where it is rapidly absorbed from the GI tract. The bioavailability via this route in dogs is ~80% and peak levels occur in 1 hour.

    b. It is rapidly and well distributed in the extracellular fluid, with 70–80% bound by albumin in dogs. CSF levels of valproic acid are ~10% of the plasma levels.

    c. It is metabolized in the liver and is conjugated with glucuronide. These metabolites and a small quantity of parent drug are excreted in the urine. The elimination $t_{1/2}$ in dogs is 1.5–3 hours.

4. Adverse effects

    a. GI disturbances and hepatotoxicity. Vomiting, anorexia, and diarrhea may be seen, which may be diminished by administration with food. Hepatotoxicity, including liver failure, is a potential adverse effect in dogs.

    b. Other potential adverse effects include CNS effects (sedation, ataxia, behavioral changes, etc.), dermatologic effects (alopecia, rash, etc.), hematologic effects (thrombocytopenia, reduced platelet aggregation, leukopenia, anemia, etc.), pancreatitis, and edema.

G. Gabapentin. It is a synthetic GABA analog that can cross BBB to exert its anticonvulsant effect.

1. Mechanism of action. GABA content in neurons is increased by gabapentin administration. However, the main effect of gabapentin is due to its inhibition of voltage-dependent Ca^{2+} channels to decrease neuronal Ca^{2+} levels, thereby inhibiting excitatory neurotransmitter release (e.g., glutamate).

2. Therapeutic uses. Gabapentin may be useful as adjunctive therapy for refractory or complex partial seizures, or in the treatment of chronic pain in dogs or cats. It is administered orally.

3. Pharmacokinetics. In dogs, oral bioavailability is ~80%. Peak plasma levels occur ~2 hours post-administration. In dogs, elimination is primarily via kidneys, but ≤40% of gabapentin is metabolized by the liver to N-methyl-gabapentin. The elimination $t_{1/2}$ is 3–4 hours in dogs. No $t_{1/2}$ information is available for cats.

4. Adverse effects. Sedation, ataxia, and mild polyphagia are noticeable side effects. Abrupt discontinuation of gabapentin may cause seizures.

H. Levetiracetam. It is used orally as an adjunctive therapy for refractory canine epilepsy. It is well tolerated in dogs and an initial prospective trial in cats was favorable.

1. **Mechanism of action.** Levetiracetam inhibits hypersynchronization of epileptiform burst firing and propagation of seizure activity. The exact mechanism is not understood. However, recent evidence suggests that it binds synaptic vesicle protein 2A in the neuron; the interaction with this neuronal vesicular protein may account for levetiracetam's anticonvulsant effect.

2. **Pharmacokinetics**
   a. It is well absorbed after oral administration and has 100% bioavailability. It is well distributed and minimally (10%) bound by albumin.
   b. While not extensively metabolized, the acetamide group of the drug is hydrolyzed to the carboxylic acid metabolite that is apparently inactive. Both the parent drug and metabolites are excreted into urine. The elimination $t_{1/2}$ in dogs, ~4 hours and in cats, ~8 hours.

3. **Adverse effects.** It has little side effects, which include changes in behavior, drowsiness, and GI disturbances (vomiting and anorexia). Withdrawal of this drug should be slow in order to prevent "withdrawal" seizures.

I. **Felbamate** is a dicarbamate drug and is used orally in dogs to treat refractory epilepsy as an adjunctive therapy or a sole anticonvulsant agent for patients with focal and generalized seizures. **At clinical doses, felbamate does not induce sedation and thus is particularly useful in the control of obtunded mental status** due to brain tumor or cerebral infarct.

1. **Mechanism of action**
   a. Blockade of NMDA receptor-mediated neuronal excitation.
   b. Potentiation of GABA-mediated neuronal inhibition.
   c. Inhibition of voltage-dependent Na^+ and Ca^{2+} channels.

2. **Pharmacokinetics**
   a. It is readily absorbed from the GI tract after oral administration, but bioavailability in pups is only 30% that of adult dogs.
   b. In dogs, ~70% of felbamate is excreted in the urine unchanged; the remainder undergoes liver metabolism by cytochrome P450 enzymes and conjugation.
   c. The elimination $t_{1/2}$ is 5–6 hours in adult dogs and 2.5 hours in pups.

3. **Adverse effects.** Side effects of felbamate are infrequently seen.
   a. The most noticeable side effect is **liver dysfunction**. Thus, it should not be given to dogs with a liver disease. Because of the potential for hepatotoxicity, it is recommended that serum biochemistry be performed every 6 months for dogs on felbamate therapy.
   b. Reversible bone marrow depression is rarely seen in dogs receiving felbamate. These dogs may have thrombocytopenia and leucopenia.
   c. Keratoconjunctivitis sicca and generalized tremor are rarely seen side effects of felbamate in dogs.

J. **Zonisamide** is a sulfonamide-based anticonvulsant drug that can be used as a sole anticonvulsant or an adjunctive therapy to control refractory epilepsy in dogs with minimal adverse effects. It is administered orally twice a day. However, the cost could be a problem for using this drug in dogs. The drug has not been studied sufficiently in cats to be recommended for this species.

1. **Mechanism of action.** Zonisamide inhibits voltage-dependent Na^+ and Ca^{2+} channels of neurons to induce hyperpolarization and decreased Ca^{2+} influx.

2. **Pharmacokinetics**
   a. It is well absorbed from the GI tract after oral administration to dogs.
   b. It is evenly distributed in the body after GI absorption and has low protein binding.
   c. Most of zonisamide is excreted in the urine, but ~20% is metabolized by the liver. In humans, it is metabolized to acetylzonisamide, 2-sulfamoylacetyl phenol, and glucuronide.
   d. The elimination $t_{1/2}$ in dogs is ~15 hours.

3. **Adverse effects.** Zonisamide has high safety margin in dogs. The reported side effects include sedation, ataxia, and anorexia.

III. CNS STIMULANTS (ANALEPTICS)

A. **Doxapram** is used most frequently in veterinary medicine as a CNS stimulant.

1. **Mechanism of action.** Doxapram stimulates respiration, which is a result of direct stimulation of the medullary respiratory centers and probably via activation of carotid and aortic chemoreceptors. Transient increases in respiratory rate and tidal volume occur. Detailed mechanism by which doxapram stimulates respiratory center transiently is not known.

2. **Therapeutic uses**
   a. Doxapram is used to arouse animals from inhalant and parenteral anesthesia or anesthetic overdose. The depth of anesthesia is reduced, but the effect could be transient.
   b. Doxapram is used for respiratory stimulation in neonates after assisted birth or C-section, and in lightly anesthetized adult dogs to evaluate laryngeal function. Low doses of doxapram increase the respiratory minute volume by stimulating the carotid bodies.
   c. Doxapram is not effective in reviving a severely depressed neonate and is not a good substitute for endotracheal intubation and ventilation.

3. **Pharmacokinetics.** The drug is well distributed into tissues. In dogs, doxapram is rapidly metabolized by the liver and most is excreted as metabolites in the urine within 24–48 hours of administration.

4. **Administration**
   a. IV administration produces an effect for 5–10 minutes.
   b. IM administration and topical application to the buccal mucosa are also effective in neonates.

5. **Adverse effects.** High doses of doxapram may induce seizures. Hypertension, arrhythmias, seizures, and hyperventilation leading to respiratory alkalosis can happen. These effects are most probable with repeated or high doses of doxapram.

IV. TRANQUILIZERS, ATARACTICS, NEUROLEPTICS, AND SEDATIVES. These

terms are used interchangeably in veterinary medicine to refer the drugs that calm the animal and promote sleep but do not necessarily induce sleep, even at high doses. Ataractic means "undisturbed"; neuroleptic means "to take hold of nerves." **Tranquilized animals are usually calm and easy to handle, but they may be aroused by and respond to stimuli in a normal fashion (e.g., biting, scratching, kicking).** When used as preanesthetic medications, these drugs enable the use of less general anesthetic.

A. **Phenothiazine derivatives include acepromazine, promethazine, chlorpromazine, fluphenazine, prochlorperazine, and trimeprazine.**

1. **Mechanism of action.** Phenothiazine derivatives affect the CNS at the basal ganglia, hypothalamus, limbic system, brain stem, and reticular activating system. **They block dopamine, α_1-adrenergic and serotonergic receptors.**

2. **Pharmacologic effects**
   a. **CNS effects**
      (1) The tranquilizing effects are due to depression of the brain stem and connections to the cerebral cortex (reticular activating system), probably via blockade of dopamine and 5-HT receptors.
      (2) All phenothiazines decrease spontaneous motor activity. At high doses, animals will be immobilized in a fixed position for long periods (extrapyramidal symptoms).
      (3) **The phenothiazine-induced tranquilization is not accompanied by analgesia.**
   b. **Cardiovascular effects**
      (1) Hypotension may develop as a result of α_1-adrenergic receptor blockade and a decrease in the sympathetic tone. Animals with high sympathetic

tone from hypovolemia may become profoundly hypotensive following phenothiazine administration, owing to **epinephrine reversal**. Treatment for this hypotension should include IV fluids and possibly an α_1-agonist drug (e.g., phenylephrine).

- **(2)** Sinus bradycardia and second-degree heart block may occur with high doses.
- **(3)** Reflex sinus tachycardia may occur if hypotension develops.
- **(4)** Antiarrhythmic effects may be seen with phenothiazine tranquilizers. A combination of the following could be responsible.
  - **(a)** α_1-Receptor blockade in the myocardium.
  - **(b)** Local anesthetic-like effect on the myocardial cells.
  - **(c)** Reduced systemic blood pressure.
- **(5) Inotropic effect.** Myocardial contractility is either unaffected or slightly reduced (due to α_1-receptor blockade in the myocardium).

c. **Respiratory effects**
- **(1)** Respiratory depression. It is induced by large doses of phenothiazine, which suppresses the respiratory center. Opioids can potentiate this effect of phenothiazine.
- **(2)** Phenothiazines depress the maximal ventilatory response to an elevated CO_2 partial pressure, although the threshold for this response remains normal.

d. **GI effects**
- **(1)** Motility is inhibited, probably due to activation of β-receptors, resulting in GI muscle relaxation. In addition, phenothiazines have weak atropine-like effects.
- **(2)** Emesis is suppressed because phenothiazines block dopamine receptors in the cells of the chemoreceptor trigger zone in the area of postrema of the medulla oblongata.

e. **Effects on blood.** Packed cell volume decreases as a result of splenic sequestration of red blood cells owing to vasodilatation.

f. **Metabolic effects**
- **(1)** Hypothermia/hyperthermia
  - **(a)** Body temperature tends to decrease after tranquilization because of increased heat loss from vasodilatation and decreased heat production from a lack of muscular activity.
  - **(b)** Phenothiazine-induced depression of the thermoregulation center in the hypothalamus may lead to hypothermia/hyperthermia, which depends on ambient temperature. This effect is probably due to blockade of dopamine and 5-HT receptors.
- **(2) Hyperglycemia.** This is due to increased epinephrine release, in response to phenothiazine-induced hypotension. Epinephrine, in turn, promotes liver glycogenolysis by activating β_2-receptors.
- **(3) Hyperprolactinemia.** This is due to increased prolactin secretion from the anterior pituitary gland. Blockade of D_2-receptors on the lactotropes increases prolactin secretion.

3. **Therapeutic uses**
a. Phenothiazines are primarily used for tranquilization. They generally do not have analgesic effects. **They should be used cautiously as a restraining agent in aggressive dogs, as it may make the animal more prone to startle and react to noises or other sensory inputs.** There is an individual variability with regard to the sensitivity to phenothiazines.
b. Most of these drugs are effective as **antiemetics.**
c. Administration of a phenothiazine prior to use of inhalant anesthetics can reduce the incidence of arrhythmias caused by myocardial sensitization to catecholamines.
d. Promethazine and trimeprazine are used to control allergy, because they block H_1-receptors.

4. Pharmacokinetics
a. In general, these tranquilizers have duration of action of 3–6 hours. They are well distributed in the circulation and >80% of circulating phenothiazines are bound by albumin.

b. They are metabolized by an oxidative process via cytochrome P450 enzymes, which is followed by conjugation. The metabolites are mostly inactive and are excreted by the kidneys along with small quantity of parent compounds over several days. The elimination $t_{1/2}$ is ~3 hours in equine.

c. Acepromazine withdrawal periods in cattle and swine. Since acepromazine is not approved by FDA to be used in these two species, the extralabel withdrawal intervals recommended by the Food Animal Residue Avoidance Databank (FARAD) are 7-day preslaughter and 48-hour milk periods.

5. Administration. Phenothiazines can be administered orally, IV, IM, or SC.

6. Adverse effects. There is no reversal agent for this class of drugs.
a. Accidental intracarotid administration in horses results in the immediate onset of seizure activity and, sometimes, death.

b. They inhibit cholinesterase (ChE) and may worsen the clinical signs of anti-ChE poisoning. They should not be given to animals within 1 month of treatment with an organophosphate compound.

c. The H_1-antagonistic effect makes phenothiazines an undesirable drug for sedation of animals prior to allergy testing.

d. Paraphimosis may occur in stallions, which is due to relaxation of retractive penis muscles via α_1-receptor blockade. Thus, phenothiazines should be used cautiously or avoided altogether in breeding stallions.

7. Contraindications
a. Anti-ChE poisoning or suspected treatment with anti-ChE antiparasitic drugs.

b. History of blood loss and hypotension.

c. Avoid in animals with moderate to severe liver dysfunction or portacaval shunt.

B. Benzodiazepine derivatives (see also II D)

1. Preparations. Diazepam, midazolam, clonazempam, and zolazepam are four drugs in this group that are used in veterinary medicine.

2. Mechanism of action (See II D)

3. Pharmacokinetics (see II D)

4. Pharmacologic effects
a. Cardiovascular effects are minimal.

b. Respiratory effects. Depressed ventilation may occur in an additive manner when the benzodiazepines are administered with other respiratory depressants (e.g., opioids, barbiturates, α_2-agonists). These drugs inhibit the respiratory centers in the medulla.

c. Muscular effects. Relaxation is mediated by benzodiazepine's inhibitory effects in the spinal cord.

5. Therapeutic uses
a. General
  (1) They are used as anticonvulsant in all the domestic species.

  (2) Benzodiazepines can be given with ketamine or tiletamine (Telazol®) to provide muscle relaxation. This combination is very convenient for short examinations and surgical procedures.

  (3) When used alone, benzodiazepine derivatives are not reliable tranquilizers in horses, dogs, or cats, but they provide satisfactory **tranquilization** in **sheep,** goats, and **neonatal foals.**

b. Diazepam
  (1) Diazepam is used orally, rectally, or IV as an anticonvulsant for the control of seizures and status epilepticus.

  (2) It can be used IV in combination with opioids (e.g., butorphanol) for **neuroleptanalgesia** or with cyclohexylamines (e.g., ketamine) or barbiturates (e.g., thiopental) for the **induction of general anesthesia.**

    c. Midazolam
- **(1)** It is used in combination with an opioid (e.g., butorphanol or oxymorphone) as a neuroleptanalgesic in older or debilitated dogs and cats.
- **(2)** It can be used as part of the drug protocol for induction of anesthesia. Mixed with ketamine, it provides muscle relaxation. Midazolam, injected IV, reduces the total thiobarbiturate dose needed for intubation in dogs and cats.

    d. Zolazepam is used exclusively with tiletamine (Tilazol®) for anesthesia in dogs, cats, and other domestic and wild animals.

6. Adverse effects (see also II D 1 e)
- **a. Benzodiazepines may produce excitement** rather than tranquilization in some animals. Animals that are mentally depressed or sedated prior to the administration of a benzodiazepine are less likely to become excited.
- **b. Ataxia, weakness,** and **muscle fasciculations** may occur in horses.
- **c. Reversal. Flumazenil** is a specific competitive antagonist for benzodiazepine receptors and has minimal agonist activity. Flumazenil is given IV at 0.01–0.02 mg/kg.

C. α_2-**Adrenergic agonists** These drugs activate α_2-adrenergic receptors in the CNS, thereby causing analgesia, sedation, and skeletal muscle relaxation. These effects of α_2-agonists make them useful as preanesthetics. The dosages of anesthetics usually can be reduced by ≥70%. Because of their nature in activating α_2-adrenergic receptors, they have many untoward effects, including hypertension, bradycardia, and decreased GI motility. However, the safety of these drugs can be greatly increased by the use of α_2- antagonists to reverse their effects.

1. Mechanism of action. α_2-Agonists activate α_2-receptors that are $G_{i/o}$-coupled receptors; $G_{i/o}$ mediates many inhibitory effects on the nervous systems and endocrine glands (see Chapter 1 for G-proteins and Figure 2-3 of Chapter 2 for α_2-receptor location). High doses of xylazine, detomidine, and romifidine also activate α_1-receptors.

2. Pharmacological effects
- **a. Analgesia.** Centrally active α_2-agonists exert a powerful analgesic action over head, neck, and body, but is minimal in extremities. These drugs may play a role modulating spinal pain processing.
  - **(1)** α_2-Receptors are located on the dorsal horn neurons of the spinal cord, where they can inhibit the release of nociceptive neurotransmitters, for example, substance P and calcitonin gene-related peptide (CGRP).
  - **(2)** α_2-**Adrenergic mechanisms do not work through opioidergic mechanisms, because cross-tolerance is not usually present.** α_2-Agonist-mediated analgesia is not reversed by opioid antagonists.
- **b. Sedation.** α_2-Agonists induce potent sedation.
  - **(1)** The degree of sedation varies among species and compounds. Ruminants are most sensitive to α_2-agonists, followed by cats, dogs, and horses. Pigs are least sensitive to α_2-agonists in domestic animals.
  - **(2)** Among available α_2-agonists, following clinical doses, medetomidine causes the greatest sedation, which is followed by xylazine. Romifidine and detomidine cause least sedation among the four.
  - **(3)** Locus coeruleus is among the structures responsible for the α_2-agonist-induced sedation and the α_2-receptors in this structure mediate the sedation.
  - **(4)** High doses of α_2-agonists may induce CNS excitation, which is attributable to activation of α_1-receptors.
- **c. Skeletal muscle relaxation.** α_2-Agonists produce skeletal muscle relaxation by inhibiting intraneuronal transmission of impulses in the CNS. These drugs do not work at the neuromuscular junction. At the clinical doses, romifidine exerts less muscle relaxant (head drop) and ataxia than other α_2-agonists used in veterinary medicine, probably because of its additional α_1-agonistic (excitatory) activity.
- **d. Emesis.** It is induced in carnivores and omnivores, and is commonly seen in the cat, and less frequently in the dog. Emesis is induced more frequently by IM

than IV administration. These drugs activate the α_2-receptors in the chemoreceptor trigger zone of the area postrema to induce emesis.

e. GI effects. α_2-Agonists reduce both GI motility and secretions and these effects make them useful for the treatment of diarrhea. α_2-Agonists may cause these GI effects by inhibiting the release of acetylcholine from parasympathetic nerves.

f. Cardiovascular effects. The IV administration of α_2-agonists causes mild hypertension for ≤ 10 minutes, which is followed by hypotension lasting several hours. The IM administration of α_2-agonists usually causes only hypotension.

   (1) Bradycardia accompanied by sinus arrhythmia and/or second-degree heart block is usually seen during hypotension and hypertension.

   (2) The hypertension is due to activation of the postsynaptic α_2-receptors of vascular smooth muscle.

   (3) The hypotension is caused by reduced norepinephrine release by the sympathetic nerve at the vascular smooth muscle. This is due to the decreased sympathetic outflow from the CNS as well as activation of presynaptic α_2-receptors in the sympathetic terminal.

   (4) Bradycardia (with or without sinus arrhythmia) is due to decreased norepinephrine release to the myocardium, particularly the SA node. An increase in baroreceptor reflex during hypertension may also contribute to bradycardia. Therefore, administration of an anticholinergic agent may change the α_2-agonist-induced bradycardia into tachycardia, while potentiating the α_2-agonist-induced hypertension.

g. Renal effects. α_2-Agonists induce diuresis through inhibiting vasopressin release and/or inhibiting vasopressin's action on free water reabsorption from the collecting duct of the kidney.

h. Respiratory effects. α_2-Agonists cause hypoxemia (and sometimes pulmonary edema) in ruminants, especially sheep. This effect is not seen in other species. Hypoxemia is most severe after IV administration of the drug. Postural changes (lateral recumbency) during CNS depression probably contribute to impaired oxygenation. The hypoxemia is due to activation of peripheral α_2-receptors at

   (1) vascular and bronchial smooth muscle, causing bronchospasm and vasospasm;

   (2) blood platelets, causing transient platelet aggregation with pulmonary microembolism; and

   (3) pulmonary intravascular macrophage, causing activation followed by cytokine and inflammatory mediator release.

i. Neuroendocrine effects. α_2-Agonists inhibit sympathoadrenal outflow and decrease the release of norepinephrine and epinephrine.

   (1) α_2-Agonists inhibit insulin release; this effect is very pronounced in ruminants, which results in a moderate to severe hyperglycemia lasting up to 24 hours.

   (2) α_2-Agonists increase growth hormone release by inhibiting somatostatin release from the hypothalamus and stimulating growth hormone—stimulating hormone release from the median eminence. The α_2-agonist-induced growth hormone release is not sustained; consecutive daily drug administration can only maintain increased secretion for <1 week.

3. Therapeutic uses

α_2-Agonists are used as a sedative, analgesic, and immobilizing agent. They are also used to induce epidural analgesia, as a preanesthetic, and as a part of the anesthetic combination. In this regard, xylazine-ketamine is a commonly used, but not very safe, parenteral anesthetic combination [see 5 c (6)].

4. Antagonism of the effects of α_2-agonists. α_2-Receptor blockers have been used to reverse the pharmacological and toxicological effects of α_2-agonists. They are administered IV or IM. Yohimbine (0.1 mg/kg) and tolazoline (1–2 mg/kg) are desirable α_2-blockers for nonruminants and ruminants, respectively. Atipamezole (0.2 mg/kg) works well in all species. Atropine should not be used to antagonize the bradycardia and heart block induced by α_2-agonists, since it may cause severe hypertension, tachycardia, and GI atony in animals treated with an α_2-agonist.

5. Xylazine. It is approved by the FDA for use in the cat, dog, horses, and wildlife, for example, deer and elk. However, it is also frequently used in other species, particularly the cattle. It is administered IM, IV, or SC.

   a. Pharmacokinetics

      (1) The distribution $t_{1/2}$ of xylazine is 1–6 minutes. The $t_{1/2}$ of elimination after IV administration of xylazine is 50 minutes in the horse, 40 minutes in cattle, 25 minutes in sheep, and 30 minutes in the dog. The pharmacologic effects of xylazine may last much longer than its plasma $t_{1/2}$.

      (2) Xylazine is converted in the liver by cytochrome P450 enzymes into hydroxyl/methyl/thiourea metabolites. About 70% of metabolites are excreted into urine and 30% into feces. Although it is not reported, some forms of conjugates are expected to be found in the excreta.

      (3) In cattle, after IM administration of 0.35 mg/kg, IM, concentrations of xylazine and 2,6-dimethylaniline (a toxic metabolite of xylazine) were below the limit of quantification (10 µg/kg) by 72 hours in tissues and 12 hours in milk. Thus, the FARAD recommends a preslaughter withdrawal period of 4 days and milk withdrawal time of 24 hours in cattle.

   b. Adverse effects

      (1) Because of the GI stasis associated with xylazine administration, bloat may be a result.

      (2) Xylazine-induced bradycardia with sinus arrhythmia/arrest can be severe. Close monitoring is needed; in very severe cases, the use of an α_2-antagonist may be necessary to save the animal.

      (3) Xylazine affects the thermoregulation center in the hypothalamus, thus it produces hypothermia when the ambient temperature is low, and hyperthermia when the ambient temperature is high. Thus, the use of xylazine to immobilize wildlife should be performed with caution and the use of α_2-antagonist to control the pharmacological effects of xylazine (or other α_2-agonists) in wildlife is a must.

   c. Contraindications

      (1) Cardiac aberrations

      (2) Hypotension or shock

      (3) Renal insufficiency

      (4) Hepatic impairment

      (5) Epilepsy (because xylazine may precipitate seizures in susceptible animals).

      (6) Use of xylazine in combination with ketamine should be used only in young healthy animals because this combination synergistically suppresses cardiopulmonary function of the animal.

      (7) Immediate collapse, convulsions, and sudden death can occur in horses given xylazine into the carotid artery.

      (8) A cautious approach should be taken whenever xylazine is used in treatment of colic, because xylazine's powerful analgesic effect can mask the underlying problem and because xylazine can paralyze the GI tract.

      (9) Xylazine should not be given to animals (particularly mares and ruminants) within the last month of pregnancy, since it may induce abortion.

     (10) Xylazine should not be given to dehydrated animals or those with urinary obstruction because of its potent diuretic effect.

6. Detomidine (Dormosedan®). It is approved by the FDA for use in horses. It is administered IM or IV.

   a. Pharmacokinetics

      (1) The elimination $t_{1/2}$ is 1.2 hours for the IV dose and 1.8 hours for the IM dose.

      (2) Metabolism to detomidine carboxylic acid and hydroxydetomidine glucuronide and thereafter excretion into the urine seems to be the major elimination route.

   b. Adverse effects

      (1) Following the recommended dose, piloerection, sweating, partial penis prolapse, and salivation, and occasionally, slight muscle tremors may be seen.

(2) Excessive doses of detomidine can induce CNS excitation. The above two side effects of detomidine are also seen with the administration of other α_2-agonists.

(3) IV sulfonamides should not be used in detomidine-treated horses as potentially fatal dysrhythmias may occur.

(4) Detomidine at 400 µg/kg ($10\times$ of recommended dose of 40 µg/kg) daily for three consecutive days can produce myocardial necrosis in horses.

(5) Other adverse effects seen with xylazine administration may also occur in animals treated with detomidine.

7. **Medetomidine (Dormitor®). It is the most potent and selective α_2-agonist available for use in veterinary medicine.** It can induce light anesthesia in some individual animals; short examinations/procedures can be performed in these animals.

   a. **Pharmacokinetics**
      (1) After IV or IM administration, onset of effect is rapid (5 minutes for IV; 10–15 minutes for IM). Peak concentration after IM administration in dogs and cats is seen within 30 minutes. The elimination $t_{1/2}$ is 1–1.5 hours.
      (2) Medetomidine is metabolized by the liver cytochrome P450 enzymes into hydroxyl-medetomidine and conjugates. In addition, medetomidine has been shown to inhibit cytochrome P450 enzymes of the liver.

   b. **Adverse effects.** These are the same as stated in the xylazine section and are the extension of the pharmacological effects of the α_2-agonist. However, since medetomidine is a very potent α_2-agonist, the adverse effects can be very severe. Thus, the use of an α_2-antagonist, for example, atipamezole may be needed to reverse these adverse effects of medetomidine.

8. **Romifidine (Sedivet®).** It is for IV use in horses.

   a. **Pharmacokinetics.** Following IV administration, the elimination $t_{1/2}$ is ~50 minutes. It is metabolized by the liver (cytochrome P450 enzymes) into 4-hydroxyromifidine and further into glucuronide conjugate, which is excreted into urine.

   b. **Adverse effects.** The adverse effects of romifidine are similar to those of xylazine and detomidine.

V. OPIOIDS

A. General features

1. **Terminology**
   a. The term "**opioid**" is all-inclusive, and refers to a drug that binds to all or part of a subtype of opioid receptors. An opioid may be synthetic, semisynthetic, or naturally occurring. The drug may be an agonist or an antagonist.
   b. The term "**opiates**" applies to drugs derived from the poppy (opium) plant.
   c. The term "**narcotics**" is commonly used to refer to opioid analgesics. In pharmacology, the term refers to drugs that induce sleep, but in the legal arena, it is used to indicate any drug that causes dependence.
   d. The term "**partial agonist**" is to describe the substance that activates a receptor, but only produces a partial physiological response compared to a **full agonist** (see Figure 1-5). It produces a partial response because it has high affinity for the receptor, but has lower intrinsic activity. Thus, it displays both agonistic and antagonistic effects. Such a substance shows agonistic activity when it is given alone; however, if it is given after a full agonist, it will antagonize/reduce the effect of the full agonist. Example: Butorphanol is a partial agonist for the µ-receptor (see below).
   e. The term "**agonist-antagonist**" is to describe the substance that has agonistic effect on one kind of receptors, but has antagonistic effect on another kind of receptors. Example: Nalbuphine is an agonist for the κ-receptor, and an antagonist for the µ-receptor (see below).

TABLE 4-1. Opioid Receptor-Mediated Effects

Effects	Receptor Types		
	μ	κ	δ
Analgesia			
Supraspinal	+	+	+
Spinal	+	+	+
Sedation	+	+	0
↓Respiration	+	0	0
↓GI transit	+	0	0
Diuresis	0	+	0
NT Release			
↓Acetylcholine	+	0	0
↓Dopamine	+	0	+
Hormone Release			
Prolactin	+	0	0
Growth hormone	+	0	+
↓Vasopressin	0	+	0
Euphoria	+	0	0
Dysphoria	0	+	0
Miosis (dogs)	+	+	0
Vasodilatation	+	0	0
Bradycardia	+	0	0

Activities of drugs are given at the receptors for which the drug has an effect.
+, receptor mediates the effect; 0, no effect. NT, neurotransmitter

2. **Receptors.** Opioid receptors are naturally occurring sites in the body that respond to endogenous opioid neuropeptides (i.e., enkephalins, dynorphins, endorphins). **All opioid receptors are $G_{i/o}$-coupled receptors that mediate the inhibition of neurotransmission and endocrine secretion** (see Chapter 1 for information on G proteins).
   a. **The receptors are present in numerous cells/tissues,** including the brain, spinal cord, urinary tract, GI tract, and vas deferens.
   b. **Classification.** There are at least three receptor subtypes. The following are information on the location of the receptor and effects mediated by the receptor (see also Table 4-1).
      (1) **Mu (μ) receptors** are located throughout the brain and in laminae I and II of the dorsal horn of the spinal cord.
          Activation of μ-receptors causes supraspinal and spinal analgesia, euphoria, sedation, miosis, **respiratory depression**, chemical dependence, and inhibition of ACh and dopamine release, and decreased GI motility due to inhibition of ACh release.
      (2) **Kappa (κ) receptors** are found in the cerebral cortex, spinal cord, and other brain regions, for example, hypothalamus.
          Activation of κ-receptors results in spinal and supraspinal analgesia, mild sedation, **dysphoria, inhibition of vasopressin release to induce diuresis**, and miosis.
      (3) **Delta (δ) receptors** are located in the limbic system, cerebral cortex, and spinal cord. Activation of δ-receptors results in spinal and supraspinal analgesia, inhibition of dopamine release, and cardiovascular depression.
   c. **Drug–receptor relationship.** A drug may affect several receptors in the same way (as an agonist or an antagonist), or it may be an agonist or partial agonist for one and an antagonist for another (Table 4-2).
3. **General characteristics of opioids**
   a. **Pharmacologic effects**

TABLE 4-2. Actions and Selectivities of Some Opioid Drugs at the Three Receptor Classes

Drugs	Receptor Types		
	μ	κ	δ
Tramadol	+	0	0
Methadone	+++	0	0
Morphine	+++	+	0
Etorphine	+++	+++	+++
Fentanyl	+++	0	0
Sufentanil	+++	+	+
Butorphanol	P	+++	0
Buprenorphine	P	−−	0
Nalbuphine	−−	++	0
Naloxone	−−−	−−	−
Diprenorphine	−−−	−−−	−−

Activities of drugs are given at the receptors for which the agent has affinity.
+, agonist; −, antagonist; P, partial agonist; 0, no affinity. The number of symbols is an indication of potency.

(1) Analgesic effects. Endogenous opioids (e.g., endorphins, enkephalins, dynorphins) are released by the neuroendocrine cells to activate opioid receptors. Exogenous opioids are used to activate or antagonize these receptors.
   (a) Opioid analgesia occurs at the level of the brain (supraspinal), spinal cord, and possibly the periphery.
   (b) μ-Receptor agonists produce profound analgesia.
   (c) The duration of opioid analgesia is usually shorter than the elimination $t_{1/2}$ for reasons that are not understood.
(2) Respiratory effects
   (a) μ-Receptor agonists are respiratory depressants; therefore, they cause an increase in the arterial CO_2 tension and a decrease in the arterial O_2 tension and pH. The hypercapnia results from a reduced sensitivity of neurons in the brain stem to CO_2.
   (b) In dogs, μ-receptor agonists frequently cause panting, which may be a thermoregulatory response. The opioid resets the dog's hypothalamic temperature control point; by panting, the dog is trying to cool itself to a new set point.
(3) Cardiovascular effects. Opioids generally spare the cardiovascular system.
   (a) The heart rate may decrease in dogs following administration of a μ-receptor agonist, this is mediated via vagal stimulation.
   (b) Hypotension may develop from peripheral vasodilatation, which is also mediated by μ-receptors.
(4) GI effects. Antidiarrheal effects and constipation are caused by stimulation of central (i.e., μ) and peripheral (i.e., κ and μ) receptors.
b. Therapeutic uses. Opioids are used for
   (1) Analgesia
   (2) Preanesthetic medication
   (3) Induction and maintenance of anesthesia in dogs and cats. μ-Agonists produce a dose-dependent decrease in the minimum alveolar concentration (MAC) of inhalant anesthetic necessary to produce anesthesia, but usually they will not produce anesthesia alone.

B. Opioid agonists

1. **Morphine.** It is the prototype opioid agonist to which all others are compared (Table 4-3).

TABLE 4-3. Relative Analgesic Activities and Elimination Half-Lives of Opioids

Opioids	Elimination $t_{1/2}$ in Humans (hours)	Relative Analgesic Activity (Morphine = 1)
Tramadol	6.3–8.8	<0.5
Nalbuphine	5	0.5–1.0
Morphine	3.7	1
Butorphanol	2.1–8.8	4–7
Hydromorphone	2.6	5
Oxymorphone	1.3	10
Alfentanil	1.5–2	7.5–25
Buprenorphine	37	30
Fentanyl	4	75–125
Sufentanil	2.5	375–1,250

a. **Mechanism of action.** Morphine is a μ-agonist and a less potent κ-agonist.

b. **Pharmacologic effects**

(1) In dogs, morphine induces vomiting by stimulating the chemoreceptor trigger zone. The receptors mediating opioid-induced vomiting are thought to be the dopaminergic D_2-receptors.

(2) In dogs, morphine is generally considered to inhibit GI motility, but may initially induce defecation by increasing GI muscle contractility, which is due to an increase in Ca^{2+} release from the sarcoplasmic reticulum.

(3) In dogs and primates, morphine causes miosis, which is mediated by both μ- and κ-receptors, while in other species (especially cats), morphine causes mydriasis.

c. **Therapeutic uses**

(1) Morphine is used for the treatment of acute pain in dogs, cats, and horses.

(a) In cats, low doses of morphine can be safely used for pain relief.

(b) In horses, the addition of sedatives (e.g., xylazine or diazepam) reduces aimless walking activity and results in good analgesia for standing procedures.

(2) Morphine may be used as an anesthetic premedication in dogs.

(3) The venodilation that results from morphine administration has been used in canine heart failure therapy as a means of reducing cardiac preload.

(4) Antitussive effect in dogs is quite good.

d. **Pharmacokinetics.** Morphine can be administered parenterally and epidurally. When given orally, a sustain-release product may be used.

(1) When given orally, bioavailability of morphine is reduced, probably because of a high first-pass (liver) effect.

(2) It readily crosses the placenta. Thus, it can easily narcotize newborns. The opioid antagonist naloxone can reverse the effects of morphine and other opioids in both newborns and dams.

(3) Morphine is metabolized in the liver by glucuronidation and excreted in the urine. Because cats are deficient in this metabolic pathway, the $t_{1/2}$ of most opioids including morphine in cats is probably prolonged.

(4) The elimination $t_{1/2}$ is 1 hour in dogs and 1.5 hours in horses.

e. **Adverse effects**

(1) **Hyperexcitability** may occur in cats, pigs, cattle, and horses following high doses of μ-agonist administration. Low doses, concurrent administration of a tranquilizer/sedative, or both will eliminate this side effect.

(2) **Hypotension.** IV morphine-induced vasodilatation/hypotension; part of this effect is due to histamine release. Other opioids, except meperidine, do not increase histamine release.

(3) **Cerebral hemorrhage and edema.** Opioids should be used with caution in dogs with head injuries because if respiration is depressed and arterial CO_2 values increase (which induces vasodilatation), the resultant increased cerebral blood flow may contribute to further cerebral hemorrhage and edema.

2. **Tramadol.** It is a synthetic μ-receptor opiate agonist that also inhibits reuptake of serotonin and norepinephrine. These latter effects of tramadol contribute to the drug's analgesic efficacy. It is not a controlled drug in the United States, but has potential for human abuse.
   a. **Therapeutic uses.** It may be useful as an analgesic or antitussive. It is given orally.
   b. **Pharmacokinetics**
      (1) In dogs after oral administration, bioavailability is about 65%, but there is inter-patient variability.
      (2) Tramadol is extensively metabolized in the liver; one of the metabolites O-desmethyltramadol is active, which is 6 times more potent than tramadol as an analgesic and has 20 times more potency than tramadol in binding to μ-receptors. For this reason, naloxone only partially antagonizes the analgesic effects of tramadol.
      (3) Tramadol and O-desmethyltramadol have a plasma $t_{1/2}$ of ~2 hours in dogs.
   c. **Adverse effects.** Tramadol appears to be well tolerated in dogs and cats. It could cause a variety of adverse effects similar to morphine.
3. **Methadone.** It is a synthetic opiate, which is a μ-agonist that may be used as an alternative to morphine in dogs and cats. **Methadone causes less sedation and vomiting than do morphine.**
   a. **Therapeutic uses.** It is administered IV, IM, and SC as an alternative opioid pre-anesthetic or analgesic in dogs or cats.
   b. **Pharmacokinetics.** It is widely distributed and extensively bound to albumin (60–90%). Methadone is metabolized in the liver by cytochrome P450 enzymes into inactive metabolites. The elimination $t_{1/2}$ is 2–3 hours in dogs.
   c. **Adverse effects.** These are very similar to those of morphine. Methadone tends to cause less sedation or vomiting than does morphine.
4. **Oxymorphone**
   a. **Chemistry.** Oxymorphone is a dihydroxy derivative of morphine.
   b. **Pharmacologic effects**
      (1) **Analgesic effects.** The analgesic potency of oxymorphone is ten times that of morphine.
      (2) **GI effects.** It occasionally causes vomiting.
      (3) **Cardiovascular effects.** When administered IV to dogs, the cardiac output transiently decreases, while mean arterial pressure and systemic vascular resistance increase.
   c. **Therapeutic uses**
      (1) **Analgesia.** Oxymorphone is used as an analgesic in dogs and cats. In cats, it should be used at a low dose or in combination with a tranquilizer.
      (2) **Preanesthetic medication.** In dogs, oxymorphone is used as a preanesthetic medication.
      (3) **Neuroleptanalgesia** is a state of sedation and analgesia without losing consciousness, produced by administering a tranquilizer and an opioid. Oxymorphone combined with acepromazine is one example of a neuroleptanalgesic combination that is frequently used in dogs.
      (4) **Anesthesia.** In swine, it has been used in combination with xylazine and ketamine for IV anesthesia.
   d. **Pharmacokinetics.** It is administered via IV, IM, SC, and rectal routes. The onset of analgesic efficacy occurs within 15–30 minutes, depending on the route of administration. Plasma $t_{1/2}$ is 2–3 hours in humans. The $t_{1/2}$ information is not available for animals. Metabolism and elimination of oxymorphone follow the same way as morphine.
   e. **Adverse effects** are very similar to those of morphine.
5. **Hydromorphone.** This is an injectable opioid sedative/restraining agent, analgesic and preanesthetic similar to oxymorphone. It is less expensive than oxymorphone, but has shorter duration of action.
   a. **Pharmacokinetics.** It is administered via IV, IM, SC, and rectal routes. The onset of analgesic efficacy occurs within 15–30 minutes, depending on the route of administration. Plasma $t_{1/2}$ is 2–3 hours in humans. The $t_{1/2}$ information is

not available for animals. Metabolism and elimination of hydromorphone is the same as morphine.

   b. Adverse effects. These are similar to those of morphine.

6. Fentanyl. A synthetic opioid that is a potent μ-agonist.

   a. Therapeutic uses. Fentanyl may be used in dogs and cats as part of an **anesthetic induction** regimen or a potent analgesic to control postoperative and chronic pain.

   (1) It is difficult to induce anesthesia with fentanyl alone without the addition of another drug (e.g., midazolam, thiopental, or isoflurane).

   (2) Transdermal fentanyl patches applied topically can produce analgesia of <72 hours. Therefore, these patches are used to control chronic pain. Cats and dogs achieved effective plasma concentrations (for analgesia) 7 and 24 hours after topical application, respectively.

   b. Pharmacokinetics

   (1) Fentanyl has a more rapid onset of analgesia than morphine after IV administration because it is more lipid soluble.

   (2) It has a shorter duration of action than morphine (30–60 minutes in dogs and cats).

   (3) Fentanyl is metabolized in the liver by cytochrome P450 enzymes; the metabolites are excreted into urine.

   (4) The elimination $t_{1/2}$ is ~4 hours in dogs.

   c. Adverse effects

   (1) Auditory stimuli may evoke a motor response from the animal.

   (2) Panting, defecation, and flatulence are common.

   (3) Bradycardia and hypersalivation may warrant treatment with anticholinergic drugs (e.g., glycopyrrolate).

7. Alfentanil. It is a derivative of fentanyl, and is four times less potent than fentanyl. It is a μ-receptor agonist.

   a. Therapeutic uses. It is used as an analgesic and sedative, and is used for adjunctive anesthesia, particularly in cats.

   b. Pharmacokinetics. It is given IV, IM, or SC, and is rapidly absorbed following administration. About 90% of the drug is bound to albumin. It is primarily metabolized in the liver by cytochrome P450 enzymes to inactive metabolites that are excreted in the urine along with 1% of the unchanged drug. The elimination $t_{1/2}$ in dogs is 20 minutes.

   c. Adverse effects. These are very similar to those of fentanyl.

8. Sufentanil. It is a fentanyl derivative, which is 5–10 times more potent than fentanyl in analgesic activity.

   a. Pharmacologic effects resemble those of fentanyl.

   b. Therapeutic uses. It is administered IV, IM, SC, or epidurally in a minute dosage (3 μg/kg). It may be useful for adjunctive anesthesia, epidural analgesia, or a postoperative analgesic.

   c. Pharmacokinetics

   (1) The absorption following the parenteral administration is quick (<5 minutes). Approximately 90% is bound to albumin. The elimination $t_{1/2}$ is ~2.5 hours in humans. No $t_{1/2}$ information is available for animals.

   (2) Sufentanil is metabolized primarily in the liver and small intestine via *O*-demethylation and *N*-dealkylation. The parent drug and these metabolites are excreted in the urine.

   d. Adverse effects. Dose-related CNS and respiratory depression is the principal adverse effect.

9. Carfentanil. It is ~10,000 times more potent than morphine in analgesic activity.

   a. Therapeutic uses. It is administered IM to immobilize large/wild animals.

   (1) Carfentanil is an opioid used to immobilize large exotic animals, mostly nondomestic ungulates (e.g., elk, giraffe, and zebra) and large carnivores (e.g., black bear).

   (2) It has been used with xylazine to immobilize wild horses, but its effects in domestic horses (e.g., muscle rigidity, paddling, tachycardia, and hypertension) are unacceptable.

b. Pharmacokinetics

  (1) The $t_{1/2}$ of carfentanil is quite variable (2–24 hours). Thus, short-acting opioid reversal agents (e.g., naloxone) are eliminated faster than the carfentanil and their effects will not last as long.

c. Adverse effects. Carfentanil-induced disruption of body temperature regulation (hyperthermia/hypothermia) can be fatal in the field. Respiratory and CNS depression is another concern. Therefore, the use of a reversing agent is a must to antagonize the pharmacological effects of carfentanil. Naltrexone is usually used for this purpose, since it has a longer duration of action than naloxone (see E 1 and 2 for information on opioid antagonists).

C. Opioid partial agonists

1. Butorphanol. It is a partial agonist for μ-receptors, but a full agonist for κ-receptors.

  a. Pharmacologic effects. Butorphanol-induced analgesia and respiratory depression are dose-dependent to a certain point; further increases in the dosage do not produce more analgesia. Indeed, butorphanol can antagonize the effect of a μ-agonist that was previously administered.

  b. Therapeutic uses

  (1) Opioid reversal. Butorphanol can be used to reverse the μ effects of other opioids (e.g., morphine, oxymorphone). It allows reversal of sedation and respiratory depression, while maintaining some analgesia (κ effect).

  (2) Analgesic. Butorphanol is used as an analgesic; it has an analgesic potency 4–7 times that of morphine.

  (3) Antitussive and antiemetic. In dogs, butorphanol doses lower than those necessary to produce analgesia have antitussive and antiemetic effects. It is used for the relief of chronic nonproductive cough associated with inflammatory conditions of the upper respiratory tract.

  (4) When given as a preanesthetic, the dose of the induction anesthetic can be lowered.

  c. Pharmacokinetics

  (1) Butorphanol is given IV, IM, SC, or orally. It is completely absorbed after administration. It is well distributed in the body, and 80% of circulating butorphanol is bound by plasma proteins.

  (2) It is metabolized in the liver to hydroxybutorphanol and norbutorphanol, and these metabolites are mostly excreted into the urine along with 5% of the parent drug.

  (3) The elimination $t_{1/2}$: <1 hour in horses and <2 hours in dogs.

  (4) Following IV doses in horses, the onset of action is ~3 minutes with a peak analgesic effect at 15–30 minutes. The duration of action in horses is <4 hours after a single dose.

  d. Adverse effects

  (1) In dogs and cats, the effects include sedation, ataxia, anorexia, or diarrhea.

  (2) In horses, those include ataxia, sedation, but excitement has been noted as well. Butorphanol could decrease gut motility and induce ileus. Very high doses IV (1–2 mg/kg) can lead to the development of nystagmus, salivation, seizures, hyperthermia, and decreased GI motility. These effects are considered transitory in nature.

D. Opioid agonist-antagonist drugs

1. General information

  a. Classification. Opioid agonist-antagonists bind to several receptors (usually μ and κ) and affect each receptor in a different manner. They are subdivided into two types given as follows:

  (1) One type (e.g., nalbuphine) antagonizes μ-receptors but activates κ-receptors.

  (2) The other type (e.g., buprenorphine) is a partial agonist for μ-receptors, and an antagonist for κ-receptors.

b. Therapeutic uses

   (1) Analgesia. Agonist-antagonist drugs are used to produce analgesia through activation of the μ- or κ-receptors.

   (2) Reversal of respiratory and CNS depression. Agonist-antagonist drugs can also be used to reverse the respiratory and CNS depression of a pure μ-receptor agonist. These agents have the advantage of eliminating most of the respiratory depression without totally eliminating the analgesia.

c. Disadvantages. Agonist-antagonist opioids are **more difficult to reverse** than agonists when overdosed because of their high receptor affinity.

2. Buprenorphine. It has 30 times the analgesic potency that of morphine.

a. Mechanism of action. Buprenorphine has a strong affinity for μ-receptors, 50 times that of morphine. **It is a partial agonist at the μ-receptor and an antagonist at the κ-receptor.**

   It is resistant to antagonism by naloxone because of its strong affinity for μ-receptors.

b. Therapeutic uses. It is used as an analgesic in small animals.

c. Pharmacokinetics

   (1) It is administered IV, IM, or SC.

   (2) It is highly bound (96%) to plasma proteins (α- and β-globulins), crossing the placenta.

   (3) It has a longer duration of action than other opioids (up to 8 hours), since it has high affinity for μ-receptors. The elimination $t_{1/2}$ of 37 hours in humans is the longest among opioid analogs (Table 4-3), which is due to the binding to globulins. No $t_{1/2}$ information is available for animals.

   (4) It is metabolized in the liver by N-dealkylation and glucuronidation. These metabolites are then eliminated by biliary excretion into the feces (~70%) and urinary excretion (~27%).

d. Adverse effects. The major side effects are respiratory depression and sedation.

3. Nalbuphine is an agonist-antagonist with potency equal to that of morphine. It is an antagonist at the μ-receptor and an agonist at the κ-receptor.

a. Therapeutic uses

   (1) It is used to control mild to moderate pain only. The analgesia lasts about 45 minutes in dogs and 2–3 hours in cats.

   (2) It is used topically to control pain associated with corneal ulcer. For this purpose, 1% solution is applied topically four to six times a day.

b. Pharmacokinetics. It is administered IM. It does not bind to plasma proteins. It undergoes glucuronidation in the liver and the metabolite is excreted in the urine. The elimination $t_{1/2}$ in humans is 5 hours. No $t_{1/2}$ information is available for animals.

c. Adverse effects. These are very similar to those of morphine.

E. Opioid antagonists bind to μ-, κ-, and δ- receptors, but do not activate them. They are pure antagonists with no agonist activity.

1. Naloxone

a. Mechanism of action. Naloxone has a high affinity for μ-receptors and lower affinity for κ- and δ-receptors, which allow it to displace opioid agonists from these receptors.

b. Therapeutic uses

   (1) Reversal of respiratory depression

      (a) Naloxone is used postoperatively to reverse the respiratory depression caused by μ-receptor opioids. However, the analgesic effects will also disappear. The resultant pain may initiate undesirable behavioral and physiologic responses (e.g., excitement, tachycardia, and hypertension) that are difficult to reverse because of the strong affinity the antagonists have for the receptors.

      (b) Naloxone is used to reverse opioid-induced respiratory depression in neonates following cesarean delivery.

        (c) Since nalbuphine and butorphanol have good μ-receptor antagonistic activity, and they are more persistent than naloxone, these two drugs are probably more useful than naloxone in reversing opioid-induced respiratory depression.

    (2) Treatment of shock. High doses have been beneficial in the treatment of septic, hypovolemic, and cardiogenic shock.

  c. Pharmacokinetics

    (1) When given IV, it has a rapid onset of action of 1–2 minutes. When given IM, it has an onset of action of <5 minutes. It usually persists 45–90 minutes, but may act for up to 3 hours.

    (2) It is distributed rapidly throughout the body with high levels found in the brain, kidneys, spleen, skeletal muscle, lung, and heart. The drug also readily crosses the placenta.

    (3) It is metabolized in the liver by cytochrome P450 enzymes and excreted into the urine after the metabolite is conjugated to glucuronide. The elimination $t_{1/2}$ in humans is ~1 hour. No $t_{1/2}$ information is available for animals.

  d. Adverse effects. Naloxone itself has no adverse effects. Since naloxone's duration of action may be shorter than that of the opioid being reversed, the signs of respiratory depression should be closely monitored, as additional doses of naloxone and/or ventilatory support may be needed.

2. Naltrexone. It is a long-lasting opioid receptor antagonist, which can be used to reverse opioid-induced respiratory depression and can be used to antagonize the immobilizing effect of a potent opioid (e.g., carfentanil).

  a. Mechanism of action. Naltrexone is a long-acting μ-, κ-, and δ-receptor antagonist.

  b. Therapeutic uses

    (1) It is administered IV or IM for reversing opioid-induced immobilization/depression particularly in wildlife and large animals.

    (2) It is given orally to treat behavioral problems in dogs (e.g., constant licking, tail chasing). The mechanisms for such use are not known.

  c. Pharmacokinetics

    (1) Naltrexone circulates throughout the body. Only 20–30% is bound to plasma protein.

    (2) It is metabolized in the liver, and the primary metabolite (6-β-naltrexol) has opioid-receptor blocking activity. Naltrexone and its metabolites are excreted into the urine.

    (3) In humans, the plasma $t_{1/2}$ of naltrexone is ~4 hours and ~13 hours for 6-β-naltrexol. No $t_{1/2}$ information is available for animals.

  d. Adverse effects. Naltrexone is relatively free of adverse effects in animals.

SUGGESTED READING

Boothe DM. 2001. "Anticonvulsant drugs and analeptic agents." In *Veterinary Pharmacology and Therapeutics.* Edited by Adams HR. 8th ed., pp. 360–382. Ames, IA: Iowa State University Press.

Dewey CW. 2006. Anticonvulsant therapy in dogs and cats. *Vet Clin North Am Small Anim Pract* 36:1107–1127.

Gross ME. 2001. "Tranquilizers, α_2-adrenergic agonists, and related agents." In *Veterinary Pharmacology and Therapeutics.* Edited by Adams HR. 8th ed., pp. 534–552. Ames, IA: Iowa State University Press.

Gustein HB, Akil H. 2006. "Opioid analgesics." In *Goodman & Gilman's The Pharmacological Basis of Therapeutics.* Edited by Brunton LL, Lazo JS, Parker KL. 11th ed., pp. 547–590. New York: McGraw-Hill.

Hsu WH. 1981. Xylazine-induced depression and its antagonism by alpha-adrenergic blocking agents. *J Pharmacol Exp Ther* 218:188–192.

Hsu WH, Schaffer DD, Hansen CE. 1987. Effects of tolazoline and yohimbine on central nervous depression, bradycardia, and tachypnea in sheep. *J Am Vet Med Assoc* 190:323–326.

http://www.drugs.com

Plumb DC. 2005. *Veterinary Drug Handbook.* 5th ed. Ames, IA: Blackwell Publishing.

STUDY QUESTIONS

DIRECTIONS: Each of the numbered items or incomplete statements in this section is followed by answers or by completions of the statement. Select the **one** lettered answer or completion that is **best** in each case.

1. Which one of the following drugs will reverse the respiratory depression caused by previous oxymorphone administration, but still leave the dog with some analgesia?

(A) Tramadol
(B) Fentanyl
(C) Naloxone
(D) Morphine
(E) Nalbuphine

2. Which one of the following statements concerning buprenorphine is true?

(A) It is a partial agonist opioid with partial agonist activity at the μ-receptor and agonist activity at the κ-receptor.
(B) It is an agonist–antagonist opioid with partial agonist activity at the μ-receptor.
(C) It is a very potent μ-agonist used to immobilize nondomestic ungulates.
(D) It is an antagonist at μ-, κ-, and δ-receptors.
(E) It is an α$_2$-adrenoreceptor agonist in the central and peripheral nervous system.

3. Which of the following is a correct statement about phenothiazine tranquilizers?

(A) They also have potent analgesic activity.
(B) They stimulate α$_1$-adrenergic receptors to induce hypertension.
(C) They evoke hypoglycemia by increasing insulin secretion.
(D) Most of them are desirable restraining agents for aggressive dogs.
(E) They suppress emesis by blocking dopamine receptors in the chemoreceptor-trigger zone.

4. Which one of the following drugs is an antagonist at the μ-, κ-, and δ-receptors?

(A) Naloxone
(B) Morphine
(C) Oxymorphone

(D) Sufentanil
(E) Butorphanol

5. Compared to morphine, which one of the following drugs is most potent in terms of analgesic effect?

(A) Oxymorphone
(B) Tramadol
(C) Butorphanol
(D) Fentanyl
(E) Methadone

6. A common side effect of oxymorphone administration in the dog is

(A) panting.
(B) vomiting.
(C) defecation.
(D) hypotension.
(E) tachycardia.

7. Which one of the following opioid receptors is correctly matched with its function?

(A) μ-Supraspinal analgesia
(B) μ-Vasoconstriction
(C) δ-Respiratory depression
(D) κ-Antidiuresis
(E) κ-Respiratory depression

8. Phenobarbital can be used as an oral anticonvulsant. What other anticonvulsant drug is metabolized in the liver and produces phenobarbital as a metabolite?

(A) Primidone
(B) Phenytoin
(C) Diazepam
(D) Pentobarbital
(E) Potassium bromide.

9. A horse to be tranquilized is given an IV injection of xylazine. The horse immediately falls to the ground and goes into violent seizures. What is the probable cause?

(A) The horse was prone to seizures, and xylazine lowered the threshold enough for a seizure to occur.
(B) The injection was given into the carotid artery instead of the jugular vein.
(C) Extreme hypotension from epinephrine reversal led to cerebral hypoxia and seizures.
(D) α_2-Adrenoreceptor stimulation decreased activity at the GABA-receptors.
(E) Increased insulin release by the pancreas secondary to α_2-receptor stimulation caused acute hypoglycemia.

10. Which one of the following drugs will reverse the effects of diazepam in case there is an overdose?

(A) Butorphanol
(B) Naloxone
(C) Flumazenil
(D) Yohimbine
(E) Zolazepam

11. Which of the following statements concerning α_2-adrenergic agonists is *incorrect?*

(A) Ruminants are more sensitive to the sedative properties of these drugs than nonruminants.
(B) IM administration of these drugs induces vomiting more frequently than does IV administration.
(C) They induce antidiuresis.
(D) Concurrent administration of ketamine may synergistically suppress cardiopulmonary function.

12. The drug of choice to treat status epilepticus in dogs is

(A) diazepam.
(B) acepromazine.

(C) phenobarbital.
(D) primidone.
(E) potassium bromide.

13. IV administration of xylazine in the horse frequently results in which of the following cardiac abnormalities?

(A) Atrial fibrillation
(B) Sinus tachycardia
(C) Premature atrial contractions
(D) Second-degree atrioventricular block
(E) Premature ventricular contractions

14. Which anticonvulsant is excreted unchanged by the kidneys and acts by hyperpolarizing the neuronal membrane after entering the cell through chloride channels?

(A) Valproic acid
(B) Phenobarbital
(C) Diazepam
(D) Gabapentin
(E) Potassium bromide

15. IV administration of an α_2-agonist produces all of the following pharmacological effects, except

(A) bradycardia.
(B) increased GI motility.
(C) transient hypertension.
(D) diuresis.

16. The α_2-agonist with the most selectivity and potency for α_2-receptors is

(A) medetomidine
(B) detomidine
(C) romifidine
(D) xylazine

ANSWERS AND EXPLANATIONS

1. The answer is E.
The agonist-antagonist opioid nalbuphine will reverse the effects of oxymorphone at the μ-receptor while still providing analgesia via stimulation of the κ-receptor. Fentanyl, morphine, and carfentanil are μ-agonists, like oxymorphone. Naloxone is an antagonist at all opioid receptors and would reverse the analgesia as well as the respiratory depression.

2. The answer is B.
Buprenorphine is an agonist-antagonist opioid with partial agonist activity at the μ-receptor. Butorphanol is a partial agonist for the μ-receptor and a full agonist for the κ-receptor. Carfentanil is the very potent μ-agonist used to immobilize nondomestic ungulates. Naloxone and naltrexone are antagonists at μ-, κ-, and δ-receptors. Xylazine, detomidine, and medetomidine are α_2-adrenoreceptor agonists in the central and peripheral nervous systems.

3. The answer is E.
The antiemetic effect of phenothiazine tranquilizers is due to blockade of dopamine receptors in the chemoreceptor-trigger zone. They do not have noticeable analgesic effect. They also block α_1-adrenergic receptors to induce hypotension. They evoke hyperglycemia by promoting epinephrine release from the adrenal medulla, which increases glycogenolysis by activating hepatic β_2-receptors. Caution must be exercised when using them as restraining agents in aggressive dogs, since the aggressive dogs can bite under phenothiazine-induced tranquilization.

4. The answer is A.
Naloxone and naltrexone are pure antagonists at all three opioid receptors (μ, κ, and δ). Morphine and oxymorphone are agonists at μ- and κ-receptors. Butorphanol is a partial agonist at the μ-receptor, but a full agonist at the κ-receptor. Sufentanil is an agonist at all three opioid receptors.

5. The answer is D.
Fentanyl is 75–125 times more potent than morphine. Tramadol, which is less than 0.5 times as potent as morphine, is the least potent opioid analgesic. Methadone is slightly less potent than morphine. Butorphanol is 4–7 times as potent as morphine, and oxymorphone is 10 times as potent as morphine.

6. The answer is A.
Administration of oxymorphone to dogs commonly causes panting and bradycardia. Occasionally, dogs will vomit. Fentanyl commonly causes defecation, panting, and flatulence. Morphine may cause hypotension because of associated histamine release and vasodilatation.

7. The answer is A.
μ-Receptor stimulation causes supraspinal and spinal analgesia, euphoria, respiratory depression, decreased GI motility, miosis, and sedation. κ-Receptor stimulation causes supraspinal and spinal analgesia, mild sedation, dysphoria, diuresis, and miosis. δ-Receptor stimulation causes supraspinal and spinal analgesia.

8. The answer is A.
Primidone is a deoxybarbiturate that is metabolized by the liver to produce phenylethylmalonamide (PEMA) and phenobarbital. Primidone and its two active metabolites have anticonvulsant activity. Phenytoin, diazepam, pentobarbital, and potassium bromide are all anticonvulsants, but none of them is metabolized by the liver to form phenobarbital.

9. The answer is B.
Accidental intracarotid injection of xylazine is very uncommon, but it can occur in horses because of the anatomical proximity of the carotid artery and the jugular vein. The high concentration of xylazine delivered by the carotid artery to the brain results in convulsions and immediate collapse of the horse. Most horses survive with supportive therapy. Acepromazine gives a similar initial response when injected in the carotid artery, but many horses do not survive. Xylazine given by the intravenous route is not normally associated with seizure activity and has no direct effect on GABA-receptors. Blood pressure is not decreased initially. Xylazine inhibits insulin release in horses, leading to hyperglycemia, not hypoglycemia.

10. The answer is C.

Flumazenil, a specific benzodiazepine-receptor-blocking drug, will reverse the effects of diazepam. It has high affinity for the drug receptor, great specificity, and very little intrinsic activity. Flumazenil is a competitive antagonist. Naloxone is an opioid antagonist. Yohimbine is an α_2-receptor antagonist. Butorphanol is partial agonist opioid. Zolazepam is a benzodiazepine-receptor agonist (like diazepam).

11. The answer is C.

α_2-Adrenergic agonists can induce diuresis by inhibiting AVP (ADH) secretion. Ruminants are most sensitive to α_2-adrenergic agonist-induced sedation. Intramuscular administration of these drugs induces vomiting more frequently than the IV route. Concurrent administration of ketamine and an α_2-adrenergic agonist may synergistically suppress cardiopulmonary function.

12. The answer is A.

Diazepam, administered IV, is the drug of choice to treat status epilepticus in dogs. Acepromazine is a phenothiazine tranquilizer, not an anticonvulsant, and may actually lower the seizure threshold. Phenobarbital is too slow in its onset of action to be valuable in treating status epilepticus. Even with IV administration, it may take 20 minutes before phenobarbital exerts a significant anticonvulsant effect. Primidone and potassium bromide are oral anticonvulsants with slow onset of action. Primidone needs to be metabolized by the liver to produce phenobarbital before it is effective.

13. The answer is D.

IV administration of xylazine induces second-degree A-V block, which is due to the increase in blood pressure (vasoconstriction), leading to an increase in baroreceptor reflex to stimulate the vagus nerve that innervates the A-V node. The second-degree A-V block usually lasts 5-10 minutes after IV administration of xylazine. Xylazine administration can induce sinus arrhythmia (or sinus arrest in severe cases), which is due to the decrease in the sympathetic tone. Xylazine does not induce sinus tachycardia, premature atrial contractions, or premature ventricular contractions.

14. The answer is E.

Potassium bromide is not bound to plasma proteins and is not metabolized, but is excreted unchanged by the kidneys. Bromide and chloride both can enter neurons through existing chloride channels, for example, those associated with GABA receptors. Because both ions have a negative charge, their movement into the cell makes the membrane potential more negative (hyperpolarization). Apparently, when bromide enters the cell, it causes longer-lasting hyperpolarization than chloride. Thus, the neuron is less likely to fire on its own or when stimulated, thereby preventing seizures.

15. The answer is B.

Activation of α_2-adrenergic receptors decreases GI motility by inhibiting parasympathetic tone. Bradycardia, transient hyerptension, and diuresis are pharmacologic effects of α_2-agonists.

16. The answer is A.

Medetomidine is the selective α_2-adrenergic agonist used in veterinary medicine. Xylazine, detomidine, and romifidine have more α_1-adrenergic agonistic activity than medetomidine.

Chapter 5

Behavior-Modifying Drugs
Arthi Kanthasamy and Walter H. Hsu

I. GENERAL CONSIDERATIONS

A. Biochemical imbalance in the monoaminergic (5-HT and NE) and GABAergic neurotransmitter system have been implicated in behavioral problems seen in companion animals.

B. Behavioral problems most commonly encountered in animals include fear, anxiety, aggression, compulsive disorder, inappropriate elimination behavior, and cognitive dysfunction in geriatric patients.

C. Oral route of drug administration is routinely used in treating behavioral disorders.

D. There is potential for adverse effects following long-term use of behavior-modifying drugs. Before starting a rational drug therapy the animals must undergo complete laboratory analysis, thorough evaluation of background medical histories, and neurological examination to determine the physiological basis of the abnormal behavior.

E. Psychotherapeutic treatment outcomes are most effective when used in combination with behavioral modification therapy and environmental management.

F. **Phenothiazines should not be used to treat aggressive behavior because in some cases they may cause or induce aggressive behavior in animals that have no history of aggressive behavior.**

In the present chapter, focus will be on anxiolytic drugs, drugs that modulate monoaminergic and GABAergic neurotransmission, and progestins.

G. **Neurotransmitters involved in the actions of antidepressant drugs**

1. **Monoamine hypothesis of mood**
   a. According to this theory, monoamines including serotonin (5-HT) and norepinephrine (NE) are proposed to play a central role in the expression of mood. Therefore, any impairment in the activity of the amines is believed to lead to depression, while increase in activity may result in mood elevation. Accordingly, agents that enhance the actions of these neurotransmitters have proven efficacy in the management of symptoms related to depression.
   b. **Monoamines.** Monoamines include dopamine, NE, epinephrine, and 5-HT. See Chapters 2 and 3 for information on synthesis and metabolism of monoamines.
      (1) **Dopamine (DA)**
         (a) DA is the major neurotransmitter in the brain. It plays a key role in behavioral and drug reinforcement; regulates emesis, prolactin release, mood states, cognitive, and motor functions.
         (b) DA is found in several neuronal tracts including nigrostriatal, mesolimbic, and tuberoinfundibular tracts.
         (c) DA exerts inhibitory actions via G-protein-coupled receptors that facilitate the activation of K^+ channels. There are at least five DA receptor subtypes, namely, D_1, D_2, D_3, D_4, and D_5. Activation of D_1 and D_5 receptors (coupled to G_s) increases cAMP levels by stimulating adenylyl cyclase, while activation of D_2, D_3, and D_4 receptors (coupled to $G_{i/o}$) decreases cAMP levels by inhibiting adenylyl cyclase. Notably, D_2 receptors are primarily presynaptic and function as autoinhibitory receptors by inhibiting DA release.

(d) A partial list of drugs that affect dopaminergic neurotransmission include CNS stimulants (e.g., amphetamines), and monoamine oxidase-B (MAO-B) inhibitors (e.g., selegiline).

(2) Norepinephrine (NE)

(a) NE plays a key role in learning, memory, mood, sensory processing, sleep, and in the regulation of anxiety.

(b) The cell bodies of the noradrenergic neurons are located in the locus coeruleus or the lateral tegmental area of the reticular formation. Several brain regions, namely, thalamus, cerebral cortex, cerebellum, and thalamus receive diffuse noradrenergic input. For example, nor-adrenergic projections to the limbic cortex are believed to regulate emotions.

(c) The excitatory effects are mediated via activation of α_1- and β-receptors, which results in a decrease in K^+ conductance. Conversely, the inhibitory effects are mediated via activation of α_2-receptors that leads to neuronal hyperpolarization via increase in K^+ conductance. Furthermore, activation of presynaptic α_2-receptors is associated with decrease in calcium conductance, hence resulting in decreased presynaptic release of NE.

(d) Drugs that enhance noradrenergic neurotransmission include CNS stimulants, tricyclic antidepressants (TCAs), and monoamine oxidase inhibitors (MAOIs).

(3) Serotonin (5-HT)

(a) 5-HT has been proposed to play a central role in the regulation of sleep, body temperature, arousal, emotion, and higher cognitive functions. Dysfunction in the central serotonergic system is postulated to underlie mood disturbances, anxiety, aggression, restlessness, and obsessive compulsive disorder (OCD).

(b) The cell bodies of the serotonergic neurons are located in the raphe nuclei of the brain stem. They send diffuse projections to the entire CNS, including the spinal cord, cerebellum, and areas of diencephalon and telencephalon. Multiple subtypes of 5-HT receptors have been identified and to date the receptors have been categorized under seven different families including, $5-HT_1$, $5-HT_2$, $5-HT_3$, $5-HT_4$, $5-HT_5$, $5-HT_6$, and $5-HT_7$. All of them are G-protein-coupled receptors with the exception of $5-HT_3$ receptor family, which is a ligand-gated ion channel (Chapter 3 II B3).

(c) 5-HT primarily has an inhibitory role; however, depending on the receptor subtype, it can exhibit both inhibitory and excitatory effects. For example, buspirone's partial agonist effects on $5-HT_{1A}$ receptors (coupled to $G_{i/o}$) are related to elevation in K^+ conductance and associated membrane hyperpolarization.

(d) 5-HT enhancing drugs are effective modulators of behavior. For example, TCAs and selective serotonin reuptake inhibitors (SSRIs) enhance 5-HT neurotransmission by elevating synaptic levels of 5-HT.

c. Acetylcholine. (ACh, see Chapter 2 for information on synthesis and metabolism)

(1) ACh is proposed to play a key role in arousal, consciousness, memory consolidation, and motor coordination.

(2) ACh is present in the neurons of somatic and visceral motor nuclei present in the brain and spinal chord that innervates the hippocampus, cerebral cortex, and basal ganglia.

(3) Most CNS responses to ACh are mediated through G-protein-coupled muscarinic receptors. At a few sites, ACh elicits its response via activation of $G_{i/o}$-coupled M_2 receptors that leads to slowing of neuronal discharge by increasing K^+ conductance. In addition, activation of M_2 receptors inhibits adenylyl cyclase, which leads to inhibition of neurotransmitter release.

(4) A few of the undesirable side effects associated with TCAs such as dry mouth, urine retention, and decreased GI motility have been linked to their muscarinic blocking effects.

I MAJOR DRUG CLASSES

A. Anxiolytic drugs

1. **Benzodiazepines.** diazepam(Valium®), clorazepate(Tranxene®), Alprazolam (Xanax®), oxazepam (Serax®), lorazepam (Ativan®), chlordiazepoxide (Librium®)
2. **Buspirone** (Buspar®)

B. Antidepressants

1. **Tricyclic Antidepressants (TCAs).** amitriptyline (Elavil®), clomipramine (Clomicalm®), imipramine (Tofranil®), doxepin (Sinequan®)
2. **Serotonin Selective Reuptake Inhibitors (SSRIs).** fluoxetine (Prozac®), Paroxetine (Paxil®), sertraline (Zoloft®), fluvoxamine (Luvox®)
3. **Monoamine Oxidase Inhibitors (MAOIs).** selegiline (Anipryl®)
4. **Progestins.** medroxyprogesterone acetate (Depo-Provera®), megestrol acetate (Ovaban®)

II ANXIOLYTIC DRUGS

A. Benzodiazepines (BZDs) (See Chapter 4; Section II C and D for more information on BZDs.)

1. **General considerations**
   a. **Mechanism of action.** The behavioral effects are attributed to BZD's actions on the cerebral cortex, limbic system, and most notably thalamus. BZDs induce membrane hyperpolarization by facilitating GABA-mediated chloride conductance (see also Chapter 4).
   b. **Pharmacological Effects.** BZDs exhibit dose-dependent, but minimal CNS depressant effects. For example, at lower doses, they exhibit mild sedative and anxiolytic effects, whereas at higher doses, they have hypnotic effects.
   c. **Therapeutic uses**
      (1) BZDs are useful in the management of fear, phobia, and anxiety particularly in situations where rapid onset may be desirable.
      (2) BZDs are useful particularly for the management of fears induced by stimuli that can be predicted in advance. Examples include clinical management of inappropriate urination-submissive urination, urine marking behavior, storm phobia, separation anxiety in dogs; foal rejection in mares; and urine spraying, storm phobia, separation anxiety, and extreme timidity in cats.
      (3) Several of the long term effects are attributed to intermediate metabolite functions.
      (4) BZDs can be used in combination with other psychotropic drugs such as TCAs or SSRIs.
   d. **Pharmacokinetics**
      (1) BZDs include a wide array of drugs that differ in their pharmacokinetic properties.
      (2) BZDs are rapidly absorbed from the GI tract and distributed throughout the body.
      (3) BZDs bind avidly to plasma proteins, exhibit high lipophilicity, and readily cross the blood–brain barrier.
      (4) BZDs are metabolized primarily via the hepatic microsomal system and eliminated in the urine as glucuronide conjugates or oxidized metabolites. However, cats have been reported to exhibit compromised drug metabolism.

    e. Adverse effects
- **(1)** Withdrawal of BZDs should be gradual because sudden cessation of drug treatment may result in relapse of symptoms that may be more intense than that existed before drug treatment.
- **(2)** BZDs have the potential to cause physical addiction.
- **(3)** Adverse effects include ataxia, sedation, muscle relaxation, anxiety, paradoxical excitement, hallucinations, and memory deficits.
- **(4)** Owing to its ability to cross placental barrier and entry into milk, it must be used cautiously in pregnant and lactating animals.

    f. Contraindications. The use of BZDs is contraindicated in cases involving aggression. Although BZDs reduce aggression, sometimes it may disinhibit behaviors, hence resulting in increased aggressiveness.

2. Diazepam
    a. Mechanism of action. Diazepam has CNS depressant effects but lacks peripheral autonomic blocking effects.
    b. Therapeutic uses. Diazepam is a well-characterized BZD that is used for the treatment of behavioral disorders.
- **(1)** Diazepam reduces signs of fear in dogs. However, it is less effective in treating storm phobia and separation anxiety as compared to alprazolam.
- **(2)** In cats, although initially beneficial in ameliorating urine spraying behavior, resumption of urine spraying behavior (50–75%) was observed when drug treatment was discontinued.

    c. Pharmacokinetics
- **(1)** It undergoes extensive first-pass metabolism and is metabolized to desmethyldiazepam (nordiazepam), temazepam, and oxazepam. In all species, the $t_{1/2}$ of the metabolites are longer than those of the parent compound.
- **(2)** Collectively, because of the large interspecies difference, the pharmacokinetic parameters cannot be extrapolated from other species
- **(3)** Alprazolam may be used as a suitable alternative to minimize hepatic toxicosis associated with diazepam.
- **(4)** The plasma protein-binding capacity of diazepam is ~98%.
- **(5)** In cats, the $t_{1/2}$ of diazepam is ~6 hours, whereas the $t_{1/2}$ of desmethyldiazepam is ~21 hours. In dogs, diazepam is rapidly metabolized, $t_{1/2}$ is ~3 hours, while the $t_{1/2}$ of desmethyldiazepam averaged 7 hours.

    d. Adverse effects
- **(1)** In cats, behavioral changes may manifest as irritability, depression, and altered demeanor.
- **(2)** **Hepatic necrosis** is the most serious adverse event reported in cats. It is postulated that a toxic intermediate metabolite may be responsible for the hepatic toxicosis.
- **(3)** Concurrent administration with other drugs that compete for cytochrome P450 (CYP450) enzyme system, including the SSRIs, may decrease the rate of metabolism of diazepam.

3. Clorazepate
    a. Therapeutic uses. In dogs, it is used in the management of anxiety, especially when long duration of action is desired, for example, separation anxiety.
    b. Pharmacokinetics
- **(1)** Clorazepate is one of the most rapidly absorbed BZDs.
- **(2)** Clorazepate is primarily oxidized in the acidic environment of the stomach to its active metabolite desmethyldiazepam (nordiazepam) before absorption.
- **(3)** Following oral administration, mean peak levels are reached usually within 98 minutes after a single oral dose and 153 minutes after multiple oral doses, suggesting improved management when the drug is given twice daily instead of a single dose.
- **(4)** The plasma protein binding capacity of nordiazepam is high (~97%).
- **(5)** The $t_{1/2}$ is 284–355 minutes and it is the same irrespective of the frequency of dosing.

    c. Adverse effects. Diazepam can cross the placental barrier and enter into the milk. There is an increased risk of teratogenicity when administered during the first trimester of pregnancy. Therefore, it should not be used in pregnant and nursing females.

4. **Alprazolam**
   a. **Therapeutic uses**
      (1) Its rapid response makes it a good choice in treating panic disorders in dogs where a rapid resolution is essential. For example, it is effective when the drug is administered 30–60 minutes before the storm.
      (2) Higher doses of the drug are required to treat panic-like states such as separation anxiety and thunderstorm phobia as compared with generalized anxiety.
      (3) In cats, it is used in the treatment of anxiety disorders and inappropriate urination behaviors.
      (4) The combination of alprazolam and clomipramine has been proven to be beneficial in the management of storm phobia in dogs.
   b. **Pharmacokinetics**
      (1) The two common metabolites produced by CYP450 include α-hydroxy-alprazolam and benzophenone, although the latter is an inactive metabolite.
      (2) Interindividual variability in plasma steady state concentration is seen in humans.
      (3) Alprazolam is moderately plasma protein bound (80%).
      (4) In humans, it has a rapid onset of action and the $t_{1/2}$ is 6–27 hours. No information is available for animals.
   c. **Adverse effects.** Dogs receiving alprazolam at a moderately high dose to treat anxiety-related disorders are at risk for developing physical dependence, withdrawal anxiety tremors, or seizures. Hence, the drug should be withdrawn gradually over a period of several weeks.
   d. **Contraindications.** Alprazolam should not be given in conjunction with drugs that impair CYP 450 3A, including ketoconazole and itraconazole.

5. **Oxazepam**
   a. **Therapeutic uses**
      (1) Oxazepam provides longer duration of action as compared to diazepam and it has been effectively used as an appetite stimulant in cats.
      (2) In humans, it is particularly useful in treating elderly patients with compromised hepatic function because it does not produce long-acting active metabolites.
      (3) As with other benzodiazepines, oxazepam may be useful in the management of fears and phobias in cats or dogs
   b. **Pharmacokinetics**
      (1) Oxazepam does not generate active metabolites. However, in humans and pigs, the primary metabolite is the inactive glucuronide conjugate of oxazepam, which accounts for 95% of the metabolites that are eliminated in the urine.
      (2) Oxazepam has pronounced plasma protein binding (97%).
      (3) In humans, the $t_{1/2}$ is ~8 hours and peak plasma levels occur at ~3 hours. No information is available for animals.
   c. **Adverse effects.** On rare occasions, leucopenia and hepatic dysfunction have been reported in humans.

6. **Lorazepam**
   a. **Therapeutic uses**
      (1) It can be orally administered as a suitable alternative to diazepam.
      (2) It is also useful in cats because the chances of developing idiopathic hepatic necrosis are minimal.
      (3) It is used as an appetite stimulant and in the treatment of compulsive disorders.
      (4) It may be safely used in individuals with compromised liver function and in geriatric dogs, because it does not produce active metabolites.
   b. **Pharmacokinetics**
      (1) After oral administration, it is rapidly absorbed in dogs, although to a lesser degree in cats.

      (2) It is primarily metabolized via glucuronide conjugation The formation of the conjugate is much faster in dogs as compared to cats.

      (3) It is excreted primarily in the urine and to a lesser extent in the feces in dogs and pigs. In cats, the drug is excreted in equal parts in both feces and urine.

      (4) Plasma protein-binding capacity of lorazepam is $\sim$85%.

      (5) In humans, the time to peak plasma concentrations is $\sim$2 hours. The mean $t_{1/2}$ is $\sim$12 hours, whereas $t_{1/2}$ of lorazepam glucuronide is $\sim$18 hours. No information is available for animals.

   c. Adverse effects. Increased appetite, paradoxical excitation, and anxiety have been reported to occur early in therapy, although they resolve with continued use or by decreasing the dose.

  7. Chlordiazepoxide

   a. Mechanism of action. It acts on the limbic system of the brain, thereby modulating emotional responses.

   b. Therapeutic uses

      (1) It has appetite stimulant, anti-anxiety, and sedative properties.

      (2) Chlordiazepoxide is beneficial in the treatment of aggression and intense fear in a number of zoo animals.

   c. Pharmacological effects. Chlordiazepoxide lacks autonomic blocking effects at moderate doses, hence it exerts minimal effects on the blood pressure or heart rate.

   d. Pharmacokinetics

      (1) Metabolites generated via liver metabolism include desmethyldiazepam, demoxepam, desmethylchlordiazepoxide, and oxazepam. These metabolites are active and have long $t_{1/2}$.

      (2) In dogs, plasma levels peak in 7–8 hours.

      (3) Chlordiazepoxide is excreted in the urine, only 1–2% is excreted in the unchanged form.

      (4) Plasma protein-binding capacity of chlordiazepoxide is $\sim$95%.

      (5) In dogs, one of the metabolites demoxepam has a $t_{1/2}$ of 10–20 hours with considerable interindividual variability. In cats, plasma levels peak in $\sim$90 minutes when given at a dose of 1.25 mg/kg intraperitoneally (IP).

   e. Adverse effects

      (1) Side effects include sedation, ataxia, and rage.

      (2) Because chlordiazepoxide may induce leucopenia and liver dysfunction, blood cell counts and chemistry must be monitored on a regular basis, especially when the drug is administered for an extended period.

B. **Buspirone.** Buspirone is the first nonsedating anxiolytic drug to be developed and marketed.

  1. Mechanism of action. Buspirone may elicit its anxiolytic effects partly via its **partial agonistic effects on 5-HT$_{1A}$ receptors** located in the dorsal raphe nucleus of the brain. Additionally, it has been reported to exhibit moderate affinity to dopamine receptors.

  2. Pharmacological effects

   a. The CNS depressant effects are minimal.

   b. Buspirone is nonsedating and it does not produce psychomotor disturbance, or disinhibition phenomenon.

   c. Therapeutic efficacy is achieved only when the drug is administered for several weeks.

  3. Therapeutic uses

   a. In dogs, it can be used for the management of generalized anxiety although, less successful in treating storm phobia or separation anxiety.

   b. In cats, the buspirone can be used for modulating urine spraying behavior and inappropriate urination.

   c. It is used to reduce anxiety in cases involving inter-cat aggression within the same household.

d. It is used as an adjunct to improve the effectiveness of SSRIs in the management of OCD, although with limited success.

e. In dogs, the buspirone and fluoxetine combination therapy has been successfully used to treat complex behavioral problems involving anxiety, aggression, and stereotypic behaviors.

4. Pharmacokinetics. It is primarily metabolized by CYP450 enzymes to one active metabolite, 1-pyrimidinylpiperazine, and several other inactive metabolites.

   a. Buspirone is highly (95%) plasma protein bound.

   b. In humans, the $t_{1/2}$ is ~2.5 hours. Because of the short $t_{1/2}$ the drug must be administered at least two to three times/day. No such information is available for animals.

   c. Adverse effects

   (1) The incidence of side effects is very low, which is an advantage in its use as a behavior-modifying drug. Sedation does not occur in humans; however, has been reported in animals. The most common side effects reported in humans include dizziness, insomnia, nervousness, nausea, headache, and fatigue.

   (2) Unlike BZDs, long-term use of buspirone is not associated with withdrawal effects or dependence, and the potential for abuse is less likely as compared to BZDs.

IV. ANTIDEPRESSANTS

A. **General considerations.** Four classes of drugs are categorized under the antidepressants category. The list includes TCAs, selective SSRIs, monoamine oxidase inhibitors (MAOIs), and progestins. These drugs differ in their mechanism of action (Figure 5-1), side effect profile (Table 5-1), pharmacokinetic parameters, and relative therapeutic efficacy in treating certain behavioral disorders. Despite their inherent differences, all of these drugs except progestins share certain commonalities.

1. They modulate monoamine neurotransmission (mainly NE and 5-HT) and their respective target receptor sites.

2. Antidepressants have anxiolytic effects at clinical doses and are generally well tolerated in animals.

3. The pharmacological effects are elicited within hours or days following the first dose; however, may require several weeks for the onset of clinical response.

4. The delayed onset of therapeutic effects of antidepressants appears to be related to elevated levels of NE and 5-HT together with altered sensitivity of post- and presynaptic receptors, including 5-HT_{1A} and α_2-adrenergic receptors.

TABLE 5-1. Pharmacological Properties of Antidepressant Drugs

Drug	Sedative Effects	Antimuscarinic Effects	NE-Reuptake Inhibition	5-HT Reuptake Inhibition
Amitriptyline	+++	+++	+++	+++
Doxepin	+++	+++	+	++
Imipramine	++	+	+	++
Clomipramine	+++	++	+++	+++
Fluoxetine	+	+	−	+++
Fluvoxamine	−	−	−	+++
Paroxetine	+	−	−	+++
Sertraline	+	+	+	+++

−,none; +, slight; ++, moderate; +++, high.

B. **Tricyclic antidepressants (TCAs)**

1. **General considerations**

    a. The name TCAs refers to a group of compounds that have a three-ring nucleus.

    b. The drugs most commonly used in animals include amitriptyline, imipramine, clomipramine, and doxepin; and to a lesser extent nortriptyline and desipramine.

    c. In recent years, TCAs have been mostly replaced by SSRIs in human medicine because of decreased frequency of side effects. Nevertheless, their low cost has favored the use in veterinary behavioral medicine.

    d. **Mechanism of action (Figure 5-1)**

    (1) TCAs block the reuptake (transporter mechanisms) of NE and 5-HT into the presynaptic terminal at varying magnitudes.

    (2) TCAs exert antagonistic effects at α-treceptors, muscarinic, and histaminergic receptors (Table 5-1). In fact, TCAs cause desensitization of presynaptic α_2-receptors consequently leading to an increase in extrasynaptic levels of NE. Furthermore, TCA's α_2-blocking effects have been linked to drug-induced orthostatic hypotension.

    e. **Therapeutic uses**

    (1) In general, they reduce anxiety and arousal; in some circumstances, they may enhance learning. Unlike BZDs, they do not produce disinhibition phenomena.

    (2) TCAs are used in dogs for the management of mild aggression, compulsive behavior, and a variety of anxious states.

    (3) In cats, they are used for the treatment of inappropriate urination and spraying behavior, excessive grooming, anxiety states, and control of excessive vocalization.

    (4) Because of the delayed onset of therapeutic effects, improvement in behavior may not be seen until 3–4 weeks after initiation of drug therapy. Abrupt cessation of drug treatment should be avoided due to the risk of development of withdrawal responses.

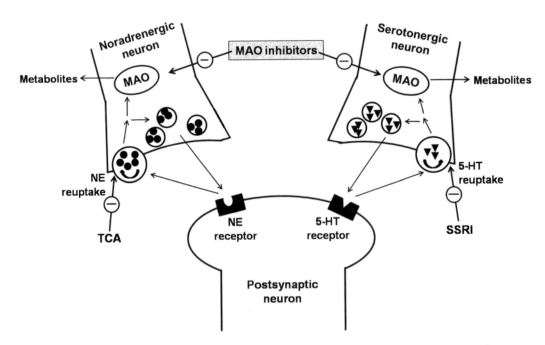

FIGURE 5-1. Schematic of potential sites of action of antidepressant drugs. TCA, tricyclic antidepressant; SSRI, selective serotonin reuptake inhibitor. (Modified from *Basic and Clinical Pharmacology*, 9th ed., by Katzung, McGraw-Hill, 2004.)

f. Pharmacokinetics
  (1) TCAs are substrates of CYP450 enzymes.
  (2) Concurrent administration of agents that inhibit CYP450 can increase serum levels of TCAs. For example, SSRIs are inhibitors of CYP450 enzymes.
  (3) Because of the risk of drug interactions, caution must be exercised when using combination drug therapy, especially drugs that modulate CYP 450 activity.

g. Adverse effects
  (1) Adverse effects are not a major concern in young healthy animals.
  (2) Geriatric patients and animals with compromised hepatic function need to be closely monitored.
  (3) Onset of side effects may be immediate or delayed depending on the duration of treatment.
  (4) Most commonly seen side effects include GI disturbance, mild sedation, constipation, dry mouth, and urinary retention.
  (5) The occurrence of side effects is partly attributed to its antagonistic effects at the above-mentioned receptors.
  (6) TCAs lower seizure threshold and may exacerbate seizures in predisposed animals.
  (7) Occasionally, agranulocytosis is seen.
  (8) It is contraindicated in the following:
    (a) Narrow-angle glaucoma and keratoconjunctivitis sicca.
    (b) Because of its cardiovascular (CV) effects (cardiomyopathies, and ECG abnormalities), ECGs should be evaluated in dogs that have a predisposition for CV events.

2. Amitriptyline. It is relatively inexpensive and is popular among veterinarians.
  a. Therapeutic uses
    (1) It is used as an antianxiety agent and as a pharmacological adjunct to behavioral therapy.
    (2) In dogs, it is commonly used for the treatment of aggression, self-induced mutilation, and separation anxiety.
    (3) In cats, it is used for the treatment of psychogenic alopecia and excessive vocalization. Most commonly, it is used for the management of urine marking behavior and inappropriate urination.
    (4) Amitriptyline has been used in the treatment of severe recurring idiopathic interstitial cystitis in cats. The beneficial effects are attributed, in part, to its analgesic effects and reduction in bladder spasms due to its antimuscarinic effect.

  b. Pharmacokinetics
    (1) It is rapidly absorbed from the GI tract.
    (2) It is metabolized in the liver and excreted in the urine.
    (3) It is metabolized into triptyline, nortriptyline (active), and various other metabolites.
    (4) Amitriptyline is ~95% plasma protein bound.
    (5) The elimination $t_{1/2}$ in dogs is 6–8 hours.

  c. Adverse effects
    (1) The most common side effects in dogs and cats include sedation, mydriasis, and urinary retention. Once daily night-time dosing may be adopted to avoid daytime sedation.
    (2) Weight gain, somnolence, and reduced grooming have been reported.
    (3) Because it is excreted in the milk and its potential for teratogenicity, it is not recommended in pregnant or lactating animals.

  d. Contraindications
    (1) Combination therapy with anticholinergic and CNS depressants may lead to additive effects; therefore, concurrent administration should be avoided.
    (2) Concomitant use with a CYP450 inhibitor such as cimetidine, ketoconazole, or chloramphenicol may inhibit the metabolism of TCAs, resulting in elevated plasma levels of the drug and toxicity.

(3) Concurrent use of the antithyroid agent methimazole can increase the potential risk of agranulocytosis in cats.

3. Clomipramine

  a. Mechanism of action. Clomipramine inhibits the reuptake of both NE and 5-HT; however, it is the most selective 5-HT uptake inhibitor among other commercially available TCAs. Additionally, recent evidences suggest that TCAs may have selective MAO-B inhibitory effects in the rat brain.

  b. Therapeutic uses

    (1) In the United States, it is approved by FDA for the treatment of separation anxiety in dogs when used in combination with behavior-modification therapy.

    (2) It can be used in the treatment of canine compulsive disorders, such as tail chasing, and acral-lick dermatitis.

    (3) It is useful in the treatment of dominance-related aggression in dogs.

    (4) Adjunct treatment with alprazolam may be necessary for the effective management of noise phobia.

    (5) In cats, it is useful for the treatment of urine spraying behavior and psychogenic alopecia.

  c. Pharmacokinetics

    (1) It is highly lipophilic and therefore readily crosses the lipid membrane barrier.

    (2) The major metabolite is desmethylclomipramine, which subsequently form conjugates that are eliminated in the urine or through the bile into feces.

    (3) In dogs, the plasma concentration of clomipramine to desmethyl-clomipramine is 3:1. The desmethyl metabolite is implicated in its antimuscarinic effects. This may partly explain the lower incidence of side effects observed in dogs. Alternatively, rapid metabolism may account for fewer side effects observed in dogs.

    (4) The plasma protein binding of clomipramine is ~96%.

    (5) The average $t_{1/2}$ in dogs is 5–7 hours after a single dose and 2–4 hours after multiple doses.

  d. Adverse effects

    (1) Side effects including sedation, mydriasis, regurgitation, appetite changes, and urinary retention have been reported.

    (2) It should not be administered to pregnant and nursing females.

  e. Contraindications

    (1) It should not be used in animals those have demonstrated hypersensitivity to clomipramine and other TCAs.

    (2) It should not be used in combination with MAOIs within 2 weeks of discontinuation of an MAO inhibitor.

    (3) It is contraindicated in patients with a history of epilepsy, cardiac arrhythmias, glaucoma, or urine and stool retention.

4. Imipramine

  a. Mechanism of action

    (1) It primarily works by blocking 5-HT reuptake at the synapses and to a lesser degree NE reuptake.

    (2) It also exerts MAO inhibitory effects on both A and B isoforms.

  b. Therapeutic uses

    (1) Imipramine has been used in the treatment of inappropriate urination (submissive and excitement related) in dogs.

    (2) In a certain population of beagles, it has been shown to improve abnormal withdrawn and depressed behavior.

    (3) In dogs and cats, it has been used to treat cataplexy and urinary incontinence. Its antimuscarinic effect may stabilize smooth muscle of the urinary bladder and activation of α_1-adrenergic receptors in the urinary sphincters also play a role in the treatment of urinary incontinence.

    (4) In stallions, it is used for the treatment of ejaculatory dysfunction. It appears that elevated extrasyaptic levels of NE induced by TCAs may facilitate the activation of α_1-adrenergic receptors that enables ejaculation.

c. **Pharmacokinetics**
(1) It is rapidly absorbed from the GI tract.
(2) The plasma drug levels peak in 1–2 hours after oral administration.
(3) Substantial amounts of the drug are metabolized by hepatic first pass metabolism, resulting in high blood levels of desipramine, an active metabolite of imipramine.
(4) Imipramine has plasma protein binding of 60–96%.
(5) In humans, it has an elimination $t_{1/2}$ of ~12 hours. It has extensive peripheral distribution presumably related to its high lipophilicity.

d. **Adverse effects**
(1) Horses and cattle may exhibit generalized weakness and ataxia. Hemolysis and discolored urine may occur.
(2) Side effects in humans, include sedation, tachycardia, GI effects, and urinary retention.

e. **Contraindications.** Concurrent use with MAOIs is not recommended.

5. **Doxepin**
a. **Mechanism of action**
(1) Doxepin exerts moderate inhibitory effects at the norepinephrine transporter (NET) and weak inhibitory effects at the serotonin transporter (SERT).
(2) Doxepin has potent H_1 and H_2 inhibitory effects possibly accounting for its antipruritic effects.

b. **Therapeutic uses**
(1) Doxepin is used as an adjunctive therapy for psychogenic dermatitis; particularly related to anxiety in small animals.
(2) Doxepin use is banned in race horses because it has been used to calm excited horses.

c. **Pharmacokinetics**
(1) In the dog, it is rapidly absorbed following oral administration. The plasma concentration peaks in 30–60 minutes.
(2) The drug undergoes extensive hepatic biotransformation to desmethyldoxepin and nordoxepin; the former being the active metabolite and it is found to accumulate in various tissues.
(3) The plasma protein binding for doxepin is ~80%.
(4) In humans, it has an elimination $t_{1/2}$ of 8–25 hours. No information is available for animals.

d. **Adverse effects**
(1) In humans, the most common antimuscarinic side effects include constipation and dry mouth. However, urine retention and blurred vision have also been reported.
(2) It can cause cardiac arrhythmias following drug overdose.

e. **Contraindications**
(1) It is contraindicated in animals with hypersensitivity to TCAs and a history of urinary retention or glaucoma.
(2) Concomitant administration with MAOIs should be avoided.

C. **Serotonin selective reuptake Inhibitors (SSRIs)**

1. **General considerations**
a. **Mechanism of action (see Figure 5-1).** As the name implies, it selectively blocks the reuptake of 5-HT by the SERT with minimal effects on NE. This leads to elevated synaptic levels of 5-HT, hence resulting in acute 5-HT_{1A} receptor desensitization. However, with chronic use, it leads to downregulation of 5-HT_{1A} autoreceptors that may explain the delay in onset (4–6 weeks) of the effects of antidepressants.

b. **Therapeutic uses**
(1) SSRIs are commonly used in domestic animals for the management of anxiety, affective aggression, certain forms of compulsive disorders, and urine marking.
(2) It is used in the treatment of generalized anxiety disorder in humans.

(3) In dogs, SSRIs are used for the treatment of separation anxiety, compulsive disorders, and dominance-type aggression.

(4) In cats, it is beneficial in treating urine spraying, aggression, and compulsive disorders such as psychogenic alopecia and fabric chewing.

c. Pharmacokinetics

(1) All SSRIs are metabolized in the liver and excreted into the urine.

(2) SSRIs are competitive inhibitors of several isoforms of CYP450 liver enzymes.

(3) The onset of therapeutic effect is slow; at least 3–4 weeks is required to observe the improvement in behavior following the initiation of drug therapy.

d. Adverse effects

(1) SSRIs have an excellent safety profile. Unlike TCAs, they exhibit lower incidence of cholinergic, histaminergic, and adrenergic side effects (see Table 5-1).

(2) Side effects in most species include sedation, tremor, constipation, diarrhea, nausea, anxiety, irritability, agitation, anorexia, seizures, and agitation. However, inappetence, and mild sedation are the most commonly observed side effects in dogs and are transient in nature.

(3) Cats, in particular, should be monitored for food intake, and urine and fecal excretion due to concerns of GI disturbances.

(4) A phenomenon known as "5-HT syndrome" resulting from excessive levels of synaptic levels of 5-HT has been reported in rare instances. Alternatively, it may also result when SSRIs are concurrently taken with other medications that interfere with 5-HT metabolism, for example, MAO inhibitors. Although the exact mechanism is unclear, it is generally believed that the excessive 5-HT_{1A} receptor stimulation may contribute to the condition. In humans, the symptoms of serotonin syndrome are changes in mental status, including confusion, anxiety, agitation, ataxia, tremor, and myoclonus; cardiovascular changes, including hypertension and sinus tachycardia; GI effects, including nausea, diarrhea, excessive salivation, and hyperpyrexia.

e. Drug Interactions

(1) Concurrent administration of medications that are metabolized by CYP450 may lead to elevated plasma levels and resulting toxicity.

(2) SSRIs produce significant inhibition of CYP2D6 that metabolizes TCAs including clomipramine, desipramine, imipramine, and nortriptyline. As a result, concurrent administration of the above-mentioned drugs may lead to "5-HT syndrome." Likewise, MAOIs should not be given concomitantly with SSRIs because they may lead to fatal drug interactions including 5-HT syndrome, diaphoresis, hyperpyrexia, and unreactive pupils.

2. Fluoxetine (Reconcile®, Prozac®)

a. Therapeutic uses

(1) In dogs, fluoxetine is used for the treatment of dominance-related aggression, intraspecies aggression, acral lick dermatitis and other compulsive disorders.

(2) In cats, it is used for the treatment of inappropriate urination, urine spraying behavior, psychogenic alopecia, and aggression.

b. Pharmacokinetics

(1) It is well absorbed following oral administration.

(2) It is extensively metabolized in the liver to norfluoxetine, the active metabolite; however, it has less potent 5-HT reuptake inhibitory properties. Both fluoxetine and norfluoxetine exhibit slow rates of renal elimination.

(3) The plasma protein binding of fluoxetine is ~95%.

(4) In dogs, the elimination $t_{1/2}$ of fluoxetine and norfluoxetine are 24 hours and 5 days, respectively. Therefore, the drug may be present in the circulation weeks after discontinuation of drug administration.

c. Adverse effects

(1) In dogs, panting, anxiety, irritability, anorexia, and aggressive behavior in previously nonaggressive animals have been reported.

(2) In cats, changes in sleep pattern, inappropriate elimination behavior, and changes in behavioral pattern (anxiety, irritability) have been reported.

d. Contraindications

(1) It exhibits high plasma protein binding (~95%); therefore, concomitant administration with drugs that compete for the protein binding sites may lead to adverse effects.

(2) Caution should be exercised when administered in patients with diabetes mellitus because it may cause hypoglycemia by increasing insulin receptor sensitivity.

3. Paroxetine

a. Therapeutic uses

(1) It is used in the management of canine aggression and stereotypic behavior.

(2) In cats, it may be used for the treatment of inappropriate urination and aggression.

b. Pharmacokinetics

(1) It is well absorbed orally and can be given alone or with food.

(2) The clinical efficacy of paroxetine is essentially from the parent compound and the contribution from the metabolites is minimal.

(3) In geriatric patients while initiating therapy, the drug should be administered at the lowest dose and should be titrated gradually upward because plasma levels of the drug may be elevated in geriatric patients due to decreased clearance time.

(4) Paroxetine inhibits CYP450 enzyme (CYP2D6); however, the magnitude of inhibition is less when compared with fluoxetine and fluvoxamine.

(5) The $t_{1/2}$ of paroxetine in animals is unavailable. In humans, the $t_{1/2}$ is ~24 hours.

c. Adverse effects

(1) Anorexia is a common side effect in dogs, although typically transient.

(2) It should not be used in patients with narrow angle glaucoma.

(3) Constipation is a common anticholinergic side effect in cats. Therefore, fecal and urinary excretion should be monitored regularly, especially during the first week of therapy.

4. Sertraline

a. Therapeutic uses. In both cats and dogs, it is used in the treatment of aggression, OCD and anxiety-related disorders.

b. Pharmacokinetics

(1) It exhibits a similar pharmacokinetic profile to that of paroxetine in humans.

(2) It is highly plasma protein bound (97%).

(3) It undergoes extensive hepatic first pass metabolism and is primarily metabolized to *N*-desmethylsertraline.

(4) The 5-HT reuptake inhibitory effects of N-desmethylsertraline are less potent than those of the parent compound.

(5) The excretion of the unchanged or original form of sertraline in the urine represents only a minor mode of elimination. Almost 50% of the metabolites of sertraline are eliminated in the feces.

(6) It exerts inhibitory effects on the liver enzyme CYP2D6, although to a lesser extent than that of paroxetine or fluoxetine.

(7) The mean $t_{1/2}$ of sertraline in humans is 26 hours; no such information is available for animals.

c. Adverse effects

(1) The side effect profile in dogs include mydriasis, hind limb weakness, hyperactivity, and anorexia.

(2) In cats, the adverse effects include sedation, anorexia, behavioral changes (anxiety, irritability, and sleep disturbance), vomiting, and diarrhea.

(3) Sertraline exerts minor inhibitory effects on the liver enzyme CYP2D6. Caution should be exercised when used with drugs such as TCAs and dextromethorphan, used in the treatment of kennel cough.

(4) Patients with chronic liver impairment metabolize sertraline more slowly as compared to patients with normal metabolism. Because of the potential for toxicity, it should be used with caution in animals with compromised liver function.

5. Fluvoxamine

a. Therapeutic uses

It can be used for the treatment of aggression and compulsive disorders in both cats and dogs. In particular, it can be used to treat maternal aggression.

b. Pharmacokinetics

(1) It is completely absorbed and only 10% of the dose is excreted in its unchanged form.

(2) Fluvoxamine is ~80% plasma protein bound.

(3) The $t_{1/2}$ of fluvoxamine is ~15 hours in dogs.

c. Adverse effects

(1) In a small percentage of animals it can cause anxiety and changes in appetite pattern, Fluvoxamine should not be concurrently administered with MAOIs. A 2-week washout period should be implemented before initiation of drug therapy with MAOIs.

(2) When fluvoxamine is given concomitantly with BZDs, it may decrease the clearance of BZDs that are metabolized via hepatic oxidation.

D. **Monoamine oxidase inhibitors (MAOIs)**

1. General considerations

a. Mechanism of action

(1) The antidepressant effects of the drugs are attributed primarily to their actions in the brain.

(2) MAOIs are drugs that work by inhibiting both isoforms of MAO, hence resulting in elevated levels of vesicular monoamines (Figure 5-1).

(3) Two isoforms of MAO have been identified, namely, MAO-A and MAO-B.

(a) **MAO-A.** Catalyzes the oxidative deamination of 5-HT, catecholamines, and exogenous amines, especially tyramine derived from a variety of food sources (wine and cheese). Therefore, MAO inhibitors should not be given concurrently with tyramine containing foods because it may cause an increase in blood pressure resulting from elevated levels of NE.

(b) **MAO-B.** Oxidatively deaminates catecholamines including DA, epinephrine, NE, phenylethylamine, and to a lesser degree 5-HT.

(c) **Species-specific difference in MAO isoforms.** MAO-B is the predominant isoform found in human platelets, whereas both isoforms are expressed in dog platelets.

b. MAO-A inhibitors and nonselective MAO inhibitors are seldom used in veterinary behavioral medicine. Therefore, the focus will be on selegiline, a selective MAO-B inhibitor.

2. Selegiline

a. Mechanism of action

(1) Selegiline is an irreversible and selective inhibitor of MAO-B.

(2) It inhibits the reuptake of NE and 5-HT into presynaptic terminals.

(3) It inhibits the presynaptic D_2 receptors, thereby promoting DA release.

(4) It acts as a free radical scavenger of DA-derived oxidative species in the CNS by promoting superoxide dismutase (SOD) and catalase activity.

b. Therapeutic uses

(1) Selegiline can be used to manage the emotional behavioral disorders in cats, including territorial and fear-related aggression, reduced appetite, compulsive licking, house soiling, and excessive vocalization.

(2) It is useful in treating "rage syndrome" in cocker spaniels.

(3) It is approved by FDA for the treatment of canine cognitive dysfunction (CCD), a disorder observed in elderly dogs. CCD is characterized by decreased social interaction, changes in sleep cycle, confusion, disorientation, loss of prior house training, and obedience commands. Furthermore, histological lesions reminiscent of Alzheimers' β-amyloid plaques have been

identified in the postmortem brains of geriatric dogs that exhibited behavioral problems before death.

(4) Selegiline appears to exhibit beneficial effects on learning in both young and geriatric patients.

(5) Selegiline is used to treat cognitive dysfunction in geriatric cats.

(6) Selegiline may suppress cataplexy in canine narcolepsy. Aberrant MAO activity or an imbalance in 5-HT and other neurotransmitter transmission has been implicated in the pathogenesis of human cataplexy.

c. **Pharmacokinetics**

(1) In dogs, selegiline exhibits rapid absorption from the GI tract but has low bioavailability (10%). In humans, it exhibits high plasma protein binding (~85%). Plasma concentrations peak around 20–30 minutes.

(2) The three major metabolites of selegiline include l-(–) amphetamine, l-(–) methamphetamine, and N-desmethylselegiline. A few of the sympathomimetic effects observed with selegiline might be partly attributed to its metabolites.

(3) In dogs, the elimination $t_{1/2}$ is ~80 minutes.

(4) Therapeutic responsiveness may require at least 3–4 weeks following initiation of drug therapy.

(5) Most MAOIs are used for the treatment of progressive irreversible neurodegeneration and therefore it should not be discontinued in responsive patients.

(6) In the event of treatment failure, a washout period of 2 weeks is recommended after termination of MAOI therapy and initiation of a new antidepressant therapy.

d. **Adverse effects.** The occurrence of side effects is rare. However, at high doses, it can cause hyperactivity and stereotypy in dogs. Since the levels of phenylethylamine are increased in the CNS of treated dogs, it may produce amphetamine-like stimulant effects. For example, in dogs, restlessness, agitation, vomiting, disorientation, diarrhea, and decreased hearing have been reported.

e. **Contraindications**

(1) Severe CNS toxicity can occur when given in combination with TCAs, namely, amitriptyline, clomipramine, and SSRIs—fluoxetine and paroxetine. In severe cases, it may lead to 5-HT syndrome.

(2) Selegiline should not be concurrently administered with potential MAO inhibitors such as amitraz, a topical ectoparasiticide.

(3) Use of selegiline, in conjunction with α_2-agonists, may lead to large fluctuations in blood pressure. Periodic monitoring of blood pressure is recommended.

E. | **Hormonal therapy**

1. **General considerations.** Synthetic progestins have been used for the alleviation of behavioral problems. However, the low therapeutic efficacy, potentially serious side effect profiles, and availability of more specific agents have made synthetic progestins almost obsolete. Synthetic progestins are used as a last resort only when other therapeutic interventions and behavioral therapy have failed, and euthanasia, abandonment, or relinquishment is probable. Only the two most frequently used synthetic progestins in veterinary behavioral medicine will be discussed, namely, megestrol acetate (MA) and medroxyprogesterone acetate (MPA).

a. **Mechanism of action**

(1) The behavioral improvement mediated by progestins is attributed to both antiandrogenic and calming effect on the limbic system.

(2) Progestins elicit a wide array of actions including inhibition of secretion of pituitary gonadotropins, inhibition of production of sex steroids, and activation of $GABA_A$ receptors similar to BZDs.

b. **Therapeutic uses**

(1) Progestins have been commonly used in the management of sexually dimorphic behavior including roaming, dominance aggression in dogs and cats, urine marking, excessive vocalization, and persistent mounting in neutered male cats.

(2) MA is FDA approved for the postponement of estrus and the alleviation of pseudo-pregnancy in dogs.

(3) Occasionally, MPA is used to treat feline psychogenic alopecia and dermatitis, although tranquilizing agents may be preferable.

(4) In parrots, progestins have been used to treat feather-picking behavior.

c. **Adverse effects**

(1) MA has profound adrenocortical suppressing effects at therapeutic doses, which is due to the inhibition of ACTH secretion; however, symptoms of adrenocortical insufficiency are rare (for further information please refer to Chapter 12). If the animal, however, demonstrates clinical signs of stress (vomiting, lethargy), exogenous steroid support should be instituted. The most prevalent side effects include sedation, polyphagia, and polydipsia—attributed to the glucocorticoid activity of progestins.

(2) Various pathological changes including endometritis, cystic endometrial hyperplasia, mammary hypertrophy, and neoplasia have been identified in the uterus of both dogs and cats depending on the dose and the duration of drug therapy.

(3) Neuroendocrine problems such as diabetes mellitus and iatrogenic Addison's syndrome may develop at therapeutic doses. However, they are transient and have been shown to be resolved within 3 months of discontinuation of drug therapy.

d. **Contraindications**

(1) MPA should not be used in prepubescent cats, especially intact females due to increased risk of mammary hypertrophy.

(2) In dogs, it may precipitate underlying endocrine and uterine conditions including diabetes and endometrial hyperplasia.

2. **Medroxyprogesterone acetate (MPA)**

a. **Pharmacokinetics.** MPA sterile parenteral suspension (Depo-Provera®) is administered IM or SC once a month, since in cats, one treatment will have a duration of action of 30 days. This is because MPA in suspension is absorbed very slowly from the injection site.

(1) Approximately 90% of the drug is reported to be bound to plasma proteins (refer to Chapter 12 for more information).

(2) It is extensively metabolized in the liver followed by conjugation and elimination in the urine (in humans).

3. **Megestrol acetate (MA)**

a. **Pharmacokinetics.** MA is administered orally.

(1) MA has a rapid onset of action.

(2) In dogs, feces (~87%) is the major route of elimination and urine (~9%) represents the minor mode of elimination.

(3) Almost 90% of the drug is eliminated by the end of 1 week. Information on plasma protein binding is unavailable.

(4) In humans, the plasma $t_{1/2}$ averaged ~35 hours.

SUGGESTED READING

Crowell-Davis S, Murray T. 2006. *Veterinary Psychopharmacology.* Ames, IA: Blackwell Publishing. http://www.drugs.com

Katzung BG, Trevor AJ, Masters SB. 2005. *Katzung and Trevor's Pharmacology.* 7th ed. New York: McGraw-Hill.

Landsberg G, Hunthausen W, Ackerman L. 2003. *Handbook of Behavior Problems of the Dog and Cat.* 2nd ed. Oxford: Elsevier Saunders.

Plumb DC. 2005. *Veterinary Drug Handbook.* 5th ed. Ames, IA: Blackwell Publishing.

STUDY QUESTIONS

DIRECTIONS: Each of the lettered items or incomplete statements in this section is followed by answers or by completions of the statement. Select the **one** lettered answer or completion that is **best** in each case.

1. Which one of the following antidepressant drugs is most effective in the treatment of psychogenic dermatitis?

(A) Doxepin
(B) Fluoxetine
(C) Imipramine
(D) Desipramine
(E) Sertraline

2. Which of the following behavior-modifying drugs is most likely to produce pronounced antimuscarinic side effects and cardiac disturbances?

(A) Fluoxetine
(B) Sertraline
(C) Alprazolam
(D) Diazepam
(E) Imipramine

3. Which of the following drugs should not be concurrently administered with fluoxetine due to the risk of "serotonin syndrome" and cardiovascular disturbances?

(A) Imipramine
(B) Selegiline
(C) Clomipramine
(D) Amitriptyline
(E) All of the above

4. Which of the following is the most commonly seen adverse effect in cats administered diazepam for the treatment of noise phobia?

(A) Endometrial hyperplasia
(B) Urinary retention
(C) Orthostatic hypotension
(D) Hepatic necrosis
(E) Blurred vision

5. Which of the following drugs can be used for the treatment of anxiety-related disorders in geriatric animals or in patients with impaired liver function?

(A) Oxazepam
(B) Diazepam
(C) Lorazepam
(D) Chlordiazepoxide
(E) Both A and C

6. Which of the following drugs is most likely to produce dis-inhibition phenomenon, manifested as increased aggressiveness?

(A) Imipramine
(B) Clomipramine
(C) Fluoxetine
(D) Sertraline
(E) Diazepam

7. Which of the following behavior-modifying drugs may precipitate diabetes mellitus?

(A) MPA
(B) Imipramine
(C) Selegiline
(D) Clomipramine
(E) Fluoxetine

8. Which of the following drugs is FDA-approved for the treatment of separation anxiety in dogs?

(A) Clomipramine
(B) Amitriptyline
(C) Imipramine
(D) Doxepin
(E) Diazepam

9. Which of the following drugs exerts its actions through selective inhibition of serotonin transporter?

(A) Fluoxetine
(B) Imipramine
(C) Medroxyprogesterone
(D) Buspirone
(E) Doxepin

10. According to the monoamine theory of depression imbalances, which of the following neurotransmitter(s) play a key role in the disease pathogenesis?

(A) Norepinephrine
(B) Serotonin
(C) Acetylcholine
(D) GABA
(E) Both A and B

11. Which of the following drugs is useful in providing rapid relief from anxiety associated with noise phobia?

(A) Amitriptyline
(B) Imipramine
(C) Fluoxetine
(D) Sertraline
(E) Alprazolam

12. Which of the following drugs is a partial 5-HT_{1A} receptor agonist and is effective when used in combination with fluoxetine for the treatment of aggression and stereotypical behavior in dogs?

(A) Buspirone
(B) Imipramine
(C) Diazepam
(D) Medroxyprogesterone
(E) Alprazolam

13. Which of the following drugs is a selective irreversible MAO-B inhibitor and is useful in the treatment of canine cognitive dysfunction (CCD)?

(A) Selegiline
(B) Medroxyprogesterone
(C) Sertraline
(D) Alprazolam
(E) Fluoxetine

ANSWERS AND EXPLANATIONS

1. The answer is A.
Doxepin, which is categorized under TCAs, exhibits moderate inhibitory effects at the NET and weak inhibitory effects at the SERT. In addition, doxepin has potent H_1-antihistaminic effects which may partially account for its potent antipruritic effects. This pharmacological aspect has been particularly useful as an adjunct therapy for the treatment of psychogenic dermatitis in companion animals. However, TCAs such as imipramine and desipramine have moderate H_1-antihistaminic effect which may account for its sedative effects observed, especially during the first few weeks of drug therapy. SSRIs such as fluoxetine and sertraline, however, have very little H_1-antihistamine effect. Furthermore, SSRIs produce fewer adverse effects than do other nonselective antidepressants.

2. The answer is E.
Unlike SSRIs—fluoxetine and sertraline— TCAs (e.g., imipramine) produce undesirable side effects at therapeutic doses. In addition to their transporter inhibiting properties, they exhibit potent antimuscarinic effects which is manifested as dry mouth, constipation, urinary retention, tachycardia, and blurred vision. In order to improve tolerability to the antimuscarinic effects of TCAs, the dose is normally increased with gradual increments during the first few weeks of therapy. However, blurred vision and GI disturbance are among the less common side effects observed with BZDs such as alprazolam and diazepam. SSRIs exhibit little or no affinity for the cholinergic and histaminergic receptors and exhibit minimal effects on cardiac conduction. SSRIs are well tolerated by patients with heart diseases and in geriatric patients who are more susceptible to orthostatic hypotension and antimuscarinic effects.

3. The answer is E.
Fluoxetine, an SSRI, should not be concurrently administered with MAOIs and TCAs, because the aforementioned drugs have the ability to increase synaptic levels of 5-HT which may lead to a fatal condition known as "serotonin syndrome," which is characterized by agitation, restlessness, confusion, seizures, GI disturbance, and profound hypertension. In addition, when MAOIs are coadministered with TCAs, they can cause potentially life-threatening severe hypertensive crisis. Thus, a 2-week washout period should be instituted between the discontinuation of MAOI and initiation of drug therapy with an SSRI or TCA.

4. The answer is D.
Diazepam differs from other BZDs in that it can cause idiopathic hepatic necrosis in cats, the most serious adverse event in this species. Toxic intermediates play a role in the disease pathogenesis. Therefore, it is essential to rule out any underlying liver condition; complete blood count and blood chemistries need to be performed to ensure the well-being of the cat. TCAs exert anti-muscarinic effects, which are characterized by urinary retention and blurred vision, tachycardia, dry mouth, and constipation. In addition, ventricular arrhythmias may be seen in animals that have an underlying cardiac conduction abnormality. On the contrary, progestins which are seldom used in veterinary behavior medicine because of their unfavorable side effect profile can cause endometrial hyperplasia and, therefore, should not be used in intact females.

5. The answer is E.
Both oxazepam and lorazepam are particularly useful in the treatment of anxiety disorders in geriatric animals and in animals with compromised liver function because, unlike diazepam and chlordiazepoxide, they do not generate long-acting metabolites.

6. The answer is E.
Diazepam, a benzodiazepine, is used for the treatment of anxiety-related disorder, especially when the stimuli can be predicted in advance, for example, storm phobia. However, it may cause loss of inhibition, hence resulting in aggressiveness. Thus,

benzodiazepines should be avoided or used cautiously in aggressive animals. On the contrary, TCAs such as imipramine and clomipramine and SSRIs such as fluoxetine and sertraline do not produce disinhibition phenomenon, because they have little or no GABA-modulating effects. In fact, combination therapy involving SSRIs and BZDs have demonstrated improved clinical outcome in the treatment of abnormal behavior.

7. The answer is A.
Progestins may precipitate an underlying diabetes mellitus condition, which is due to their glucocorticoid activity. Studies in humans have shown that depressed patients receiving TCAs may have decreased fasting blood glucose levels. Conversely, SSRIs may cause an increase in fasting blood glucose levels in depressed individuals. Thus, blood glucose levels needs to be monitored in animals placed on TCAs and SSRIs.

8. The answer is A.
Clomipramine is approved by the FDA for the treatment of separation anxiety in dogs.

9. The answer is A.
Fluoxetine, an SSRI that is used in the treatment of separation anxiety, obsessive compulsive disorder, and dominance type aggression. Fluoxetine works by selectively blocking the SERT, hence resulting in elevated synaptic levels of 5-HT. This acute increase in 5-HT leads to the activation of 5-HT$_{1A}$ autoreceptors, thereby resulting in decreased synaptic release of 5-HT. Conversely, during chronic administration, it leads to the downregulation of 5-HT$_{1A}$ receptors, thereby facilitating an increase in 5-HT neurotransmission. This may partly explain the delayed onset of action of SSRIs (4–6 weeks). Buspirone elicits therapeutic effects via its partial agonistic effects on 5-HT$_{1A}$ receptors. In addition, stimulation of feedback inhibitory effect on 5-HT release may account for buspirone's anxiolytic effects. On the contrary, the therapeutic effects of TCAs are attributed to their varying degree of selectivity for the SERT and the NET. All of the above-mentioned drugs share one thing in common, that is, delayed onset of action, which may take several weeks to develop an improvement in behavior.

10. The answer is E.
According to the monoamine theory of depression, impairments in both 5-HT and NE neurotransmission have been implicated in the disease process. Deficiency of certain monoamines such as NE and 5-HT in certain key regions of the brain may account for the depression. Conversely, the theory proposes that elevation of the monoamines may account for the mania. However, the monoamine theory of depression is considered to be over simplistic, because it does not provide an explanation as to why the pharmacological effects occur immediately whereas the clinical therapeutic response requires at least several weeks. Downregulation of feedback inhibitory receptors allows increased synthesis of the neurotransmitter and enhanced release of the neurotransmitter into the synaptic cleft, resulting in increased activation of the postsynaptic signaling events, which may partially account for the delayed therapeutic response. The undesirable side effects associated with TCAs are attributed to antimuscarinic effects.

11. The answer is E.
Unlike SSRIs and TCAs, alprazolam, a fast-acting benzodiazepine, attains maximal plasma levels within 1–2 hours and therefore has a rapid onset of action. Although it causes CNS depression and the potential for physical dependence is quite high, it has proven efficacy in the management of anxiety-related behavior that can be predicted in advance, for example, noise phobia. SSRIs and TCAs may be used in combination with BZDs to limit the tolerance and dependence associated with long-term use of BZDs. Furthermore, both TCAs and SSRIs require several weeks to develop an improvement in behavior and therefore may not be suitable to provide acute relief from storm phobia.

12. The answer is A.
Buspirone acts as a full agonist at presynaptic receptors, resulting in a decrease in 5-HT biosynthesis and inhibition of neuronal firing. Additionally, it acts as a partial agonist at postsynaptic 5-HT$_{1A}$ receptors, resulting in an increase in 5-HT- mediated cell signaling. Thus, buspirone exhibits dual effects on serotonergic neurotransmission. Unlike BZDs, it does not cause sedation, cognitive impairment, or psychomotor disruption. Thus, it serves as a therapeutic adjunct to either

SSRIs or benzodiazepines for the treatment of behavioral disorders in companion animals. Progestins, such as MPA, should be used only as a last resort, especially when the animal is refractory to other behavior-modification therapy.

13. The answer is A.

Selegiline is a selective reuptake inhibitor of DA and an irreversible inhibitor of MAO-B. The neuroprotective effects of the drug have been shown to be beneficial in the treatment of CCD, characterized by decreased social interaction, confusion, disorientation, and failure to adhere to previous house training and obedience commands. SSRIs such as fluoxetine and sertraline exhibit selective inhibitory effects on the SERT. BZDs enhances GABA-mediated chloride conductance, hence resulting in the blockade of neuronal firing. The behavioral improvement observed following MPA administration is primarily attributed to its antiandrogenic effects and modulatory effects on the limbic system. Unfortunately, the low therapeutic efficacy and potentially serious side effect profile have limited its use in the treatment of behavioral disorders.

Chapter 6

Anesthetics

Dean H. Riedesel

I. **INTRODUCTION.** Anesthesia is a reversible process resulting in the total loss of sensation in a body part or the whole body. Anesthesia may be induced by a drug or drug combination that depresses nervous tissue activity peripherally (local and regional anesthesia) or centrally (general anesthesia). General anesthesia implies that the animal is experiencing unconsciousness, hyporeflexia, analgesia, and has skeletal muscle relaxation.

A. Local anesthetics block nerve impulse conduction and render an area or region of the body insensitive to painful stimuli. These agents do not induce unconsciousness. Local anesthetics may be administered in the following ways:

1. Topically
2. By injection
   a. Into the tissues in the vicinity of peripheral nerve endings that are to be anesthetized (i.e., infiltration)
   b. Around major nerves to desensitize the tissues they innervate
   c. Into the epidural or subarachnoid space to desensitize a large region of the body bilaterally
   d. Into joint spaces

II. LOCAL ANESTHETICS

A. Introduction

1. Action potentials are changes in the resting membrane potential that convey information within the nervous system. The resting membrane potential (approximately -60 to -90 mV) results from the difference between the intracellular and extracellular concentration of K^+ and the selective permeability of the cell membrane to Na^+ and K^+. This concentration difference is maintained by an ion pump within the cell membrane that is fueled by ATP. The Na^+, K^+-ATPase pump transports three Na^+ out of the cell for every two K^+ transported into the cell.
   a. **Phases of the action potential**
      (1) **Threshold.** The resting membrane potential must reach a specific threshold value before an action potential results.
         (a) Small decreases in the membrane potential (toward zero potential) that do not reach the threshold value do not lead to the propagation of an action potential.
         (b) Action potentials are an all-or-none response to a stimulus (i.e., they do not reflect the strength of the stimulus).
      (2) Depolarization results from a rapid transient change in the cell's permeability to Na^+. Positively charged Na^+ rapidly stream into the cell through Na^+ channels, altering the membrane potential.
      (3) **Repolarization.** The channels that allow Na^+ to move into the cell close after a few milliseconds at the peak of the action potential. K^+ then rapidly diffuses out of the cell, returning the membrane potential to its resting level.
      (4) **Return to resting potential.** After repolarization, the Na^+-K^+-ATPase pump reestablishes the normal concentration difference of Na^+ and K^+ across the membrane of the cell, readying it to fire again.

b. Propagation of action potentials. Action potentials self-perpetuate along the length of the nerve fiber.

    (1) Unmyelinated nerves develop a flow of current from the depolarized region into the resting segment. The current flow reduces the membrane potential of the resting segment to a value that exceeds threshold and the action potential is propagated.

    (2) In myelinated nerves, action potentials are generated only at the nodes of Ranvier. Action potentials appear to "jump" from node to node. Nerve impulse conduction velocity is much faster in myelinated nerves, as compared with unmyelinated nerves.

2. **Classification of nerves.** Nerves are classified according to their size, myelination, and function.

    a. Historically, the unmyelinated C fibers and small diameter myelinated A-δ fibers (i.e. pain fibers) have been shown to be easier to block with local anesthetics than myelinated, large fibers (i.e. sensory and motor fibers).

    b. More recent studies have shown that the small unmyelinated C (pain) fibers are the last fiber type to be blocked by lidocaine. Thus, controversy exists concerning the susceptibility of the various nerve types to local anesthetics and results also vary depending on the nerve and lipid solubility of the drug studied.

B. **Mechanism of action**

1. **Local anesthetics block the propagation of an action potential by inhibiting the flux of Na^+ through voltage-gated Na^+ channels.**

2. The exact site of action of local anesthetics is unknown. One popular theory is that the uncharged base form of the local anesthetic molecule diffuses through the nerve cell membrane, becomes protonated (i.e. binds with H^+) inside the cell, and then binds to the Na^+ channel and essentially "plugs" the channel.

C. **Chemistry**

1. **Structure.** Local anesthetics have three structural components: an aromatic group, an intermediate bond, and a tertiary amine (Figure 6-1).

    a. The intermediate bond is a connecting hydrocarbon chain that is either an ester or an amide.

    b. The addition of carbon atoms to the aromatic region or the amine end of the molecule increases its lipid solubility and, therefore, its potency.

2. **Characteristics**

    a. Local anesthetic drugs are weak bases; therefore, they are usually water insoluble. Commercial products are prepared as hydrochloride salt solutions, which

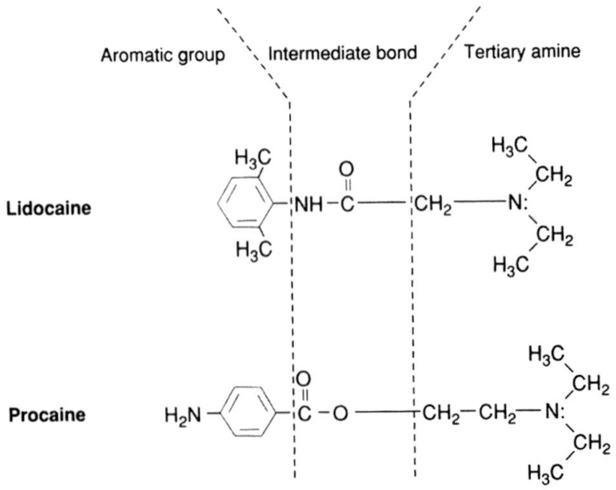

FIGURE 6-1. Structures of lidocaine and procaine. Lidocaine is amide-linked and procaine is ester-linked.

TABLE 6-1. Properties of Local Anesthetics

Drug	Lipid Solubility	pK_a	Relative Potency	Duration
Ester Linked				
Procaine	1	8.9	1	Short
Amide Linked				
Lidocaine	3.7	7.86	2	Intermediate
Mepivacaine	1.3	7.7	2	Intermediate
Bupivacaine	34	8.1	8	Long

    are acidic. The acidity increases the stability and water solubility of the local anesthetic solution.

  b. Local anesthetics exist in solution as uncharged and charged molecules.

$$B + H^+ \leftrightarrow BH^+, \text{ where}$$

B is the basic uncharged form of the local anesthetic; BH^+ is the positively charged cation form; and H^+ is the hydrogen ion.

    (1) The relative proportions of uncharged and charged molecules depend on the pH of the solution and the dissociation constant (pK_a) of the drug (Table 6-1).

      (a) If the local anesthetic is injected into an acidic environment, the increased [H^+] produces more ionized drug (BH^+), thus, decreasing the effectiveness of the local anesthetic.

      (b) Conversely, if the local anesthetic is injected into an alkaline environment, which has low [H^+], greater amounts of the drug will exist in the base form, increasing the effectiveness of the local anesthetic.

    (2) The uncharged molecule (B) diffuses more rapidly across the nerve sheath than the ionized or charged molecule (BH^+). The charged molecule, however, is thought to be the active form of the drug in the axoplasm.

D. Pharmacokinetics

  1. Absorption and speed of onset (Table 6-1)

    a. Lipid solubility is directly proportional to potency and duration of action. The higher the lipid solubility, the more potent the agent and the longer its duration of action.

    b. The pK_a correlates with the speed of onset.

      (1) Drugs with a pK_a closest to the body's pH of 7.4 (e.g., 7.6–6.9) have a rapid onset of action.

      (2) Drugs with a high pK_a (e.g., 8.1–8.9) have a slower rate of onset.

  2. Distribution

    a. Protein binding correlates with the duration of action. The binding site for the local anesthetic within the Na^+ channel is thought to be a protein (receptor).

    b. Epinephrine is added to some local anesthetics (e.g., lidocaine) to prolong the duration of action. The local vasoconstriction induced by the epinephrine limits systemic absorption of the local anesthetic, maintaining the local tissue concentration. When epinephrine is combined with drugs that already have a long duration of action (e.g., bupivacaine), the effect is less dramatic.

  3. Metabolism

    a. Ester-linked local anesthetics undergo hydrolysis by cholinesterase in the plasma and, to a lesser extent, in the liver.

    b. Amide-linked local anesthetics are metabolized in the liver which requires conjugation with glucuronic acid. Cats are more likely to develop toxicity from these drugs because they glucuronidate drugs less than other species.

E. **Therapeutic uses**

1. **Anesthesia**
    a. **Topical anesthesia.** Local anesthetics are used to desensitize the mucous membranes of the eye, nose, and larynx.
        (1) Lidocaine is commonly used to desensitize the larynx of cats prior to endotracheal intubation.
        (2) Proparacaine is used to desensitize the cornea.
        (3) Topical application of lidocaine (2.5%) and prilocaine (2.5%) in a eutectic mixture can be used to penetrate intact skin. After 45–60 minutes of contact time the skin is anesthetized enough for painless venipuncture.
        (4) Lidocaine (5%) transdermal patches do not desensitize the skin or interfere with normal motor function but may provide local analgesia by blocking abnormally functioning Na^+ channels and are used to treat dermal (e.g., incision) pain.
    b. **Infiltrative anesthesia.** Local anesthetics are used to desensitize tissues in a limited area (e.g., in order to debride and suture a laceration).
    c. **Peripheral nerve blocks are used to desensitize larger areas.** For example, a paravertebral nerve block would be used to desensitize the paralumbar fossa of a cow prior to a laparotomy.
    d. **Epidural injection** of a local anesthetic desensitizes the spinal cord or cauda equine and is useful for procedures such as caudal abdominal, pelvic limb, or perineal surgery.
    e. **Neurolytic anesthesia.** Ethyl alcohol, which is neurolytic, has been used in veterinary medicine to produce a prolonged nerve blockade in animals. Loss of nerve function can last as long as 1 year (i.e., as long as it takes the nerve to regenerate).

2. **Control of arrhythmias.** Lidocaine infused or injected IV is used to control premature ventricular contractions.

3. Constant rate IV infusion of lidocaine produces analgesia which facilitates general anesthesia and may be part of a multimodal approach to pain control postoperatively.

4. IV infusion of lidocaine in the horse may increase intestinal motility and be useful in treating some forms of hypomotility. The mechanism of action is unknown but thought to involve anti-inflammatory, analgesia, or altering the sympathetic inhibitory reflexes by suppressing the nerve transmission in afferent sensory pathways.

F. **Adverse effects** can occur if the plasma concentration of the local anesthetic reaches certain threshold values. The relative toxicity of the local anesthetics closely follows their anesthetic potency. For example, bupivacaine is toxic at a lower plasma concentration than lidocaine.

1. **Central nervous system (CNS).** Skeletal muscle twitches are the first sign of toxicity, but tonic-clonic seizures are imminent and often the first clinical sign.

2. **Cardiovascular system.** Signs of toxicity usually occur at higher plasma concentrations than those associated with CNS signs. Plasma concentration of lidocaine that produces cardiovascular toxicity may be lower for cats than in other species.
    a. Prolongation of the PR and QRS intervals may result from slowed impulse conduction.
    b. Hypotension and decreased myocardial strength (i.e., a negative inotropic effect) may occur.

3. **Methemoglobinemia** may occur following use of prilocaine or benzocaine in cats and rabbits.

4. **Tissue damage** from the injection of local anesthetics is rare. But, neurotoxicity and myotoxicity have been reported.

III. **INHALANT ANESTHETICS.** The primary site of action of these agents is the brain and spinal cord. Analgesia and unconsciousness are produced when the concentration of the anesthetic reaches a specific level in the CNS.

A. **Mechanism of action.** Because the physiologic mechanism of consciousness is unknown, it is not surprising that the mechanism of action of inhalant anesthetics is also unknown. The following are two current hypotheses regarding the mechanism of action of inhalant anesthetics:

1. **Single mechanism.** The observation that anesthesia has been produced using the gaseous phase of a wide variety of chemically unrelated compounds has led to the unitary hypothesis, which holds that all general anesthetics act through one basic mechanism.
   a. The fact that increasing the atmospheric pressure reverses the anesthetic effect of all inhalant anesthetics tested seems to support a single mechanism of action.
   b. In 1908, Meyer and Overton observed that anesthetic potency is correlated with the solubility of the drug in olive oil. This observation has been cited as support for a common mechanism of action.
2. **Multiple mechanisms.** Each anesthetic may have a unique mechanism of action.

B. **Pharmacokinetics.** Through ventilation of the lungs, an anesthetic partial pressure is established within the alveoli. **Increasing either the inspired concentration of anesthetic or alveolar ventilation will increase the partial pressure in the alveolus. The drug diffuses from the alveoli into the blood and is circulated to all parts of the body.** Anesthetic molecules move from areas of high partial pressure to areas of low partial pressure. Removal of anesthetic from the alveolus is affected by the solubility of the anesthetic in blood (i.e., the blood:gas partition coefficient), cardiac output, and the difference in partial pressure between the alveolus and the venous blood entering the lung.

1. **Minimum alveolar concentration (MAC). The MAC of an inhalant anesthetic is the alveolar concentration that prevents gross purposeful movement in 50% of patients in response to a standardized painful stimulus.** The MAC is used as a measure of potency. MAC values for the most frequently used inhalant anesthetics are listed in Table 6-2.

TABLE 6-2. Minimum Alveolar Concentration (MAC) for Inhalant Anesthetics

Anesthetic	Canine (%)	Feline (%)	Equine (%)
Isoflurane	1.28	1.28	1.28
	1.30	1.50	1.31
	1.31	1.61	1.43
	1.39–1.50	1.90	1.44
		2.21	1.64
Sevoflurane	2.10	2.58	2.31
	2.36	3.07	2.84
		3.41	
Desflurane	7.2	9.79	7.02
	7.68–8.19	10.27	8.06
	10.3		
Nitrous oxide	188	255	205
	222		
	297		

Each line represents the results of a published study.
Data from E. P. Steffey and K. R. Mama. Inhalation anesthetics. In *Lumb and Jones's Veterinary Anesthesia and Analgesia*, 4th ed., Edited by W. J. Tranquilli, J. C. Thurmon, and K. A. Grimm. Blackwell Publishing, Ames, IA, 2007.

TABLE 6-3. Inhalant Anesthetics in Decreasing order of Lipid Solubility

Inhalant Anesthetic	Oil/Gas Partition Coefficient	Potency Rank	Blood/Gas Partition Coefficient
Isoflurane	91.0	1	1.46
Sevoflurane	47.0	2	0.68
Desflurane	18.7	3	0.42
Nitrous oxide	1.4	4	0.47

(1) The anesthetic dose required to anesthetize 95% of animals is ~1.2–1.4 times the MAC. Surgical anesthesia levels are achieved by obtaining alveolar concentrations equal to 1.4–1.8 times the MAC.

(2) If two anesthetics are administered simultaneously, the MAC multiples are additive.

b. **Factors affecting MAC values**

(1) Hypothermia, severe hypotension, advanced age, pregnancy, severe hypoxemia, severe anemia, or the concurrent administration of certain drugs (e.g., opioids, tranquilizers) may decrease the MAC value for a particular patient.

(2) Hyperthermia or hyperthyroidism may increase the MAC value for a particular patient.

(3) The duration of anesthesia, patient gender, acid–base balance, and hypertension have no effect on the MAC value.

c. Relationship to lipid solubility. The Meyer–Overton Observation states that the oil:gas partition coefficient correlates inversely with anesthetic potency. The more lipid soluble the anesthetic, the lower the MAC and the higher the potency. Conversely, the lower the lipid solubility, the higher the MAC and the lower the potency (Table 6-3).

2. **Blood:gas partition coefficient.** The solubility of an agent is most commonly expressed in terms of a blood:gas partition coefficient. Solubility of the agent in blood correlates with the speed of induction and recovery. Table 6-3 contains the blood:gas partition coefficients for the inhalant anesthetics.

a. A high blood:gas partition coefficient indicates that the blood can hold a large amount of the anesthetic. Therefore, it will take longer to raise the alveolar partial pressure because the blood will keep absorbing the anesthetic as it is brought by ventilation to the alveolus.

b. In addition, it takes a long time before the blood is saturated with enough drug to cause diffusion of an adequate amount into the tissues. Therefore, induction and recovery are slow.

3. A plot of the ratio of concentration of anesthetic in the alveolus (F_A) to the concentration inspired (F_I) provides information about the various inhalant anesthetics (Figure 6-2).

C. **Administration**

1. By controlling the anesthetic concentration in the alveolus, the anesthetist is controlling the anesthetic concentration in the brain. Because the inhalant anesthetics move in the body by diffusion, it is necessary to administer high concentrations to the lungs initially in order to establish the necessary partial pressure in the brain.

2. Most inhalant anesthetics are liquid at room temperature and require a vaporizer to form a safe and accurate vapor concentration to be inhaled by the patient.

a. The boiling point indicates what physical state the drug will be in at room temperature. If the boiling point is below room temperature (20°C), then the drug exists as a gas at room temperature (Table 6-4).

b. The vapor pressure of a liquid compound indicates how volatile it is and the maximum concentration that can be achieved (see Table 6-4).

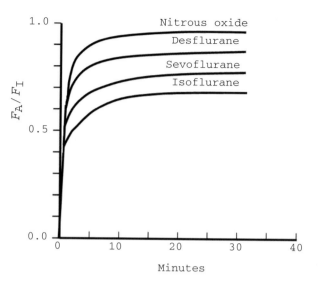

FIGURE 6-2. The rise in the alveolar anesthetic concentration (F_A) toward the inspired concentration (F_I). The less soluble the anesthetic, the faster the rise in the ratio toward 1.0. Nitrous oxide has a more rapid rise than desflurane because of its greater inspired concentration.

TABLE 6-4. Physical–Chemical Properties of the Inhalant Anesthetics

Inhalant Anesthetic	Boiling Point (°C)	Vapor Pressure 20°C (mm Hg)	Maximum Concentration 20°C (%)
Isoflurane	48	240	32
Sevoflurane	58.5	160	21
Desflurane	23.5	700	87
Nitrous oxide	−89	−	100

(1) The higher the vapor pressure, the easier it is to vaporize the compound.
(2) The maximum concentration that can be achieved is calculated by dividing the vapor pressure by the atmospheric pressure (760 mm Hg at sea level) and multiplying by 100.
(3) To determine the volume of gaseous anesthetic that will result from the vaporization of a liquid anesthetic, the following formula can be used:

$$\frac{(X)(SG)}{GMW} \times 22,400 = V_1, \text{ where}$$

X is volume of liquid anesthetic (mL); SG is specific gravity (g/mL); GMW is gram molecular weight (g/mole); and V_1 is the volume of anesthetic gas produced (mL).

The resultant volume (V_1) assumes standard conditions of 1 atm of pressure (760 mm Hg) and 0°C. To convert the volume to room temperature (20°C) requires Charles's law, which states that if pressure is held constant,

TABLE 6-5. Physical–Chemical Properties of the Liquid Inhalant Anesthetics

Inhalant Anesthetic	Molecular weight (g)	Specific Gravity at 20°C (g/mL)	Vapor (mL) from 1 mL of liquid 20°C
Isoflurane	185	1.49	195
Sevoflurane	200	1.52	183
Desflurane	168	1.47	210

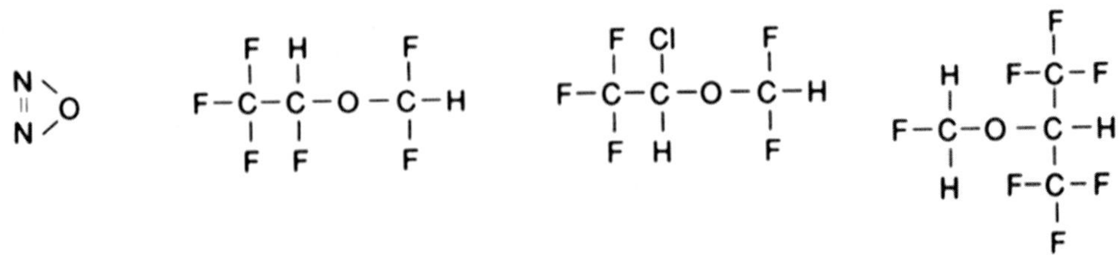

Nitrous oxide   **Desflurane**   **Isoflurane**   **Sevoflurane**

FIGURE 6-3. Chemical structures of the inhalant anesthetics.

volume and temperature will vary directly.

$$\frac{V_1}{T_1} = \frac{V_2}{T_2}, \text{ where}$$

V_1 is the volume of gas at 0°C (273°K); T_1 is 273°K; V_2 is the volume at room temperature; and T_2 is the room temperature (293°K, 20°C).

Table 6-5 contains the specific gravity, gram molecular weight, and volume at room temperature for some of the common inhalant anesthetics.

D. **Preparations.** When selecting an anesthetic agent, physical examination and clinical test results, as well as the underlying condition necessitating anesthesia, are factors that must be considered when selecting an anesthetic agent.

1. **Nitrous oxide**
   a. **Chemistry** (Figure 6-3). Nitrous oxide is an odorless, nonflammable, inorganic gas at room temperature. It will support combustion by dissociating into nitrogen and oxygen.
   b. **Pharmacokinetics**
      (1) Induction and recovery from anesthesia are rapid because of nitrous oxide's extremely low solubility—the body quickly becomes saturated with the inhaled concentration.
      (2) **Second gas effect.** The physical movement of nitrous oxide out of the alveolus into the blood stream tends to concentrate the other components of the alveolus, enhancing their absorption.
         (a) The second gas effect can be advantageous during mask induction, decreasing the length of time that the animal may struggle before unconsciousness and relaxation occur.
         (b) It may be a liability during recovery when the nitrous oxide in the blood quickly moves from the blood into the alveolus. This physical movement of gas dilutes the other components of the alveolus (e.g., oxygen) and may lead to diffusion hypoxia. To prevent hypoxemia, 100% oxygen should be administered to all patients for at least 5 minutes after nitrous oxide is discontinued.
   c. **Pharmacologic effects**
      (1) **The cardiopulmonary effects of nitrous oxide are minimal.**
         (a) Nitrous oxide directly depresses myocardial function. However, because nitrous oxide also directly stimulates the sympathetic nervous system, depression of myocardial function is minimal.
         (b) Nitrous oxide does not sensitize the myocardium to epinephrine.
      (2) **Hepatic and renal effects.** Liver and kidney function are unaffected by nitrous oxide.
      (3) **Effects during pregnancy and delivery.** Nitrous oxide readily crosses the placenta; hypoxemia may develop if a neonate is allowed to breathe room air immediately after cesarean delivery.
   d. **Therapeutic uses.** Nitrous oxide is not a very potent anesthetic; **surgical anesthesia is not obtainable in animals with nitrous oxide alone.** Concentrations of

50–66% are commonly used and the remainder of the anesthetic dose is provided by some other inhalant drug (e.g., isoflurane). The analgesic effect of nitrous oxide allows the anesthetist to administer lower concentration of more potent anesthetics, minimizing the cardiopulmonary effects of these agents.

 e. **Administration.** Nitrous oxide is administered quantitatively using flowmeters. A mixture of oxygen and nitrous oxide is determined by the respective flowmeters so that the desired percent of nitrous oxide is delivered to the anesthetic circuit. For example, if the ratio of oxygen to nitrous oxide is 1:1, then the mixture consists of 50% nitrous oxide and 50% oxygen.

 f. **Adverse effects**

   (1) **Hypoxemia** in anesthetized animals is frequently the result of ventilation-perfusion (V/Q) mismatch in the lung. A high percentage of inhaled oxygen usually prevents the arterial oxygen from becoming dangerously low, whereas a low percentage predisposes animals to hypoxemia.

     (a) Large domestic animals frequently develop V/Q mismatch during anesthesia/recumbency, and reducing the inhaled oxygen percentage with typical concentrations of nitrous oxide further predisposes them to hypoxemia. Therefore, **nitrous oxide is seldom used in adult horses and cattle because it may increase the incidence and severity of hypoxemia.**

     (b) Administration of nitrous oxide at concentrations greater than 70% is discouraged because it places any anesthetized animal at risk of developing hypoxemia.

   (2) **Distention of gas-filled spaces.** The blood solubility of nitrous oxide is 35 times greater than that of nitrogen. Because room air is 79% nitrogen, nitrous oxide will accumulate in and distend closed, gas-filled spaces (such as those that occur with pneumothorax or intestinal blockage). Nitrous oxide is contraindicated in animals with pockets of trapped gas.

   (3) **Pernicious anemia and neurologic dysfunction** have been reported in humans following chronic exposure to nitrous oxide, which inhibits the activity of vitamin B_{12}-dependent enzymes in the body.

2. **Isoflurane** is a halogenated methyl ethyl ether inhalant anesthetic cleared for veterinary use in dogs and horses.

 a. **Chemistry**

   (1) **Structure.** Isoflurane is halogenated ether (see Figure 6-3).

   (2) **Characteristics**

     (a) A colorless liquid with a characteristic, pungent odor. It is a stable compound that does not require additives to maintain shelf life; however, it is supplied in a brown bottle.

     (b) The specific gravity and the vapor pressure are similar to those of halothane, which is rarely used today.

 b. **Pharmacokinetics**

   (1) **Induction and recovery.** Because of its low blood:gas partition coefficient, isoflurane rapidly induces anesthesia, patients change levels of anesthesia quickly, and recovery is rapid.

   (2) **Elimination.** Metabolism of isoflurane is very low (~0.17% is metabolized); consequently, it has not been associated with organ toxicity. Thus, isoflurane can be considered for anesthesia in animals with hepatic or renal disease.

 c. **Pharmacologic effects with organ toxicity**

   (1) **Cardiovascular effects**

     (a) Isoflurane depresses cardiovascular function and decreases arterial blood pressure in a dose-dependent manner because of a decreased stroke volume and decreased systemic vascular resistance. However, isoflurane-anesthetized animals maintain a higher cardiac output at deeper levels of anesthesia than halothane-anesthetized animals because the decrease in stroke volume is counteracted by an increase in heart rate.

     (b) Heart rhythm remains relatively normal.

     (c) Catecholamine sensitization and resultant cardiac arrhythmias occur with isoflurane, but to a lesser extent than with other inhalant anesthetics.

(2) Ventilatory effects. In most species, the respiratory rate and tidal volume are decreased, leading to an increase in the arterial carbon dioxide partial pressure. Apnea occurs in most species at around 2.5 MAC.

(3) CNS effects

    (a) Isoflurane is a dose-dependent CNS depressant that produces general anesthesia by an unknown mechanism.

    (b) Body temperature usually decreases unless a supplemental heat source is provided.

    (c) Cerebral blood flow is unchanged at doses of less than 1.2 MAC. Cerebral blood flow increases at high multiples of MAC, but the vessels are still responsive to carbon dioxide. Thus, controlled ventilation to decrease the arterial carbon dioxide partial pressure will counteract the cerebral vasodilation of deep levels of isoflurane anesthesia.

(4) Muscular effects. Isoflurane potentiates the nondepolarizing muscle relaxant drugs (e.g., atracurium).

(5) Hepatic effects. Hepatic function is reversibly depressed. No cases of hepatic necrosis resulting from the use of isoflurane have been reported.

(6) Renal effects. Renal function is reversibly depressed, causing a decrease in renal blood flow, glomerular filtration rate, and urine production.

    d. Therapeutic uses. Isoflurane is widely used in dogs, cats, birds, and horses and is not contraindicated in any species. It is the current agent of choice for animals with suspected increases in intracranial pressure.

    e. Adverse effects. Because of its inertness, isoflurane has not been associated with any organ toxicities. Malignant hyperthermia can be triggered by isoflurane.

3. Desflurane is a new inhalant anesthetic agent that is approved for use in humans. Its use in veterinary medicine has been very limited.

    a. Chemistry (see Figure 6-3). Desflurane's fluorinated methyl ethyl ether structure is similar to that of isoflurane.

    b. Pharmacokinetics. Induction and recovery are rapid with desflurane, which has a blood:gas partition coefficient similar to that of nitrous oxide. Compared with other inhalants that are currently in use, desflurane's potency is low.

    c. Biotransformation in the body is very low in humans at 0.02% metabolized.

    d. Pharmacologic effects. Cardiovascular effects are similar to those produced by isoflurane.

    e. Administration. The vapor pressure of desflurane is high; therefore, a sophisticated vaporizer is necessary in order to accurately control the vaporization.

4. Sevoflurane has been approved for veterinary use in the dog.

    a. Chemistry. Sevoflurane is polyfluorinated methyl isopropyl ether inhalant anesthetic (see Figure 6-3).

    (1) Sevoflurane is degraded by many carbon dioxide absorbents (i.e., soda lime) and the resulting alkene (pentafluoroisopropenyl fluoromethyl ether, or compound A) has been shown to be nephrotoxic in rats. **Renal damage related to clinical sevoflurane usage in dogs has not been reported** and safety studies in this species found no toxicity.

    (2) Desiccated soda lime in an anesthetic machine will react with sevoflurane and result in excessive heat production and formation of carbon monoxide. Extremely rare cases of spontaneous fire in the breathing circuit of human anesthetic machines have been reported.

    b. Pharmacokinetics

    (1) Induction and recovery. Sevoflurane has a low blood:gas partition coefficient; therefore, induction and recovery are rapid.

    (2) Elimination. Sevoflurane is primarily exhaled but 2–5% is metabolized by the liver to fluoride ion and hexafluoroisopropanol (HFIP). The HFIP is rapidly conjugated with glucuronic acid and eliminated by the kidney.

    c. Pharmacologic effects

    (1) Cardiovascular effects

    (a) Cardiac output is decreased due to a decrease in stroke volume and depression of myocardial contractility.

(b) Dose-dependent decrease in arterial blood pressure due to the decreased stroke volume and, in some cases, a decrease in peripheral vascular resistance.

(c) Renal blood flow and glomerular filtration rate decrease in a dose-dependent manner. These effects are rapidly reversed after anesthesia.

(d) Hepatic blood flow is decreased and hepatic clearance of drugs is reduced. All potent inhalant anesthetics have the potential to cause hepatocellular damage from reduced oxygen delivery. Hepatotoxicity from sevoflurane has not been reported.

(2) Ventilation is depressed in a dose-dependent fashion.

(a) At low doses, the tidal volume decreases but the respiratory frequency remains normal.

(b) At high doses, the respiratory frequency also decreases.

(c) Hypercapnia (increased $PaCO_2$) occurs but the normal increase in minute ventilation from such a stimulant does not occur with sevoflurane anesthesia and ventilation is often controlled during anesthesia.

d. Malignant hyperthermia can be triggered by sevoflurane.

IV. INJECTABLE ANESTHETICS

A. Barbiturates and barbituric acid derivatives

1. General information

a. Chemistry. Barbituric acid is formed by combining urea and malonic acid.

(1) Substitutions at the various carbon and nitrogen atoms produce drugs with varying characteristics (Figures 6-4 and 6-5).

(a) Oxybarbiturates have an oxygen molecule bound to C2.

(b) Thiobarbiturates have a sulfur molecule bound to C2. Thiobarbiturates are generally more lipid soluble and more highly protein bound than the oxybarbiturates.

(2) The resulting weak acids are supplied as sodium salts. Solutions consisting of barbiturate salts dissolved in water are very alkaline (pH 10–11.5).

b. Mechanism of action

(1) Barbiturates bind to γ-aminobutyric acid (GABA)-gated Cl^- channels and increase the frequency that these Cl^- channels open resulting in hyperpolarization of the neurons.

Drug	X	R_1	R_2	R_3	Duration of action
Pentobarbital	O	Ethyl	1-Methylbutyl	H	Short
Phenobarbital	O	Ethyl	Phenyl	H	Long
Methohexital	O	Allyl	1-Methyl-2-pentynyl	CH_3	Ultrashort
Thiopental	S	Ethyl	1-Methylbutyl	H	Ultrashort

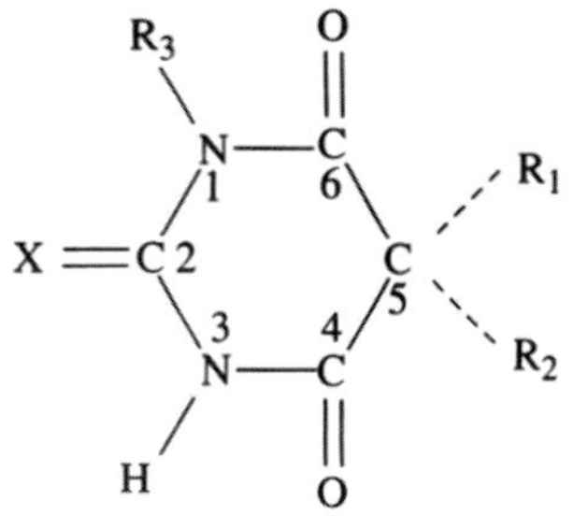

FIGURE 6-4. Barbiturates commonly used in veterinary medicine.

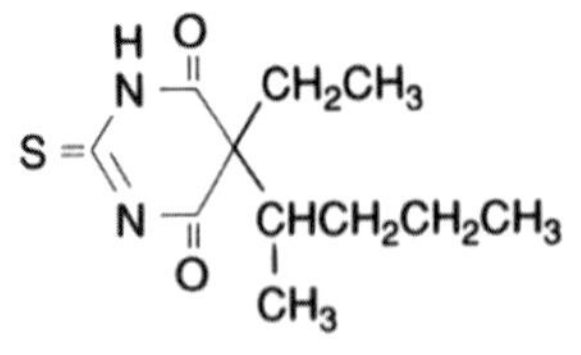

Thiopental 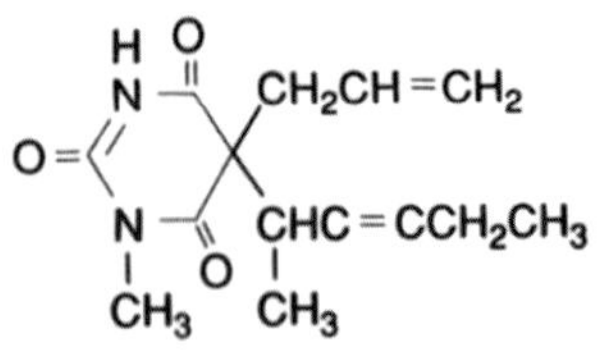 **Methohexital**

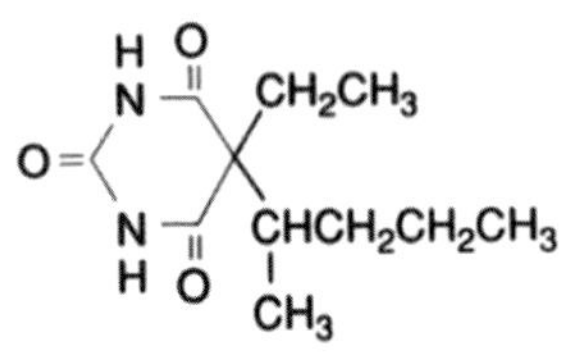

Pentobarbital 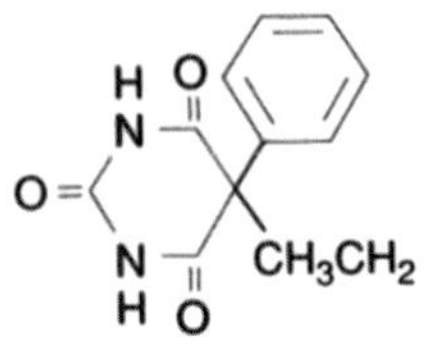 **Phenobarbital**

FIGURE 6-5. Chemical structures of the injectable anesthetics.

(2) Barbiturates decrease the excitatory effects of the neurotransmitter glutamate.

(3) They suppress synaptic transmission by inhibiting Na^+ and Ca^{2+} channels and opening K^+ channels.

c. Pharmacokinetics

(1) Distribution depends on the lipid solubility of the agent, protein binding, and ionization. Only non-protein-bound and nonionized molecules cross the blood–brain barrier.

  (a) Lipid solubility

   i. Oxybarbiturates are less lipid soluble and slower to enter the brain than thiobarbiturates, but their duration of action is longer.

   ii. Thiobarbiturates are rapid in onset because of their high lipid solubility and ultrashort in duration because they redistribute in the body to muscle tissue (Figure 6-6).

  (b) Protein binding parallels lipid solubility. Barbiturates bind to plasma proteins. Decreased protein binding (e.g., as a result of uremia or hypoalbuminemia) will increase the clinical effect of a dose of a thiobarbiturate.

  (c) Ionization. The degree of ionization in the blood stream depends on the pK_a of the particular drug and the pH of the blood. The nonionized form of the drug has greater lipid solubility and will penetrate the CNS quickly.

(2) Metabolism and redistribution (see Figure 6-6) are important in determining early recovery from anesthesia with these drugs.

  (a) Initially, metabolism is quite high when plasma levels are elevated and delivery of the drug to the liver is high, but after plasma levels decrease, the metabolism of these drugs is quite slow. The fat compartment of the body slowly accumulates these drugs because of their high lipid solubility; however, blood flow to fat is low and rapid redistribution to this compartment does not occur (see Figure 6-6). Repeat doses of thiobarbiturates may result in high drug concentrations in the fat compartment. When drug administration is stopped, the accumulated stores return to the blood stream, resulting in a prolonged elevation of plasma drug levels and prolonged recovery from anesthesia.

d. Pharmacologic effects

(1) Cardiovascular effects. IV injection in the normovolemic patient causes transient hypotension and an increase in heart rate.

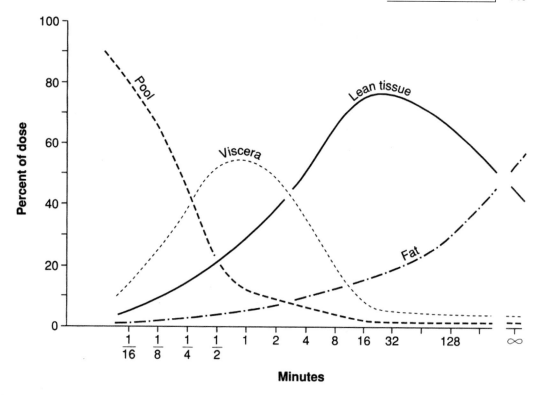

FIGURE 6-6. Distribution of a thiopental dose following IV injection. Initially, the drug is primarily in the central blood pool, but it rapidly redistributes to the viscera, lean tissue (muscle), and adipose tissue. At the time of recovery (10–15 minutes postinjection), most of the drug is in the lean tissue compartment.

    (2) Ventilatory effects. Transient apnea following the IV injection of these compounds occurs fairly commonly as a result of depression of the respiratory centers in the brain stem.

    (3) CNS effects
        (a) Barbiturates cause a dose-dependent depression of the CNS function.
            i. Low doses may cause sedation or excitement.
            ii. Moderate doses cause general anesthesia.
            iii. High doses lead to profound CNS depression.
            iv. Overdoses cause apnea and, eventually, cardiovascular depression and death.
        (b) Barbiturates decrease cerebral blood flow, cerebral oxygen consumption, cerebral blood volume, and intracranial pressure.

    (4) Effects during pregnancy and delivery. Placental transfer of barbiturates is rapid after IV injection.

    (5) Analgesic effects. Barbiturates are not analgesic in subanesthetic doses. There is evidence that some barbiturates are hyperalgesic at subanesthetic doses.

2. Preparations and therapeutic uses
    a. Ultrashort-acting barbiturates are very lipid soluble; therefore, their onset of action is rapid and their duration of action is short (10–30 minutes).
        (1) Thiopental. Thiopental is administered by IV injection for short duration anesthesia in dogs and cats. In large domestic animals (e.g., horses, cattle), the thiobarbiturates are commonly administered with guaifenesin, a central acting muscle relaxant (see V D).

(a) Therapeutic uses

i. Thiobarbiturates are considered one of the drugs of choice for induction of anesthesia in animals with suspected increased intracranial pressure.

ii. The plasma $t_{1/2}$ is 3–4 hours.

iii. These agents can be used for maintenance of anesthesia; however, repeat doses may lead to slow recovery because of saturation of the redistribution sites.

iv. Thiobarbiturates are safe for induction of anesthesia for cesarean section because these drugs redistribute rapidly in the dam and fetus. By the time the fetus is delivered, the fetal blood levels are quite low.

(b) Adverse effects

i. Prolonged recovery. Plasma clearance of these drugs is prolonged in greyhounds. Therefore, they experience a long duration of effect and slow recovery. Use of thiobarbiturates in greyhounds and other sight hounds is not recommended.

ii. Cardiac arrhythmias may occur if a large IV dose of a thiobarbiturate is administered rapidly. Premature ventricular contractions are most common. The ventricular arrhythmia is usually short in duration but potentially detrimental to the patient.

iii. Allergic reactions to these drugs have been reported but are extremely rare.

iv. Local irritation. Perivascular injection may lead to necrosis and sloughing of substantial amounts of tissue. Use of dilute solutions (2.5% thiopental), injection of saline into the area, and/or injection of lidocaine to dilute the drug and alter the pH may help prevent tissue irritation.

(2) Methohexital is more rapidly metabolized than the thiobarbiturates and the other oxybarbiturates because of its higher lipid solubility, which results from the addition of a methyl group. It is more potent than thiopental.

(a) Therapeutic uses

i. Like the thiobarbiturates, methohexital is safe for use during cesarean section.

ii. It is safe for use in greyhounds and other sight hounds. Because of methohexital's rapid redistribution and metabolism by the liver, recovery is quick.

(b) Adverse effects. Methohexital is more likely than the thiobarbiturates to cause a period of excitement during induction and recovery.

b. Short-acting barbiturates (e.g., pentobarbital) are less lipid soluble and have a longer duration of action (30–60 minutes) than the ultrashort-acting agents.

(1) Therapeutic uses

(a) Pentobarbital, which has a very low margin of safety, is the primary ingredient of euthanasia agents.

(b) Pentobarbital is occasionally used for IV anesthesia in dogs, cats, pigs, and small ruminants.

(c) Also used for seizure control when a long-acting drug is desired.

(2) Adverse effects

(a) Low doses administered IV may cause an excitement phase characterized by whining, paddling, and incoordination.

(b) Recovery is slow and characterized by paddling of the limbs and incoordination. Sedation, physical assistance, or both may be required to ensure a smooth recovery.

c. Long-acting barbiturates (e.g., phenobarbital) are the least lipid soluble and the slowest in their onset of action, but they have a long duration of action (6–12 hours). **Phenobarbital is used primarily as an anticonvulsant at subanesthetic doses**, not as a general anesthetic (see Chapter 4).

B. Cyclohexylamines

1. **Dissociative anesthesia, which is characterized by analgesia and superficial sleep, is a term used to describe the CNS state produced by these drugs. Different levels of the CNS seem to become dissociated from one another—the EEG reveals depression of the thalamoneocortical portion of the brain and enhanced activity in the limbic system.**
   a. **Many reflexes (e.g., palpebral, laryngeal, pharyngeal) are maintained** and the skeletal muscles of the eyelid are contracted, opening the orbit.
   b. **Somatic analgesia is good, but visceral analgesia is poor.**
   c. **Muscle relaxation is poor.** Animals are described as cataleptic, a state characterized by rigidity and partial extension of the limbs.

2. **Pharmacologic effects**
   a. **Cardiovascular effects.** Cyclohexylamines directly depress cardiovascular function; however, in healthy animals, they increase sympathetic tone, masking the direct effect and resulting in overall stimulation of cardiovascular function.
      (1) The heart rate is maintained or increased.
      (2) The blood pressure and cardiac output are increased.
   b. **Ventilatory effects.** Ventilation is depressed, causing the arterial O_2 tension to decrease and arterial CO_2 tension to increase. Cats and many other species develop an apneustic breathing pattern, characterized by an inspiratory hold and a very short expiratory pause.
   c. **CNS effects**
      (1) Cerebral blood flow and intracranial pressure are increased by these anesthetic drugs.
      (2) Dilation of pupils occurs.
   d. **Effects during pregnancy and delivery.** These drugs rapidly cross the placenta and affect the fetus.

3. **Preparations include ketamine and tiletamine.**
   a. Ketamine is approved by the FDA for use in cats, but numerous other species have been safely anesthetized with ketamine. It is a Schedule III drug.
      (1) Chemistry. Ketamine is commercially available as an aqueous solution with a pH of 3.5. The solution contains a racemic mixture of the two isomers of ketamine.
      (2) Mechanism of action. Ketamine inhibits the polysynaptic actions of the excitatory neurotransmitters acetylcholine (ACh) and L-glutamate in the spinal cord. It is a potent noncompetitive antagonist of the N-methyl-D-aspartate (NMDA) receptor complex.
      (3) Pharmacokinetics. Ketamine is metabolized by the cytochrome P450 enzymes of the liver, and some of the metabolites (e.g., norketamine) have anesthetic activity. Norketamine is one-fifth to one-third as potent as ketamine and slowly hydroxylated and then conjugated with glucuronide to form a water-soluble compound that is excreted by the kidneys. The metabolites and a small amount of unchanged ketamine are excreted in the urine. The cat may excrete more unchanged ketamine in the urine than other species. The plasma $t_{1/2}$ in the cat, calf, and horse is 1–1.5 hours.
      (4) Administration
         (a) Ketamine can be administered IM or IV to cats, dogs, small ruminants, and swine. In adult horses and cattle, it is only administered IV.
         (b) Ketamine combinations. Animals usually receive a tranquilizer (e.g., acepromazine, xylazine, diazepam) along with ketamine in order to provide muscle relaxation.
            i. Xylazine, guaifenesin, or both are frequently administered to horses prior to administration of ketamine. Both xylazine and guaifenesin provide muscle relaxation.
            ii. Diazepam, midazolam, or xylazine are frequently used with ketamine in dogs and cats in order to prevent seizures and provide

muscle relaxation. When xylazine and ketamine are administered together, the decreased heart rate and cardiac output from xylazine are partially reversed. But, arterial blood pressure, systemic vascular resistance, and myocardial oxygen consumption also increase in these animals. Because of these cardiovascular effects, xylazine–ketamine combinations should only be used in healthy patients and not administered to dogs or cats with reduced cardiopulmonary reserve.

  iii. Guaifenesin, diazepam, or xylazine may be used in combination with ketamine in pigs, cattle, and goats.

  (5) Adverse effects

  (a) Seizures are common in horses and dogs following administration of ketamine alone.

  (b) Profuse salivation may occur in cats. Laryngeal and pharyngeal reflexes are present, but they are not active enough to prevent life-threatening airway obstruction. Anticholinergic drugs administered before or along with ketamine will prevent excessive salivation.

  (c) Corneal ulceration. Because the eyes remain open during anesthesia, the cornea may dry out and ulcerate if not protected by an ophthalmic ointment.

  (d) Intraocular pressure increases due to increases in extraocular muscle tone. Ketamine should be avoided in cases with cornea injuries and ulcers.

  (e) Cerebral blood flow and oxygen consumption increases with ketamine. Intracranial and cerebral spinal fluid pressures increase. Ketamine should be avoided in cases with intracranial hypertension (e.g., head trauma or intracranial tumors).

b. Telazol® contains equal amounts of tiletamine, a cyclohexylamine, and zolazepam, a benzodiazepine tranquilizer. It is a Schedule III drug.

  (1) Therapeutic uses

  (a) Telazol® is used for anesthesia of short duration in dogs and cats. It is very useful in the feral cat or uncooperative dog because it can be administered IM, has a rapid onset of action, and the volume of injection is small.

  (b) Telazol® is used in many other domestic and exotic species.

    i. It has been used for short-term anesthesia in horses following administration of xylazine and butorphanol.

    ii. It is combined with xylazine and ketamine for use in pigs.

    iii. It may be used alone or in combination with xylazine in small ruminants.

  1. Administration. Telazol® can be administered IM, SC, or IV.

  2. Adverse effects

  (a) Recoveries are slow and smooth in cats, but in dogs, recoveries are sometimes accompanied by muscle tremors, paddling, and whining. Rough recoveries may occur in dogs because they metabolize the zolazepam more rapidly than the tiletamine.

  (b) Hyperthermia may result from the increased muscles activity.

  (c) Tachycardia may occur in dogs.

  3. Contraindications

  (a) Cyclohexylamines may increase intraocular pressure by inducing contraction of the extraocular muscles; therefore, they are contraindicated in animals with corneal ulcers or lacerations.

  (b) They are contraindicated in animals with head trauma or a space-occupying mass in the brain.

C. Propofol

  1. Chemistry. Propofol, a substituted isopropylphenol, is an alkylphenol derivative that is unrelated to any other anesthetic drug currently in use. It is formulated in a 1% aqueous emulsion containing 10% soybean oil, 1.2% egg lecithin, and 2.25% glycerol.

2. **Mechanism of action.** Propofol induces anesthesia by activating $GABA_A$ receptors.
3. **Pharmacokinetics**
   a. **Induction.** The onset of action is rapid and induction is smooth. Repeated doses in dogs do not accumulate.
   b. **Distribution.** Propofol is highly protein bound.
   c. **Metabolism**
      (1) The duration of anesthesia following a single IV injection is very short (2–10 minutes) because propofol is rapidly metabolized by glucuronide synthase in the liver. Cats have much less glucuronide synthase with which to metabolize propofol; therefore, prolonged infusion or consecutive day injections may not be tolerated.
      (2) The lungs have been shown to remove a significant amount of propofol from the circulating blood and may participate in drug metabolism as well.
      (3) The plasma $t_{1/2}$ is 1–2 hours.
4. **Therapeutic uses**
   a. The milky white emulsion is used primarily in dogs and cats for IV induction of anesthesia for short procedures or prior to inhalant anesthesia.
   b. Rapid redistribution and metabolism result in quick recovery of psychomotor function; therefore, propofol is ideal for outpatient cases.
   c. Propofol decreases cerebral blood flow and cerebral oxygen consumption; therefore, it is safe for use in animals with head trauma or increased intracranial pressure.
5. **Adverse effects**
   a. Myoclonic twitching and limb paddling are sometimes seen in dogs following propofol administration.
   b. Direct myocardial depression is due to a decrease in $[Ca^{2+}]_i$ and myofilament sensitivity to Ca^{2+}. Peripheral vasodilation, and venodilation occur, causing blood pressure and cardiac output to decrease. Propofol must be used cautiously in traumatized animals and those with hypovolemia or impaired left ventricular function.
   c. Transient apnea following a rapid, IV bolus dose is common is dogs and cats.
   d. **Heinz body formation.** Phenolic compounds may cause oxidative damage to erythrocytes in cats. Daily infusions resulted in the formation of Heinz bodies, anorexia, and malaise.
   e. **Septicemia.** Propofol's vehicle (soybean oil, egg lecithin, and glycerol) is supportive of bacterial growth; therefore, great care must be taken to avoid contamination of the drug prior to injection or septicemia may result.

D. **Etomidate** is a sedative hypnotic nonbarbiturate drug of ultrashort duration. It has a wide margin of safety, with a therapeutic index of 16 (as compared with thiopental, which has a therapeutic index of 4–7).

1. **Pharmacokinetics.** Etomidate undergoes rapid hepatic hydrolysis and does not accumulate, even following repeated doses. The plasma $t_{1/2}$ is 3 hours.
2. **Pharmacologic effects**
   a. Etomidate causes minimal depression of cardiovascular and respiratory function.
   b. It decreases cerebral blood flow, metabolic rate, and oxygen consumption.
   c. Etomidate inhibits adrenal steroidogenesis by inhibiting 11β-hydroxylase, reducing the normal increase in plasma cortisol levels associated with anesthesia and surgery for up to 3 hours. The clinical importance of this inhibition is unknown but has been associated with an increase in mortality of human patients with septicemia.
3. **Mechanism of action.** Etomidate is a short-acting hypnotic, which appears to have GABA-like effects. Unlike the barbiturates, etomidate reduces subcortical inhibition at the onset of hypnosis while inducing neocortical sleep. A part of the action of etomidate consists of a depression of the activity and reactivity of the brain stem reticular formation.

4. Therapeutic uses. Etomidate is administered IV to dogs and cats for induction of anesthesia for short procedures or prior to inhalant anesthesia. The commercial preparation is very hypertonic and may cause pain and hemolysis upon IV injection.

5. Adverse effects

   a. Myoclonus and excitement can occur either on induction or recovery. These effects can be prevented by adequate preinduction sedation with a tranquilizer or opioid drug.

   b. Etomidate inhibits myocardial contractility. The direct negative inotropic effect of etomidate results from a decrease in myocardial Ca^{2+} levels by inhibiting Ca^{2+} influx.

V. PREANESTHETIC MEDICATONS

V. **PREANESTHETIC MEDICATONS** facilitate anesthesia and surgery by improving the rapidity and smoothness of induction, reducing anxiety, providing analgesia and amnesia, and compensating for some of the side effects of anesthesia (e.g., salivation, bradycardia).

A. **Opioids** (see Chapter 4) are administered to provide analgesia.

B. **Tranquilizers** (see Chapter 4) provide preoperative sedation and amnesia and help to prevent or counteract the CNS stimulation caused by some anesthetics.

C. **Anticholinergic agents** (see Chapter 2) prevent profuse salivation and bradycardia.

D. **Central muscle relaxants**

   1. Guaifenesin is a central acting muscle relaxant that is used IV with thiobarbiturates and ketamine for induction of anesthesia in horses, cattle, and swine.

   a. Chemistry. Guaifenesin is a white powder that is dissolved in water, 0.9% saline, or 5% dextrose to produce a final drug concentration of 5–10%.

   b. Mechanism of action. Guaifenesin is a centrally acting muscle relaxant that blocks polysynaptic reflexes and depresses impulse transmission by internuncial neurons in the spinal cord.

   c. Pharmacokinetics. Guaifenesin is metabolized by the liver, and the conjugate metabolites are excreted by the kidney. The plasma $t_{1/2}$ is 60–80 minutes.

   d. Pharmacologic effects

   (1) Cardiovascular effects. Guaifenesin decreases arterial blood pressure in horses but has minimal effects on cardiac output or heart rate.

   (2) Respiratory effects. Diaphragmatic function and respiration are minimally depressed.

   (3) Analgesic effects. Sedation accompanies the muscle relaxation, but analgesia is minimal.

   (4) Effects during pregnancy and delivery. It readily crosses the placenta but does not adversely affect the fetus.

   e. Administration. Guaifenesin is usually mixed with either a thiobarbiturate or ketamine. This combination is then rapidly infused into the jugular vein of a tranquilized horse to induce anesthesia.

   f. Adverse effects

   (1) Perivascular injection causes acute inflammation, necrosis, and sloughing at the injection site.

   (2) Prolonged infusions will lead to drug accumulation in the body and extremely long recovery times.

   (3) Urticaria is occasionally seen in horses following guaifenesin administration. This effect is thought to be a drug-induced allergic reaction.

   (4) Overdoses can cause bradycardia, hypotension, extensor rigidity, apneustic breathing, and cardiac arrest.

(5) Concentrations exceeding 10% in cattle or 12.5% in horses are associated with intravascular hemolysis and hemoglobinuria.

2. Methocarbamol. It is a guaifenesin-analog, which bears pharmacologic effects very similar to guaifenesin.

a. Therapeutic uses. It is usually not used as a preanesthetic; instead, it is used as an adjunctive therapy for acute inflammatory and traumatic conditions of the skeletal muscle, for example, to relax muscle in canine intervertebral disk disease and equine acute rhabdomyolysis, and to reduce muscle spasms, particularly in pyrethroid toxicity.

b. Pharmacokinetics. It is used orally and IV. Limited pharmacokinetics data are available in animals.

(1) It is well absorbed from the GI tract when given orally. T_{max} in humans is 2 hours.

(2) It is widely distributed in tissues, including CNS. Approximately 50% is bound by plasma proteins.

(3) It is metabolized by hepatic cytochrome P450 enzymes. Methocarbamol metabolites are excreted mostly in the urine along with a small amount of parent compound.

(4) The plasma elimination $t_{1/2}$ of methocarbamol in humans is 1–2 hours.

c. Adverse effects. The side effects of methocarbamol are very similar to those of guaifenesin. It is irritating, and thus should avoid extravasation. Other routes of parenteral administration are prohibited.

SUGGESTED READING

Evers AS, Maze M. 2004. *Anesthetic Pharmacology: Physiologic Principles and Clinical Practice.* Philadelphia, PA: Churchill Livingston.

Plumb DC. 2005. *Veterinary Drug Handbook.* 5th ed. Ames, IA: Blackwell Publishing.

Stoelting RK, Hillier SC. 2006. *Pharmacology and Physiology in Anesthetic Practice.* 4th ed. Philadelphia, PA: Lippincott Williams & Wilkins.

Tranquilli WJ, Thurmon JC, Grimm KA. 2007. *Lumb and Jones' Veterinary Anesthesia and Analgesia.* 4th ed. Ames, IA: Blackwell Publishing.

STUDY QUESTIONS

DIRECTIONS: Each of the numbered items or incomplete statements in this section is followed by answers or by completions of the statement. Select the **one** lettered answer or completion that is **best** in each case.

1. What is the first indicator of local anesthetic toxicity?

(A) Skeletal muscle twitching
(B) Tonic-clonic convulsions
(C) Hypotension
(D) Cardiac arrhythmias
(E) Vomiting

2. Which inhalant anesthetic has the lowest vapor pressure?

(A) Isoflurane
(B) Sevoflurane
(C) Desflurane
(D) Nitrous Oxide
(E) Propofol

3. If several dogs are breathing 50% nitrous oxide, they would probably all be responsive to a painful stimuli. If the MAC of nitrous oxide is ~200%, how much isoflurane would have to be administered to render 50% of these dogs unresponsive to a painful stimulus?

(A) 1.00 MAC isoflurane
(B) 0.75 MAC isoflurane
(C) 0.66 MAC isoflurane
(D) 0.50 MAC isoflurane
(E) 0.25 MAC isoflurane

4. Inhalant anesthetics vary in how quickly the alveolar concentration (blood concentration) will approximate the inspired concentration. Which one of the following anesthetics has the fastest rate of rise in alveolar concentration?

(A) Sevoflurane
(B) Desflurane
(C) Nitrous oxide
(D) Isoflurane

5. Which one of the following anesthetics is an NMDA receptor antagonist?

(A) Thiopental
(B) Propofol
(C) Etomidate
(D) Ketamine
(E) Guaifenesin

6. Which one of the following drugs inhibits steroidogenesis in the adrenal gland for several hours after administration?

(A) Thiopental
(B) Propofol
(C) Etomidate
(D) Ketamine
(E) Guaifenesin

7. Which injectable anesthetic is best suited for use in a small animal requiring an outpatient procedure?

(A) Propofol
(B) Pentobarbital
(C) Thiopental
(D) Tiletamine-zolazepam
(E) Guaifenesin

8. Which of the following drugs is a highly lipid-soluble oxybarbiturate with an ultrashort duration of action?

(A) Methohexital
(B) Pentobarbital
(C) Thiopental
(D) Phenobarbital

9. Which local anesthetic is used topically on the cornea of animals?

(A) Lidocaine
(B) Proparacaine
(C) Bupivacaine
(D) Procaine
(E) Mepivacaine

ANSWERS AND EXPLANATIONS

1. The answer is A.
Skeletal muscle twitching is the first recognizable sign of local anesthetic toxicity. Twitching of the skeletal muscles may rapidly progress to tonic-clonic convulsions. Cardiovascular toxicity (as manifested by hypotension and arrhythmias) usually occurs at a higher dose than that necessary to produce neurologic toxicity. Gastrointestinal signs (e.g., vomiting) are not usually associated with local anesthetic toxicity.

2. The answer is B.
Sevoflurane has a vapor pressure of 160 mmHg. The vapor pressures of isoflurane and desflurane are 240 and 664 mm Hg, respectively. Nitrous oxide is a gas at room temperature and as such by definition does not have a vapor pressure. Propofol is an injectable liquid anesthetic not an inhalant.

3. The answer is B.
The MAC of nitrous oxide is ~200%. Thus, animals breathing 50% nitrous oxide will be receiving 0.25 MAC (50%/200% = 0.25). Simultaneously, inhaled anesthetics are additive; therefore, another 0.75 MAC would be required to reach a level that would be equivalent to 1.0 MAC. By definition, this is the MAC that would render 50% of the animals unresponsive to painful stimuli.

4. The answer is C.
Nitrous oxide is the least soluble gas in current veterinary use; therefore, the alveolar concentration quickly approaches the inspired concentration. In other words, the ratio of the concentration of anesthetic in the alveolus to that inhaled ($F_A:F_I$) approaches 1.0 quickly.

5. The answer is D.
Ketamine is an antagonist at the NMDA receptor and is responsible for most of this drug's anesthetic and analgesic effects. Thiopental, propofol, and etomidate bind to the GABA receptor and result in neuron inhibition through hyperpolarization of the membrane. Guaifenesin is not an anesthetic at all but rather a central acting muscle relaxant and is thought to disrupt nerve impulse transmission at the level of the internuncial neurons of the spinal cord.

6. Answer is C.
Etomidate causes a dose-dependent inhibition of the conversion of cholesterol to cortisol. 11β-Hydroxylase appears to be the enzyme inhibited by this drug. This may be important in patients that need an intact cortisol response for survival, such as sepsis. The other drugs have no inhibitor effect on the adrenal gland.

7. The answer is A.
Propofol is rapidly redistributed and metabolized in the body; therefore, the recovery time for the return of normal activity and behavior is very short. Even though thiopental is classified as an ultrashort-acting barbiturate, there is longer time period necessary for return of normal activity and behavior. Pentobarbital and Telazol are longer-acting drugs. Guaifenesin is primarily a muscle relaxant used for the induction of anesthesia in horses and cattle.

8. The answer is A.
Most oxybarbiturates, with the exception of methohexital, are less lipid soluble than thiobarbiturates. A methyl side chain increases methohexital's lipid solubility and results in an ultrashort duration of action. Pentobarbital and phenobarbital are long-acting oxybarbiturates. Thiopental is ultrashort-acting thiobarbiturates.

9. The answer is B.
Proparacaine is a rapidly acting topical anesthetic used to desensitize the cornea for measuring intraocular pressure (tonometry) or relief of corneal pain to facilitate examination. The duration of effect is short, around 5–10 minutes.

Chapter 7

Nonsteroidal Anti-inflammatory Drugs

Walter H. Hsu and Arthi Kanthasamy

I. **GENERAL CONSIDERATION.** The nonsteroidal anti-inflammatory drugs (NSAIDs) discussed in this chapter fall under two classes, namely, inhibitors of prostaglandin (PG) synthesis and miscellaneous (locally applied) anti-inflammatory drugs. The PG inhibitors induce anti-inflammation and analgesia without affecting consciousness, while locally applied drugs exert their effects directly on the local lesions. **The PG inhibitors have been used extensively to alleviate mild to moderate pain, and is also effective in treating cephalgia, myalgia, arthralgia, and other pain from the integument; although they do not relieve visceral (except flunixin), or sharp and intense pain.**

A. **Mechanisms of action of NSAIDs.** Most of the NSAIDs act by inhibiting PG biosynthesis and in some instances leukotrienes. Hence, an understanding of PG biosynthesis and its physiological functions is essential to better comprehend the mechanism of drug action of the various NSAIDs listed below:

1. **Prostaglandins, leukotrienes, and their synthesis (see Figure 3-3)**
   a. Prostaglandins are produced by a wide array of tissues including lungs, GI tract, kidney, and liver. They are metabolized primarily at the site of action hence resulting in decreased circulating levels of PGs.
   b. Prostaglandins, prostacyclins, and thromboxanes collectively known as **prostanoids** are synthesized from the same precursor, arachidonic acid (AA).
   c. AA is an important component of cell membrane and is released by the action of phospholipase A_2 and other acyl hydrolases, which are subject to regulation by hormones and other stimuli. Subsequently, AA undergoes cyclization and oxygenation to prostanoids via the cyclooxygenase (COX) pathway; and to leukotrienes via the lipooxygenase (LOX) pathway.
   d. Majority of the NSAIDs that are currently used elicit their potent **anti-inflammatory, antipyretic, and analgesic effects** through differential inhibition of COX-1 and COX-2 (see below) and to a lesser extent LOX.

2. **Cyclooxygenase (COX) pathway.** Prostanoids are synthesized primarily via the COX pathway; there are two COX isoforms, COX-1 and COX-2. In addition, the recently identified acetaminophen-inhibitable COX-3 isoform is found to be expressed in the canine brain. COX-3 participates in the pyresis processes.
   a. **COX-1 is constitutively expressed in several tissues and is termed "house keeping enzyme" because of its essential role in the maintenance of several homeostatic process including gastric mucosal cytoprotection, renal function, vascular homeostasis, platelet aggregation.**
   b. **COX-2 is an inducible form because it is expressed at the site of injury, inflammation and in certain pathological states such as osteoarthritis.** Interestingly, recent reports indicate that it may also be constitutively expressed in a tissue-specific manner including, bone, kidney, and brain and may promote delayed wound healing.
   c. Both isoforms share 60% structural homology; yet they are distinct in several aspects. For example, COX-2 has a flexible and slightly wider active site in comparison to COX-1. This has led to the burgeoning interest in developing COX-2 selective inhibitors, but with COX-1 sparing action. Although, adopting such a strategy has raised great concerns regarding their adverse effects on the heart and kidneys in recent years.

3. **Lipoxygenase (LOX) pathway.** AA is converted by 5-LOX to 5-hydroperoxyeicosatetraenoic acid, which is eventually converted to leukotriene B_4 (LTB$_4$). LTB$_4$ plays a central role in inflammation, increased microvascular

permeability, and chemotactic properties involving neutrophil–endothelial adhesion, and neutrophil aggregation and degranulation.

II. INHIBITORS OF PG SYNTHESIS

All NSAIDs have proven efficacy in reducing pain and inflammation in animals. It is particularly useful in treating clinical conditions including osteoarthritis, rheumatoid arthritis, ankylosing spondylitis, gout, and dental pain. Although NSAIDs provides effective short-term pain relief, chronic use of nonselective or traditional NSAIDs may increase the risk of GI complications.

A. Pharmacological consideration

1. **All of them exert analgesic, anti-inflammatory and antipyretic actions by inhibiting PG synthesis via blocking COX.** Some NSAIDs also inhibit LTB_4 synthesis by blocking LOX.
2. **Analgesic effects of NSAIDs** are related to blockade of PGE_2-mediated enhancement of pain sensitization produced by proinflammatory mediators such as bradykinin and substance P at the nerve endings in the CNS and at the sites of inflammation.
3. **One should exercise caution** when increasing the dose of an NSAID to induce analgesia in case of intense pain because of the emergence of their toxic effects at these levels.
4. Unlike, narcotic analgesics, **NSAIDs do not produce tolerance or physical dependence** with regards to analgesia.
5. **The antipyretic effects** or temperature-lowering action works only in the presence of a fever, because they impair the ability of pyrogens to raise the temperature set point of the thermoregulatory centers in the anterior hypothalamus, thereby promoting heat loss by sending signals through the descending system to cause cutaneous vasodilatation, sweating, and panting. The temperature-lowering action of NSAIDs do not influence normal body temperature.
6. **The anti-inflammatory effect** of NSAIDs is due to inhibition of PGE_2 synthesis, stabilization of lysosomal membranes, inhibition of the complement system, phagocytosis, leukocyte accumulation, and synthesis of mucopolysaccharide and histamine, antagonism of bradykinin's action, induction of oxygen radical scavenger action and uncoupling of oxidative phosphorylation to deprive inflammatory tissues of energy.
7. **The COX-1 inhibitors decrease blood clotting by inhibiting platelet aggregation** (they inhibit synthesis of thromboxane $A_2(TXA_2)$, which are proaggregatory). Since platelets cannot synthesize new COX, the inhibition is irreversible in these cells. This could result in prolonged bleeding time.
8. **The COX-2 inhibitors at the recommended dosages exhibit minimal GI damaging effects**, since COX-1 mediates the maintenance of GI mucosa.

B. Pharmacokinetics consideration

1. As weak acids, NSAIDs usually are readily absorbed following oral administration.
2. Injectable solutions tend to be alkaline and can cause pain and necrosis in cases of extravasation.
3. **Circulating NSAIDs are bound vividly by albumin, which decreases volume of distribution.** Unbound drugs can reach target tissues for actions and metabolism. **Displacement from albumin due to competition by other drugs for the albumin binding sites or hypoalbuminemia can lead to higher plasma levels of unbound drugs, which can predispose the patient to drug-induced adverse effects.**
4. Drug elimination rates of NSAIDs are variable, depending on drugs and species. Most NSAIDs are eliminated primarily via hepatic phases I and II metabolisms. Conjugate metabolites are then excreted in the urine/feces. However, a small amount may be excreted in their unchanged form in the urine/feces as well.

5. The use of NSAIDs in cats is a great challenge to clinicians, since there are no FDA-approved drugs available for use in this species, except the injectable meloxicam. In addition, very little pharmacokinetics information is available for cats. Since cats have inefficient cytochrome P450 and glucuronidation conjugation system; the extrapolation of NSAIDs dosages from other species needs to be carefully validated.

6. Young and old patients may require smaller doses of NSAIDs due to weak liver and kidney status, which may result in lower elimination rates.

C. Adverse effects

1. All NSAIDs can cause adverse effects particularly at large doses and when used for longer periods. **The ones that are used most commonly in human medicine can cause poisoning in animals, for example, aspirin, acetaminophen, ibuprofen, indomethacin, and naproxen. Cats and dogs are more vulnerable to adverse effects of NSAIDs than humans.**

2. The following are the commonly seen adverse effects of NSAIDs in animals: vomiting, diarrhea, **GI ulceration, hepatotoxicity, renal toxicity**, CNS depression, and circulatory disturbances. The GI ulceration is the most common and serious adverse effect of NSAIDs. **Underlying nephrotoxicity, hepatotoxicity, or impaired cardiac conditions may exaggerate the adverse effects associated with NSAIDs.**

3. **Under normal conditions, PGE_2 (activating G_s-coupled EP2 and EP4 receptors) and $PGF_{2\alpha}$ (activating G_q-coupled FP receptors) confer cytoprotective effects on the gastric mucosa.** Blockade of COX results in excessive secretion of gastric acid with a concomitant decrease in gastric mucosal cytoprotective substances; hence, resulting in **GI hemorrhage, ulceration, and perforation**. Impaired platelet activity may cause pronounced GI hemorrhage. Gastric cotherapy with misoprostol, a synthetic PGE_1 analog which activates both EP2 and EP4 receptors, may lower the risk of GI damage in patients. Misoprostol also inhibits gastric acid secretion (Figure 11-2).

4. **NSAID-induced renal toxicity reflects inhibition of vasodilatory PGs.** The prostanoids PGE_2 and PGI_2 play a key role in the regulation of renal blood flow since their G_s-coupled receptors mediate vasodilatation. They promote natriuresis and diuresis in the kidney. These mechanisms are critical especially when the systemic levels of vasoconstrictors, renin, angiotensin, and norepinephrine are elevated under stress. NSAID-mediated inhibition of PGE_2 and PGI_2 biosynthesis may cause edema, hyperkalemia, and acute renal failure. **Patients with compromised renal function could be seriously affected.**

5. **NSAID-induced hepatotoxicity.** The mechanisms underlying the hepatotoxic effects of NSAIDs are presently unclear.

D. Drug interactions

1. Concurrent use of glucocorticoids and other NSAIDs should be avoided due to increased risk of GI adverse effects.

2. Concurrent use of high protein-binding drugs or drugs that share the same metabolic pathway including anticonvulsant drugs, behavior-modifying drugs, and warfarin requires careful monitoring.

3. Concurrent use of aminoglycosides warrants careful monitoring, due to increased risk of nephrotoxicity.

E. Guidelines for the safe use of NSAIDs

1. Individualized dosing based on the drug's efficacy, age of the animal, and duration of action.

2. Screen patients for underlying renal and hepatic dysfunction by performing routine diagnostic procedures.

3. Monitor the hydration status of patients. Hypovolemic animals should not be placed on NSAIDs before improving the hydration status.

4. An adequate wash out period should be allowed prior to administering a new NSAID.

5. Administer the lowest possible effective dose for the shortest period to minimize risk of injury.
6. **Concurrent use of glucocorticoids and NSAIDs should be avoided due to increased risk of GI complications.**

III. INDIVIDUAL NSAIDs

A. Classification of NSAIDs

1. **Nonselective COX inhibitors:**
   a. **Enolic acids**
      Oxicams: Meloxicam
      Pyrazolones: Phenylbutazone
   b. **Carboxylic acid**
      Nicotinic acid: Flunixin meglumine
      Fenamates: Meclofenamic acid
      Salicylates: Aspirin
      Propionates: Ibuprofen, Naproxen, Ketoprofen, Carprofen
      Acetic acid: Etodolac
2. **COX-2 selective inhibitors:**
   Coxibs: Deracoxib, Firocoxib
3. **Dual inhibitors: (COX/and 5-LOX):**
   Propanamide: Tepoxalin

B. Aspirin (Acetylsalicylate). Aspirin is a prototypical NSAID that is effective and inexpensive.

1. **Mechanism of action.** Aspirin elicits its effects via acetylation and irreversible inhibition of COX; hence, resulting in decreased PG synthesis. Irreversible inhibition of platelet COX-1 by aspirin is responsible for the blockade of TXA_2 production and its associated anticoagulant effects. In contrast, inhibition produced by other NSAIDs are reversible.
2. **Therapeutic uses**
   a. In general, aspirin is useful as an analgesic and an NSAID in dogs and cats, particularly in the control of osteoarthritis. However, it is not effective in treating colic. As an analgesic, aspirin is given orally in cats at 10 mg/kg, every 48 hours, and the same dose is given every 12 hours in dogs.
   b. It can be an adjunct therapy for septic and endotoxic shocks in animals having a heavy infection.
   c. Sulfasalazine, an oral salicylate-sulfonamide, is used to treat chronic inflammatory conditions of bowel, for example, ulcerative colitis. After oral administration, the intestinal flora metabolize it into sulfapyridine and 5-aminosalicylic acid; the latter stays in bowel to exerts its anti-inflammatory effect and the former is absorbed from the intestine (see Chapter 11).
3. **Pharmacokinetics**
   a. Aspirin is readily absorbed from both the stomach and upper intestine. Gastric acidity enhances absorption by favoring deionization, while high blood flow through the upper intestine compromises the higher ionization of aspirin due to higher pH.
   b. Buffered aspirin. Since the acidity of regular aspirin can irritate stomach, particularly in dogs and cats, buffered aspirin is preferred for these two species. Although buffered aspirin is more ionized, and thus less rapidly absorbed from the GI tract, the total GI absorption of buffered aspirin is similar to that of regular aspirin.
   c. A total of 70–90% of circulating aspirin is bound by albumin.
   d. Aspirin is inactive, but is rapidly metabolized to salicylic acid to elicit its effects.

  e. In animals, salicylate metabolism is primarily through glucuronidation; there is extensive species variation, plasma $t_{1/2}$ is 25–45 hours in cats, $\sim$8 hours in dogs, 5 hours in horses, and 1.5 hours in humans.

  f. Cats have very limited glucuronidation (by glucuronide transferase), and thus are most sensitive to aspirin toxicity. After the exhaustion of glucuronidation, salicylate then form conjugates with glutathione.

4. Adverse effects

  a. Aspirin-induced signs of GI upset including vomiting, anorexia, GI ulceration, diarrhea may be seen even at therapeutic doses.

  b. Aspirin-induced paradoxical hyperpyrexia is due to an increase in O_2 consumption, leading to increased metabolic rate and increased heat production due to uncoupling of oxidative phosphorylation.

  c. In the early phase aspirin-induced acid–base disturbances may be manifested as respiratory alkalosis due to direct stimulation of the medullary receptor center, leading to hyperventilation. This may be followed by respiratory acidosis as a result of CNS depression during the late phase.

  Metabolic acidosis may arise from:

  (1) Salicylic acid induced release of H^+,

  (2) Uncoupling of oxidative phosphorylation, may lead to build up of pyruvate and lactate,

  (3) An increase in fat metabolism, leading to ketoacidosis,

  (4) A depression of renal function, resulting in the accumulation of sulfuric and phosphoric acid.

  d. **Dehydration** due to vomiting, sweating, and hyperpyrexia, may be life threatening.

  e. **Pulmonary edema** is seen in sheep.

  f. In animals that are placed on chronic aspirin therapy, drug treatment must be **discontinued 7 days before surgery to minimize the risk of bleeding during surgery**.

  g. **Caution must be exercised when placing dogs with joint diseases on long-term therapy. In particular, aspirin can inhibit PG synthesis by canine chondrocytes that may result in the aggravation of joint disease**.

  h. **Drug interactions** of aspirin happen most often due to salicylate-mediated displacement of other drugs that compete for the same albumin-binding site, for example, warfarin (in this case the end effect is aggravated due to the additive anticoagulant effects of both drugs).

  i. **Treatment of aspirin toxicity**

  (1) Induce emesis in the case of acute toxicity.

  (2) Increase removal of the drug, for example, gastric lavage followed by administration of activated charcoal, and peritoneal dialysis.

  (3) Increase urinary excretion of aspirin by administering an alkalinizing agent (e.g., $NaHCO_3$), which may serve to correct the underlying metabolic acidosis.

  (4) Initiate IV fluid therapy to address dehydration and metabolic acidosis that accompany drug overdose.

C. **Meclofenamic acid**

1. Mechanism of action. It is a derivative of anthranilic acid, which, in turn, is a salicylic acid analog. The human product is for extra-label use, since the veterinary product has become obsolete. Nonselective inhibition of both COX-1 and COX-2 is the primary mechanism of action. Additional effects may include prostaglandin receptor blockade.

2. Therapeutic uses. It is for oral use in the dog and horse. It is used in treatment of osteoarthritis in the horse as well as soft tissue inflammation, (e.g., laminitis) that affects the locomotor system. To a lesser extent, it is also used in dogs to improve mobility in hip dysplasia. It is effective in the control of anaphylaxis attributed to kinins, PGs, and leukotrienes in particular. For long-term use of the drug, the lowest effective dosage that maintains a satisfactory anti-inflammatory effect should be the objective. The onset of action is slow, taking from 36 to 96 hours to develop.

3. **Pharmacokinetics.** After oral dosing, plasma level peaks within 1–4 hours. The elimination $t_{1/2}$ in horses is 1–8 hours. It can be detected in urine 96 hours after the final dose. It is metabolized in the liver primarily by oxidation to an active hydroxymethyl metabolite that may be further oxidized to an inactive carboxyl metabolite. The information for dogs is not available.

4. **Adverse effects. In dogs, chronic administration (>48 hours) has been shown to be associated with increased incidence of GI events, including hemorrhage and diarrhea**. Overdose in horses may induce buccal erosions, anorexia, GI disturbances, lower packed cell volume of blood. Therapeutic dose may induce colic and diarrhea in horses heavily infested with GI parasites. Chronic use of the drug in dogs can induce vomiting, tarry stools, leukocytosis, low hemoglobin levels, and small intestinal erosions.

D. **Acetaminophen.** This drug is unsafe in small animals.

E. **Phenylbutazone. The safety and efficacy profile in addition to its affordability makes it the most commonly used NSAID in the horse.**

1. **Mechanism of action. Phenylbutazone, which belongs to the enolate class shows COX-2 inhibitory effects and COX-1 sparing effect in both horses and dogs.**

2. **Therapeutic uses.** It is approved by the FDA for oral and IV administration in the dog and horse. One should avoid perivascular injection due to the risk of phlebitis. It is used to treat various forms of lameness as well as osteoarthritis and other painful conditions of the limbs including soft tissue or nonarticular rheumatism. It reduces nonspecific inflammation in other conditions, for example, thrombophlebitis, pericarditis, and pleurisy. **Its misuse by unscrupulous individuals to mask lameness in horses has created serious ethical concerns in the racing industry.**

3. **Pharmacokinetics**
   a. After IV administration of the clinical doses, the plasma $t_{1/2}$ is 2.5–6 hours in the dog and horse.
   b. The long duration of action (24–72 hours) may be due to the following reasons:
      (1) Irreversible binding of the drug to COX. Thus, new enzyme production at the inflammation site needs to occur before PGs can be synthesized.
      (2) The albumin that binds phenylbutazone may penetrate into inflamed tissues; consequently, the plasma levels of phenylbutazone may be underestimated in inflamed tissues.
      (3) The active metabolite oxyphenbutazone persists in the body.
   c. Binding of phenylbutazone to albumin in the animals exceeds 99%.
   d. Phenylbutazone is almost completely metabolized in the horse, two major metabolites being oxyphenbutazone and γ-hydroxyphenylbutazone.
   e. In the horse, 25% of phenylbutazone is eliminated via renal excretion over 24 hours.
   f. In the dog, oxyphenbutazone persists in urine for ≥48 hours following oral dosing of phenylbutazone, but the unchanged drug could not be detected in urine at the end of 36 hours.
   g. Phenylbutazone induces the production of hepatic microsomal enzymes, resulting in progressively lower plasma levels during chronic administration of the drug.

4. **Adverse effects**
   a. The following signs/lesions may be seen: Anorexia, depression, colic, hypoproteinemia, diarrhea, petechial hemorrhages of mucous membranes, oral and GI tract erosions and ulcers, renal papillary necrosis and anuria, and death.
   b. Death is attributable to a protein-losing enteropathy that can result in a decrease in blood volume, hemoconcentration, hypovolemic shock, and circulatory collapse. If GI tract ulceration is prominent, the shock syndrome may possibly be intensified by a septic component.

    c. Phenylbutazone must not be administered to animals afflicted with serious cardiac, renal, hepatic injury, or hematocytologic disorder.

    d. Phenylbutazone must not be administered to female dairy cattle ≥ 20 months of age. The Food Animal Residue Avoidance Databank (FARAD) discourages the use of phenylbutazone in any food animals because of its prolonged excretion.

F. **Flunixin meglumine (Banamine®, etc.).** It is a nicotinic acid derivative. It has potent anti-inflammatory and analgesic effects and is indicated for the treatment of acute and surgical pain.

  1. Mechanism of action. Flunixin shows greater COX-2 inhibitory effects than COX-1 in horses. In dogs, it appears to exhibit preferential COX-1 inhibitory effects.

  2. Therapeutic uses. NSAIDs are effective in alleviating pain that is of somatic and integumental origin, although less effective in relieving visceral pain. Flunixin is an exception; it alleviates visceral pain related to colic. Furthermore, in horses flunixin is effective in producing the longest duration of postoperative analgesia ($\sim$13 hours) followed by carprofen ($\sim$12 hours) and phenylbutazone ($\sim$8 hours). In cattle, it is used for the control of pyrexia associated with respiratory disease and endotoxemia, and for the control of inflammation in endotoxemia and mastitis.

  3. Pharmacokinetics

    a. It is administered IV or IM. When administered IV, it has a plasma $t_{1/2}$ of 2–4 hours in horses, 3–6 hours in cattle, 4 hours in dogs, and 1–1.5 hours in cats. It can be detected in plasma for 8 hours and in urine for >48 hours.

    b. After parenteral administration, onset of pharmacologic action is ≤ 2 hours, the peak effect is seen at 12–16 hours, and the duration of action is 24–36 hours. Accumulation of the drug at the sites of inflammation may be responsible for the longer duration of action, despite a shorter $t_{1/2}$. Its anti-inflammatory action after a single IV dose results in the abolition of PGE_2 in exudate for 12–24 hours.

    c. Renal excretion contributes extensively to elimination of flunixin from the body. Urine concentration of the drug in both conjugate and free form is $\sim$40 times higher than that of plasma.

    d. Withdrawal periods in cattle. Since flunixin is not approved by FDA for cattle, the extralabel withdrawal intervals recommended by FARAD are: 4-day preslaughter and 72-hour milk periods.

  4. Adverse effects

    a. Myonecrosis when administered via the IM route.

    b. Overdose of flunixin in horses may cause multiple ulcers on the tongue, gingiva, palate, lips, and stomach. CNS depression, listlessness, and anorexia may also occur. Rare anaphylactic-like reactions may occur particularly after rapid IV administration.

    c. Acute renal failure and GI damage have been reported in dogs treated with flunixin.

    d. Hematochezia and hematuria can be seen in cattle treated for longer than 3 days.

G. **Naproxen.** It is a nonselective COX inhibitor.

  1. Therapeutic uses. It is used orally in horses for soft tissue problems, for example, myositis. Naproxen can be used to treat inflammatory swelling associated with lameness. **Naproxen is too toxic to be used in small animals**.

  2. Pharmacokinetics

    a. The plasma $t_{1/2}$ is 4 hours in horses. It may take 5–7 days to see a beneficial response after starting treatment.

    b. It is metabolized into a glucuronide conjugate and excreted into urine for ≥ 48 hours.

  3. Adverse effects. The following effects are uncommon in horses, which include GI ulcers and diarrhea, hypoproteinemia, anemia, nephrotoxicity, and CNS depression.

H. **Ibuprofen and indomethacin.** These two drugs are not routinely used in veterinary medicine due to its low safety profile.

I. Ketoprofen (Ketofen®). It is a propionic acid derivative. Commercially available form of ketoprofen is a racemic mixture containing both S (+) and R (−) enantiomers. The S (+) enantiomer is responsible for majority of the drug's anti-inflammatory effects, whereas the R (−) enantiomer imparts analgesic effects with minimal ulcerogenic potential.

1. **Mechanism of action.** Ketoprofen is a nonselective inhibitor of COX. Additionally, it also blocks LTB_4 biosynthesis via the LOX pathway, which may broaden its efficacy as an anti-inflammatory agent. It may also promote proteoglycan biosynthesis, thereby enhancing synovial membrane activity and increasing the viscosity of synovial fluid. The potent anti-inflammatory effects associated with ketoprofen may be due to its sequestration at the sites of inflammation, for example, inflamed synovial joint.

2. **Therapeutic uses.** It is approved for use in horses for the alleviation of inflammation and pain associated with acute and chronic musculoskeletal disorders.

3. **Pharmacokinetics.** The drug has excellent bioavailability of 80–100% with a short elimination $t_{1/2}$ of ~1 hour in horses, 1.5 hours in dogs and cats. It is eliminated via the kidneys. Ketoprofen appears relatively safe to be used in horses and may have a lower incidence of adverse effects than either phenylbutazone or flunixin.

4. **Adverse effects.** Upon oral administration, it can cause GI injury including ulceration, bleeding, and vomiting. Preoperative use of ketoprofen in animals with hemostatic disorders warrants caution due to the risk of decreased platelet aggregation. Careful monitoring is required when used in patients with compromised renal function including renal insufficiency or failure.

J. Carprofen (Rimadyl®). It is a propionic acid derivative that is related to ketoprofen. Carprofen exhibits greater ability to inhibit (100 times) COX-2 as compared to COX-1.

1. **Therapeutic uses.** Carprofen is approved for use as an analgesic and anti-inflammatory drug in dogs. It can be used in both short-term and long-term pain management in musculoskeletal conditions. In addition, it provides excellent pain relief when used as a part of preemptive analgesia.

2. **Pharmacokinetics.** The pharmacokinetics in dogs and cats are considerably different. The elimination $t_{1/2}$ is ~20 hours in cats, whereas 5–9 hours in dogs. Following oral administration in dogs, the T_{max} occurs 1–3 hours. The drug is highly bound to albumin (99%). It is metabolized in the liver via oxidation followed by glucuronidation. The metabolites undergo extensive enterohepatic recycling. About 70–80% of drug is eliminated in the feces; the remaining 10–20% is excreted in the urine.

3. **Adverse effects.** The COX-1 sparing effect may account for lower frequency of GI ulceration and hemorrhage. The most commonly encountered adverse events include anorexia, vomiting, and diarrhea. It should be used with caution in animals with an underlying hepatic or renal condition due to increased risk of hepatotoxicity and nephrotoxicity. Carprofen is not recommended in animals with hemostatic disorders; pregnant, lactating, or breeding bitches.

K. Etodolac (EtoGesic®). Etodolac is an indole acetic acid derivative. In dogs, it preferentially inhibits COX-2.

1. **Therapeutic uses.** It is for the control of pain and inflammation associated with osteoarthritis in dogs. It may be used as an analgesic and anti-inflammatory drug for many other conditions.

2. **Pharmacokinetics.** Etodolac is rapidly absorbed following oral administration with a rapid onset of action of 30–60 minutes in majority of the cases. The drug is primarily excreted via the bile into the feces as glucuronide conjugates. It undergoes enterohepatic recycling, which leads to a long plasma $t_{1/2}$ (10–14 hours) and allows once daily dosing.

3. **Adverse effects.** Like other NSAIDs, etodolac can cause GI disturbances, CNS depression, hepatotoxicity, and nephrotoxicity, probably at a lower rate than COX-1 inhibitors (see II C). Caution must be exercised when using in animals with hepatic, renal, and hematological impairment. Etodolac may induce

keratoconjunctivitis sicca in dogs; therefore, tear production must be monitored before and during treatment.

L. **Deracoxib** (Deramaxx®). It is a diaryl-substituted pyrazole that is chemically related to others in the "coxib" class. **Deracoxib is a COX-2 inhibitor**.

1. **Therapeutic uses**. It is used in dogs for the treatment of pain and inflammation associated with osteoarthritis (1–2 mg/kg, PO, once a day), and for the management of postoperative pain and inflammation (3–4 mg/kg, PO, once a day, 7 days maximum) associated with orthopedic surgery.
2. **Pharmacokinetics.** Deracoxib is administered orally, and postprandial administration is preferred to protect GI mucosa. In dogs, following oral administration, the elimination $t_{1/2}$ is 3 hours and T_{max} is ~2 hours. The drug is highly protein bound (90%), thus concurrent use of other protein binding drugs warrants close monitoring. The drug is primarily excreted via the bile into the feces as glucuronide conjugates. Although a small quantity (20%) of the drug may be excreted in the urine.
3. **Adverse effects.** Like other NSAIDs, the most commonly reported side effects include GI disturbances, CNS depression, hepatotoxicity, and nephrotoxicity (see II C).

M. **Firocoxib (Previcox®).** It is a dimethylfuranone that is chemically related to other "coxibs." Firocoxib is one of the most selective COX-2 inhibitors used in veterinary medicine.

1. **Therapeutic uses**. It is used in dogs for the treatment of pain and inflammation associated with osteoarthritis (5 mg/kg, PO, once a day).
2. **Pharmacokinetics**.
   a. The oral drug absorption process is highly variable among subjects. Coadministration with food delays firocoxib absorption (T_{max} from 1 to 5 hours) and decreases peak concentrations (C_{max} from 1.3 to 0.9 µg/mL). However, food does not affect the overall bioavailability of firocoxib.
   b. The absolute bioavailability of firocoxib is ~40% when administered as a 5 mg/kg oral dose to fasted adult dogs. Firocoxib is rapidly cleared from the blood via hepatic metabolism and fecal excretion.
   c. Despite a high level of plasma protein binding (96%), firocoxib exhibits a large volume of distribution (V_d of total drug = 4.6 L/kg) and a terminal elimination $t_{1/2}$ of ~8 hours.
3. **Adverse effects.** Despite the fact that firocoxib is a highly selective COX-2 inhibitor, like other NSAIDs, firocoxib still can cause GI disturbances. Vacuolization without inflammatory cell infiltrates is seen in the thalamic region of the brain when administered at 3–5 times the recommended dose.

N. **Meloxicam (Metacam®).** It is an oxicam derivative, which is a preferential COX-2 inhibitor.

1. **Therapeutic uses.** Meloxicam is approved in dogs and cats for the treatment of chronic pain and inflammation associated with osteoarthritis. Meloxicam is effective in controlling postoperative pain. Improved analgesia is seen in dogs given a combination of meloxicam with epidural morphine–mepivacaine.
2. **Administration and pharmacokinetics**
   a. Meloxicam is absorbed well after oral administration. Food does not alter rates of absorption. Peak plasma levels occur in ~8 hours after oral administration. It can be administered SC as a single one-time dose in cats. Repeated use of meloxicam in cats can evoke acute renal failure and death. Do not follow meloxicam dose with any other NSAID in cats.
   b. A total of 97% of meloxicam is bound to albumin.
   c. It is metabolized in the liver to form glucuronide conjugates. Majority of these metabolites are eliminated in the feces. The plasma $t_{1/2}$ appears to be species-specific: 12–24 hours in dogs, 15 hours in cats, and ~3 hours in horses.
3. **Adverse effects.** Meloxicam is a relatively safe NSAID in dogs. GI distress (vomiting, anorexia, and diarrhea) is the most commonly reported adverse effect along

with lethargy and behavioral changes as well as anemia. However, such problems still occur rarely and are transient in nature. Caution is needed when administering in hypovolemic animals because decreased renal blood flow may increase the risk of nephrotoxicity.

When given SC, meloxicam can cause pain in injection site(s).

Meloxicam is not recommended for use in pregnant, lactating, or in animals that are <4 months of age.

4. **Drug interactions.** Meloxicam may decrease the clinical efficacy of angiotensin converting enzyme inhibitors. For other drug interactions see II C.

O. **Tepoxalin (Zubrin®).** Tepoxalin belongs to the class of dual inhibitors. It is a nonselective COX inhibitor with additional pronounced and unique inhibitory effect on LOX.

1. **Mechanism of action**
   a. Tepoxalin is a dual inhibitor of both COX and LOX. By inhibiting both COX-1 and COX-2 and 5-LOX at the approved recommended dosage in dogs it may have fewer adverse effects on GI tract.
   b. Tepoxalin reduces the production of PGs associated with pain, hyperpyrexia, and inflammation.
   c. Its inhibition of LOX may reduce leukotrienes synthesis, including LTB_4. Since LTB_4 contributes to increased GI tract inflammation by increasing cytokine production, neutrophil longevity and release of proteases, the reduction of LTB_4 will help protect GI mucosa. Leukotrienes may also contribute to inflammatory responses seen in osteoarthritis and their inhibition could reduce clinical signs seen with the disorder.

2. **Therapeutic uses.** It is used to control the pain and inflammation associated with osteoarthritis in dogs. Because it inhibits leukotrienes synthesis, it might benefit allergic conditions in dogs. It is useful to control postoperative pain associated with soft tissue surgery.

3. **Pharmacokinetics**
   a. Tepoxalin is readily absorbed after oral administration. T_{max} is 2–3 hours after oral administration.
   b. It is rapidly metabolized to several metabolites, including one that is active (tepoxalin pyrazole acid). Tepoxalin and tepoxalin pyrazole acid are highly bound to albumin (98–99%). Plasma elimination $t_{1/2}$ for tepoxalin and tepoxalin pyrazole acid are 2 hours and 13 hours, respectively. Metabolites are eliminated in the feces.

4. **Adverse effects**
   a. GI distress (anorexia, vomiting, diarrhea, ulceration) and CNS depression, hepatotoxicity, and nephrotoxcity may occur.
   b. Its effect in dogs <6 months of age, lactating, and pregnant dogs has not been determined and therefore not recommended for use.
   c. The rise for tepoxalin-induced GI stress is less than other NSAIDs, since it inhibits LOX. For other NSAIDs, shunting of prostaglandin biosynthesis via the LOX pathway following COX inhibition may increase the production of vasoconstrictors (LTC_4 and LTD_4) and the chemoattractant (LTB_4), which might contribute to the ulcerogenic actions of these NSAIDS.
   d. Its wide safety margin is attributed, in part, to its low bioavailability at higher than recommended doses and its poor water solubility facilitates fecal excretion.

IV. **MISCELLANEOUS ANTI-INFLAMMATORY DRUGS**

A. **Dimethyl sulfoxide (DMSO)**

1. **Chemistry.** DMSO is a solvent for many aromatic and unsaturated hydrocarbons as well as organic nitrogen compounds and inorganic salts.
   a. DMSO is a clear, colorless to straw-yellow liquid.

    b. Because of its hygroscopic characteristics, DMSO can absorb >70% of its weight in water from the air at a temperature of 70°F and 65% relative humidity. Therefore, the container should be tightly sealed.

2. Pharmacologic effects. DMSO possesses anti-inflammatory, analgesic, antimicrobial, antifungal, anticholinesterase, and diuretic activity. In addition, DMSO is able to rapidly penetrate the skin (but not nail or tooth enamel) following topical application.

3. Mechanisms of action

    a. Anti-inflammatory effect. DMSO and its metabolite dimethyl sulfide trap free radicals such as superoxide.

    b. Analgesic effect. DMSO produces a thermal effect that may account for its alleviation of muscle and joint pain.

    c. Skin penetrating effect. DMSO increases the permeability of the skin by altering the plasma membrane of the epithelial cells. As it rapidly penetrates the membrane barriers, DMSO carries dissolved compounds (e.g., another drug) with it, regardless of the size and characteristics of the molecule.

    d. Other effects. DMSO inhibits synthesis of prostaglandins. In addition, DMSO has diuretic, anticholinesterase, and weak antibacterial and antifungal effects (when use topically). The mechanisms by which DMSO exerts these effects are not understood.

4. Therapeutic uses

    a. DMSO is used to reduce acute swelling resulting from musculoskeletal trauma.

    b. Other possible indications include:

        (1) Acute traumatic conditions of the CNS including cerebral edema and posterior paralysis resulting from spinal cord trauma.

        (2) Cystitis associated with urethral obstruction in the cat.

        (3) Superficial burns.

        (4) Skin grafts.

        (5) Transient ischemic conditions.

        (6) Edema of the limbs resulting from fractures.

        (7) Swelling and engorgement of the mammary glands in the nursing bitch.

        (8) Severe inflammation resulting from the extravascular injection of irritating drugs or lick granuloma.

        (9) While the potential indications for DMSO are numerous, unfortunately, the lack of well-controlled study design leave many more questions than answers regarding this drug.

5. Pharmacokinetics

    a. Absorption. DMSO is well absorbed after topical application.

    b. Fate

        (1) DMSO is extensively and rapidly distributed to every part of the body.

        (2) The $t_{1/2}$ in horses is ~9 hours following IV administration.

        (3) DMSO is rapidly metabolized to dimethyl sulfide, methyl sulfinic acid, and dimethyl sulfone.

    c. Excretion. DMSO and its metabolites are excreted primarily by the kidneys; some biliary and respiratory excretion also occurs. DMSO and methyl sulfinic acid are believed to be responsible for the obnoxious oyster-like odor detectable on the breath seconds after the application of DMSO to the skin.

6. Administration. DMSO is administered topically. Only technical grade, but not industrial grade, of DMSO should be used in animals. Rubber gloves should be worn during application, and DMSO should be applied only to clean and dry areas to avoid carrying other chemicals into the systemic circulation.

7. Adverse effects. When used as labeled, DMSO appears to be a safe drug.

    a. Local effects (e.g., a burning sensation, erythema, vesiculation, dry skin, and allergic reactions) and a garlicky or oyster-like breath odor are the most likely adverse effects. These effects are transient and quickly resolve when therapy is discontinued.

    b. Lenticular changes, which may result in myopia, have been noted when high doses of DMSO are used chronically (i.e., longer than 14 days in dogs or 30 days in horses).

    c. When administered IV, DMSO may cause hemolysis and hemoglobinuria. These effects can be minimized by slowly administering ≤20% DMSO.

    d. Hepatic and renal damages, and pulmonary edema.

    e. CNS disturbances, for example, sedation, coma, seizures, and opisthotonus.

8. Contraindications

    a. DMSO must not be used in animals that are being treated concurrently with anticholinesterases.

    b. DMSO must be used cautiously in animals with mast cell tumors, since it degranulates these cells.

    c. DMSO must not be used in animals with severe dehydration and shock; DMSO-induced vasodilatation may exacerbate the conditions.

B. **Polysulfated glycosaminoglycan (Adequan®) (PSGAG)**

    1. Chemistry. PSGAG belongs to a new class of drugs termed disease-modifying osteoarthritis (OA) drugs (DMOADs). This antiarthritic compound is chemically similar to mucopolysaccharides of cartilage. PSGAG is a glycosaminoglycan extracted from the bovine trachea, which is then subjected to esterification to be sulfated.

    2. Mechanisms of action

        a. PSGAG inhibits or delays the progression of the appearance of morphological cartilaginous lesions associated with OA.

        b. PSGAG modulates clinical signs of OA by indirectly promoting chondroprotective effects while preventing the deleterious effects of proinflammatory mediators including PGs and cytokines on the articular cartilage.

        c. PSGAG through proteolytic enzyme inhibition decreases or reverses the mechanisms that result in the loss of cartilaginous mucopolysaccharides associated with OA.

        d. PSGAG improves joint articular function by enhancing synovial membrane activity and by increasing the viscosity of synovial fluid.

        e. Anti-inflammatory effects are due to:

            (1) Inhibition of PGE_2 biosynthesis that is induced following joint injury,

            (2) Inhibition of leukocyte migration and elevated interleukin levels at the site of inflamed joints,

            (3) Elevation of hyaluronate levels at the joints is believed to improve joint function.

    3. Therapeutic uses. PSGAG is used in horses to treat traumatic joint dysfunction and noninfectious degeneration of the carpal joint and in dogs to treat OA and prevention of hip dysplasia.

    4. Pharmacokinetics. No information regarding the pharmacokinetics of PSGAG is available.

    5. Administration. PSGAG is administered intra-articularly (IA) or IM. Occasionally, IA administration may cause joint infections. Thus, when administered intra-articularly, the joint area must be shaved, cleansed, and sterilized prior to injection to avoid complications associated with infection.

    6. Adverse effects. When used according to label instructions, PSGAG is safe. However, a few adverse drug events are associated with PSGAG administration:

        a. Rarely, animals show inflammatory joint reactions consisting of joint pain, effusion, swelling, and lameness (aseptic arthritis). This reaction may result from hypersensitivity, trauma sustained during injection, overdose or excessively frequent administration, or drug interactions.

        b. Septic arthritis may be induced if the sterile injection procedure is not followed.

    7. Contraindications. Intra-articular injections must not be administered when the overlying skin shows lesions of infection, or in cases of septic arthritis.

C. **Hyaluronate sodium**

    1. General aspects

        a. Hyaluronate sodium (HS), sodium salt of hyaluronic acid (HA), is a prototype of naturally occurring mucopolysaccharide. It is a nonsulfated glycosaminoglycan consisting of repeating disaccharide units of d-glucuronic acid and *N*-acetyl-D-glucosamine.

   b. HA is synthesized primarily by the Type B synoviocytes in the synovial membrane. It is also an important component of articular cartilage matrix. HA is found naturally in the connective tissue of animals. High concentrations of HA are found in the synovial fluid, vitreous humor of the eye, and umbilical cord. Surfaces of articular cartilage are covered with a thin layer of a protein–hyaluronate complex; hyaluronate is also found in the cartilage matrix.

2. **Mechanism of action**
   a. HS has the following effects in joints:
      (1) A cushioning effect, elicits a chemotactic response by reducing cell migration and decreasing cellular influx into the joint.
      (2) A lubricating effect on the articular soft tissues.
      (3) A scavenging effect, by removing oxygen-derived free radicals and autacoids from the joint.
   b. Exact mechanism of action of HS is unknown, but:
      (1) It is suggested to replenish the depleted or depolymerized endogenous HA in the synovial fluid.
      (2) It is hypothesized that injection of HS into an inflamed arthritic joint promotes the biosynthesis of higher molecular weight HA.
      (3) Hs might decrease PGs biosynthesis and release from macrophages during phagocytosis.
3. **Therapeutic uses**. Hs can be administered intra-articularly to dogs and horses to treat synovitis that is not associated with severe degenerative joint disease. It may be helpful to treat secondary synovitis in conditions where full thickness cartilage has been lost. **Horses treated with Hs exhibited reduced lameness, thinning of the articular cartilage, and reduced surface fibrillation as compared to saline injected joints. However, currently it is unclear whether HS's anti-inflammatory effects or secondary chondroprotective effects contributes to its beneficial effects in the management of clinical signs associated with OA.**
4. **Pharmacokinetics.** No information is available in animals.
5. **Adverse effects.** These are usually local effects, which are manifested by heat, swelling and/or effusion in the joint. Effects generally subside within 24–48 hours, but may continue up to 96 hours for resolution. No treatment for these adverse effects is recommended. When used in combination with other drugs, incidence of flares may actually be higher. Synovial infection can occur if the injection is not administered under aseptic conditions.

SUGGESTED READING

Boothe DM. 2001. "The analgesic, antipyretic, anti-inflammatory drugs." In *Veterinary Pharmacology and Therapeutics*. Edited by Adams HR. 8th ed., pp. 433–451. Ames, IA: Iowa State University Press.

Clark TP. 2006. The clinical pharmacology of cyclooxygenase-2 selective and dual inhibitors. *Vet Clin North Am Small Anim Pract* 36:1061–1085.

http://www.drugs.com

McCann ME, Andersen DR, Zhang D, Brideau C, Black WC, Hanson PD, Hickey GJ. 2004. In vitro effects and in vivo efficacy of a novel cyclooxygenase-2 inhibitor in dogs with experimentally induced synovitis. *Am J Vet Res* 65:503–512.

Plumb DC. 2005. *Veterinary Drug Handbook*. 5th ed. Ames, IA: Blackwell Publishing.

Streppa HK, Jones CJ, Budsberg SC. 2002. Cyclooxygenase selectivity of nonsteroidal anti-inflammatory drugs in canine blood. *Am J Vet Res* 63:91–94.

STUDY QUESTIONS

DIRECTIONS: Each of the numbered items or incomplete statements in this section is followed by answers or by completions of the statement. Select the **one** lettered answer or completion that is **best** in each case.

1. Which one of the following enzymes influences the $t_{1/2}$ of aspirin in domestic animals?

(A) Glutathione reductase
(B) Cyclooxygenase
(C) *N*-acetyl transferase
(D) Glucuronide transferase
(E) Cytochrome P450 oxidase

2. Bioavailability of carprofen can be increased by

(A) increasing urine pH.
(B) using enteric-coated tablets.
(C) administering sodium bicarbonate orally.
(D) maintaining a low pH in the stomach.

3. Most widely used analgesic in racehorses in the United States is

(A) aspirin.
(B) phenylbutazone.
(C) naproxen.
(D) xylazine.
(E) mecloflenamic acid.

4. Which one of the following anti-inflammatory drugs acts through proteolytic enzyme inhibition to reverse the loss of cartilaginous mucopolysaccharides that occurs in arthritis?

(A) Carprofen
(B) Dimethyl sulfoxide
(C) Polysulfated glycosaminoglycan
(D) Phenylbutazone
(E) Flunixin meglumine

5. Which of the following is the most frequently seen adverse effect of the prostaglandin inhibitors?

(A) Agranulocytosis
(B) Gastric ulcers
(C) Renal papillary necrosis

(D) Anemia
(E) Hepatitis

6. Meloxicam alleviates all of the following types of pain *except*:

(A) headache.
(B) muscle pain joint pain.
(C) joint pain.
(D) colic.

7. The antipyretic effect of an NSAID can result from all of the following *except*:

(A) inhibition of prostaglandin synthesis in the central nervous system.
(B) dilation of the peripheral vasculature.
(C) sweating.
(D) lowering body temperature in both normal and febrile animals.

8. Which of the following NSAIDs is approved by FDA to be used in cats?

(A) Carprofen
(B) Etodolac
(C) Firocoxib
(D) Meloxicam
(E) Tepoxalin

9. Which of the following NSAIDs is the most selective in inhibiting COX-2 among the ones approved for use in dogs?

(A) Carprofen
(B) Etodolac
(C) Firocoxib
(D) Meloxicam
(E) Tepoxalin

10. All of the following concerning the pharmacological actions of aspirin are true, *except*:

(A) reversible inhibition of COX-1.
(B) significant drug interaction with anticoagulants.

(C) GI ulceration and hemorrhage.

(D) antiplatelet effects.

11. Which of the following NSAIDs exerts its actions through dual inhibition of cyclooxygenase (COX) and 5-lipooxygenase (5-LOX)?

(A) Deracoxib

(B) Carprofen

(C) Phenylbutazone

(D) Tepoxalin

12. Which of the following NSAID(s) is used for the alleviation of visceral pain associated with colic in horses?

(A) Flunixin meglumine

(B) Phenylbutazone

(C) Aspirin

(D) Carprofen

(E) Meclofenamic acid

13. Which of the following is the correct statement concerning COX-2 inhibitors?

(A) They decrease platelet function.

(B) They have greater analgesic activity than other NSAIDs.

(C) Their anti-inflammatory activity is better than that of other NSAIDs.

(D) They do not affect the kidney.

(E) They cause less gastric ulceration than other NSAIDs.

14. Which of the following is an incorrect statement concerning the drug interactions of NSAID?

(A) Concurrent use of a glucocorticoid is encouraged, since this practice will ensure better anti-inflammatory activity.

(B) Concurrent use of diazepam may increase the activity of both drugs.

(C) Concurrent use of gentamicin can increase nephrotoxicity of NSAID.

(D) Concurrent use of two NSAIDs should be avoided.

15. Which of the following is a correct statement regarding DMSO?

(A) It is more useful in the treatment of chronic inflammatory conditions than acute ones.

(B) It has potent antidiuretic effect.

(C) DMSO traps free radicals and inhibits prostaglandin synthesis, which may account for its anti-inflammatory effects.

(D) The adverse effects include CNS and respiratory disturbances, but not hepato- or nephrotoxicity.

ANSWERS AND EXPLANATIONS

1. The answer is D.
Glucuronidation is the main biotransformation process for aspirin and dictates the plasma half-life of the compound. Aspirin is primarily metabolized by glucuronidation. Because the ability to conjugate glucuronic acid varies among species, the plasma $t_{1/2}$ of aspirin also varies. Aspirin irreversibly binds cyclooxygenase to inhibit the formation of prostaglandins. When glucuronidation capabilities are exhausted, salicylates form conjugates with glutathione. *N*-Acetyl transferase and cytochrome P450 enzyme are not involved in the biotransformation of aspirin.

2. The answer is D.
Carprofen is a weak acid that crosses biologic membranes most readily in an acidic environment and least readily in an alkaline environment. Increasing the pH of the urine or administering sodium bicarbonate decreases the bioavailability of aspirin because these measures induce an alkaline environment.

3. The answer is B.
Phenylbutazone is widely used as an equine analgesic because it is effective against many types of lameness and because of its low cost.

4. The answer is C.
Polysulfated glycosaminoglycan is chemically similar to the mucopolysaccharides of cartilage; therefore, it can reverse the mechanisms that cause the loss of these mucopolysaccharides. DMSO exerts anti-inflammatory effects mainly by scavenging free radicals. Phenylbutazone and flunixin meglumine inhibit prostaglandin synthesis.

5. The answer is B.
GI erosions and ulcers are the most frequently seen adverse effects of the prostaglandin inhibitors.

6. The answer is D.
The inhibitors of prostaglandin synthesis do not relieve deep visceral pain, such as colic. They usually alleviate pain from the integument, including skeletal muscles and joints.

7. The answer is D.
Prostaglandin synthesis inhibitors lower the set point of the thermoregulatory center of the hypothalamus in febrile animals (but not normal animals), causing vasodilatation and panting.

8. The answer is D.
Meloxicam is approved for dogs and cats for the treatment of chronic pain and inflammation associated with osteoarthritis. None of the other NSAIDs are approved for use in cats.

9. The answer is C.
Firocoxib is one of the most selective COX-2 inhibitors used in veterinary medicine.

10. The answer is A.
Aspirin exerts its pharmacological actions through acetylation and irreversible inhibition of COX-1 active site. The COX-1 inhibitory effects may account for the increased frequency of GI ulceration and bleeding.

11. The answer is D.
Tepoxalin, the newly introduced NSAID for the treatment of osteoarthritis, is categorized under dual inhibitors. Dual inhibitors act by inhibiting both COX and 5-LOX pathways. Its inhibitory effects on both branches of the arachidonic acid metabolism pathway have been shown to produce fewer GI damages in dogs.

12. The answer is A.
It is well established that NSAIDs work by alleviating pain that is of somatic and integument origin; although less effective in relieving visceral pain. Flunixin is an exception; it alleviates visceral pain related to colic in horses. In addition, it provides the longest duration of postoperative analgesia in comparison to carprofen and phenylbutazone in horses.

13. The answer is E.
COX-2 inhibitors cause less gastric damages than other NSAIDs; this is the reason that they are widely used in both veterinary and human medicine. They do not decrease platelet activity; they do not have greater analgesic or anti-inflammatory activity than other NSAIDs. Their nephrotoxic effect is not less than other NSAIDs.

14. The answer is A.
Concurrent use of a glucocorticoid with an NSAID should be avoided, since this practice will increase the risk of GI ulceration. Since NSAIDs are bound vividly by plasma protein (albumin), any drugs that are bound by albumin will cause drug interactions with an NSAID. Many drugs affecting CNS, including diazepam, fall into this category.

Concurrent use of NSAIDs is discouraged, since this practice will increase the free form of both drugs in the plasma, increasing the pharmacological and toxicological effects of both drugs.

Aminoglycoside antibiotics are potentially nephrotoxic, and thus concurrent use of an aminoglycoside with an NSAID will increase the risk of nephrotoxicity.

15. The answer is C.
DMSO traps free radical oxidants that evoke inflammatory processes. This is why it is more useful in treating acute than chronic conditions. DMSO has potent diuretic effect. The adverse effects of DMSO are many, which include CNS and respiratory disturbances as well as hepatotoxicity and nephrotoxicity.

Chapter 8

Drugs Acting on the Cardiovascular System

Wendy A. Ware

I. DRUGS USED IN HEART FAILURE THERAPY

A. Introduction

1. **Heart failure** occurs when abnormal cardiac function causes inadequate blood delivery to the tissues or adequate delivery only with elevated cardiac filling pressures. It can involve abnormalities of systolic or diastolic function, or both.

   a. **Congestive heart failure** (CHF) is characterized by high cardiac filling pressure which leads to venous congestion (behind the affected side of the heart) and tissue fluid accumulation. It is a complex clinical syndrome rather than a specific etiologic diagnosis. Although poor contractility often underlies CHF, chronic cardiac overload (volume or pressure) or other injury can also stimulate a cascade of neurohormonal and cardiac responses that eventually lead to congestive signs and further deterioration in function.

   (1) **Left-sided congestive signs** include pulmonary venous congestion and edema (resulting in cough, tachypnea, dyspnea, orthopnea, pulmonary crackles, tiring, hemoptysis, cyanosis). Chronic pulmonary congestion can lead to varying degrees of pulmonary hypertension and sometimes, right-sided CHF signs.

   (2) **Right-sided congestive signs** include systemic venous hypertension, with resulting jugular venous distension, hepatic (and abdominal visceral) congestion, pleural effusion (resulting in dyspnea, orthopnea, cyanosis), ascites, small pericardial effusions, and sometimes, subcutaneous edema.

   b. **Forward (low output) failure** causes tiring, exertional weakness, syncope, prerenal azotemia, and peripheral cyanosis (from poor cutaneous circulation). Cardiac arrhythmias frequently occur with all manifestations of heart failure. These signs can occur with either left or right heart disease.

2. **Pathophysiology** of heart failure

   a. **Cardiac remodeling** involves changes in myocardial size, shape and stiffness that occur in response to various mechanical, biochemical, and molecular signals induced by the underlying injury or stress.

   (1) **Myocardial hypertrophy.** Changes include myocardial cell hypertrophy, cardiac cell dropout (apoptosis), excess interstitial matrix formation, fibrosis, and abnormal collagen binding between individual myocytes. Increased mechanical forces (ventricular wall stress), as well as various neurohormones (e.g., angiotensin II, norepinephrine, endothelin, aldosterone) and cytokines (e.g., a tumor necrosis factor-α), are stimuli for cardiac remodeling. Myocardial hypertrophy helps normalize wall stress. Systolic pressure loads mainly cause "concentric" hypertrophy, with myocardial fiber thickening; volume loads mainly cause "eccentric" hypertrophy, with myocardial fiber elongation. Hypertrophy can interfere with diastolic function by making the ventricle "stiffer."

   (2) **Frank–Starling mechanism.** Acutely increased filling pressure and end diastolic volume (preload) induce greater force of contraction and help increase overall cardiac output. Valvular insufficiency, arterial hypertension, and ventricular outflow obstruction as well as volume retention lead to increased preload. Compensatory hypertrophy lessens the importance of the Frank–Starling mechanism in stable, chronic heart failure.

   b. **Neurohormonal mechanisms.** Neurohormonal responses contribute to cardiac remodeling and have systemic effects. Excessive activation of neurohormonal "compensatory" mechanisms leads to the clinical syndrome of CHF.

171

(1) Increased sympathetic nervous tone. Short-term effects of increased contractility, heart rate, and venous return can increase cardiac output. But over time, increased afterload stress and myocardial oxygen requirement, contribute to cellular damage, myocardial fibrosis, and increased potential for cardiac arrhythmias.

(2) Activation of the renin–angiotensin–aldosterone system. Angiotensin II stimulates potent vasoconstriction and aldosterone secretion, and has other important effects. Aldosterone promotes Na^+ and Cl^- reabsorption in the kidney; it also contributes to pathologic remodeling and myocardial fibrosis.

(3) Antidiuretic hormone (vasopression). This hormone directly causes vasoconstriction and also promotes free water reabsorption.

(4) Other substances. Cytokines (e.g., TNF-α), endothelins, and other substances also play a role in abnormal myocardial hypertrophy and/or fibrosis in heart failure.

(5) Endogenous vasodilatory mechanisms. These oppose the vasoconstrictor responses in heart failure and include natriuretic peptides (atrial NP and brain NP, nitric oxide, and vasodilatory prostaglandins). Normally, a balance between vasodilator and vasoconstrictor effects maintains circulatory homeostasis. As heart failure progresses, the influence of the vasoconstrictor mechanisms predominates.

c. Pathophysiologic groups of heart failure. As an aid to choosing therapy, the causes of heart failure can be viewed according to major underlying pathophysiologic mechanism. Nevertheless, several pathophysiologic abnormalities usually coexist; both systolic and diastolic function abnormalities are common in advanced failure.

(1) Myocardial (systolic pump) failure. Dilated cardiomyopathy is the most common cause. Valvular insufficiency may or may not be present initially, but usually develops as the affected ventricle dilates.

(2) Volume overload. A leaky valve or abnormal systemic-to-pulmonary connections are common causes. Cardiac pump function is often maintained well initially, but myocardial contractility deteriorates over time.

(3) Systolic pressure overload. Congenital ventricular outflow obstruction, and systemic or pulmonary hypertension are common causes. Concentric hypertrophy increases ventricular wall thickness and stiffness, and predisposes to ischemia; eventually myocardial contractility declines.

(4) Reduced ventricular compliance with impaired filling (diastolic dysfunction). Examples include hypertrophic and restrictive myocardial disease and pericardial disease. Contractile ability is usually normal initially, but elevated filling pressure leads to congestion and may diminish cardiac output.

B. **Overview of heart failure therapy**

1. Treatment strategies are aimed at modifying either the results of neurohormonal activation (i.e., Na^+ and water retention) or the activation process itself (e.g., angiotensin-converting enzyme inhibition). Goals are to control edema and effusions, improve cardiac output, reduce cardiac workload, support myocardial function, and manage concurrent arrhythmias. The clinical severity of heart failure influences the treatments used. Animals with heart failure caused by systolic dysfunction (e.g., dilated cardiomyopathy or advanced valvular insufficiency) benefit most from arteriolar vasodilation (reduced afterload) and also positive inotropic support.

a. Acute CHF. Acute CHF is characterized by severe cardiogenic pulmonary edema, with or without pleural and/or abdominal effusions or poor cardiac output. Therapy is aimed at rapidly clearing pulmonary edema, improving oxygenation, and optimizing cardiac output (see Table 8-1).

b. Chronic heart failure. Therapy is tailored to the individual's needs by adjusting dosages, adding or substituting drugs, and modifying lifestyle or diet. Pleural effusion and large-volume ascites that accumulate despite medical therapy are drained to improve respiration. As heart disease progresses, more aggressive

TABLE 8-1. Management of Acute Decompensated Congested Heart Failure*

- Avoid stress!
- Provide cage rest
- Enhance oxygenation:
  - Check airway patency
  - Give supplemental O_2 (avoid >50% for >24 hours)
  - If frothing is evident, suction airways
  - Intubate and mechanically ventilate if needed
  - Perform thoracocentesis if pleural effusion suspected
- Remove alveolar fluid:
  - Initiate diuresis:
    - Furosemide (dogs: 2–5 [–8] mg/kg IV or IM q1–4 hours until respiratory rate decreases, then 1–4 mg/kg q6–12 hours, or 0.6–1 mg/kg/h CRI (see cited text for more information); cats: 1–2 (–4) mg/kg IV or IM q1–4 hours until respiratory rate decreases, then q6–12 hours)
  - Redistribute blood volume:
    - Vasodilators (sodium nitroprusside: 0.5–1 mcg/kg/min (initial) CRI in D5W, titrate upward as needed to 5–15 mcg/kg/min, monitor arterial pressure (see cited text for more information); or 2% nitroglycerin ointment (+/– with hydralazine): dogs: $^1/_2$–1 $^1/_2$ inch cutaneously q6 hours; cats: $^1/_4$–$^1/_2$ inch cutaneously q6 hours.
    - (± morphine [dogs only, see below])
    - (± phlebotomy [6–10 mL/kg])
- Reduce bronchoconstriction:
  - Aminophylline (dogs: 4–8 mg/kg slow IV, IM, SC or 6–10 mg/kg PO q6–8 hours; cats: 4–8 mg/kg IM, SC, PO q8–12 hours) or similar drug
- Mild sedation to reduce anxiety:
  - Butorphanol (dogs: 0.2–0.3 mg/kg IM; cats: 0.2–0.25 mg/kg IM); or
  - Morphine (dogs: 0.025–0.1 mg/kg IV boluses q2–3 minutes to effect, or 0.1–0.5 mg/kg single IM or SC dose)
  - Acepromazine (cats: 0.05–0.2 mg/kg SC; or 0.05–0.1 mg/kg IM with butorphanol), or
  - Diazepam (cats: 2–5 mg IV; dogs: 5–10 mg IV)
- Reduce afterload:
  - Hydralazine: dogs: initial 0.5–1.0 mg/kg PO, repeat in 2–3 hours (until systolic arterial pressure is 90–110 mm Hg), then q12 hours (avoid nitroprusside); or
  - Enalapril (0.5 mg/kg PO q12–24 hours) or other ACE inhibitor (avoid nitroprusside); or
  - Amlodipine (dogs: 0.1–0.3 mg/kg PO q12–24 hours)
- Increase contractility (if myocardial failure present):
  - Dobutamine[†] (1–10 mcg/kg/min CRI; start low), or dopamine[‡] (dogs: 1–10 mcg/kg/min CRI; cats: 1–5 mcg/kg/min CRI; start low).
  - Amrinone (1–3 mg/kg IV; 10–100 mcg/kg/min CRI), or milrinone (50 mcg/kg IV over 10 minutes initially; 0.375–0.75 mcg/kg/min CRI [human dose]).
  - Pimobendan (PO, see Appendix II), or
  - Digoxin (see Appendix II for PO maintenance dosage); loading dose (see cited text for indications): PO—1 or 2 doses at twice calculated maintenance; dog IV: 0.01–0.02 mg/kg—give $^1/_4$ of this total dose in slow boluses over 2–4 hours to effect; cat IV: 0.005 mg/kg—give $^1/_2$ of total, then 1–2 hours later give $^1/_4$ dose bolus(es), if needed.
- Monitor and manage abnormalities as possible:
  - Respiratory rate, heart rate and rhythm, arterial blood pressure, body weight, urine output, hydration, attitude, serum biochemistry and blood gas analyses, and pulmonary capillary wedge pressure (if available).
- Diastolic dysfunction (e.g., cats with hypertrophic cardiomyopathy):
  - General recommendations, O_2 therapy, and furosemide as above.
  - +/– Nitroglycerin and mild sedation.
  - Consider IV esmolol (200–500 mcg/kg IV over 1 minute, followed by 25–200 mcg/kg CRI) or diltiazem (0.15–0.25 mg/kg over 2–3 minutes IV).

*Adapted from Wendy A. Ware. *Cardiovascular Disease in Small Animal Medicine.* 2007, London, UK, Manson Publishing, p. 171.

[†]Dilution of 250 mg dobutamine into 500 mL of fluid yields 500 mcg/mL; infusion at 0.6 mL/kg/h yields 5 mcg dobutamine/kg/min.

[‡]Dopamine is diluted in saline solution, 5% dextrose in water, or lactated Ringer's solution; 40 mg of dopamine into 500 mL of fluid provides 80 mcg/mL; infusion at 0.75 mL/kg/h provides 1 mcg dopamine/kg/min.

therapy is usually needed. Support of myocardial function with pimobendan (or digoxin) is helpful for many dogs, and some cats.

   c. Treatment implications for diastolic dysfunction
   (1) Hypertrophic cardiomyopathy (HCM). Disease such as HCM, which impairs ventricular filling, is treated with drugs that slow heart rate (to increase filling time and reduce ischemia). Improved cardiac relaxation is also a goal. Diltiazem (Ca^{2+} blocker), a β-adrenergic blocker and/or an angiotensin converting enzyme inhibitor (ACEI) are most commonly used.
   (2) Cardiac tamponade. Impaired filling caused by cardiac tamponade or pericardial restriction is treated by pericardiocentesis or pericardiectomy rather than drugs.

C. **Diuretics.** Diuretic therapy is indicated to control edema and effusions that occur in CHF. Excessive use of diuretics in heart failure exacerbates neurohormonal activation. Diuretics are discussed in more detail in Chapter 9.

   1. **Furosemide.** This loop-diuretic is used almost exclusively for animals with cardiogenic edema or effusion.
      a. Acute CHF. Although aggressive furosemide therapy is indicated for acute, fulminant pulmonary edema, the smallest effective doses are used for chronic heart failure therapy.
      b. Chronic heart failure. Furosemide should not be used as monotherapy for chronic heart failure management.
      c. Adverse effects are usually related to excessive fluid and/or electrolyte losses.
   2. **Spironolactone.** This K^+-sparing diuretic may be a useful adjunct therapy for chronic refractory heart failure, although it appears to have little diuretic effect in normal dogs.
      a. Aldosterone release can occur despite ACE inhibitor use. Spironolactone's antialdosterone effect may mitigate aldosterone-induced cardiovascular remodeling.
      b. Spironolactone must be used cautiously in patients receiving an ACEI or K^+ supplement, and is absolutely contraindicated in hyperkalemic patients.
      c. Adverse effects relate to excess K^+ retention and GI disturbances. Spironolactone may decrease digoxin clearance.
   3. **Thiazide diuretics.** Chlorothiazide or hydrochlorothiazide is occasionally used in combination with furosemide and other therapy for refractory CHF.
      a. Thiazide diuretics decrease renal blood flow and should not be used in the presence of azotemia.

D. **Angiotensin converting enzyme inhibitors (ACEIs).** This is a group of drugs that, by inhibiting the action of ACE, block the conversion of an inactive precursor peptide (angiotensin I) into the active angiotensin II. In this way, the effects of the renin–angiotensin–aldosterone cascade are opposed. ACE also degrades certain vasodilator kinins, including bradykinin. Most ACEIs (except captopril and lisinopril) are prodrugs which are converted to their active form in the liver. Severe liver dysfunction can interfere with this conversion.

   1. **Pharmacologic effects and mechanism of action**
      a. The main benefits of ACEIs arise from reducing the effects of neurohormonal activation (Figure 8-1).
      b. Arteriolar and venous vasodilation
         (1) Inhibition of locally produced ACE within vascular walls may produce a local vasodilatory response, even in the absence of high circulating renin levels.
         (2) The vasodilating effects of ACEIs may be enhanced by vasodilatory kinins normally degraded by ACE.
      c. Inhibition of angiotensin II production decreases aldosterone secretion, a hormone that promotes renal Na^+ retention. ACEI's diuretic effect is modest.
      d. ACEIs may also (potentially) oppose abnormal CV remodeling changes.

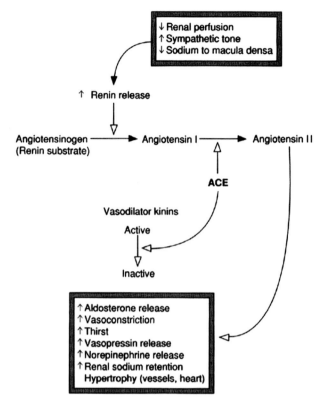

↑ Renin release

Angiotensinogen ⟶ Angiotensin I ⟶ Angiotensin II
(Renin substrate)

ACE

Vasodilator kinins

Active

Inactive

↑ Aldosterone release
↑ Vasoconstriction
↑ Thirst
↑ Vasopressin release
↑ Norepinephrine release
↑ Renal sodium retention
  Hypertrophy (vessels, heart)

↓ Renal perfusion
↑ Sympathetic tone
↓ Sodium to macula densa

FIGURE 8-1. The renin–angiotensin cascade and effects of angiotensin II. Angiotensin converting enzyme (ACE) catalyzes the conversion of angiotensin I to angiotensin II and degrades vasodilator kinins (e.g., bradykinin). Open arrows—enzymatic reaction.

2. Therapeutic uses and administration

   a. An ACEI is indicated for the chronic management of most causes of chronic heart failure, especially dilated cardiomyopathy, chronic valvular insufficiency, and HCM.

   b. An ACEI is considered the first choice agent in the management of systemic arterial hypertension in dogs. An ACEI may also be useful in cats with hypertension.

   c. An ACEI may help slow progression of chronic renal failure in cats, and possibly dogs.

3. Adverse effects of ACEIs include hypotension, GI upset, renal function deterioration, and hyperkalemia (especially when used with a K^+-sparing diuretic or K^+ supplement).

   a. Azotemia. If azotemia develops, the diuretic dosage is decreased first. If necessary, the ACEI dose is reduced or the drug discontinued.

4. ACEI used commonly for CHF management

   a. Enalapril is the only ACEI licensed for veterinary use.

   (1) Enalapril is well absorbed orally; bioavailability is not decreased by food.

   (2) Enalapril is hydrolyzed in the liver to its most active form, enalaprilat.

   (3) Peak ACE-inhibiting activity occurs within 4–6 hours in dogs. Duration of action is 12–14 hours; effects are minimal by 24 hours after once daily dosing.

   (4) Maximal activity in cats occurs within 2–4 hours after an oral dose; some ACE inhibition (50% of control) persists for 2–3 days.

   (5) Enalapril and its active metabolite are excreted in the urine.

      (a) Significant adverse effects on renal function in dogs with advanced mitral regurgitation are generally not a concern.

      (b) Renal failure and severe CHF prolong the drug's elimination, so reduced dosage or benazepril are used in this situation.

b. Benazepril is often chosen in animals with preexisting renal disease. Benazepril may also slow renal function deterioration and partially mitigate hypertension in cats with renal disease.

   (1) Oral administration is absorbed at rate of ~40%, which is not affected by feeding.

   (2) Benazepril is metabolized to its active form (benazeprilat) in the liver.

   (3) Peak ACE inhibition occurs within 2 hours of PO administration in dogs and cats. Complete ACE inhibition occurs in cats at doses of 0.25–0.5 mg/kg. There is >90% ACE inhibition at 24 hours.

   (4) Repeated dosing moderately increases drug plasma concentrations.

   (5) Benazepril is eliminated equally in urine and bile in dogs. In cats, ~85% is excreted in the feces and only 15% in the urine.

c. Other ACEIs sometimes used for CHF include captopril, lisinopril, ramipril, quinipril, fosinopril, and imidapril.

   (1) Captopril is well absorbed orally (75% bioavailable), but **feeding decreases bioavailability by 30–40%.**

      (a) Hemodynamic effects appear within 1 hour, peak in 1–2 hours, and last <4 hours in dogs.

      (b) Captopril is excreted in the urine.

   (2) Lisinopril is a lysine analog of enalaprilat with direct ACE-inhibiting effects.

      (a) Lisinopril is 25–50% bioavailable; absorption is not affected by feeding.

      (b) Time to peak effect is 6–8 hours. Once daily dosing appears to be effective.

E. **Other vasodilators** can further improve cardiac output and reduce edema and effusions in selected heart failure patients. Agents that reduce arteriolar resistance are also used in the treatment of hypertension. Vasodilators can affect arterioles, venous capacitance vessels, or both ("balanced" vasodilators).

1. Introduction

   a. Arteriolar dilators decrease systemic vascular resistance, arterial blood pressure, and afterload on the heart by relaxing arteriolar smooth muscle. This helps improve forward cardiac output and can reduce (mitral) regurgitant flow, thereby decreasing left atrial pressure and pulmonary congestion. **An arteriolar or mixed vasodilator drug should be initiated cautiously to avoid hypotension and reflex tachycardia.**

   b. Venodilators relax systemic veins, increase venous capacitance, decrease cardiac filling pressures (preload), and reduce pulmonary congestion. They are used mainly in treating acute CHF.

2. Hydralazine

   a. Preparation and chemistry. Hydralazine (Apresoline®) is a phthalazine-derivative vasodilating agent.

   b. Pharmacologic effects and mechanism of action. Hydralazine directly relaxes arteriolar smooth muscle with little effect on the venous system. Cerebral, coronary, splanchnic, and renal circulations are affected more than skeletal muscle or skin vasculature. Its effect is dependent on intact vascular endothelium.

   c. Therapeutic uses and administration. Hydralazine, in combination with furosemide, is especially useful for dogs with mitral insufficiency and severe pulmonary edema by rapidly reducing arterial resistance (afterload). This helps reduce regurgitant volume and pulmonary venous pressure and increase forward cardiac output. Hydralazine has also been used in the treatment of myocardial failure and hypertension.

   d. Pharmacokinetics. The drug is rapidly absorbed orally, with onset of action within 1 hour. Peak effect occurs within 3–5 hours and lasts up to 12 hours in dogs. There is extensive first-pass hepatic metabolism of this drug. However, in dogs, increased doses saturate this mechanism and increase bioavailability. A small amount of the drug is excreted unchanged in the urine. The $t_{1/2}$ is 2–4 hours in people. The Cl_T is about 70 mL/min/kg and V_d is 9 L/kg; bioavailability is decreased by over 60% with food.

    e. Adverse effects. Hypotension is most common. Hydralazine causes significant reflex tachycardia in some animals. The dose should be reduced if this occurs; sometimes adding digoxin or a β-blocker is also necessary. Hydralazine can exacerbate the increased neurohumoral response in heart failure, and enhance Na^+ and water retention. GI upset may also occur, especially in cats.

3. Amlodipine

    a. Preparation and chemistry. Amlodipine besylate (Norvasc®) is dihydropyridine Ca^{2+} channel blocker.

    b. Pharmacologic effects and mechanism of action. Ca^{2+} channel blockers as a group block Ca^{2+} influx across cardiac and vascular smooth muscle cell membranes. Amlodipine mainly has vasodilating effects, with no appreciable cardiac effects.

    c. Therapeutic uses and administration. Amlodipine is the drug of first choice for systemic arterial hypertension in cats. It can be a useful adjunct therapeutic agent in hypertensive dogs, and may be effective as a single agent in some. It also is used as adjunct therapy in dogs with refractory CHF (especially from mitral valve disease). It is administered PO.

    d. Pharmacokinetics. Plasma $t_{1/2}$ of amlodipine is ~30 hours in dogs, and maximal effects occur 4–7 days after initiating therapy. Oral bioavailability is high (88% in dogs) and peak plasma concentrations are reached 3–8 hours after oral administration; plasma concentrations increase with chronic therapy. The drug undergoes hepatic metabolism, but there is no extensive first-pass elimination; caution is warranted in animals with poor liver function. Excretion is through the urine and feces. Amlodipine's effect on blood pressure lasts ≥24 hours in cats. Amlodipine generally does not have significant effects on serum creatinine concentration or body weight in cats with chronic renal failure.

    e. Adverse effects. Hypotension is possible, but less likely than with hydralazine because of the slower onset of action. Infrequently, inappetence, azotemia, lethargy, hypokalemia, reflex tachycardia, or weight loss may occur.

4. Nitrates

    a. Preparation and chemistry. Commonly used nitrates include **sodium nitroprusside** (for IV infusion), **nitroglycerine** topical ointment (2%), and oral **isosorbide dinitrate.**

    b. Pharmacologic effects and mechanism of action. Nitrates cause peripheral vasodilation.

        (1) Nitroprusside is a potent direct dilator of both arteriolar and venous smooth muscle; it reduces afterload as well as preload on the heart. The infused dosage should be titrated to maintain mean arterial pressure above 70 mm Hg.

        (2) Nitroglycerin and isosorbide dinitrate act mainly on the venous system and reduce cardiac filling pressures (preload) by their venodilating effects. They are metabolized in vascular smooth muscle to produce nitric oxide, which indirectly mediates vasodilation via activation of guanylyl cyclase to produce cyclic GMP, which in turn activates protein kinase G to open K^+ channels and close Na^+ channels, thereby inducing hyperpolarization of the muscle.

    c. Therapeutic uses and administration

        (1) Sodium nitroprusside is mainly administered IV in the treatment of fulminant CHF; it is sometimes used for acute hypertensive crisis. This agent should only be used when arterial blood pressure and IV infusion rate can be constantly monitored.

        (2) Nitroglycerin. The major indication for nitroglycerin is acute cardiogenic pulmonary edema. Nitroglycerin ointment (2%) is usually applied to the skin of the groin, axillary area, or ear pinna, although the efficacy of this in heart failure is unclear. An application paper or glove is used to avoid skin contact by the person applying the drug. Nitroglycerin ointment or isosorbide dinitrate are used occasionally in chronic CHF management, either combined with standard therapy for refractory CHF, or with hydralazine or amlodipine in animals that cannot tolerate ACEIs.

d. Pharmacokinetics

    (1) **Sodium nitroprusside's** effect on blood pressure last less than 10 minutes, so the drug must be given by intravenous infusion. Nitroprusside is metabolized to a cyanide radical, and then further metabolized in the liver; elimination is via the urine, feces, and exhaled air.

    (2) **Other nitrates.** Because of extensive first-pass hepatic metabolism after oral administration, the transcutaneous route is used most often in animals for other nitrates, although **nitroglycerine** is also well absorbed sublingually. Nitroglycerine ointment (2%) is applied to the patient's skin (usually the groin, axillary area, or ear pinna) every 4–6 hours using application papers or gloves. Onset of action is within 1 hour, with variable duration of effect (e.g., 2–12 hours). The $t_{1/2}$ in dogs is unclear; it is <5 minutes in people, but metabolites have some activity. Dosage and absorption are variable. The self-adhesive, sustained-release preparations may be useful, but have not been systematically evaluated in small animals.

e. Adverse effects.
Profound hypotension is the major side effect of sodium nitroprusside. Cyanide toxicity can result from excess or prolonged use (e.g., over 48 hours). Hypotension may result from excessive or inappropriate use of other nitrates as well. Chronic high dosages and frequent application or long acting formulations are most likely to be associated with the development of drug tolerance.

F. Positive inotropic drugs

1. Pimobendan (Vetmedin®)

  a. Preparation and chemistry. Pimobendan is a benzimidazole–pyridazinone derivative, nonsympathomimetic, nonglycoside inotropic drug that also has vasodilating properties.

  b. Pharmacologic effects and mechanism of action. This drug increases myocardial contractility by increasing myofilament sensitivity to Ca^{2+} and by inhibiting phosphodiesterase III (which breaks down cyclic AMP). The latter mechanism is responsible for pimobendan's vasodilating properties. The drug also appears to have some anticytokine and antithrombotic properties.

  c. Therapeutic uses and administration. Pimobendan is approved for use in dogs with CHF from dilated cardiomyopathy or chronic mitral valve disease. It is used in combination with diuretic and other therapy (sometimes including digoxin) as appropriate for the individual case. The total daily oral dose (0.5 mg/kg) is divided (not necessarily equally) and administered BID using a combination of whole and half chewable tablets (or capsules where available).

  d. Pharmacokinetics. Pimobendan is metabolized in the liver to an active metabolite. Excretion is mainly through the feces. There is >90% protein binding of both drug and active metabolite. The elimination $t_{1/2}$ for pimobendan and its metabolite are ~0.5 and 2 hours, respectively. There is a wide tissue distribution and there is a delay from the time of peak plasma concentrations to maximal effect on myocardial contractility (dP/dt_{max}). Increased dP/dt_{max} is observed for ≥ 8 hours after dosing. Inotropic effect may be attenuated by concurrent use of a β- or Ca^{2+}-blocker.

  e. Adverse effects. About a third of patients may experience reduced appetite, lethargy, diarrhea, and dyspnea, with fewer dogs exhibiting azotemia, weakness and other signs; however, these signs may be due to the underlying CHF. Sporadic mild increase in serum alkaline phosphatase has occurred, and hyperactivity, hemorrhage, drooling, constipation, and diabetes mellitus have been reported as suspected adverse reactions.

2. Digoxin

  a. Preparation and chemistry. Digoxin is a cardiac glycoside. It is essentially the only digitalis glycoside still in clinical use.

  b. Pharmacologic effects and mechanism of action

    (1) **Positive inotropic effect (Figure 8-2).** Digoxin competitively binds to and inhibits Na^+, K^+-ATPase at the myocardial cell membrane. Decreased

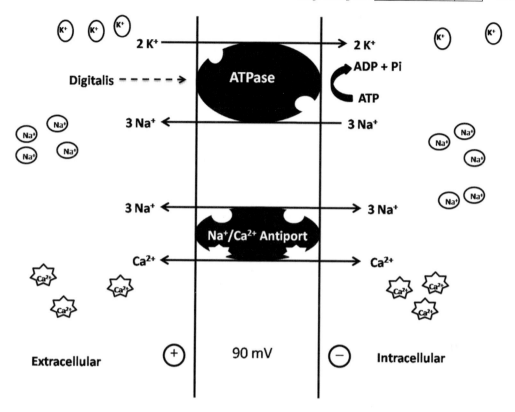

FIGURE 8-2. Digoxin mechanism of action in myocardium. Digoxin-induced inhibition of Na^+, K^+-ATPase leads to an increase in myocardial Na^+ concentration. Through Na^+–Ca^{2+} exchanger, an increase in Ca^{2+} influx is reached. The increase in myocardial Ca^{2+} concentrations enhances the muscle contractility.

extracellular Na^+ transport causes intracellular accumulation, which promotes Ca^{2+} entry via the Na^+–Ca^{2+} exchange. The drug's modest positive inotropic effect results from increased Ca^{2+} available to the contractile proteins.

(2) **Antiarrhythmic effects.** Digoxin also has some antiarrhythmic effects against supraventricular tachyarrhythmias which are mediated primarily via increased parasympathetic tone to the sinus and A-V nodes and atria. The drug also has some direct effects, which further prolong the conduction time and the refractory period of the A-V node.

(3) Digoxin also improves arterial baroreceptor sensitivity in heart failure, which helps counteract excessive neurohormonal activation.

c. **Therapeutic uses and administration**

(1) Digoxin is used for its modest positive inotropic effect. Digoxin has generally been used in the treatment of heart failure caused by or associated with myocardial failure, such as dilated cardiomyopathy and advanced, chronic pressure or volume overloads (e.g., aortic insufficiency, long-standing patent ductus arteriosus, mitral, or tricuspid insufficiency). However, this use is being supplanted by pimobendan.

(2) Digoxin is used for its antiarrhythmic effect against supraventricular arrhythmias. It is only moderately effective in slowing the ventricular response rate in atrial fibrillation and does not cause conversion to sinus rhythm.

(3) Digoxin is usually contraindicated in HCM, where it may worsen existing ventricular outflow obstruction; although it has been used when clinical signs of right heart failure develop. Digoxin is generally not useful for patients with pericardial disease. Digoxin is usually contraindicated when sinus

or A-V nodal disease is present; it is relatively contraindicated with most serious ventricular arrhythmias because the drug may exacerbate them.

(4) **Factors affecting dosage.** Conservative doses should be used. Therapy is almost always begun using oral maintenance (rather than IV or loading) doses. There is only a weak correlation between digoxin dose and serum concentration in dogs with heart failure, indicating that other factors are important in determining the serum concentrations of this drug.

(a) **Renal function.** Serum digoxin concentrations are increased in dogs and cats with renal dysfunction because of reduced total body clearance and volume of distribution. There appears to be no correlation between degree of azotemia and serum concentration.

(b) **Body condition.** Since much of the drug is bound to skeletal muscle, animals with reduced muscle mass or cachexia, as well as those with compromised renal function can easily become toxic at the usual calculated doses. In addition, because digoxin has poor lipid solubility the dose should be based on the calculated lean body weight; this is especially important in obese animals.

(c) **Serum concentration measurement.** After 1 week of therapy (or dosage alteration) serum concentrations should be measured.

i The sample is drawn 8–10 hours after the previous dose. If serum concentration is <0.8 ng/mL, the digoxin dose can be increased by ≤30%, and the serum concentration measured the following week.

ii If serum concentration cannot be measured and toxicity is suspected, the drug should be discontinued for 1–2 days, then reinstituted at half of the original dose.

(d) **Therapeutic serum concentration** is considered to be between 0.8 and 2.0 ng/mL. This is reached within 2–4.5 days (with PO dosing every 12 hours) in dogs. In cats, therapeutic serum concentration is achieved with low doses given every 48 hours; concentrations are ∼50% higher with the alcohol-based (less palatable) elixir than with tablets. In horses, serum concentrations of 0.5–2.0 ng/mL are achieved within 1–2 hours. Significant enterohepatic recycling may produce a second peak serum concentration in horses.

d. **Pharmacokinetics**

(1) **Absorption** is ∼60% for the tablet form and 75% for the elixir. Absorption is decreased by food, kaolin–pectin compounds, antacids, and malabsorption syndromes. Steady state serum concentrations are achieved in ∼7 days for dogs, in ∼10 days for cats, and in 3–5 days for horses.

(2) **Fate.** About 27% of the drug in serum is protein bound. Elimination is mainly renal. There is minimal hepatic metabolism. Digoxin $t_{1/2}$ is reported to be 23–39 hours in dogs, 25–78 hours in cats, and 13–23 hours in horses.

e. **Adverse effects.** Myocardial toxicity is of greater concern than GI toxicity. Fatal myocardial toxicity may occur before other signs develop, especially in patients with myocardial failure. **P-R interval prolongation or signs of GI toxicity should *not* be used to guide progressive dosing of digitalis.** Serum concentration measurement should be used to guide dosing. Loading doses should not be used in myocardial failure.

(1) **Myocardial toxicity** can cause almost any cardiac rhythm disturbance, including ventricular tachyarrhythmias, supraventricular premature complexes and tachycardia, sinus arrest, Mobitz type I second-degree A-V block, and junctional rhythms.

(a) **Calcium overload.** Diastolic sequestration and systolic release of Ca^{2+} may be impaired in diseased myocardial cells. Digoxin use can lead to cellular Ca^{2+} overload and electrical instability.

(b) Toxic levels of digoxin also **increase sympathetic** tone to the heart causing increased automaticity. In addition, the parasympathetic effects of slowed conduction and altered refractory period facilitate the occurrence of re-entrant arrhythmias.

(c) Digoxin also can stimulate spontaneous automaticity of myocardial cells by inducing and potentiating **late after-depolarization**; this is enhanced by cellular stretch, calcium overloading, and hypokalemia.

(2) GI toxicity. GI upset is the other major toxicity and may occur before signs of myocardial toxicity develop, especially in patients without myocardial failure. Its signs include anorexia, depression, vomiting, borborygmus, and diarrhea. Direct effects of digitalis on chemoreceptors in the area postrema of the medulla may be the cause of some of the GI signs (e.g., vomiting).

(3) Factors predisposing to digoxin toxicity

   (a) Hypokalemia predisposes to myocardial toxicity by leaving more available binding sites on membrane Na^+, K^+-ATPase for digitalis.

   (b) Renal dysfunction (see above)

   (c) Hypercalcemia and **hypernatremia** potentiate both the inotropic and toxic effects of the drug.

   (d) Abnormal thyroid hormone levels can lead to digitalis toxicity (hyperthyroidism increases the drug's myocardial effects and hypothyroidism reduces its clearance); therefore, dosage reduction may be needed.

   (e) Hypoxia sensitizes the myocardium to the toxic effects of digitalis.

   (f) Certain drugs increase digoxin serum concentration. Quinidine displaces the drug from skeletal muscle binding sites and reducing its renal clearance. Verapamil and amiodarone also can increase serum digoxin concentration; other drugs possibly do as well (including diltiazem, prazosin, spironolactone, and triamterene). Drugs affecting hepatic microsomal enzymes may also have effects on digoxin metabolism. Neomycin and sulfasalazine decrease bioavailability.

(4) Therapy for digitalis toxicity depends on the signs manifested.

   (a) GI signs usually respond to drug withdrawal and correction of fluid or electrolyte disturbances.

   (b) Atrioventricular conduction abnormalities also usually resolve with drug withdrawal, although sometimes an anticholinergic agent is needed.

   (c) Ventricular tachyarrhythmias in dogs are treated with lidocaine or phenytoin.

   i Other therapy includes IV K^+ supplementation (if serum K^+ is <4.0 mEq/L), IV fluid to correct dehydration and maximize renal function, and in some cases, propranolol to help control ventricular tachyarrhythmias (as long as no conduction blocks are present).

   ii Oral administration of the steroid-binding resin cholestyramine is only useful very soon after accidental overdosage of digoxin, since this drug undergoes minimal enterohepatic circulation. A preparation of digoxin-specific antigen binding fragments (Digoxin immune Fab; Digibind®) derived from ovine antidigoxin antibodies have been used occasionally for digoxin overdose in dogs.

3. **Dobutamine and dopamine (sympathomimetic agents).** See Chapter 2 for more information.

   a. **Preparation and chemistry. Dopamine** (Intropin®) is an endogenous catecholamine that is a precursor to norepinephrine. **Dobutamine** (Dobutrex®) is a synthetic analog of dopamine.

   b. **Pharmacologic effects and mechanism of action.** Catecholamines increase contractility and heart rate, especially at higher doses. Stimulation of cardiac β_1-adrenergic receptors (coupled to G_s) activates adenylyl cyclase to increase cyclic AMP synthesis, which stimulates a protein kinase A that in turn activates Ca^{2+} channels, leading to increased Ca^{2+} influx and greater contractility.

   (1) Dopamine stimulates β- and α-receptors at higher doses. Peripheral vasoconstriction occurs at 10–15 mcg/kg/min. At low doses (less than 2–5 mcg/kg/min IV infusion), it also stimulates vasodilator dopaminergic receptors in the renal, mesenteric, coronary, and cerebral circulations.

   (2) Dobutamine stimulates β_1-receptors, but has only weak action on β_2- and α-receptors; it does not stimulate dopaminergic receptors. The drug increases contractility, with minimal effects on heart rate and blood pressure at lower infusion rates (3–7 μg/kg/min).

   c. **Therapeutic uses and administration**
      (1) **Myocardial failure.** Dopamine and dobutamine are used, in conjunction with other therapy, for short-term inotropic and blood pressure support in dogs and cats with myocardial failure. Use of catecholamines for heart failure is limited by the development of β-receptor downregulation. Generally these drugs are given for no more than 3 days.
      (2) **Hypotension** that is not responsive to fluid loading.
      (3) Dopamine is also used to increase renal blood flow in acute oliguric renal failure.
   d. **Pharmacokinetics.** The very short $t_{1/2}$ (less than 2 minutes) and extensive hepatic metabolism of the catecholamines used clinically makes them suitable only for IV administration, usually by constant infusion.
   e. **Adverse effects.** At higher doses, dopamine and dobutamine increase heart rate, myocardial oxygen demand, and the risk of inducing ventricular arrhythmias. Development of sinus tachycardia or tachyarrhythmias should prompt a decrease in infusion rate.
      (1) Dobutamine is less arrhythmogenic than other catecholamines, but may precipitate supraventricular and ventricular arrhythmias at higher infusion rates (10–20 mcg/kg/min). Cats are more sensitive to dobutamine than dogs and may exhibit seizures or other adverse effects at relatively low dosages.
      (2) By increasing renal blood flow, dopamine may enhance the renal clearance of other drugs.

4. **Amrinone** and **Milrinone** (phosphodiesterase inhibitors)
   a. **Preparation and chemistry. Amrinone** is also known as inamrinone. Amrinone and milrinone are bipyridine cardiac inotropic agents.
   b. **Pharmacologic effects and mechanism of action.** These agents inhibit phosphodiesterase III, an intracellular enzyme that degrades cAMP. They produce vasodilation as well as an increase in myocardial contractility.
   c. **Therapeutic uses and administration.** Amrinone and milrinone are sometimes used for short-term inotropic support in dogs and cats with severe myocardial failure. The drugs are available for IV injection. They can be used concurrently with other types of inotropic agents.
   d. **Pharmacokinetics.** Effects begin within 3 minutes and peak in 10 minutes after IV bolus injection, but are short-lived in normal dogs (<30 minutes). Constant infusion is required for sustained effect. Peak effect using constant rate infusion occurs in ~45 minutes in dogs.
   e. **Adverse effects**
      (1) These agents may exacerbate ventricular tachyarrhythmias.
      (2) Higher dosages result in greater vasodilation, with reduction of blood pressure and increases in heart rate.
      (3) Other adverse effects could include vomiting/diarrhea, hepatotoxicity, thrombocytopenia (with prolonged use).

G. **Drugs used in heart disease causing diastolic function.** Agents that increase diastolic filling time, reduce myocardial O_2 requirements, and/or facilitate myocardial relaxation are used in the treatment of HCM and other causes of severe hypertrophy.

1. **β-Blockers** such as atenolol (propranolol, metoprolol, and others) are often used to slow heart rate and reduce myocardial O_2 consumption. See II D and Chapter 2 for more information.
   a. Certain β-blockers (e.g., carvedilol, metoprolol) may also be useful in the long-term management of dilated cardiomyopathy and chronic valve disease, but further study is needed.
2. **Calcium entry blockers**, as a group, cause coronary and systemic vasodilation, enhanced myocardial relaxation, and sometimes, reduced cardiac contractility. **Diltiazem** has been used commonly in cats with HCM (see II D for additional information).

3. **ACE inhibitors** (e.g., enalapril, benazepril) are being increasingly used in the management of CHF from HCM (see above and also Chapter 3).

II. ANTIARRHYTHMIC DRUGS

A. Introduction

1. **Multiple factors underlie the development of cardiac rhythm disturbances.**
   a. Both overt and subclinical changes in cardiac structure or function can alter cell electrophysiologic characteristics in ways that predispose to arrhythmia formation.
      (1) Changes in normal cellular conduction properties or automaticity caused by cardiac structural or physiologic remodeling can predispose to arrhythmia development. Genetic factors and environmental stresses can contribute.
      (2) Additional triggering (e.g., premature stimulus or abrupt change in heart rate) and/or modulating factors (e.g., changes in autonomic tone, circulating catecholamines, ischemia, or electrolyte disturbances) also appear necessary to provoke and sustain rhythm disturbances.
   b. Abnormal rhythms, as well as normal sinus node activity, are influenced by the autonomic nervous system. Many conditions affect prevailing autonomic tone.
2. In general, underlying mechanisms are categorized as disorders of impulse formation, disorders of impulse conduction, or combinations of both. Identifying the specific mechanism for an arrhythmia in the individual patient is often difficult.
   a. Disorders of impulse conduction can cause bradyarrhythmias when conduction fails in the AV node, atria, or SA node, causing asystole or a slow escape rhythm.
   b. Disorders of impulse conduction can also cause tachyarrhythmias when re-entry (re-entrant excitation, circus movement, reciprocating tachycardia) occurs.
   c. Re-entry is a common arrhythmia mechanism.
      (1) It involves an area where conduction is blocked or delayed, but which recovers excitability in time to transmit the depolarizing wave back around so that tissue that had been previously depolarized becomes activated again.
      (2) Re-entry can occur within defined anatomic pathways (anatomic re-entry) or because of functional electrophysiologic changes in adjacent tissues (functional re-entry).
3. The clinical context of the arrhythmia is important.
   a. Some arrhythmias are benign and do not require treatment.
      (1) Ventricular ectopy that develops after thoracic trauma in previously healthy animals generally resolves without therapy.
      (2) Occasional ventricular premature contractions (VPCs) have also been identified in clinically normal animals.
   b. While some arrhythmias are of no clinical consequence, others cause weakness, syncope, or sudden death, especially in animals with underlying disease.
   c. Arrhythmias that compromise cardiac output, arterial blood pressure, and coronary perfusion can promote myocardial ischemia, deterioration of cardiac pump function, and, sometimes, sudden death.
      (1) These arrhythmias tend to be either very rapid (e.g., sustained ventricular or supraventricular tachyarrhythmias) or very slow (e.g., advanced AV block with a slow or unstable ventricular escape rhythm).
      (2) Rapid sustained tachycardia of either supraventricular or ventricular origin reduces cardiac output acutely, and eventually leads to myocardial dysfunction and CHF (tachycardia-induced cardiomyopathy).
4. An arrhythmia may be suspected from the animal's history or identified on physical examination.
   a. An accurate ECG diagnosis is important.

B. Overview of cardiac arrhythmia therapy

1. Therapy is indicated for arrhythmias that cause clinical signs of hemodynamic compromise, and when the patient has a disease known to be associated with sudden arrhythmic death.
   a. Ideal goals of antiarrhythmic drug therapy might be to totally suppress all abnormal beats, and prevent further arrhythmias and sudden death, but these are not often realistic goals.
   b. Successful therapy usually is sufficient reduction in frequency (e.g., by ≥70–80%) or repetitive rate of ectopic beats to restore normal hemodynamic status and eliminate clinical signs.
   c. Even apparently complete arrhythmia suppression does not remove the risk of a lethal arrhythmia and sudden death.

2. Antiarrhythmic drugs may slow the rate of tachycardia, terminate a re-entrant arrhythmia, or prevent abnormal impulse formation or conduction.
   a. These effects can occur through modulation of tissue electrophysiologic properties and/or autonomic nervous system effects.
   b. The traditional (Vaughan Williams) antiarrhythmic drug classification system consists of four classes based on the drug's predominant cardiac electrophysiologic effects (Table 8-2), but this system has shortcomings.
      (1) Class I agents have membrane-stabilizing effects that tend to slow conduction as well as decrease automaticity and excitability.

TABLE 8-2. Antiarrhythmic Drug Classification*

Class	Drug	Mechanism and ECG Effects
I		Decrease fast inward Na^+ current; membrane-stabilizing effects (slowed conduction, decreased excitability and automaticity)
IA	Quinidine, procainamide	Moderately slows conduction, increases action potential duration; can prolong QRS complex and Q-T interval
IB	Lidocaine, mexiletine, phenytoin	Little change in conductivity, decreases action potential duration; QRS complex and Q-T interval unchanged
IC	Flecainide, propafenone	Markedly slows conduction without change in action potential duration
II	Atenolol, propranolol, esmolol, metoprolol, carvedilol, others	β-adrenergic blockade, reduces effects of sympathetic stimulation (no direct myocardial effects at clinical doses)
III	Sotalol, amiodarone, others	Selectively prolongs action potential duration and refractory period; antiadrenergic effects; Q-T interval prolonged
IV	Diltiazem, verapamil	Decreases slow inward Ca^{++} current (greatest effect on SA and AV nodes)
Other agents with antiarrhythmic effects include	Digoxin	Antiarrhythmic action results mainly from indirect autonomic effects, especially increased vagal tone
	Atropine and other anticholinergic drugs	Oppose vagal effects on SA and AV nodes

*Adapted from Wendy A. Ware. *Cardiovascular Disease in Small Animal Medicine.* 2007, London, UK, Manson Publishing, p. 199.

(2) Class II consists of β-adrenergic antagonists, which act by inhibiting catecholamine effects on the heart.

(3) Class III drugs prolong the effective refractory period of cardiac action potentials without decreasing conduction velocity.

(4) Class IV contains calcium-entry blocking drugs. These are most useful for supraventricular tachyarrhythmias; ventricular arrhythmias usually are unresponsive to them.

c. Suggested drug dosages are listed in Appendix II.

3. Therapy for supraventricular tachyarrhythmias

a. Supraventricular premature complexes:

(1) Occasional premature beats do not require antiarrhythmic therapy.

(2) Predisposing factors should be minimized as far as possible.

b. Frequent atrial premature contractions or brief paroxysmal supraventricular tachycardia (SVT):

(1) Digoxin (Table 8-2) is used first in dogs with heart failure and in cats with dilated cardiomyopathy.

(2) A β-blocker or the Ca^{2+} blocker diltiazem can be added if the arrhythmia is not sufficiently controlled with digoxin (along with an ACE inhibitor and furosemide for heart failure).

(3) For cats with HCM or hyperthyroidism a β-blocker (e.g., atenolol or propranolol) is used, although diltiazem could be an alternative.

(4) Recurrent supraventricular tachyarrhythmias that are refractory to these drugs may respond to amiodarone, sotolol, procainamide, quinidine, or a Class IC agent.

c. Acute therapy for sustained or persistent paroxysmal SVT:

(1) A vagal maneuver is tried initially for sustained SVT.

(2) When SVT persists, a Ca^{2+} channel blocker is usually administered next.

(a) Diltiazem (IV or PO loading) is preferred.

(b) Verapamil (IV) is also effective, but is not recommended for dogs with myocardial dysfunction or heart failure because of its greater negative inotropic effect.

(3) A β-blocker given slowly IV (propranolol, esmolol) is an alternative, but also has negative inotropic effects.

(4) IV digoxin is another alternative, but it is generally less effective than Ca^{2+} channel blockers.

(a) Digoxin is not used in pre-excitation syndrome because it can decrease the refractory period of the accessory pathway, although it slows AV conduction.

(5) Lidocaine (IV) can be effective in some cases of SVT caused by an accessory pathway or ectopic atrial focus, although it is most often used for wide-QRS tachyarrhythmias.

(6) If Ca^{2+} channel- or β-blocker or lidocaine therapy does not control persistent SVT, IV procainamide may.

(7) Refractory SVT (AV node-independent) may respond to sotalol or amiodarone.

(8) Once the rhythm is controlled, PO maintenance digoxin and/or diltiazem or a β-blocker are used most often for long-term therapy.

(a) Amiodarone or sotalol are alternative agents in cases refractory to conventional drugs.

(b) Procainamide, quinidine, or a Class IC drug have also been used

d. Atrial fibrillation (AF) is usually associated with marked atrial enlargement, except in large/giant breeds of dog and in large animal species. Because permanent conversion to sinus rhythm is unlikely in most animals with atrial enlargement, the usual goals of therapy are to slow AV conduction and to manage underlying disease.

(1) If rapid HR reduction is indicated, IV diltiazem is recommended because it has less negative inotropic effect than verapamil and propranolol.

    (2) Long-term oral therapy usually includes digoxin in dogs (and cats with my-ocardial failure). But **digoxin alone often does not adequately slow the heart rate animals with heart failure or during exercise.** Either a β-blocker or dil-tiazem can be added to further slow AV conduction; low initial doses are used and titrated upward to effect.

    (3) Amiodarone can be used if additional rate control is needed.

    (4) For cats with HCM and AF, diltiazem or a β-blocker is used without digoxin.

    (5) When ventricular pre-excitation is present in a patient with AF, AV nodal blocking drugs (Ca^{2+} blockers, digoxin, and possibly β-blockers) should not be used because they can paradoxically increase the ventricular response rate. Amiodarone is recommended in these cases; sotalol or procainamide can also be used.

  e. AF in larger animals without signs of heart disease or failure may convert to si-nus rhythm, either spontaneously or with drug treatment or electrical cardiover-sion. Conversion is more likely with AF of recent onset and normal atrial size.

    (1) Pharmacologic cardioversion is sometimes achieved with quinidine, but this is only used where this is no or only mild underlying disease.

    (2) Alternatively, high-dose diltiazem alone (PO for 3 days) has sometimes been effective in dogs, as has amiodarone, propafenone, and sotolol. Acute onset AF associated with high vagal tone may convert with IV lidocaine.

4. Therapy for ventricular tachyarrhythmias

  a. Occasional ventricular premature complexes (VPCs) are usually not treated, es-pecially in an otherwise asymptomatic animal. Moderately frequent, single VPCs of uniform configuration may also not require antiarrhythmic drug treatment, especially if underlying heart function is normal.

  b. Acute therapy for ventricular tachycardia

    (1) Lidocaine (IV) is usually the first-choice drug for controlling serious ventricu-lar tachyarrhythmias in dogs.

    (2) PO sotalol, or mexiletine, or IV amiodarone, can be more effective in some cases. IV amiodarone must be given cautiously because marked hypotension can occur.

    (3) Alternatively, procainamide (given IV, IM, or PO) or quinidine (given IM or PO) can be tried. If a single IM or PO loading dose of either drug is effective (within 2 hours), lower doses can be given every 4–6 hours IM or PO.

    (4) Addition of a β-blocker or other combination therapy is sometimes effective.

    (5) Cats with frequent ventricular tachyarrhythmias are usually given a β-blocker first. Alternatively, low doses of lidocaine can be tried, but cats, are sensitive to the neurotoxic effects of this drug. Procainamide or sotolol can also be used.

  c. Chronic oral therapy for ventricular tachyarrhythmias

    (1) The same, or similar, drug that was most effective during acute therapy is often continued PO in cases where long-term therapy is needed.

    (2) Sustained-release procainamide or mexiletine (Class I agents) can be used alone, or with a β-blocker. β-Blockers may confer some protection against ventricular fibrillation.

    (3) Sotolol or amiodarone (Class III agents) may provide greater antifibrillatory protection.

5. Therapy for bradyarrhythmias

  a. If the arrhythmia is the result of a drug effect, discontinuation or dosage reduc-tion is also used, as appropriate.

  b. Symptomatic bradyarrhythmias (e.g., sinus bradycardia, sick sinus syndrome, atrial standstill, high grade AV block) are initially treated with atropine (or at-ropine challenge test).

  c. If the arrhythmia is responsive to atropine challenge, oral anticholinergic therapy may be useful.

  d. An emergency infusion of dopamine or isoproterenol may increase the ventricu-lar escape rate in animals with high-grade AV block, although ventricular tach-yarrhythmias may also be provoked

e. Temporary or permanent artificial pacing is indicated when there is inadequate increase in heart rate with medical therapy.

C. **Class I agents (membrane stabilizers)**

1. **Class I agents (local anesthetics)** slow conduction and decrease automaticity and excitability by their membrane stabilizing effects. Most of these agents are dependent on extracellular K^+ concentration for their effects.
   a. Drugs in Class I have also been subclassified (see Table 8-2).
   b. Concurrent use of a Class I drug and a drug of another class (or even subclass) may increase antiarrhythmic efficacy in cases refractory to a single agent.
   c. Contraindications. All these drugs are contraindicated in the presence of complete heart block, and should be used only cautiously in patients with sinus bradycardia, sick sinus syndrome, and first- or second-degree A-V blocks.
   d. Adverse effects. All antiarrhythmic drugs may cause exacerbation of arrhythmias (proarrhythmic effect), especially the Class IC agents.

2. **Lidocaine**
   a. **Preparation and chemistry.** Lidocaine HCl is available as an injectable solution of various concentrations. The 2% concentration is most commonly used.
   b. **Pharmacologic effects and mechanism of action.** Lidocaine has little effect on sinus rate, AV conduction rate, and refractoriness. See Table 8-2, Class IB.
      (1) The electrophysiologic effects of lidocaine (and other Class I drugs) are very dependent on extracellular K^+ concentration; hypokalemia may make the drug ineffective, while hyperkalemia intensifies the drug's depressant effects on cardiac membranes.
      (2) Lidocaine suppresses automaticity in both normal Purkinje fibers and diseased myocardial tissue, slows conduction, and reduces the supernormal period. It has greater effects on diseased and hypoxic cardiac cells.
      (3) Lidocaine produces minimal hemodynamic effects and little to no depression of contractility at therapeutic doses when given slowly IV. Hypotension can be associated with toxic levels.
   c. **Therapeutic uses and administration.** Lidocaine is used IV mainly to suppress frequent ventricular premature contractions and ventricular tachycardia, although it may convert some cases of SVT.
   d. **Pharmacokinetics**
      (1) Because of almost complete first-pass hepatic elimination, lidocaine is administered IV, usually as slow boluses followed by constant rate infusion. Antiarrhythmic effects after an IV bolus occur within 2 minutes and disappear within 10–20 minutes.
      (2) Constant rate infusion without a loading dose results in steady state levels in 4–6 hours.
      (3) Lidocaine undergoes rapid hepatic metabolism; some metabolites are active. The $t_{1/2}$ after IV injection is <1 hour in the dog (similar in the cat).
      (4) A V_d of 5.7 L/kg and Cl_T of 62 mL/min/kg are reported for the dog. A V_d of 1.7 L/kg, Cl_T of 64.4 mL/min/kg, and a $t_{1/2}$ of 3.1 hours are reported for the horse.
      (5) Therapeutic plasma concentrations are 2–6 mcg/mL.
      (6) Propranolol, cimetidine, and other drugs which decrease liver blood flow slow the metabolism of lidocaine. Reduced hepatic blood flow associated with heart failure can also predispose to toxicity.
   e. **Adverse effects.** Central nervous system (CNS) excitation is the most common toxic effect. Signs include agitation, disorientation, muscle twitches, nystagmus, and generalized seizures. Nausea may also occur. Cats are particularly sensitive to the drug's toxic effects and may suffer respiratory arrest along with seizures. Horses are also very sensitive to CNS toxic effects. QRS widening can occur.

3. **Mexiletine**
   a. **Preparation and chemistry.** Mexiletine HCl is available as oral capsules.

b. **Pharmacologic effects and mechanism of action.** Mexiletine is similar to lidocaine in its electrophysiologic, hemodynamic, and antiarrhythmic properties (see Table 8-2).

c. **Therapeutic uses and administration.** Mexiletine is used to suppress frequent ventricular premature contractions and ventricular tachycardia.

d. **Pharmacokinetics**
   (1) Mexiletine appears to have good oral absorption.
   (2) The drug is highly protein bound. It undergoes liver metabolism (influenced by liver blood flow) and some renal excretion (which is slower with alkaline urine). The $t_{1/2}$ in dogs is 4.5–7 hours (depending to some degree on urine pH).
   (3) Therapeutic serum concentration is thought to be 0.5–2.0 mcg/mL.

e. **Adverse effects.** Toxic effects are similar to lidocaine. Vomiting, anorexia, tremor, ataxia, disorientation, sinus bradycardia, and thrombocytopenia have been reported in dogs.

4. **Procainamide**
   a. **Preparation and chemistry.** Procainamide HCl is similar in structure to procaine. It is available as an injectable solution and in tablets or capsules as well as extended release tablets.

   b. **Pharmacologic effects and mechanism of action** (see Table 8-2). Procainamide has both direct (Class IA) and indirect (vagolytic) effects similar to quinidine.
      (1) Oral and IM administrations of this drug are not associated with marked hemodynamic effects; however, rapid IV injection can cause significant hypotension and cardiac depression (but less than with IV quinidine).

   c. **Therapeutic uses and administration.** Procainamide is used mainly for frequent ventricular premature contractions and ventricular tachycardia; it also may be effective against some supraventricular tachyarrhythmias.

   d. **Pharmacokinetics**
      (1) Procainamide is well absorbed orally in the dog. Procainamide is thought to be 20% protein bound in the dog. The V_d is 1.4–2.1 L/kg in dogs.
      (2) Constant IV infusion may be used; steady state is reached in 12–22 hours.
      (3) Elimination is by hepatic metabolism as well as renal excretion in proportion to the creatinine clearance. The $t_{1/2}$ is 2.5–4 hours; the sustained release form has a slightly longer $t_{1/2}$ of 3–6 hours in dogs.
      (4) The metabolite N-acetylprocainamide is found in horses, but is not present to any significant degree in dogs. In the horse, a V_d of 2.4 L/kg, Cl_T of 3.9 mL/min/kg, and a $t_{1/2}$ of 3–7 hours are reported.
      (5) Therapeutic plasma range in dogs is 4–12 mcg/mL.

   e. **Adverse effects.** Procainamide may exacerbate hypotension or heart failure.
      (1) The toxic effects are similar to those of quinidine but usually milder. GI upset and prolongation of the PR, QRS, or Q-T intervals can occur.
      (2) Increased ventricular response rate to atrial fibrillation can result when used without digoxin, β-blocker, or Ca^{2+} entry blocker.
      (3) More serious toxic effects include hypotension, depressed A-V conduction, and worsening of arrhythmias (may result in syncope or ventricular fibrillation).

5. **Quinidine**
   a. **Preparation and chemistry.** Quinidine is an alkaloid derived from quinine or the cinchona (or related) plants. Gluconate, polygalacturonate, and sulfate salts have been used clinically PO. The gluconate salt is available for injection.

   b. **Pharmacologic effects and mechanism of action.** Quinidine is a Class IA agent (see Table 8-2). The drug's actions result from both direct electrophysiologic and vagolytic effects.
      (1) Its indirect (vagolytic) effects, at low doses, may increase sinus node rate or the ventricular response rate to atrial fibrillation by antagonizing the drug's direct effects.
      (2) As with other Class I agents, hypokalemia reduces the antiarrhythmic effectiveness of quinidine.

(3) Vasodilation (via α-receptor blockade), cardiac depression, and hypotension result from IV administration. Oral and IM administrations are usually not associated with adverse hemodynamic effects, but could be in patients with underlying cardiac disease.

c. **Therapeutic uses and administration.** Quinidine is used less commonly than other antiarrhythmic agents now. It can be effective against frequent ventricular tachyarrhythmias; it also may be effective against some supraventricular tachyarrhythmias.

(1) Quinidine may successfully convert recent-onset atrial fibrillation to sinus rhythm in horses, cattle, and large dogs with normal heart size and function.

d. **Pharmacokinetics**

(1) Quinidine is well absorbed orally with little first-pass hepatic elimination. The sulfate salt is more rapidly absorbed than the gluconate. Peak effect is usually achieved 1–2 hours after oral administration.

(2) The drug is highly protein bound in dogs and cats. In the dog, a V_d of 2.9 L/kg and a Cl_T of 6 mL/min/kg are reported. In the cat, a V_d of 2.2 L/kg and Cl_T of 14.8 mL/min/kg are reported.

(3) There is extensive hepatic metabolism that is not greatly dependent on liver blood flow. Quinidine has a $t_{1/2}$ of ~6 hours in the dog, and ~2 hours in the cat. Anticonvulsants and other drugs which induce hepatic microsomal enzymes can speed the drug's metabolism.

(4) Therapeutic blood levels (2.5–5 mcg/mL) are usually reached in 12–24 hours after PO and IM administration.

(5) Slow-release sulfate, gluconate, and polygalacturonate salts prolong the drug's absorption and elimination. Administration of these q8 hours is probably adequate for dogs, while standard quinidine sulfate should be given q6 hours.

(6) In the horse, a V_d of 2.9–6.3 L/kg, Cl_T of 6–16 mL/min/kg, and a $t_{1/2}$ of 4–7 hours are reported. The drug is usually given by nasogastric tube every 2 hours for up to 5–6 doses to convert atrial fibrillation. From 10 to 50% absorption occurs within 2 hours.

(7) A plasma concentration of 2–4 mcg/mL is thought to be therapeutic.

e. **Adverse effects.** Quinidine may exacerbate hypotension or heart failure. It should not be administered IV.

(1) Toxicity occurs as an extension of the drug's electrophysiologic and hemodynamic actions. Prolongation of ECG intervals occurs as plasma concentration increases. Marked Q-T prolongation, development of bundle branch block, or QRS widening greater than 25% of the pretreatment value suggest toxicity. All degrees of A-V block and ventricular tachyarrhythmias can also result.

(2) Lethargy, weakness, and CHF can result from the drug's negative inotropic and vasodilatory effects and subsequent hypotension.

(3) Cardiotoxicity and hypotension may be partially reversible by sodium bicarbonate therapy. This temporarily decreases serum K^+ concentration and increases quinidine's binding to albumin. Because of its extensive protein binding, severe hypoalbuminemia can predispose to toxicity.

(4) GI signs (nausea, vomiting, and diarrhea) are common with oral quinidine therapy. Apprehension, depression, diarrhea, and anorexia are common in horses.

(5) Quinidine can precipitate digoxin toxicity when both drugs are used together, as it displaces digoxin from skeletal muscle-binding sites and decreases digoxin's renal clearance.

6. **Phenytoin**

a. **Preparation and chemistry.** Phenytoin Na^+ is a hydantoin-derivative available as an injectable solution in a propylene glycol/alcohol vehicle.

b. **Pharmacologic effects and mechanism of action.** Phenytoin is similar to lidocaine, but it also has some slow calcium channel inhibitory and CNS effects that may contribute to its effectiveness against digitalis-induced arrhythmias.

    c. Therapeutic uses and administration. Phenytoin is used in dogs only for the therapy of digitalis-induced ventricular arrhythmias that are not responsive to lidocaine; phenytoin is not used in cats.

    d. Pharmacokinetics

      (1) Oral bioavailability is poor; the drug is administered slowly IV.

      (2) The drug is metabolized in the liver and, by stimulating hepatic microsomal enzymes, may speed its own elimination.

      (3) The $t_{1/2}$ of phenytoin is only about 3 hours in the dog; the V_d is 1.2 L/kg and the Cl_T is 4 mL/min/kg. The drug is not used in cats, as the $t_{1/2}$ is very long (>40 hours).

      (4) Therapeutic plasma range is 10–16 μg/mL.

    e. Adverse effects. The drug has been associated with bradycardia, A-V blocks, ventricular tachycardia, and cardiac arrest.

      (1) Rapid IV injection is avoided because the propylene glycol vehicle can depress myocardial contractility and cause vasodilation, hypotension, exacerbation of arrhythmias, and respiratory arrest. Slow IV infusion and oral administration do not cause significant hemodynamic disturbances.

      (2) Other toxicity signs include depression, nystagmus, disorientation, and ataxia.

      (3) Even low doses can produce toxic serum concentrations in cats.

  7. Other Class I drugs. Flecainide and propafenone (Class IC) markedly reduce cardiac conduction velocity; they may depress automaticity in the sinus node and specialized conducting tissues at high doses. Proarrhythmia is a serious potential adverse effect of these Class IC agents. Bradycardia, intraventricular conduction disturbance, and consistent (although transient) hypotension have occurred in dogs, as well as nausea, vomiting, and anorexia. Hypotension from vasodilation and myocardial depression after IV administration can be significant.

D. **Class II agents (β-blockers)** act by inhibiting catecholamine effects on the heart. They slow heart rate, reduce myocardial oxygen demand, and increase AV conduction time and refractoriness.

  1. β-blockers are indicated for supraventricular tachyarrhythmias (including paroxysmal atrial tachycardia and frequent atrial premature complexes) and to slow the ventricular response rate in atrial fibrillation (usually in combination with digoxin).

    a. A β-blocker is the drug of first choice in cats for both supra- and ventricular tachyarrhythmias.

    b. In dogs, the combination of a β-blocker with a Class I agent often provides better arrhythmia suppression than either alone.

    c. β-blockers are also used to decrease heart rate and myocardial O_2 demand in HCM and other causes of myocardial hypertrophy, as well as in the therapy of hypertension.

  2. The antiarrhythmic effect of β-blockers relates to β_1-receptor blockade rather than direct electrophysiologic effects.

    a. Although β-receptor blockers cause little negative inotropic effect in normal animals, in those with severe underlying myocardial disease (and dependent on increased sympathetic drive to maintain cardiac output) depression of cardiac contractility, conduction, and heart rate can result.

      (1) Because the drug's effects are dependent on the level of sympathetic activation, individual response is quite variable.

      (2) Initial dosages should be low and titrated upward as needed.

    b. β-blockers enhance the depression of A-V conduction produced by digoxin, Class I antiarrhythmic drugs, and calcium entry blockers.

      (1) Using a β-blocker and calcium entry blocker simultaneously is not recommended and can lead to marked decreases in heart rate and myocardial contractility.

      (2) β-blockers can decrease liver blood flow, leading to reduced elimination of drugs that are highly dependent on liver blood flow for clearance (e.g., lidocaine, phenytoin).

    c. Toxicity is usually related to excessive β-blockade, and can lead to bradycardia, heart failure, and hypotension.

        (1) Bronchospasm or increased vascular resistance can occur with nonselective β-blockers (β_1 and β_2).

        (2) Lipophilic β-blockers (e.g., propranolol) can cause depression and disorientation via CNS effects.

        (3) Because of possible β-receptor "up-regulation" (increased number and/or affinity of receptors) during chronic β-blockade, abrupt cessation of therapy could result in serious arrhythmias.

        (4) β-blockers may also prevent the appearance of early signs of acute hypoglycemia in diabetics (e.g., tachycardia and blood pressure changes). These drugs also reduce the release of insulin in response to hyperglycemia.

3. Atenolol

    a. Preparation and chemistry. Tablets are used most often; an injectable is available.

    b. Pharmacologic effects and mechanism of action. Atenolol has β_1-receptor selectivity.

    c. Therapeutic uses and administration. See **II D 1**, above. Atenolol is the agent used most often for chronic oral β-blockade.

    d. Pharmacokinetics

        (1) Oral bioavailability in dogs and cats is about 90%.

        (2) Atenolol is excreted in the urine; renal impairment delays clearance. The $t_{1/2}$ of atenolol is slightly over 3 hours in dogs and about 3.5 hours in cats.

        (3) Atenolol's β-blocking effects are evident for 12 hours but are gone by 24 hours in normal cats.

    e. Adverse effects. Weakness or exacerbation of heart failure can be observed, as with other β-blockers. Adverse CNS effects are unlikely because atenolol is hydrophilic and does not readily cross the blood–brain barrier.

4. Propranolol

    a. Preparation and chemistry. Propranolol HCl is available as an injectable solution as well as oral tablets and solution.

    b. Pharmacologic effects and mechanism of action. Propranolol is a nonselective β-blocker.

    c. Therapeutic uses and administration. Propranolol can be used for acute (IV) or chronic (oral) β-blockade.

    d. Pharmacokinetics

        (1) Feeding delays the rate of oral absorption and increases the clearance of an intravenous dose (by increasing liver blood flow).

        (2) Propranolol has extensive first-pass hepatic metabolism; however, chronic administration and higher doses cause hepatic enzyme saturation and increased bioavailability. Propranolol lowers hepatic blood flow, thereby prolonging its own elimination and that of other drugs dependent on liver blood flow for their metabolism.

        (3) The $t_{1/2}$ of propranolol in the dog is only 1.5 hours or less (0.5 to over 4.2 hours in cats), but active metabolites exist. A V_d of 3.3–6.5 L/kg and Cl_T of 34–70 mL/min/kg are reported in the dog. Dosing q8 hours appears to be adequate in both dogs and cats.

        (4) In the horse, a V_d of 2.3 L/kg, Cl_T of 12–21 mL/min/kg, and a $t_{1/2}$ of 1.2–1.7 hours are reported. Bioavailability is low.

    e. Adverse effects. Propranolol toxicity is usually related to excessive β-blockade. Propranolol and other lipophilic β-blockers can cause depressed attitude and disorientation because of CNS effects.

5. Esmolol

    a. Preparation and chemistry. Esmolol HCl is used as an IV injection.

    b. Pharmacologic effects and mechanism of action. Esmolol is an ultra-short acting agent that selectively blocks β_1-adrenergic receptors.

    c. Therapeutic uses and administration. Esmolol is useful as short-term treatment for acute (usually supraventricular) tachyarrhythmias and CHF from hypertrophic obstructive cardiomyopathy. Esmolol can be used to test whether a β-blocker would be an effective therapeutic strategy in such cases.

   d. Pharmacokinetics
   (1) Esmolol is rapidly metabolized by blood esterases. The $t_{1/2}$ is less than 10 minutes.
   (2) Steady state occurs in 5 minutes with, or 30 minutes without, a loading dose. Effects dissipate within 10–20 minutes of discontinuing infusion.
   e. Adverse effects are minimal because of the drug's brief $t_{1/2}$.

   6. Metoprolol
   a. Preparation and chemistry. Metoprolol tartrate is available as oral tablets and an injectable. Metoprolol succinate extended release tablets are also available.
   b. Pharmacologic effects and mechanism of action. Metoprolol is a β_1-selective agent.
   c. Therapeutic uses and administration. Metoprolol (a second-generation β-blocker) has been used as an antiarrhythmic drug. It may be useful as well for long-term heart failure therapy in dogs with stable DCM and chronic valvular disease (see carvedilol, below).
   d. Pharmacokinetics
   (1) Metoprolol is well absorbed PO, but bioavailability is reduced by a large first-pass effect. There is minimal protein-binding.
   (2) The drug is metabolized in the liver and excreted in the urine. $t_{1/2}$ is 1.6 hours in dogs and 1.3 hours in cats.
   e. Adverse effects. As for other β-blockers, including exacerbation of CHF.

   7. Carvedilol
   a. Preparation and chemistry. Carvedilol is available in oral tablet form.
   b. Pharmacologic effects and mechanism of action. Carvedilol blocks β_1-, β_2-, and α_1-adrenergic receptors, but is without intrinsic sympathomimetic activity. It also has some other effects (including antioxidant activity, some Ca^{2+} blocking effect, and also promotes vasodilation).
   c. Therapeutic uses and administration. This third-generation β-blocker has been effective in people with chronic in heart failure in modulating pathologic cardiac remodeling and reducing mortality with long-term use. It is hoped that carvedilol (or metoprolol) might play a similar beneficial role in dogs; studies to evaluate this are ongoing.
   d. Pharmacokinetics
   (1) Peak plasma concentrations appear to be quite variable after oral administration.
   (2) The drug is eliminated mainly through hepatic metabolism. The $t_{1/2}$ is short (<2 hours) in dogs; but an active metabolite is thought to account for the nonselective β-blocking effect which lasts for 12–24 hours.
   e. Adverse effects. As for other β-blockers, including exacerbation of CHF.

   8. Other β-blockers are available. Their basic effects are similar, although their relative selectivity for β_1-receptors as well as their pharmacologic characteristics vary.

E. **Class III agents** prolong action potential duration and effective refractory period without decreasing conduction velocity. They act mainly by inhibiting the repolarizing K^+ channel I_K (delayed rectifier).

   1. Sotolol
   a. Preparation and chemistry. Sotolol HCl is available as a tablet containing a racemic mixture of the d- and l- isomers.
   b. Pharmacologic effects and mechanism of action. Sotalol is a nonselective β-blocker with Class III effects at higher doses. β-Blocking effects (from the l-isomer) occur at lower doses and are about 30% of propranolol's potency. d-Sotalol alone prolongs repolarization but has no β-blocking effect.
   c. Therapeutic uses and administration. Sotalol is used mainly for ventricular tachyarrhythmias in dogs. Sotalol has also been used in cats with severe ventricular tachyarrhythmias.

d. Pharmacokinetics
  (1) The oral bioavailability of sotalol is high with negligible first-pass effect, but absorption is reduced with food.
  (2) Sotolol is eliminated unchanged by the kidneys; renal dysfunction prolongs elimination. The $t_{1/2}$ is about 5 hours in dogs.
  (3) Sotalol's β-blocking effects last longer than its plasma $t_{1/2}$.

e. Adverse effects. The drug has minimal hemodynamic effects, although it can cause hypotension.
  (1) Although it has less negative inotropic effect than propranolol, sotolol may exacerbate myocardial failure in dogs with DCM.
  (2) Other adverse effects of sotalol can include hypotension, depression, nausea, vomiting, diarrhea, and bradycardia.
  (3) Slowed sinus rate and first-degree heart block can occur. Sotalol can be proarrhythmic (as can all antiarrhythmic agents).

2. Amiodarone
a. Preparation and chemistry. Amiodarone HCl is an iodinated benzofuran. It is available as an oral tablet and injectable solution.

b. Pharmacologic effects and mechanism of action. Although classified as a Class III agent, it also shares properties with all three other antiarrhythmic drug classes. Besides prolonging the action potential duration and effective refractory period in both atrial and ventricular tissues, it has effects on Na^+, K^+, and Ca^{2+} channels, and has noncompetitive α_1- and β-blocking properties.
  (1) Amiodarone's β-blocking effects occur soon after administration, but maximal Class III effects (and prolongation of the action potential and QT interval) are not achieved for weeks with long-term administration.

c. Therapeutic uses and administration. Amiodarone is indicated for refractory tachyarrhythmias of both atrial and ventricular origin.

d. Pharmacokinetics. Amiodarone's pharmacokinetics are complex.
  (1) There is a delayed onset of action, and prolonged time (>10 weeks) to steady state. With long-term PO use, the drug concentrates in myocardial and other tissues (especially fat), and an active metabolite (desethylamiodarone) accumulates.
  (2) The drug is metabolized in the liver. The $t_{1/2}$ in dogs after a single PO dose is ~7.5 hours, but increases to 3.2 days with long-term use.
  (3) Therapeutic serum concentration is thought to be 1–2.5 mcg/mL.

e. Adverse effects
  (1) IV use can cause marked hypotension and bradycardia; hypersensitivity-type reactions (with acute angioedema formation) and tremors have also occurred.
  (2) Long-term use can be associated with many adverse effects, including depressed appetite, GI upset, pneumonitis leading to pulmonary fibrosis, hepatopathy, thyroid dysfunction, positive Coombs test, thrombocytopenia, and neutropenia. Other adverse effects noted with long-term use in people include corneal microdeposits, photosensitivity, bluish skin discoloration, and peripheral neuropathy.
  (3) Amiodarone can increase the serum concentrations of digoxin, diltiazem, and possibly, procainamide and quinidine.

F. **Class IV agents (Ca^{2+} channel blockers)** reduce cellular Ca^{2+} influx (the slow inward current) by blocking transmembrane L-type Ca^{2+} channels. As a group they can cause coronary and systemic vasodilation, as well as reduced myocardial contractility; but individual agents differ in these effects. Some calcium entry blockers (such as the nondihydropyridine Ca^{2+} channel blockers diltiazem and verapamil) have antiarrhythmic effects. These effects involve tissues dependent on the slow inward Ca^{2+} current. They cause dose-related slowing of the sinus node rate and A-V conduction. Contraindications to Ca^{2+} channel blocker use include sinus bradycardia, AV block, sick sinus syndrome, digoxin toxicity, and myocardial failure (for agents with pronounced negative inotropic effect). They are generally not used with a β-blocker.

1. **Diltiazem**
   a. **Preparation and chemistry.** Diltiazem HCl is a benzothiazepine Ca^{2+} channel blocker. It is available as oral tablets and injectable solution, as well as extended release tablets and capsules.
   b. **Pharmacologic effects and mechanism of action.** Diltiazem slows the sinus node rate, increases AV nodal refractory period, and can block some arrhythmias caused by abnormal automaticity, triggered mechanisms, and re-entry. Diltiazem also causes potent coronary and mild peripheral vasodilation. It has less negative inotropic effect than verapamil.
   c. **Therapeutic uses and administration.** Diltiazem is indicated for supraventricular tachyarrhythmias. It is often combined with digoxin to further slow the ventricular response rate to atrial fibrillation in dogs. **Diltiazem is the Ca^{2+} channel blocker recommended in cats with HCM.**
   d. **Pharmacokinetics**
      (1) Diltiazem's bioavailability is only about 43% in dogs because of extensive first-pass effect. Bioavailability of conventional diltiazem is greater in cats than in dogs.
      (2) Diltiazem is metabolized in the liver; active metabolites exist. Drugs that inhibit hepatic microsomal enzymes (e.g., cimetidine, ketoconazole, chloramphenicol) reduce diltiazem's metabolism.
      (3) Effects peak within 2 hours after PO dosing and last ≥6 hours in dogs. The $t_{1/2}$ in dogs is >2 hours, but is longer with chronic PO use because of its enterohepatic circulation.
      (4) The $t_{1/2}$ in cats is 2–3 hours; plasma concentrations peak within 30–90 minutes and effects last for 8 hours.
      (5) The therapeutic range is 50–300 ng/mL.
      (6) A sustained-release preparation (Cardizem-CD®) produces plasma concentrations that peak in 6 hours and remain in the therapeutic range for 24 hours in cats.
      (7) Diltiazem XR is another sustained-release preparation. The 240-mg capsule contains four tablets of 60 mg each. There appears to be much pharmacokinetic variability among individual cats. Sustained-release diltiazem may have lesser efficacy in preventing sinus tachycardia compared with atenolol. Adverse effects may also be more frequent, including anorexia, vomiting, lethargy, and evidence of hepatopathy in cats.
   e. **Adverse effects** are uncommon at therapeutic doses, but anorexia, nausea, bradycardia, and, rarely, other GI, cardiac, or neurologic effects may occur.
      (1) Cats sporadically develop liver enzyme elevation with anorexia. Anorexia and other GI signs are more likely at higher doses. Anecdotally, some cats become aggressive or show other personality change when treated with diltiazem.
      (2) The concurrent use of diltiazem (or verapamil) and a β-blocker can cause a sudden fall in the sinus rate or complete heart block.
      (3) Toxic effects can include reduced myocardial contractility, hypotension, depression, lethargy, bradycardia, and AV block.
2. **Other Ca^{2+} blocker drugs**
   a. **Verapamil** HCl (a phenylalkylamine) has the most potent cardiac effects of the clinically used Ca^{2+}-entry blockers.
      (1) Verapamil's $t_{1/2}$ in dogs is ~2.5 hours. It is poorly absorbed and undergoes first-pass hepatic metabolism, resulting in low oral bioavailability. The pharmacokinetics in cats are similar to dogs but are reportedly more variable.
      (2) Verapamil has marked negative inotropic, and some vasodilatory effects which can cause decompensation, hypotension and even death if underlying myocardial disease is present. Verapamil is not used in patients with heart failure.
      (3) Toxic effects of verapamil include sinus bradycardia, AV block, hypotension, reduced myocardial contractility, and cardiogenic shock. The

negative inotropic effects of verapamil may be reversed with IV Ca^{2+} salts, sympathomimetic drugs, or amrinone. Atropine may mitigate bradycardia or AV block precipitated by verapamil. Verapamil reduces the renal clearance of digoxin.

b. Other Ca^{2+} channel blockers (the dihydropyridines) are used for their vasodilating effect in hypertension or chronic heart failure management. Amlodipine besylate is used most often (see p. 197).

G. Other drugs with antiarrhythmic effects

1. **Anticholinergic drugs.** Atropine sulfate and glycopyrrolate are anticholinergic agents that act by antagonism of ACh at muscarinic receptors. They increase sinus rate and AV conduction when excessive vagal tone is present.

   a. Parenteral atropine or glycopyrrolate is indicated for sinus bradycardia or AV block induced by anesthesia, CNS lesions, and certain other diseases or toxicities. See Chapter 2 for more information. An atropine response test is often used in dogs and cats presented with a bradyarrhythmia to determine the extent of vagal influence.

   b. Bradyarrhythmias responsive to parenteral atropine or glycopyrrolate may also respond to oral anticholinergic agents such as propantheline bromide and hyoscyamine sulfate.

   c. Adverse effects of vagolytic drugs include aggravation of paroxysmal supraventricular tachyarrhythmias (as in sick sinus syndrome). Other side effects of anticholinergic therapy include vomiting, diarrhea, dry mouth, keratoconjunctivitis sicca, and drying of respiratory secretions.

2. **Sympathomimetic drugs** (see Chapter 2 for more information)

   a. Isoproterenol is a β-receptor agonist that has been used to treat symptomatic AV block and bradycardia refractory to atropine, although artificial pacing is safer and more effective. Because of its affinity for β_2-receptors, it can cause hypotension and it is not used for treating either heart failure or cardiac arrest. Isoproterenol can be arrhythmogenic, like other catecholamines. Oral administration is not usually effective because of marked first-pass hepatic metabolism. Isoproterenol can cause serious tachyarrhythmias.

   b. Oral terbutaline sulfate, a β_2-receptor agonist, may have a mild stimulatory effect on HR.

   c. The methylxanthine bronchodilators aminophylline and theophylline can increase heart rate in some dogs with sick sinus syndrome when used at higher doses.

3. **Digoxin** is commonly used to treat frequent supraventricular or atrial premature beats and tachycardias. It is also used to slow A-V conduction in atrial fibrillation. See I F 2 for more information.

III. ANTIHYPERTENSIVE DRUGS

A. Introduction

1. Systemic arterial hypertension is often associated with renal disease or hyperadrenocorticism in dogs; other associated conditions include pheochromocytoma, diabetes mellitus, hypothyroidism, and liver disease. Renal disease and hyperthyroidism are the most common associated conditions in cats. Idiopathic (essential) hypertension is uncommon in dogs and cats.

   a. Certain drugs can increase blood pressure, such as glucocorticoids, mineralocorticoids, NSAIDs, phenylpropanolamine, NaCl, and even topical ocular phenylephrine.

   b. High blood pressure can damage capillary beds. The eye, kidney, heart, and brain are particularly vulnerable to damage from chronic hypertension.

2. Systemic arterial hypertension is most often recognized in middle-aged to older dogs and cats, presumably because of the associated disease conditions.
   a. Signs of hypertension relate either to underlying disease or to end-organ damage caused by the hypertension itself. Ocular signs, especially sudden blindness, are the most common presenting complaint.
   b. A diagnosis of arterial hypertension should be confirmed by measuring BP multiple times and on different days. Blood pressure measurements are indicated not only when signs compatible with hypertension are found, but also when a disease associated with hypertension is diagnosed.

B. Overview of antihypertensive therapy

1. Antihypertensive therapy is indicated for animals with severe hypertension and those with clinical signs presumed to be caused by hypertension.
   a. Measured BP in such animals is generally over 180/120 mm Hg.
   b. Some cases are hypertensive emergencies, requiring immediate therapy and intensive monitoring, but most hypertensive animals can be managed more conservatively with oral therapy.
   c. Patients with high BP that persists after treatment for the primary disease, as well as those with evidence of end-organ damage, should be treated.
   d. The goal of therapy is to reduce BP to below 150/95 mm Hg.
2. Several drugs are used as antihypertensive agents in dogs and cats:
   a. Usually one drug is administered at a time, at initially low doses. The animal is monitored to assess efficacy; two or more weeks may be needed to assess whether a significant decrease in BP has occurred.
   b. The drugs used most often are angiotensin-converting enzyme inhibitors (ACEI), the Ca^{2+}-blocker amlodipine, and β-blockers.
      (1) An ACEI is recommended as the initial antihypertensive drug in dogs.
      (2) Amlodipine is recommended as the drug of first-choice in cats, unless hyperthyroidism is the underlying cause. For hyperthyroid-induced hypertension, atenolol or another β-blocker is used first.
      (3) Therapy with a single agent is effective in some cases.
      (4) Combination therapy may be needed for adequate BP control in others.
   c. Hypotension is a potential adverse effect of antihypertensive drugs.
      (1) This usually is evident as periods of lethargy or ataxia.
      (2) Reduced appetite can be another adverse effect.
   d. Ancillary strategies may be helpful, although alone they are unlikely to markedly reduce BP.
      (1) Moderate dietary salt reduction (e.g., ≤0.22–0.25% Na^+ on a dry matter basis) is advised for all cases. Although not expected to normalize BP by itself, it may enhance antihypertensive drug effectiveness.
      (2) Weight reduction is usually advised for obese animals.
      (3) Drugs that can potentiate vasoconstriction (e.g., phenylpropanolamine and other α_1-adrenergic agonists), as well as glucocorticoids and progestins should also be avoided when possible.
      (4) A diuretic may help by reducing blood volume in individuals with volume expansion.
         (a) A diuretic alone is rarely effective.
         (b) Diuretics are avoided or used only with caution. in animals with renal disease.
   e. The ability to monitor BP is important when antihypertensive drugs are used. Serial measurements are needed to assess treatment efficacy and avoid hypotension.

C. Vasodilator drugs

1. **Angiotensin converting enzyme inhibitors.** ACEI may help control BP by reducing angiotensin II formation, vasodilator kinin degradation, and/or aldosterone secretion (with its effects on vascular volume).

a. An ACEI is generally the drug of first choice in hypertensive dogs.

b. Hypertension in cats with chronic renal failure is often not responsive to ACEI. But, an ACEI may help mitigate further hypertensive renal damage by preferentially reducing efferent arteriolar constriction and reducing glomerular hypertension

c. See I D for more information about ACEI.

2. Calcium-entry blockers

a. Amlodipine besylate is a long-acting dihydropyridine Ca^{2+}-blocker that causes vasodilation without appreciable cardiac effects.

(1) Amlodipine is the drug of first choice in most hypertensive cats.

(a) Oral bioavailability is high and peak plasma concentrations are reached 3–8 hours after administration (in people); plasma concentrations increase with chronic therapy.

(b) There is no extensive first-pass elimination. The drug undergoes hepatic metabolism; caution is warranted when liver function is poor.

(c) No specific pharmacokinetic data are available in cats. However, transdermal application produces measurable blood levels and pharmacologic effect, although to a lesser degree than with oral dosing. Bioavailability appears lower than with oral dosing.

(d) Amlodipine's $t_{1/2}$ is ~30 hours in dogs; maximal effects occur 4–7 days after initiating therapy.

(2) Amlodipine can be used as adjunctive therapy (or alone) in dogs if an ACEI does not sufficiently control BP.

b. Other agents, such diltiazem (see II F 1) and nifedipine might be useful in hypertensive animals.

3. Other vasodilators

a. Direct-acting vasodilator agents generally produce faster reduction in BP (e.g., nitroprusside, hydralazine).

(1) Nitroprusside can be dosed to effect by constant IV infusion, but arterial pressure should be closely monitored to avoid hypotension (see I E 4).

(2) Hydralazine given IV or PO is an alternative, especially for dogs (see I E 2).

b. α_1-Blockers oppose the vasoconstrictive effects of these α-receptors. **Their main use is for hypertension caused by pheochromocytoma.** After an α-blocker is administered, adjunctive therapy with a β-blocker can help control reflex tachycardia or arrhythmias.

(1) Phenoxybenzamine is a noncompetitive α-blocker used most often for pheochromocytoma-induced hypertension.

(2) Prazosin also has been used in some dogs.

(3) Phentolamine is used IV when hypertensive crisis is related to pheochromocytoma or other cause of catecholamine excess.

(4) Addition of a β-blocker can help mitigate pheochromocytoma-induced tachyarrhythmias, but it should not be administered alone or before an α-blocker is given.

D. **Other drugs used for hypertension**

1. β-Blockers may reduce blood pressure by slowing heart rate, and decreasing cardiac output and renal renin release (see II D).

a. Atenolol and propranolol have been used most often.

b. A β-blocker is recommended for cats with hyperthyroid-induced hypertension. **But β-blockers are often ineffective as the sole antihypertensive agent in cats with renal disease.**

c. An IV β-blocker (propranolol, esmolol, or labetolol) can be used for emergency treatment.

2. Diuretics may reduce blood pressure by promoting Na^+ and water excretion. Furosemide is usually tried, although hydrochlorothiazide may be helpful in nonazotemic dogs. See Chapter 9 for more information.

IV. DRUGS USED IN THE TREATMENT OF THROMBOEMBOLISM

A. Introduction

1. General situations that promote thrombosis include abnormal endothelial structure or function, slowed or static blood flow, and hypercoagulability (either from increased procoagulant substances or decreased anticoagulant or fibrinolytic substances).
   a. Widespread endothelial injury interferes with endothelial antiplatelet, anticoagulant, and fibrinolytic functions. An increase in coagulability and platelet activation favor thrombosis.
   b. Many common diseases are associated with thromboembolism, including sepsis, neoplasia, pancreatitis, immune-medited disease, protein-losing nephropathy, hyperadrenocorticism, shock, severe hepatopathy, and heatstroke.
2. Systemic arterial thromboembolism in cats is most often associated with cardiomyopathy, although neoplastic and systemic inflammatory disease may sometimes be the underlying condition.
3. Systemic arterial thromboembolic disease in dogs is relatively uncommon compared with cats.
   a. Thromboembolic disease (systemic as well as pulmonary) is associated with a number of conditions, including protein-losing nephropathies, hyperadrenocorticism, neoplasia, gastric dilatation–volvulus, and others.
   b. Vegetative endocarditis is the most common cardiac disease associated with systemic thromboembolism.

B. Overview of therapy for thromboembolic disease

1. The goals of therapy are to stabilize the patient by supportive treatment as indicated, prevent extension of the existing thrombus and additional thromboembolic events, reduce the size of the thromboembolus (if possible) and restore perfusion.
   a. Supportive care is given to improve or maintain tissue perfusion and optimize organ function, and to minimize further endothelial damage and blood stasis, while collateral circulation develops.
   b. Treatment for underlying or associated disease conditions is also provided, as possible.
2. Anticoagulant therapy is used to prevent extension of existing thromboemboli.
3. Although fibrinolytic therapy is used in some cases, dosage uncertainties, the need for intensive care, and the potential for serious complications limit its use.
4. Antiplatelet therapy is used to reduce platelet aggregation and growth of existing thrombi.
5. Prophylactic therapy with an antiplatelet or anticoagulant drug is commonly used in animals thought to be at increased risk for thromboembolic disease.
   a. The efficacy of thromboembolic prophylaxis is unclear and no strategy consistently prevents thromboembolism (TE).
   b. Drugs used for arterial TE prophylaxis include aspirin, clopidogrel, warfarin (coumadin), and low molecular weight heparin (LMWH).
      (1) No survival benefit has been shown for warfarin compared with aspirin in cats.
      (2) Warfarin is associated with greater expense and a higher rate of fatal hemorrhage.
      (3) Clopidogrel or LMWH prophylaxis may be more efficacious, with less risk of hemorrhage, but more experience with this therapy is needed.

C. Anticoagulant drugs

1. **Heparin**
   a. Unfractionated heparin and a number of LMWH products are available.
   b. **Pharmacologic effects and mechanism of action**
      (1) Heparin's main anticoagulant effect is produced through antithrombin activation, which in turn inhibits factors IX, X, XI, XII, and thrombin (factor II).

(2) Heparin also stimulates release of tissue factor inhibitors from vascular sites, which helps reduce (extrinsic) coagulation cascade activation.

c. Therapeutic uses and administration. Heparin is indicated to limit extension of existing thrombi and to prevent further thromboembolic episodes.

d. Pharmacokinetics

(1) Heparin must be given parenterally to be effective. It can be initially given IV, followed by subsequent SC doses.

(2) Anticoagulant activity is immediate after IV injection, but is delayed up to an hour after SC injection.

(3) Doses are adjusted to prolong the activated coagulation time to 1.5–2.5 times pretreatment level.

(4) There is extensive protein binding. Metabolism is thought to be via the liver as well as inactivation by the reticuloendothelial system.

(5) The $t_{1/2}$ in people is 1–2 hours.

e. Adverse effects

(1) Bleeding and thrombocytopenia are most common.

(2) Hypersensitivity reactions are possible.

(3) Heparin is contraindicated in patients with severe thrombocytopenia, uncontrolled bleeding, or previous hypersensitivity.

2. Low molecular weight heparins (LMWHs)

a. LMWHs are a diverse group of depolymerized heparin.

(1) These agents vary in size, structure, and pharmacokinetics.

(2) The LMWHs have differences in biological and clinical effects and are not interchangeable.

b. Pharmacologic effects and mechanism of action

(1) The smaller size of LMWH, compared to unfractionated heparin, prevents simultaneous binding to thrombin and AT III. LMWHs have more effect against factor Xa through their inactivation of AT III.

(2) LMWHs have minimal ability to inhibit thrombin, so are less likely to cause bleeding.

(a) LMWH do not markedly affect coagulation times, so monitoring aPTT is generally unnecessary.

(b) LMWH effect can be monitored indirectly by anti-Xa activity. Optimal anti-Xa activity level in cats is not known; the target range in people is reported as 0.5–1.0 U/mL, although 0.3–0.6 U/mL has also been used.

c. Therapeutic uses and administration

(1) LMWHs are indicated to limit extension of existing thrombi and prevent further thromboembolic episodes.

(a) They present a safer alternative to unfractionated heparin.

(b) But the most effective dosage for the various LMWHs is not clearly established in dogs and cats.

d. Pharmacokinetics

(1) Dalteparin sodium (Fragmin®) and enoxaparin (Lovenox®) are used most often.

(2) LMWHs have greater bioavailability and a longer $t_{1/2}$ than unfractionated heparin when given SC, because of lesser binding to plasma proteins as well as endothelial cells and macrophages.

(3) The pharmacokinetics are not clear in dogs and cats.

(a) Doses have been extrapolated from human use.

(b) There is evidence that the traditional doses do not produce a (human) target level of anti-Xa activity in cats.

i It appears that cats should be given somewhat higher doses at 4-hour intervals for dalteparin, and at 6-hour intervals for enoxaparin.

ii The optimal therapeutic range in cats, as well as the most effective dosage in sick cats, is not yet established.

(c) Optimal canine dosing guidelines are not available.

e. Adverse effects can include excessive bleeding.

3. Warfarin
  a. Warfarin is a coumadin derivative available in tablet and injectable forms as a racemic mixture.
  b. Pharmacologic effects and mechanism of action. Warfarin is an indirect-acting anticoagulant.
    (1) It inhibits the enzyme (vitamin K epoxide reductase) responsible for activating the vitamin K-dependent factors (II, VII, IX, and X).
    (2) Its effect can be overcome by sufficient amounts of vitamin K_1.
    (3) Warfarin causes a transient hypercoagulability, related to the shorter $t_{1/2}$ of anticoagulant proteins compared to most procoagulant factors.
  c. Therapeutic uses and administration. Warfarin has been used as prophylactic therapy in animals thought to be at increased risk for thromboembolic disease. There is wide variability in dose response.
  d. Pharmacokinetics
    (1) Warfarin is rapidly absorbed after oral administration.
    (2) It is highly protein bound, although there is species variability in this; concurrent use of other protein-bound drugs or change in serum protein concentration can markedly alter the anticoagulant effect because only unbound warfarin is active.
    (3) The drug is metabolized in the liver; the metabolites are inactive and are excreted through the urine.
    (4) The $t_{1/2}$ is variable (hours to days).
  e. Adverse effects relate mainly to hemorrhage and its consequences.

D. Fibrinolytic drugs

  1. Streptokinase is a nonspecific plasminogen activator that promotes the breakdown of fibrin as well as fibrinogen. It also degrades factors V, VIII, and prothrombin.
    a. The $t_{1/2}$ is ~30 minutes, but fibrinogen depletion continues for much longer.
    b. Because it is a nonspecific plasminogen activator it can cause systemic fibrinolysis, coagulopathy, and bleeding.
    c. No survival benefit has been shown for streptokinase compared to "conventional" (aspirin and heparin) treatment in cats.
    d. Adverse effects include the potential for serious hemorrhage. Acute hyperkalemia (secondary to thrombolysis and reperfusion injury), metabolic acidosis, bleeding, and other complications may lead to death. Streptokinase can increase platelet aggregability and induce platelet dysfunction.
  2. Recombinant tissue plasminogen activator (rt-PA)
    a. rt-PA is a single-chain polypeptide serine protease with a higher specificity for fibrin within thrombi and a low affinity for circulating plasminogen.
    b. Experience with rt-PA is very limited and the optimal dosage is not known. A high mortality rate in a small series of cats was thought to be related to reperfusion injury.
    c. The $t_{1/2}$ of t-PA is 2–3 minutes in dogs, but effects persist longer because of binding to fibrin.
    d. Although the risk of hemorrhage is less than with streptokinase, there is potential for serious bleeding as well as other side effects. rt-PA is also potentially antigenic in animals because it is a human protein.

E. Antiplatelet drugs. Aspirin and clopidogrel have low risk for serious hemorrhage, and require less monitoring, compared to warfarin.

  1. Aspirin (acetylsalicylic acid) is an NSAID.
    a. Aspirin irreversibly inhibits cyclooxygenase, which reduces prostaglandin and thromboxane A_2 synthesis and, therefore, subsequent platelet aggregation.
    b. Aspirin is often used to block platelet activation and aggregation in patients with, or at risk for, thromboembolic disease. The optimal dose for preventing thromboembolism is unclear. Aspirin is also used for its analgesic and antipyretic effects.

c. Aspirin is rapidly absorbed orally. It is partially hydrolyzed to salicylic acid which is widely distributed. Protein binding is extensive.

d. Salicylate is metabolized in the liver mainly by conjugation with glycine and glucuronic acid (via glucuronyl transferase). Cats lack this enzyme and therefore the $t_{1/2}$ is prolonged in this species and less frequent dosing (q2–3 days) is required compared with dogs.

e. Salicylate and its metabolites are excreted by the kidney.

f. Adverse GI effects (vomiting, inappetence, ulceration, hematemesis) occur in some animals. Buffered aspirin formulation or aspirin–Maalox combination product may be helpful. The drug can cause serious GI bleeding.

2. Clopidogrel

a. Clopidogrel (Plavix®) is a thienopyridine. These agents inhibit ADP-binding at platelet receptors and subsequent ADP-mediated platelet aggregation.

b. Clopidogrel appears to have significant antiplatelet effects. Further evaluation of its potential for thromboembolism prophylaxis in cats (and dogs) is ongoing.

SUGGESTED READING

Alwood AJ, Downend AB, Brooks MB, Slensky KA, Fox JA, Simpson SA, Waddell LS, Baumgardner JE, Otto CM. 2007. Anticoagulant effects of low-molecular-weight heparins in healthy cats. *J Vet Intern Med* 21:378–387.

Brown S, Atkins C, Bagley R, Carr A, Cowgill L, Davidson M, Egner B, Elliott J, Henik R, Labato M, Littman M, Polzin D, Ross L, Snyder P, Stepien R. 2007. Guidelines for the identification, evaluation, and management of systemic hypertension in dogs and cats. ACVIM Consensus Statement. *J Vet Intern Med* 21:542–558.

Cote E, Ettinger SJ. 2005. "Electrocardiography and cardiac arrhythmias." In *Textbook of Veterinary Internal Medicine*. Edited by Ettinger SJ, Feldman EC. 6th ed., pp. 1040–1076. Philadelphia, PA: Saunders.

http://www.drugs.com

Plumb DC. 2005. *Veterinary Drug Handbook*. 5th ed. Ames, IA: Blackwell Publishing.

Ware WA. 2007. *Cardiovascular Disease in Small Animal Medicine*. London: Manson Publishing.

◼ S T U D Y   Q U E S T I O N S

DIRECTIONS: Each of the numbered items or incomplete statements in this section is followed by answers or by completions of the statement. Select the **one** lettered answer or completion that is **best** in each case.

1. A purely venous vasodilator would be most useful in treating which of the following conditions?

(A) Chronic, stable dilated cardiomyopathy
(B) Aortic regurgitation from endocarditis
(C) Cardiac tamponade with ascites
(D) Mitral regurgitation with acute pulmonary edema
(E) Pulmonic stenosis with syncope

2. A middle-aged cat is diagnosed with HCM. Which of the following drugs would be most effective for treating the diastolic dysfunction caused by this disease?

(A) Furosemide
(B) Lidocaine
(C) Digoxin
(D) Hydralazine
(E) Diltiazem

3. All of the following angiotensin converting enzyme inhibitors are excreted mainly by the kidney, EXCEPT:

(A) Captopril.
(B) Enalapril.
(C) Lisinopril.
(D) Benazepril.

4. Which of the following statements regarding hydralazine is TRUE?

(A) Hydralazine acts to dilate both arterioles and veins.
(B) Hydralazine directly dilates arteriolar smooth muscle.
(C) Vasodilation is more pronounced in skeletal muscle and skin with hydralazine.
(D) Hypotension and reflex tachycardia are uncommon side effects.
(E) Hydralazine dampens the neurohumoral compensatory response in heart failure.

5. In general, digoxin would be indicated for a dog with _____.

(A) dilated cardiomyopathy and atrial fibrillation
(B) heartworm disease
(C) pericardial effusion
(D) hypertrophic cardiomyopathy
(E) constrictive pericarditis

6. A dog is being given oral digoxin for heart failure. Which of the following would yield the best absorption?

(A) Use of the tablet form
(B) Use of the elixir form
(C) Giving the drug with food
(D) Concurrent kaolin–pectin use
(E) Concurrent antacid use

7. The mechanism of action of digoxin's positive inotropic effect is

(A) direct stimulation of the Na^+–Ca^{2+} exchanger.
(B) competitive inhibition of Na^+, K^+-ATPase.
(C) activation of G_s protein.
(D) peripheral and central sympathetic stimulation.
(E) inhibition of phosphodiesterase activity.

8. Regarding pimobendan, all the following are true, EXCEPT:

(A) Elimination in the dog is primarily via hepatic metabolism.
(B) There is an active metabolite.
(C) The drug is often called an inodilator.
(D) The drug has phosphodiesterase III inhibiting effects.
(E) The drug substantially increases myocardial oxygen requirement while increasing contractility.

9. All the following predispose to digoxin toxicity, EXCEPT:

(A) Use of loading doses.
(B) Hypokalemia.
(C) Renal disease.
(D) Quinidine.
(E) Cholestyramine.

10. A dog is presented in severe heart failure from dilated cardiomyopathy; you decide to institute therapy with a catecholamine. Regarding dopamine and dobutamine, all the following are true, EXCEPT:

(A) Both agents have a $t_{1/2}$ between 10 and 20 minutes.
(B) Both agents have extensive hepatic metabolism.
(C) Long-term use is limited by β-receptor down-regulation.
(D) Dopamine, but not dobutamine, stimulates vasodilatory dopaminergic receptors.
(E) Dopamine is more arrhythmogenic than dobutamine.

11. In the same dog as above, you also consider amrinone therapy. All of the following are true regarding amrinone, EXCEPT:

(A) It acts by inhibiting phosphodiesterase.
(B) Peak effects occur after 45 minutes of infusion in dogs.
(C) It can be used orally twice a day.
(D) Vasodilation is also an effect.
(E) It may worsen ventricular arrhythmias.

12. Drugs which act by blocking β-adrenergic receptors comprise which class of antiarrhythmic agents?

(A) Class I
(B) Class II
(C) Class III
(D) Class IV

13. Which antiarrhythmic drug is INCORRECTLY matched with its classification?

(A) Lidocaine—Class IA
(B) Procainamide—Class IA
(C) Tocainide—Class IB
(D) Quinidine—Class IA
(E) Flecainide—Class IC

14. When used IV, lidocaine has all of the following effects, EXCEPT:

(A) It usually suppresses premature ventricular contractions.

(B) It consistently abolishes atrial arrhythmias.
(C) It decreases Na^+ conductance in automatic cells.
(D) It has little to no effect on sinus node pacemaker function.
(E) It is rapidly metabolized by hepatic microsomal enzymes.

15. The drug generally used for converting atrial fibrillation in horses without heart failure is

(A) procainamide.
(B) quinidine.
(C) propranolol.
(D) diltiazem.
(E) phenytoin.

16. Regarding the adverse effects of Class I antiarrhythmic drugs, which statement is INCORRECT?

(A) Central nervous system excitement is the most common toxic effect of lidocaine.
(B) Cats and horses are very sensitive to the toxic effects of lidocaine.
(C) Exacerbation of arrhythmias is not a problem with Class IA drugs.
(D) GI upset can occur with quinidine and procainamide.
(E) Marked Q-T interval prolongation can occur with quinidine.

17. A 9-year-old beagle has an irregular heartbeat and lethargy. Radiographs show moderate cardiomegaly; ECG shows second-degree heart block. Based on the information given, appropriate therapy would include

(A) digoxin.
(B) propranolol.
(C) procainamide.
(D) propantheline Bromide.
(E) diltiazem.

18. Heparin is used in cats after acute thromboembolism because of its inhibitory effects on coagulation. In combination with antithrombin III, it neutralizes all the following factors, EXCEPT:

(A) XII
(B) XI
(C) X
(D) IX
(E) VIII

ANSWERS AND EXPLANATIONS

1. The answer is D (I C 3 a).
Cases of acute, fulminant cardiogenic pulmonary edema are most likely to benefit from preload reduction with a venodilator. In general, a mixed or arteriolar vasodilator is of more benefit in most other cases and would be of benefit here, too. Preload reduction would be harmful in cardiac tamponade.

2. The answer is E (I A 2 c and I E 2).
Treatment of diastolic dysfunction centers on slowing heart rate, decreasing myocardial O_2 consumption, and enhancing relaxation. Hydralazine can contribute to increased heart rate and possibly worsen any outflow obstruction. Digoxin can also do the latter by increasing contractility and increases O_2 consumption. Furosemide and captopril may be indicated but would not address the diastolic abnormality.

3. The answer is D (I C 1 c).
Benazepril has approximately equal biliary and renal excretion.

4. The answer is B (I C 2).
Hydralazine is a direct arteriolar dilator. Vasodilation is more pronounced in cerebral, coronary, and splanchnic circulations. Hypotension and reflex tachycardia are common side effects. Enhancement of the neurohumoral response is thought to occur.

5. The answer is A (I A 2 d and I D 1 a).
Digoxin is most often used in the treatment of myocardial failure, especially when atrial fibrillation exists. Other diseases listed do not have systolic dysfunction.

6. The answer is B (I D 1 d).
Absorption is better with the elixir than the tablet form. The other factors listed decrease absorption.

7. The answer is B (I D 1 b).
Digoxin inhibits Na^+, K^+-ATPase at the myocardial cell membrane which allows Na^+ to build up inside the cell; this enhances its exchange with extracellular Ca^{2+}. The resulting increase in intracellular Ca^{2+} leads to a positive inotropic effect.

8. The answer is E (I F 1 b).
The drug sensitizes the contractile filaments to calcium ion, so can increase contractility with minimal impact on myocardial O_2 requirement.

9. The answer is E (I D 1 e).
Cholestyramine will bind digoxin in the gut and may be helpful immediately after oral overdose. All the other conditions predispose to toxicity.

10. The answer is A (I D 2).
The $t_{1/2}$ of these agents is less than 2 minutes; that, as well as their rapid hepatic metabolism, means they are effectively given only by IV infusion.

11. The answer is C (I D 3).
Amrinone's short $t_{1/2}$ necessitates IV administration, usually by constant infusion.

12. The answer is B (II B 2).
Beta-blockers are considered Class II agents (Vaughn-Williams classification system). Class I drugs are the local anesthetics, Class III drugs prolong action potential duration, Class IV drugs are the Ca^{2+} entry blockers.

13. The answer is A (II B and Table 8-2).
Lidocaine is a Class IB drug, like tocainide.

14. The answer is B (II B 1 a).
Lidocaine is generally effective for ventricular, but not usually for supraventricular (atrial) tachyarrhythmias. It decreases Na^+ conductance in automatic cells and does not affect sinus pacemaker discharge. It undergoes rapid metabolism by hepatic microsomal enzymes.

15. The answer is B (II B 1 a).
Quinidine is often successful in converting atrial fibrillation in horses without heart failure or significant underlying cardiac disease. Procainamide is much less effective for supraventricular arrhythmias. Propranolol

along with digoxin is sometimes used if heart failure is present; these drugs would be expected to slow the ventricular response rate but not convert the rhythm to sinus rhythm. Likewise, diltiazem might slow the ventricular response rate but it is usually not used clinically. Phenytoin is not used in horses.

16. The answer is C (II B 1 e).
All antiarrhythmic drugs can have proarrhythmic effects.

17. The answer is D (I D 1 a, II B 1 a, and II B 4 a).
Anticholinergic therapy is initially indicated for symptomatic second-degree heart block. The other agents listed are relatively or absolutely contraindicated with A-V nodal disease.

18. The answer is E (V A 1).
The heparin–antithrombin III complex neutralizes factors XII, XI, X, IX, and II (thrombin).

Chapter 9

Diuretics

Franklin Ahrens

I. INTRODUCTION

A. Diuretics are drugs that increase urinary loss of sodium ions (Na$^+$) and water. By shrinking extracellular fluid (ECF) volume, they mobilize edema fluid from the interstitial space and restore normal tissue perfusion and organ function. Their primary clinical use in veterinary medicine is in the prevention and treatment of generalized edema or severe local edema. Causes of generalized edema include congestive heart failure, liver disease, renal disease, or protein-losing enteropathies. The latter three conditions are characterized by low levels of plasma albumin because of the impaired synthesis (liver disease) or excess loss (renal or intestinal disease). The resulting fall in plasma oncotic pressure results in transudation of fluid from plasma to the interstitial space.

Cerebral, pulmonary, ocular, and udder edema are examples of local edema that arises from infection, inflammation, trauma, or poisons.

B. All diuretics act directly on renal tubular epithelia at specific sites in the nephron (Table 9-1). A brief review of ion and water transport in nephron segments is useful in understanding the action of diuretic drugs.

1. **Proximal convoluted tubule** (Figure 9-1). Sixty-five percent of the filtered sodium and water is reabsorbed from this segment. Sodium is absorbed by active transport, coupled transport with glucose and amino acids, and passive diffusion. High concentrations of carbonic anhydrase (CA) in tubule cells generate hydrogen ions ($CO_2 + H_2O \leftrightarrow H_2CO_3 \leftrightarrow H^+ + HCO_3^-$) which exchange for luminal sodium ions (Na$^+$–H$^+$ antiport). Filtered bicarbonate is reabsorbed from the lumen by a reversal of the above reaction (catalyzed by brush border CA) and the diffusion of CO_2 into the proximal tubule cell. Chloride and potassium are passively reabsorbed. Absorption is isosmotic since water is reabsorbed with ions. Activation of the renin–angiotensin system in response to volume depletion or a fall in blood pressure increases sodium and water reabsorption from this segment.

2. **Descending loop of Henle.** Sodium and chloride ions are not reabsorbed but become progressively concentrated in luminal fluid as water is osmotically removed into the hypertonic medullary interstitium.

3. **Thick portion of the ascending loop of Henle** (Figure 9-2). Twenty-five percent of the filtered sodium is reabsorbed in this segment. Sodium, potassium, and chloride are actively transported out of the lumen by a coupled mechanism (Na$^+$–K$^+$–2Cl$^-$ symport). The tubule epithelium is impermeable to water. The movement of ions but not water out of the lumen in this segment is essential to the countercurrent multiplier system of the kidney which generates the hypertonic-medullary interstitium. Calcium (Ca^{++}) and magnesium (Mg^{++}) are passively reabsorbed via the paracellular pathway. Luminal fluid is hypotonic as it leaves this segment.

4. Early **distal convoluted tubule** (Figure 9-3). Ten percent of filtered sodium is reabsorbed in this segment. Chloride ion is cotransported with sodium. Calcium reabsorption is increased by parathyroid hormone (PTH) acting at this segment of the nephron. The tubule epithelium is impermeable to water and thus there is further dilution of tubular urine.

5. **Late distal tubule and collecting duct** (Figure 9-4). Four percent of filtered sodium is actively reabsorbed in this part of the nephron. Potassium and hydrogen ions are secreted. An increase in the sodium load reaching this segment tends to increase K$^+$ and H$^+$ secretions as Na$^+$ is reabsorbed. Therefore, loop and thiazide diuretics indirectly increase urinary loss of K$^+$ and H$^+$ and tend

TABLE 9-1. Site of Actions of Diuretics

Nephron Segment	Diuretic
Proximal convoluted tubule	CA inhibitors (e.g., acetazolamide) Osmotic agents (e.g., mannitol) Xanthines (e.g., aminophylline)
Ascending loop of Henle	Loop diuretics (e.g., furosemide) Osmotic agents
Early distal convoluted tubule	Thiazides (e.g., hydrochlorothiazide)
Late distal tubule and collecting duct	K$^+$-sparing diuretics (e.g., triamterene or spironolactone)

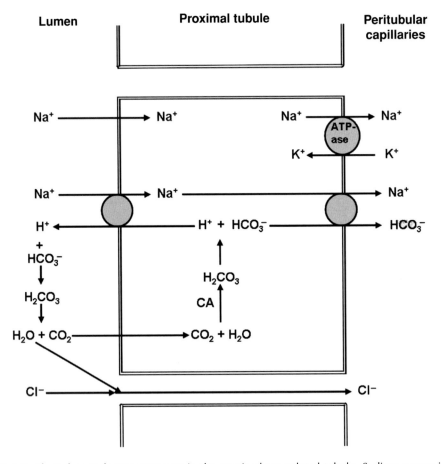

FIGURE 9-1. Electrolyte and water transport in the proximal convoluted tubule. Sodium moves into the cell down its concentration gradient—maintained by the Na$^+$–K$^+$-ATPase pump on the basolateral membrane. Sodium is also absorbed by exchange with H$^+$ at the luminal membrane (antiport). Hydrogen ion combines with filtered bicarbonate to form H$_2$CO$_3$, which is converted to H$_2$O and CO$_2$ by brush border carbonic anhydrase (CA). The reaction is reversed intracellularly. Diuretics that inhibit CA, such as acetazolamide, increase excretion of Na$^+$ and HCO$_3^-$.

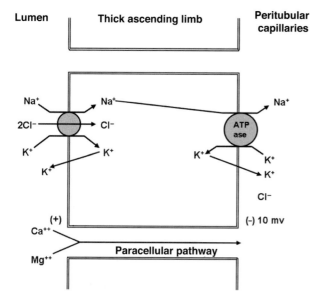

FIGURE 9-2. Electrolyte and water transport in the thick ascending limb of the loop of Henle. The Na^+–K^+–$2Cl^-$ symporter at the luminal membrane moves these ions into the cell. Part of the K^+ diffuses back to the lumen via conductance channels to maintain the lumen-positive transepithelial potential, which provides the driving force for the paracellular absorption of Ca^{++} and Mg^{++}. Inhibition of the symporter by loop diuretics, such as furosemide, increase excretion of Na^+, K^+, Cl^-, Ca^{++}, and Mg^{++}.

to produce hypokalemia and metabolic alkalosis. Aldosterone acts at this segment to increase luminal sodium channels resulting in increased sodium absorption and potassium excretion. Water is reabsorbed only if antidiuretic hormone (ADH) is present.

II. LOOP (HIGH-CEILING) DIURETICS

A. **Preparations and chemistry.** Furosemide and bumetanide are structurally related to sulfonamides. Ethacrynic acid is a derivation of phenoxyacetic acid. All are carboxylic acids. Furosemide is the most commonly used loop diuretic in veterinary medicine.

B. **Mechanism of action.** Loop diuretics inhibit electrolyte reabsorption in the thick ascending limb of the loop of Henle. They act at the luminal face of the epithelial cell

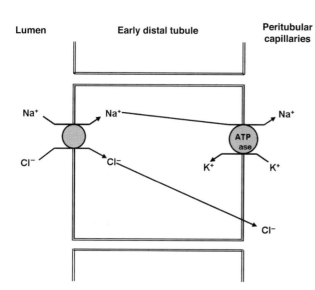

FIGURE 9-3. Absorption of sodium and chloride in the distal convoluted tubule is linked by a Na^+–Cl^- symporter in the luminal membrane. Thiazide diuretics inhibit the symporter and increase excretion of Na^+ and Cl^-.

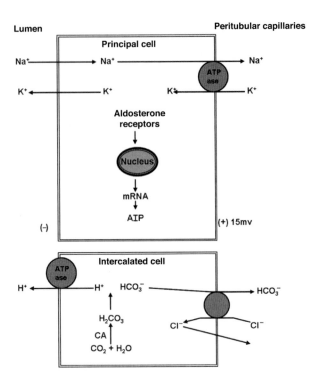

FIGURE 9-4. Electrolyte transport in the distal tubule and collecting duct. In the principal cell, sodium moves down its electrochemical gradient into the cell through Na^+ channels in the luminal membrane. Potassium moves from the cell into the lumen via K^+ channels in the luminal membrane driven by the lumen-negative transepithelial potential. This potential also aids the transport of H^+ into the lumen by the H^+-ATPase pump in the intercalated cell. Potassium-sparing diuretics such as triamterene and amiloride block luminal sodium channels to reduce Na^+ absorption and K^+ excretion. Aldosterone stimulates the production of aldosterone-induced proteins (AIP), which increases luminal sodium channels to increase Na^+ absorption.

to inhibit Na^+–K^+–$2Cl^-$cotransport into the cell. They have a rapid onset of action with peak diuresis greater than other classes of diuretics. Calcium and magnesium ion absorption from the ascending loop of Henle are also inhibited because of the decreased lumen-positive transepithelial potential. Diuretic action is independent of urinary pH. Loop diuretics produce an increase in systemic venous capacitance which may be due to their ability to stimulate prostaglandin release by the juxtaglomerular apparatus.

C. Therapeutic uses

1. Loop diuretics are the drugs of choice for the rapid mobilization of edema fluid arising from congestive heart failure, liver disease, or other causes of generalized edema, and for pulmonary, cerebral, or udder edema.
2. Furosemide increases urinary calcium excretion and is used in the treatment of hypercalcemia and hypercalcuric nephropathy in dogs and cats.
3. Furosemide may be combined with osmotic diuretics such as mannitol to maintain urine flow in severe oliguria and acute renal failure.
4. Furosemide is used for the prevention of exercise-induced pulmonary hemorrhage (EIPH) and epistaxis in racehorses. Its efficacy in this condition may be related to increased blood vessel capacitance and decreased left atrial pressure.

D. Pharmacokinetics. Furosemide, bumetanide, and ethacrynic acid are well absorbed orally. They are actively secreted into urine by the organic acid transport system of the proximal convoluted tubule and thus rapidly reach their site of action in the loop of Henle. Furosemide is excreted in the urine as unchanged drug (80%) or as the glucuronide (20%). The plasma $t_{1/2}$ is 1–2 hours for most species and the duration of diuresis is 3–6 hours for a single oral dose. If administered intravenously, the onset of diuresis is 2–20 minutes with a duration of 2 hours.

E. Administration

1. For the treatment of edema, furosemide is administered orally or intravenously three times a day for diuresis in dogs and cats and twice a day in cattle and

horses. Treatment for udder edema in cattle should not exceed 48 hours postpartum.

2. For the treatment of oliguric renal failure, furosemide is administered intravenously at hourly intervals until diuresis occurs.
3. For the prevention of EIPH, furosemide is administered intravenously to horses 1–2 hours prior to a race for EIPH prevention. Rules of use are governed by state racing authorities.
4. For the treatment of hypercalcemia or hypercalcuric nephropathy in dogs and cats, furosemide is administered in KCl-supplemented saline, intravenously, once or twice a day.

F. Adverse effects

1. Fluid and electrolyte imbalances (especially hypokalemia) are the most common adverse effects. High or prolonged doses may produce dehydration, muscle weakness, CNS depression, volume depletion, and cardiovascular collapse. Cats are more sensitive than dogs to the effects of loop diuretics and lower doses are used in this species.
2. Loop diuretics may alter electrolyte balance in the endolymph of the inner ear. Deafness is a risk if a potentially ototoxic drug (e.g., an aminoglycoside antibiotic) is administered concomitantly. In such circumstances, another class of diuretic should be employed.
3. Transient granulocytopenia and thrombocytopenia may occur.

III. THIAZIDE DIURETICS (BENZOTHIADIAZIDES)

A. Preparations and chemistry.
The thiazides are heterocyclic compounds whose structure includes a benzene ring with an unsubstituted sulfonamide group ($-SO_2NH_2$).

Chlorothiazide and hydrochlorothiazide are the most common thiazides used in veterinary medicine.

B. Mechanism of action

1. The thiazide diuretics block Na^+–Cl^- cotransport in the early part of distal tubule. Sodium, chloride, magnesium, and potassium ion excretion are increased. Calcium ion excretion is decreased because thiazides increase Ca^{++} absorption in the early distal tubule. Thiazide diuresis tends to be moderate since 90% of the filtered sodium has been reabsorbed from the nephron by the time it reaches the distal segment. Urinary excretion of ions tends to be in physiological ratios and thus distortion of ECF ion balance is minimal.
2. Thiazides are weak inhibitors of CA but at normal doses this does not contribute to their diuretic action.
3. Paradoxically, thiazides *reduce* urine output in diabetes insipidus. The mechanism of this action is unknown but is related to their natriuretic effect.
4. Thiazides may induce hyperglycemia and glycosuria in diabetic or prediabetic states by inhibiting the conversion of proinsulin to insulin.

C. Therapeutic uses

1. Chlorothiazide and hydrochlorothiazide are useful for long-term diuretic therapy in dogs and cats as adjuncts to cardiac drugs in the treatment of congestive heart failure. Hydrochlorothiazide and trichlormethiazide are used in the treatment of udder edema in cattle.
2. Thiazide diuretics are effective in reducing urine output in nephrogenic diabetes insipidus in dogs.
3. Hydrochlorothiazide reduces urinary calcium ion excretion and is used for the treatment of calcium oxalate uroliths in dogs.

D. **Pharmacokinetics.** Pharmacokinetics studies of thiazides in animals have not been reported. In man, oral absorption is 10–20% and 65–75% for chlorothiazide and hydrochlorothiazide, respectively. Onset of diuresis occurs in 2 hours and peaks in 4–6 hours. Duration of action is 6–12 hours. They are not metabolized and are excreted in the urine by active tubular secretion.

E. **Administration**

1. For the treatment of edema in heart failure, chlorothiazide or hydrochlorothiazide is administered orally twice a day in dogs and cats. A diuretic response occurs in 2–3 hours and lasts 6–12 hours.
2. For the treatment of recurrent calcium oxalate uroliths in dogs with hypercalcuria, hydrochlorothiazide is administered orally twice a day.
3. For the treatment of udder edema in cattle, hydrochlorothiazide is administered intravenously or intramuscularly twice a day. Trichlormethiazide is combined with dexamethasone in a proprietary preparation (Naquasone) administered orally once a day.
4. For the treatment of nephrogenic diabetes insipidus, chlorothiazide or hydrochlorothiazide is administered orally twice a day.

F. **Adverse effects.** The moderate diuresis produced by thiazide results in less disturbance of ECF electrolyte balance than other classes of diuretics. Hypokalemia and hypochloremia may develop with high or prolonged doses. Hyperglycemia may occur and may aggravate preexisting diabetes mellitus.

IV. OSMOTIC DIURETICS

A. **Preparations and chemistry.** Mannitol is a six-carbon sugar alcohol prepared as a 20–25% aqueous solution. It is the most important member in this class of diuretics. Glycerol and urea are used less frequently. Dimethyl sulfoxide (DMSO) prepared as a 10% solution in 5% dextrose has been used to treat edema in horses.

B. **Mechanism of action**

1. Osmotic diuretics are filtered at the glomerulus but are poorly reabsorbed from the lumen of the nephron. The presence of these unabsorbed solutes in the proximal tubule causes decreased reabsorption of water, resulting in a large volume of urine. There is a small increase in Na^+ and Cl^- excretion. Mannitol causes an increase in renal medullary blood flow via a prostaglandin-mediated mechanism. This reduces medullary tonicity, decreases extraction of water in the descending loop of Henle, and thus lowers the concentration of NaCl and the passive reabsorption of NaCl in the thick ascending loop of Henle.

C. **Therapeutic uses**

1. For the nonspecific treatment of poisoning in dogs and cats, mannitol is used to induce forced diuresis which hastens the elimination of poisons excreted by the kidney.
2. For the treatment of oliguric renal failure in dogs and cats mannitol is used as an adjunct to furosemide therapy. The osmotic expansion of the plasma increases glomerular filtration volume and maintains urine flow. Urine output must be monitored.
3. For the treatment of increased intraocular pressure of acute glaucoma in dogs and cats, osmotic diuretics such as mannitol or glycerin are used to reduce intraocular pressure.
4. For the treatment of cerebral edema in large and small animals, mannitol is used as an adjunct to furosemide to mobilize edema fluid. In addition to its diuretic

effect, mannitol may prevent the hypovolemic shock commonly observed in cerebral edema.

D. **Pharmacokinetics.** Mannitol is administered intravenously for osmotic diuresis since oral absorption is poor. It distributes to the ECF, is not metabolized, and is excreted by renal glomerular filtration. The plasma $t_{1/2}$ is 1–2 hours.

E. **Administration.** Mannitol solutions (5–20%) are administered by slow intravenous infusions over 15–30 minutes in all species. Doses may be repeated every 6–8 hours.

F. **Adverse effects.** Toxicity is rare but fluid and electrolyte balance and urine output should be monitored, especially in the treatment of oliguric renal failure. Mannitol should not be used in generalized edema or acute pulmonary edema because its saluretic effect is small and because it produces an initial expansion of the ECF which may exacerbate the edema and may cause decompensation in patients with congestive heart failure.

V. CARBONIC ANHYDRASE INHIBITORS

A. **Preparations and chemistry.** Acetazolamide, methazolamide, and dichlorphenamide are sulfonamide derivates.

B. **Mechanism of action.** These agents reversibly inhibit CA enzyme predominantly in the proximal convoluted tubules, causing a reduction in hydrogen ions available for Na^+–H^+ exchange. Carbon dioxide (CO_2) reabsorption from the glomerular filtrate is suppressed, and Na^+–HCO_3^- excretion is increased, resulting in an alkaline urine. To maintain ionic balance, Cl^- is retained by the kidney, resulting in a hyperchloremic acidosis. The resulting metabolic acidosis (low plasma HCO_3^-) eventually induces a refractory state and decreased diuresis.

High concentrations of CA occur in the ciliary process of the eye and the enzyme is involved in aqueous humor formation. CA inhibitors reduce intraocular pressure in glaucoma by decreasing the production of aqueous humor.

C. **Therapeutic uses.** The primary use of CA inhibitors is for reducing the rate of aqueous humor formation in the treatment of glaucoma. They are occasionally used as adjuncts in the treatment of metabolic alkalosis. Their diuretic action is weak and they are seldom used for this purpose now.

D. **Pharmacokinetics.** Acetazolamide and dichlorphenamide are absorbed orally, distributed to tissues with high CA concentrations (renal cortex, eye, and erythrocytes), and excreted by the kidney by active secretion and passive reabsorption. Onset of diuretic action is 30 minutes with a duration of 6–12 hours in small animals. In horses, after IV administration, the distribution $t_{1/2}$ is 60 minutes, and the elimination $t_{1/2}$ is ~7.5 hours. After oral administration in horses, the time to reach peak plasma level is ~2 hours. Bioavailability of acetazolamide in horses is only ~25%.

E. **Administration.** For glaucoma, acetazolamide, methazolamide, ethazolamide, or dichlorphenamide are given orally 2–3 times daily. In acute cases, a single intravenous dose of acetazolamide is given followed by an oral dosage regimen.

F. **Adverse effects.** Toxicity is rare. Gastrointestinal disturbances, especially vomiting, may occur with oral administration. CA inhibitors are contraindicated in the presence of liver disease because they may precipitate hepatic coma by diverting ammonia produced in the kidney from the urine to the systemic circulation as a result of urine alkalinization.

VI. POTASSIUM-SPARING DIURETICS

A. **Preparations and chemistry.** Triamterene and amiloride are cyclic amidines and are organic bases. Spironolactone is a steroid analog of the mineralocorticoid aldosterone.

B. **Mechanism of action.** Triamterene and amiloride inhibit active Na^+ reabsorption in the distal convoluted tubule and collecting duct. This reduces the net driving force for K^+ secretion. They cause a small increase in Na^+ and Cl^- excretion without increasing K^+ excretion. Their action is independent of aldosterone.

Spironolactone is a competitive antagonist of the mineralocorticoid aldosterone. It reduces the aldosterone-mediated Na^+–K^+exchange at the late distal convoluted tubule, increasing Na^+ loss while decreasing K^+ loss. Spironolactone is most effective when circulating aldosterone levels are high.

C. **Therapeutic uses.** Triamterene or amiloride is occasionally used in combination with thiazides or loop diuretics in chronic edema. The combination augments the natriuretic effect while attenuating K^+ loss.

Spironolactone is occasionally used as an adjunct to other diuretics in the treatment of refractory edema if excessive K^+ loss is a concern. Spironolactone is also used to treat adrenal gland tumors to counter the excess mineralocorticoid effects of aldosterone (sodium retention and potassium excretion).

D. **Pharmacokinetics.** Triamterene and amiloride are absorbed orally. Amiloride is excreted unchanged by the kidney. Triamterene is converted by the liver to an active metabolite—hydroxytriamterene. Both drugs are transported by the organic base secretory mechanism in the proximal tubule. Hydroxytriamterene can further form the sulfate conjugate. Peak onset of diuresis is 6–8 hours with a duration of 12–15 hours.

Spironolactone is absorbed orally, bound to plasma proteins, and is extensively metabolized by the liver. The active metabolite, canrenone, has a long half-life (16–20 hours). Diuretic action is prolonged with a duration of 2–3 days.

E. **Administration.** Triamterene is administered orally twice a day in dogs and cats. Amiloride is administered orally once a day.

Spironolactone is administered orally twice a day in dogs and cats.

F. **Adverse effects.** Hyperkalemia can occur and thus K^+ diuretics are not given in combination with one another and are contraindicated in hyperkalemic patients. Hyperkalemia is especially likely in the presence of diabetes mellitus, renal disease, or thromboembolic disease. Gastrointestinal disturbances, including nausea and vomiting, may occur.

VII. METHYLXANTHINES

A. **Mechanism of action.** The methylxanthines include aminophylline, theophylline, caffeine, and theobromine. Their diuretic effect is due to increased renal blood flow and glomerular filtration rate and to inhibition of sodium reabsorption in the proximal convoluted tubule. Diuresis is enhanced by an alkaline urine and thus greater in herbivores than carnivores. They also produce bronchodilation by inhibition of adenosine receptors and are CNS stimulants.

B. **Therapeutic uses.** Methylxanthines are rarely used as diuretics but increased urine output is observed when aminophylline or theophylline is employed as a bronchodilator in respiratory disease therapy.

C. **Pharmacokinetics of theophylline**

1. **Absorption.** Theophylline bioavailability after oral administration is ~100% when nonsustained release products are used, but is 30–75% if sustained release products are used.

2. **Distribution.** Theophylline is distributed throughout the ECF and body tissues. Because of the low volumes of distribution (0.5–1 L/kg) and theophylline's low lipid solubility, obese patients should be dosed on a lean body weight basis.

3. **Elimination.** Theophylline is metabolized primarily in the liver (in humans) to 3-methylxanthine, an active metabolite. Renal clearance contributes only about 10% to the overall plasma clearance of theophylline. The reported elimination $t_{1/2}$ are: dogs, ~6 hours; cats, ~8 hours, pigs, 11 hours; and horses, 12–17 hours.

D. **Adverse effects.** Methylxanthine may produce excitement, skeletal muscle fasciculation, vomiting, and cardiovascular toxicity including palpitations and hypotension with high or prolonged dosage.

VIII. ACIDIFYING SALTS

A. **Mechanism of action.** Acidifying salts such as ammonium chloride (NH_4Cl) lower the pH of ECF and urine. The liver converts NH_4Cl to urea, H^+ and Cl^-. Hydrogen ion is buffered by HCO_3^- in plasma and this leads to acidosis. The increased chloride load to the kidney produces urinary loss of Na^+ and Cl^- and a mild diuresis.

B. **Therapeutic uses.** Ammonium chloride is used for urinary acidification to dissolve uroliths or to prevent their formation. It is also used to enhance the renal excretion of ionizable drugs or poisons by ion trapping in the urine.

C. **Administration.** Ammonium chloride is administered orally two to three times a day or added to the diet in dogs and cats.

D. **Adverse effects.** Severe, uncompensated acidosis may result if renal function is impaired. Nausea and gastric irritation may occur with oral dosing. Ammonium chloride is contraindicated in the presence of decreased liver function because of the requirement for its hepatic conversion to urea described under mechanism of action above.

SUGGESTED READING

http://www.drugs.com

Jackson EK. 2006. "Drugs affecting renal and cardiovascular function." In *Goodman & Gilman's The Pharmacological Basis of Therapeutics*. Edited by Brunton LL, Lazo JS, Parker KL. 11th ed., pp. 737–769. New York: McGraw-Hill.

Kochevar DT. 2001. "Diuretics." In *Veterinary Pharmacology and Therapeutics*. Edited by Adams HR. 8th ed., pp. 534–552. Ames, IA: Iowa State University Press.

Plumb DC. 2005. *Veterinary Drug Handbook*. 5th ed. Ames, IA: Blackwell Publishing.

STUDY QUESTIONS

DIRECTIONS: Each of the numbered items or incomplete statements in this section is followed by answers or by completions of the statement. Select the **one** lettered answer or completion that is **best** in each case.

1. In cases of severe generalized edema, which of the following fluid compartments is increased in volume?

(A) Intracellular
(B) Interstitial
(C) Transcellular
(D) Plasma

2. Hypoalbuminemia underlies the edema arising from all of the following EXCEPT

(A) hepatic disease.
(B) congestive heart failure.
(C) renal disease.
(D) protein-losing enteropathy.

3. In the presence of renal disease, *hyper-kalemia* may occur after the administration of

(A) mannitol.
(B) triamterene.
(C) furosemide.
(D) chlorothiazide.

4. Which of the following statements concerning furosemide *is not true?*

(A) It tends to produce a metabolic alkalosis via urinary loss of hydrogen, potassium, and chloride.
(B) It decreases calcium reabsorption in the loop of Henle and increases urinary calcium loss.
(C) It may increase capacitance of pulmonary blood vessels and reduce epistaxis (nosebleed) in racehorses.
(D) It blocks $Na^+–K^+–2Cl^-$-coupled transport in the ascending loop of Henle.
(E) It is less potent than agents which act at the proximal convoluted tubule.

5. An alkaline urine and a decreased rate of aqueous humor formation in glaucoma is produced by

(A) ethacrynic acid.
(B) dichlorphenamide.
(C) mannitol.
(D) triamterene.

6. A veterinarian is presented with a dog exhibiting signs of diabetes insipidus which does not respond to desmopressin (synthetic analog of pituitary ADH). Paradoxically, urine output may *decrease* following treatment with

(A) amiloride.
(B) aminophylline.
(C) chlorothiazide.
(D) acetazolamide.
(E) ammonium chloride.

7. The high-ceiling or loop diuretics such as furosemide, ethacrynic acid, or bumetanide

(A) have a slow onset of action since they are bound to plasma albumin.
(B) are the diuretics of choice in acute pulmonary edema.
(C) are useful in treating aminoglycoside antibiotic toxicity since they increase renal excretion of this class of antimicrobials.
(D) are potentiated by CA inhibitors such as acetazolamide or dichlorphenamide because they require an alkaline urine for their diuretic action.

8. Excessive sodium retention and potassium excretion resulting from aldosterone-secreting adrenal gland tumors may be treated with

(A) furosemide.
(B) chlorothiazide.
(C) triamterene.
(D) spironolactone.

9. Intravenous mannitol (5%) would be indicated in all of the following clinical situations EXCEPT

(A) oliguria arising from traumatic shock.

(B) ingestion of toxic amounts of cleaning solution containing potassium oxalate.
(C) generalized edema arising from congestive heart failure.
(D) cerebral edema resulting from trauma.
(E) increased intraocular pressure of narrow angle glaucoma.

10. A diuretic which *decreases* calcium excretion via increased absorption in the distal tubule and is thus used to prevent calcium oxalate bladder stones, is

(A) hydrochlorothiazide.

(B) ethacrynic acid.
(C) urea.
(D) spironolactone.
(E) triamterene.

11. Hyperglycemia via inhibition of the conversion of proinsulin to insulin may occur with

(A) thiazides.
(B) loop diuretics.
(C) CA inhibitors.
(D) methylxanthines.

DIRECTIONS: The group of items in this section consists of lettered options followed by a set of numbered items. For each item, select the one lettered option that is most closely associated with it. Each lettered option may be selected once, more than once, or not at all.

Questions 12–15
For each of the following diuretic agents, choose the anatomic site in the renal nephron where the principal action of the agent occurs.

(A) Glomerulus
(B) Proximal tubule
(C) Ascending limb of the loop of Henle
(D) Distal tubule—early part
(E) Late distal tubule and collecting duct

12. Acetazolamide

13. Spironolactone

14. Furosemide

15. Chlorothiazide

16. Which of the following is contraindicated in patients with liver disease because of the danger of precipitating hepatic coma?

(A) Hydrochlorothiazide
(B) Acetazolamide
(C) Furosemide
(D) Spironolactone

17. Fluid and electrolyte imbalance leading to dehydration, muscle weakness, hypokalemia, and CNS depression may result from high or prolonged dosage with

(A) chlorothiazide.
(B) amiloride.
(C) furosemide.
(D) theophylline.

ANSWERS AND EXPLANATIONS

1. The answer is B.
Generalized edema results from accumulation of fluid in the interstitial space. In severe edema, this compartment may nearly double in volume. Intracellular, transcellular, and plasma volumes are minimally affected.

2. The answer is B.
Renal disease and protein-losing enteropathy result in loss of plasma proteins and plasma protein synthesis by the liver is decreased in hepatic disease. These conditions result in hypoalbuminemia, decreased plasma oncotic pressure, and transudation of fluid from blood vessels to the interstitial space. Plasma albumin concentrations are not changed in congestive heart failure.

3. The answer is B.
Triamterene is a potassium-sparing diuretic that inhibits active sodium reabsorption in the distal tubule and collecting duct. Potassium retention may produce hyperkalemia in the presence of renal disease. Mannitol, furosemide, and chlorothiazide are not potassium-sparing diuretics.

4. The answer is E.
Furosemide increases hydrogen, potassium, and chloride ion excretion rates which produces a metabolic alkalosis. Calcium reabsorption in the loop of Henle is decreased because of the loss of transcellular potential produced by blockade of Na^+–K^+–$2Cl^-$ cotransport. Blood vessel capacitance is increased and this may prevent exercise-induced pulmonary hemorrhage in horses. Loop diuretics are more potent than agents which act at the proximal tubules because compensatory mechanisms for sodium reabsorption are limited beyond the loop of Henle.

5. The answer is B.
Dichlorphenamide is a CA inhibitor which reduces Na^+–H^+ exchange in the proximal convoluted tubule and thus HCO_3^- ion is excreted and the urine becomes alkaline. CA activity is required for aqueous humor formation and thus the inhibition of this enzyme by dichlorphenamide reduces intraocular pressure in glaucoma. Ethacrynic

acid, mannitol, and triamterene do not inhibit CA.

6. The answer is C.
The thiazide diuretics decrease urine volume in nephrogenic diabetes insipidus. The mechanism is not completely understood but sodium depletion, increased Na^+ and Cl^- absorption in the proximal tubule and reduced volume delivered to the distal nephron, may enhance the action of ADH. This effect is not observed with other classes of diuretics.

7. The answer is B.
Loop diuretics may potentiate the ototoxicity of the aminoglycoside antibiotics and should not be used with this class of antimicrobials. They have a rapid onset of action and produce peak diuresis which is greater than other classes of diuretics. They are useful in the rapid mobilization of edema fluid in life-threatening conditions such as pulmonary edema. Their action is independent of urinary pH.

8. The answer is D.
Mineralocorticoid such as aldosterone is secreted in large amounts by adrenal gland tumors and produce excessive sodium retention and potassium excretion by the kidneys. Spironolactone is a competitive antagonist of aldosterone and ameliorates the effects of the hormone. Furosemide, chlorothiazide, or triamterene do not affect aldosterone actions.

9. The answer is C.
Osmotic diuretics produce an initial increase in blood volume which can cause decompensation in patients with congestive heart failure. In addition, they are not effective in generalized edematous states because their saluretic action is weak. They are effective in oliguria, forced diuresis in cases of poisoning, cerebral edema, and glaucoma.

10. The answer is A.
The thiazide diuretics stimulate Ca^{++} reabsorption in the early distal tubule and reduce urinary calcium concentrations. This

action may aid in preventing the formation of calcium oxalate uroliths. Loop diuretics increase calcium excretion. Spironolactone, triamterene, or urea does not affect calcium excretion.

11. The answer is A.
Thiazides may produce hyperglycemia by slowing the conversion of proinsulin to insulin. The effect is most prominent in the diabetic or prediabetic state. This effect does not occur with loop diuretics, CA inhibitors, or the methylxanthines.

12–15. The answers are: 12-B, 13-E, 14-C, 15-D.
Although acetazolamide acts on both the proximal and distal convoluted tubules, its effects on the proximal tubules are quantitatively most important for its diuretic actions because CA concentrations are highest in this segment. Spironolactone, a K^+-sparing diuretic, acts as a competitive antagonist of aldosterone. The receptor for aldosterone is located in the distal convoluted tubule and thus this is the site of action for spironolactone. Furosemide is a high-ceiling diuretic and, like ethacrynic acid, it inhibits reabsorption in the ascending limb of the loop of Henle. Chlorothiazide is one of several thiazide diuretics. The thiazides act primarily on the early part of the distal convoluted tubule to block Na^+ and Cl^- reabsorption.

16. The answer is B.
CA inhibitors, such as acetazolamide, increase urinary bicarbonate excretion and produce an alkaline urine. This eliminates the driving force for ammonia excretion into the urine to eliminate H^+ by forming NH_4^+ which is excreted. The ammonia produced by distal tubules is reabsorbed to the blood instead of excreted in urine. Ammonia is converted to urea by the liver and if liver function is impaired, blood levels of ammonia rise and may precipitate hepatic coma.

17. The answer is C.
The toxic effects of loop diuretics such as furosemide are an extension of their therapeutic effects. Their potent diuretic action may deplete the body of water and electrolytes and lead to dehydration, hypokalemia, muscle weakness, and CNS depression if administered in high or prolonged dosage. These adverse effects are less likely to occur with less potent diuretics such as chlorothiazide, amiloride, or theophylline.

Chapter 10

Respiratory Pharmacology

Dean H. Riedesel

I. **INTRODUCTION.** The primary function of the respiratory system is gas exchange between the inspired air and the pulmonary artery blood. Because of the large surface area of the alveoli and exposure to the environment, this organ system is prone to antigen–allergy responses and infection. The defenses of the respiratory system include hypersecretion of mucus, sneezing and coughing reflexes, bronchoconstriction, and macrophage activation and inflammation. Pharmacology of the respiratory system centers around these defense mechanisms and can be simplified into seven categories: (1) elimination of excess secretions and membrane congestion, (2) bronchiole dilation when excessive constriction has occurred, (3) cough suppression when it is nonproductive and detrimental to the animal, (4) control of infection and inflammation, (5) decrease pulmonary hypertension, (6) stimulate the peripheral chemoreceptors and the central respiratory center, and (7) exogenous surfactant.

II. **SECRETIONS.** A thin layer of mucus coats the surface of all airways from the bronchioles to the larynx. This mucus is secreted by Clara cells, goblet cells, and submucosal bronchial glands located within the respiratory epithelium. Mucus protects airways by entrapping inhaled particles, humidifying inspired air, and maintaining mucosal hydration. Cilia, on the apical surface of respiratory epithelial cells, propel mucus out of smaller airways into the trachea and up to the larynx to be swallowed or expectorated. The mucociliary escalator is essential for the removal of airway secretions, pathogens, cellular debris, and inhaled particulate matter from the respiratory tract. Mucoprotein content of the mucus and transepithelial movement of water and ions determine the viscosity of normal mucus. Thick mucus can also be due to the presence of bacterial and neutrophil cellular debris. The cough reflex is very important for clearance of viscous mucus. Too much mucus narrows the lumen of bronchi restricting airflow and stimulates coughing. If coughing does not rid the airway of mucus, there are several pharmacologic options in addition to treating the underlying respiratory disease.

A. **Increasing or facilitating the removal of excess, accumulated secretions. By decreasing the viscosity of these bronchial secretions, the normal action of the cilia and reflex coughing may be more effective.**

1. Methods designed to loosen secretions by hydration of the mucus.
   a. Nebulizer (aerosol) therapy with sterile or bacteriostatic water or saline produces a liquid particle suspension within a carrier gas (room air or oxygen) which, when inhaled, will add water to the airway mucus layer.
   b. Always use physiotherapy in conjunction with nebulization.
      (1) Improve tidal ventilation by mild-forced exercise after nebulization.
      (2) Manually stimulating a cough reflex via chest wall coupage, vibration, or tracheal manipulation.
   c. Efficacy is debatable.
   d. Small volume jet or ultrasonic nebulizers produce particles of 0.5–3 microns, which are best for deposition in the lower respiratory tract.

    e. Large volume aerosol therapy may be beneficial in lobar pneumonia. Done with a bland aerosol (sterile saline) in an enclosed cage with a large ultrasonic nebulizer for 30–45 minutes 2–4 times per day.

2. *N*-Acetylcysteine (*N*-acetyl-l-cysteine) is a derivative of l-cysteine and acts as a mucolytic drug.

    a. **N-Acetylcysteine** (NAC) breaks the disulfide bonds within the mucus molecules and decreases the viscosity.

    b. NAC will not only alter the viscosity of normal mucus but also the thick mucus that results from the addition of bacterial and neutrophil cellular debris.

    c. This drug is usually aerosolized and inhaled by the patient, but a powder form is available and can be formulated for oral use.

    d. **Proven benefits from NAC have not been demonstrated in veterinary patients and aerosolized, it may cause airway irritation and bronchoconstriction.**

3. **Bromhexine** HCl is a frequently prescribed mucolytic.

    a. Enhances the hydrolysis of acid mucopolysaccharides that significantly contributes to mucus viscosity.

    b. Does not alter protein in the mucus, which originates from bacteria or neutrophil cellular debris.

    c. May increase the concentration of certain antibiotics in the alveoli by altering the permeability of the alveolar/capillary membranes.

B. **Expectorants theoretically make the bronchiole secretions less viscous but their efficacy is questionable.**

1. **Potassium iodide** is an oral saline expectorant, which causes irritation to the gastric mucosa that in turn increases bronchiole secretion through a vagal reflex.

2. **Guaifenesin** is a guaiacol (wood tar) derivative that acts as an expectorant and increases airway particle clearance in humans.

    a. Guaifenesin may stimulate the gastric mucosa and increase respiratory tract secretions via reflex.

    b. The volume and viscosity of secretions does not appear to change.

    c. This compound is primarily found in over-the-counter human cough preparations.

C. **Decongestants** shrink the nasal mucosa and allow air to pass more freely. Sinusitis or reverse sneezing are other indications for decongestants.

1. H_1-antihistamines are commonly used for allergic-induced symptoms and chronic rhinitis in people but efficacy in animals is not documented. (See Chapter 3 for the pharmacology of H_1-antihistamines.)

    a. **Diphenhydramine**

    b. **Dimenhydrinate**

    c. **Chlorpheniramine**

    d. **Hydroxyzine**

2. Sympathomimetic drugs (α-receptor agonists) may be given orally or topically as nasal sprays to avoid their systemic effects. However, nasal sprays are not well tolerated in animals. Their primary effect is to constrict the precapillary arterioles, reduce blood flow, and reduce the extracellular fluid in the nasal mucosa. Nasal discharge consequently will be reduced and resistance to airflow through the nasal cavity will decrease. (See Chapter 2 for information on the pharmacology of sympathomimetics.)

    a. **Ephedrine**

    b. **Pseudoephedrine**

    c. **Phenylephrine.** This drug has been used to relieve anesthesia (recumbency)-induced nasal congestion and edema in horses. About 30 minutes before anesthetic recovery and removal of the endotracheal tube, phenylephrine is sprayed or squirted into the ventral meatus of each nostril with the external nares elevated.

III. **CONTROL OF INFECTION AND INFLAMMATION.** Antibiotic choice should ideally be based on culture and sensitivity or cytology with a Gram's stain.

A. **Antibacterial drugs** that have a good spectrum of activity. (See Chapter 15 for information on the pharmacology of antibacterial drugs.)

1. **Upper airway disease—Gram-positive spectrum is best.**
2. **Lower airway disease—Gram-negative spectrum is best.**
   a. **Cephalosporins**
   b. **Potentiated sulfonamides**
   c. **Amoxicillin**
   d. **Amoxicillin/clavulanate**
   e. **Fluoroquinolones**
3. Aerosolized antibiotics may be helpful in selected cases of infectious tracheobronchitis.

B. **Glucocorticoids**

1. Corticosteroids are important for the treatment of antigen-induced inflammatory bronchial disease such as chronic obstructive pulmonary disease (heaves) in horses and feline bronchial disease (asthma), as well as chronic bronchitis in dogs. Glucocorticoids reduce mucus hypersecretion, bronchial mucosal thickening, and airway smooth muscle constriction. (See Chapter 12 for more information on glucocorticoids.)
   a. Oral intermediate-acting steroids are preferred for ease of dosage adjustments.
      (1) Prednisolone
      (2) Prednisone
   b. Fluticasone is an inhaled glucocorticoid that is being used more frequently in animals.
      (1) It is available in a multidose inhaler (MDI) for human inhalation.
      (2) An animal mask and spacer are needed for administration.
      (3) It has 18× the affinity of dexamethasone for human glucocorticoid receptors.
      (4) Only 30% of the administered dose reaches the airways of the lung.
      (5) It may take 1–2 weeks of administration to see the maximum effects.
   c. For other inhaled glucocorticoid aerosol drugs see Table 10-1.

C. **Leukotriene receptor antagonists** are a new type of therapy. Leukotrienes are potent bronchoconstrictors and trigger inflammatory responses such as edema formation.

1. These modulators of inflammation can be used instead of corticosteroids.
2. Drugs that antagonize leukotriene receptors are zafirlukast, zileuton, and montelukast.
3. Zafirlukast has been tested in cats with experimental asthma and found not to be beneficial.
4. Whether these drugs are of any use in respiratory therapy is yet to be determined.

D. **Nonsteroidal anti-inflammatory drugs** are seldom used to treat inflammatory respiratory diseases because they tend to inhibit cyclooxygenase more than lipooxygenase enzymes. Aspirin has been used in the treatment of thromboembolism in cases of heartworm disease.

E. **Serotonin receptor inhibition** may be beneficial for feline "asthma." Cyproheptadine is the only drug in this category currently thought to be beneficial. (See Chapter 3 for information on cyproheptadine.)

F. **Cyclosporine** is an immunosuppressant drug but has been shown to be beneficial in experimental models of feline bronchial disease "asthma."

G. **Mast cell stabilizers** are used in human medicine to treat allergic asthma. These cromones, cromoglycate and nedocromil, prevent the release of inflammatory

TABLE 10-1. Drugs Available as Metered Dose Inhalers (MDI)

Drug Class	Generic Name	Indication	Comments
Bronchodilator—β₂-agonists	Albuterol	Immediate relief	Effect is short lived (<4 hours)
	Pirbuterol	Immediate relief	No animal data
	Salmeterol	Long-term (12-hour) control	Onset of action >1 hour
	Bitolterol	Immediate relief	No animal data
	Metaproterenol	Immediate relief	No animal data
	Terbutaline	Immediate relief	No animal data
	Pirbuterol	Immediate relief	No animal data
Anticholinergic agent	Ipratropium bromide	Additive bronchodilation with β₂-agonists	No animal data
Anti-inflammatory corticosteroids	Fluticasone propionate	Long-term control of inflammation	Takes 10–14 days to reach peak effect
	Flunisolide	Long-term control of inflammation	No animal data
	Budesonide	Long-term control of inflammation	No animal data
	Beclomethasone dipropionate	Long-term control of inflammation	No animal data
	Triamcinolone	Long-term control of inflammation	No animal data
Mast cell stabilizer	Cromolyn sodium	Long-term control of inflammation	No animal data
	Nedocromil sodium	Long-term control of inflammation	No animal data

JAAHA 42:165–169, 2006, Use of inhaled medications to treat respiratory diseases in dogs and cats, by P. Padrid.

mediators from mast cells by inhibiting the influx of calcium. They are administered by inhalation and efficacy in animals is not documented. (See Chapter 3 for information on cromolyn sodium.)

IV. COUGH SUPPRESSION and normalization of other respiratory reflexes. Sneezing and reverse sneezing, coughing, and airway narrowing reflexes that result in laryngospasm and bronchospasm are reflexes that are part of the normal pulmonary defenses and should not be suppressed unless they are excessive or debilitating.

A. **Coughing** is the sudden and loud ejection of air from the lungs. It is a normal protective reflex that is necessary in the diseased animal. The sensory receptors for the reflex cough are subepithelial irritant or stretch receptors that are numerous in large airways and innervated by the vagus nerve. Foreign bodies or excessive amounts of mucus on the surface of the airways can mechanically deform a sensory receptor and stimulate the cough reflex. Inflammation of the airway, for example, a viral infection, may result in the receptors becoming hyperresponsive. During a cough, the intrapleural pressure rises dramatically against a closed glottis and as a result the intrathoracic airways are compressed. Air is expelled with considerable noise through a narrowed airway and material is dislodged from the walls of large airways. Coughing is usually a good way for the animal to clear mucus from large bronchi and the trachea, but not from the smaller distal bronchi and bronchioles. Coughing is frequently a beneficial reflex and should not be suppressed unless it is dry (nonproduction) or physically tiring to the animal. Initial treatment of the coughing animal is aimed at eliminating the underlying cause and not suppressing the cough.

1. **Antitussives** decrease the severity and frequency of coughing.
   a. Peripherally acting antitussives include anti-inflammatory drugs, mucolytics, and bronchodilators.
   b. Central acting opioid and nonopioid drugs reduce the sensitivity of the cough center to afferent stimuli. The opioid cough suppressants may cause sedation, nausea, and constipation. (See Chapter 4 for more information about opioids.)
      (1) **Codeine**—dogs and cats. One of the most effective with an antitussive effect that is much greater than its analgesic effect.
      (2) **Hydrocodone**—commonly used in the dog. More potent antitussive than codeine.
      (3) **Butorphanol**—100× more effective as an antitussive than codeine. Can be given orally or parenterally to dogs and cats. It has a short duration analgesia but longer sedative effect and minimal respiratory depression with a half-life of 1.7 hours.
      (4) **Dextromethorphan** is a semisynthetic opioid that is found in many over-the-counter human cough preparations but its efficacy in animals is not documented.

V. BRONCHIAL DILATION

V. **BRONCHIAL DILATION** is beneficial to decrease resistance to airflow when excessive constriction is present. The normal bronchi have a small amount of smooth muscle tone (constriction) due to the vagus nerve activity. The airway smooth muscle tone controls airway caliber and establishes a balance between resistance to airflow (constriction) and physiological dead space (dilation). Bronchial smooth muscle is regulated by local homeostatic mechanisms, plus neural and humoral control. Equine airways receive cholinergic, adrenergic, and nonadrenergic–noncholinergic inhibitory (iNANC) and excitatory (eNANC) innervation. Similar innervation has been observed in most domestic animal species. A variety of stimuli to the airway surface can initiate the bronchoconstrictive reflex arc, including mechanical (e.g., bronchoscopy, particulates) and chemical-autacoids (e.g., acid, histamine, and secretions) factors, pulmonary edema, pulmonary embolism, and pneumothorax.

A. **Bronchodilators** are common treatments for airway disease. The horse benefits the most from these drugs.

B. **Parasympathetic system**—provides innervation to the entire tracheobronchial tree. These cholinergic nerves arise in the brain stem and course through the vagus nerve to synapse in local ganglia within the walls of the alveoli. From these ganglia, postganglionic fibers travel to airway smooth muscle and submuscosal glands. Ganglionic transmission is mediated by acetylcholine via neuronal nicotinic receptors, whereas smooth muscle contraction is mediated by acetylcholine via muscarinic receptors. M_3 muscarinic receptor subtypes mediate airway smooth muscle constriction, plus vasodilation and mucus secretion. Anticholinergic drugs will cause bronchodilation even in the normal healthy animal. (See Chapter 2 for more information about anticholinergic drugs).

1. **Atropine**—injectable
2. **Glycopyrrolate**—injectable
3. **Ipratropium**—aerosol by metered dose inhaler (MDI)
4. The parenterally administered anticholinergic drugs have significant side effects, including decreased GI peristalsis, dry mucous membranes, tachycardia, and urinary bladder relaxation. These side effects limit the chronic use of parenteral anticholinergic drugs and favor the aerosol administration of ipratropium directly to the lungs.

C. **Adrenergic system**—The sympathetic innervation plays an important role in the pathophysiology of airway diseases and treatment of bronchoconstriction. This system includes not only the sympathetic innervation but also the adrenal medulla. Norepinephrine is the principal neurotransmitter of sympathetic nerves and epinephrine is secreted by the adrenal medulla and functions as a hormone. The sympathetic innervation of the bronchi is sparse when compared to the parasympathetic system. Response to the adrenergic nervous system primarily involves the activation of β_2-adrenoreceptors that are distributed throughout the lung in all species. In vitro β_2-agonists suppress the tone of airway smooth muscle both when the tone is of spontaneous origin and when induced by an exogenous spasmogen. Relaxation is mediated by the intracellular accumulation of cAMP, which inactivates myosin light chain kinase. There are α_1- and α_2-adrenergic receptors in the lung of several species. The α_1-receptors mediate airway muscle contraction in the guinea pig, rabbit, and dog. The α_2-receptors are inhibitory to cholinergic nerves and are responsible for a decrease in acetylcholine release. The selective β_2-agonists are used clinically as bronchodilators but they are not 100% selective for β_2-receptors and concurrently stimulate some β_1-receptors. Since β_1- and β_2-receptors are distributed throughout the body, including the heart, overdosing these drugs may cause tachycardia, excitement, and sweating (horses). These drugs may transiently decrease systemic arterial blood pressure, which increases heart rate via the baroreceptor reflex. The β_2-receptor stimulation in the respiratory tract also increases the ciliary beat frequency and mucociliary clearance rate. They have some anti-inflammatory activity and can decrease the release of mediators from mast cells. The use of metered dose inhalers (MDIs) in human medicine has led to more β_2-agonist therapy and products available. These products can be used in animals with a spacer and mask.

1. **Adrenergic agonists**
    a. **Nonselective ($\alpha+\beta_1+\beta_2$) agents** may be used for the acute treatment of bronchoconstriction.
        (1) **Epinephrine**
        (2) **Ephedrine**
        (3) **Isoproterenol**
    b. **β_2-Selective agonists** produce fewer undesirable α- and β_1-effects.
        (1) **Terbutaline**—orally or parenterally for severe bronchoconstriction in cats.
        (2) **Isoetharine**—has been aerosolized and used in small animals.
        (3) **Albuterol**—has been aerosolized and used in horses and small animals.
            (a) It has a β_2/β_1 selectivity of 4.0.
            (b) Reported to be beneficial for the treatment of hypoxemia in anesthetized horses.
        (4) **Clenbuterol**
            (a) Approved in the United States for use in horses with airway obstruction such as chronic obstructive pulmonary disease (heaves).
            (b) β_2/β_1 Selectivity is 4.0.
            (c) Administered orally.
            (d) The $t_{1/2}$ in the horse is ~12 hours and the duration of effect is 6–8 hours.
            (e) Also inhibits the release of proinflammatory cytokines IL1β and tumor necrosis factor from macrophages.
            (f) Adverse effects include muscle tremors, sweating, restlessness, urticaria, and tachycardia.
        (5) Use these drugs cautiously in animals with concurrent diabetes, hyperthyroidism, hypertension, seizure disorders, or cardiac disease with arrhythmias.
        (6) For other selective β_2-agonistic aerosol drugs see Table 10-1.

D. **Methylxanthines** have been used for many years in veterinary medicine as a bronchodilator.

1. **Mechanism of action.** Methylxanthines are phosphodiesterase inhibitors, which induce bronchodilation by blocking the degradation of cAMP by phosphodiesterase in airway smooth muscle cells and inhibition of light chain myosin kinase. The increase of cAMP levels in mast cells inhibits the release of histamine and other autacoids, for example, leukotrienes which may reduce ongoing

bronchoconstriction. The increase of cAMP levels in the chromaffin cells of the adrenal medulla promotes the release of catecholamines which bronchodilate by stimulating noninnervated β_2-receptors in the lung. The other benefits of the methylxanthines are increased mucociliary clearance, improvement in diaphragmatic contractility, decreased pulmonary artery pressure, increased CNS sensitivity to $PaCO_2$, and stabilization of mast cells. In addition, methylxanthines are adenosine receptor antagonists. Adenosine receptors are coupled to $G_{i/o}$ protein, which mediate the decrease in cAMP formation by inhibiting adenylyl cyclase. Thus, adenosine receptor antagonists increase cAMP levels as well. Inhibition of adenosine receptors in the CNS may cause excitation, muscle tremors, and seizures. Increased cAMP levels in the myocardium can induce cardiac arrhythmias and the increased circulating catecholamine levels from the adrenal medulla can make the cardiac side effects worse by stimulating α- and β_1-receptors.

2. **Theophylline**
   a. **Therapeutic uses.** Theophylline is administered orally. It is used primarily to induce bronchodilation for the treatment of obstructive small airway diseases. It is advisable to use only theophylline products that are sustain-released and have suitable pharmacokinetics in animals. It is used often in patients with heart failure and/or pulmonary edema. Theophylline must be used cautiously because of its adverse effects (see below).
   b. **Pharmacokinetics**
      (1) The GI absorption is ~100% after oral administration of a nonsustained-release product. The GI absorption of sustained release products yielded 30–80% bioavailability.
      (2) Theophylline is distributed widely in the body and penetrates the blood–brain barrier. The plasma binding activity of theophylline is low (<14%). Because of low volume of distribution in cats (0.46 L/kg), obese feline patients should be dosed on a lean body weight basis.
      (3) It is metabolized in the liver to 3-methylxanthine and caffeine among other metabolites. 3-methylxanthine has weak bronchodilatory activity.
      (4) Theophylline and its metabolites are excreted via the kidneys; only 10% of a theophylline dose is excreted unchanged in urine.
      (5) The elimination $t_{1/2}$: ~8 hours in cats, ~6 hours in dogs, and 12–17 hours in horses.
   c. **Adverse effects**
      (1) Side effects in dogs and cats include nausea and vomiting, restlessness, increased gastric acid secretion, diarrhea, polyphagia, polydipsia, and polyuria.
      (2) Side effects in horses include nervousness, excitability (auditory, tactile, and visual), tremors, diaphoresis, tachycardia, and ataxia.
   d. Seizures or cardiac arrhythmias may occur in severe cases.
   e. Beware of other drugs that may inhibit hepatic CYP450 enzymes (e.g., cimetidine and fluoroquinolones) because their concurrent administration may elevate plasma levels of theophylline.

E. **Aerosol administration of drugs** is new to veterinary medicine and their efficacy is yet to be documented, although numerous case reports support their use.

1. Optimal particle size for delivery to the trachea is 2–20 microns and to the distal airways is 0.5–5 microns.
2. The benefits of aerosol therapy are that of limiting systemic absorption of the drug and introducing the drug close to the site of the problem.
3. Used primarily to treat chronic obstructive airway disease of horses, lower airway disease in felines, chronic bronchitis in dogs, and kennel cough complex in young dogs.
4. Small animal and equine specific products for administering these agents using a facemask and spacer are commercially available.
5. Bronchodilators, an anticholinergic, corticosteroids, and some antibiotics (e.g., aminoglycosides) are the primary drugs administered by this route.

VI. **Sildenafil decreases pulmonary hypertension**. Pulmonary artery blood pressure may elevate due to an increase in vascular resistance. Pulmonary hypertension has been reported in dogs with many respiratory diseases with *Dirofilaria immitis* infestation being most common. The pathophysiologic reasons for pulmonary vascular hypertrophy and remodeling are not well understood in animals and probably multifactorial. Treatment of the underlying respiratory disease is important when pulmonary hypertension is discovered, but sildenafil, a phosphodiesterase type V inhibitor, has been administered orally to induce vasodilation and reduce pulmonary hypertension in dogs and humans.

A. **Mechanism of action.** Sildenafil decreases pulmonary arterial pressure by inducing potent relaxation of arterial smooth muscle. Cyclic GMP is a potent vascular smooth muscle relaxant; sildenafil increases cyclic GMP levels in vascular smooth muscle cells, which is due to its inhibition of degradation of cyclic GMP by phosphodiesterase V.

B. **Pharmacokinetics**

1. GI absorption after oral administration is nearly complete. T_{max} is ≤ 60 minutes.
2. It is well distributed after GI absorption and 84% of the circulating level is bound by plasma proteins.
3. It is metabolized by CYP450 to many metabolites, which are excreted in the feces.
4. Its elimination $t_{1/2}$ in dogs is ~6 hours.

C. **Adverse effects.** These effects are not well defined in dogs. However, systemic hypotension can occur, particularly if combined with other medications that lower blood pressure (e.g., nitrates).

VII. **Doxapram** hydrochloride is an analeptic and a centrally acting **respiratory stimulant** that also increases the sensitivity of the peripheral chemoreceptors located in the carotid bodies. When injected IV to dogs, the respiratory rate and tidal volume (minute ventilation) increase.

A. Used to aid in the visual evaluation of laryngeal paralysis in the lightly anesthetized dog. The larynx normally abducts on inspiration because of the reflex contraction of laryngeal muscles. Dogs and cats with laryngeal paralysis, however, have reduced or no abduction on inspiration. Evaluation of laryngeal motion requires deep sedation, which unfortunately also reduces laryngeal movement making visual evaluation difficult and frequently incorrect. Injecting doxapram IV while observing the larynx of a deeply sedated dog significantly enhances laryngeal movement but has no effect on the paralyzed larynx making evaluation more reliable.

B. May stimulate respiratory effort in newborn animals but is not a substitute for endotracheal intubation and mechanical ventilation for resuscitation.

VIII. **EXOGENOUS SURFACTANT** can be administered directly into the respiratory tract of foals or calves that are born prematurely and show signs of respiratory distress. Surfactant is normally produced by the alveolar type II cells and is a complex mixture of phospholipids and protein. Surfactant is necessary in the alveoli to reduce the surface tension during inspiration and stabilizes alveoli during the resting phase after expiration. Animals born prematurely may lack surfactant production, and breathing requires an increase in effort and work. One treatment option is to inject exogenous surfactant into the lungs. Several products for human use are derived from animals.

A. Beractant is lipid extract of bovine lung with synthetic lipids.

B. Calfactant is a lipid extract of calf lung lavage fluid.

SUGGESTED READING

Boothe DM. 2001. "Drugs affecting the respiratory system." In *Veterinary Pharmacology and Therapeutics*. Edited by Adams HR. 8th ed., pp. 1105–1119. Ames, IA: Iowa State University Press.

Boothe DM. 2004. "Drugs affecting the respiratory system" In *Textbook of Respiratory Disease in Dogs and Cats*. Edited by King LG. pp. 229–252. St. Louis, MD: Saunders.

http://www.drugs.com

Padrid P. 2006. Use of inhaled medications to treat respiratory diseases in dogs and cats. *J Am Anim Hosp Assoc* 42:165–169.

Plumb DC. 2005. *Veterinary Drug Handbook*. 5th ed. Ames, IA: Blackwell Publishing.

Rozanski EA, Bach JF, Shaw SP. 2007. Advances in respiratory therapy. *Vet Clin North Am Small Anim Pract* 37:963–974.

STUDY QUESTIONS

DIRECTIONS: Each of the numbered items or incomplete statements in this section is followed by answers or by completions of the statement. Select the **one** lettered answer or completion that is **best** in each case.

1. Which one of the following drugs would be efficacious when you wanted to provide emergency bronchodilation in an "asthmatic" cat with few detrimental side effects?

(A) Terbutaline
(B) Fluticasone
(C) Propranolol
(D) Epinephrine
(E) Theophylline

2. Which one of the following drugs is a phosphodiesterase type V inhibitor used in dogs to decrease the pulmonary artery pressure?

(A) Nedocromil sodium
(B) Pirbuterol
(C) Metaproterenol
(D) Sildenafil
(E) *N*-acetylcysteine

3. Which one of the following drugs is an anticholinergic agent, which when administered with a multidose inhaler, spacer, and mask would cause bronchodilation in a horse with chronic obstructive pulmonary disease (i.e., heaves)?

(A) Clenbuterol
(B) Ipratropium
(C) Glycopyrrolate
(D) Triamcinolone
(E) Atropine

4. Which one of the following adrenergic drugs is a nonselective bronchodilator (i.e., $\alpha + \beta + \beta_2$ agonist) compared to the others (which are β_2-selective agonists)?

(A) Isoetharine
(B) Terbutaline
(C) Clenbuterol
(D) Albuterol
(E) Epinephrine

5. Which one of the following describes the mechanism of action of theophylline?

(A) It stimulates the M_3 receptor to induce vasodilatation.
(B) It blocks the release of interleukin-1β and tumor necrosis factor.
(C) It blocks the degradation of cyclic AMP in the smooth muscle cells.
(D) It increases the sensitivity of the peripheral chemoreceptors.

6. Which one of the following drugs would be useful in visually evaluating the laryngeal motion of the deeply sedated dog?

(A) Doxapram
(B) Theophylline
(C) Sildenafil
(D) Zafirlukast

7. Which expectorant, when nebulized and inhaled, breaks the disulfide bonds within the tracheal mucus molecules?

(A) Guaifenesin
(B) *N*-acetylcysteine
(C) Potassium iodide
(D) Saline
(E) Terbutaline

8. Which one of the following drugs will, when injected or sprayed into the ventral meatus of the nose, reduce nasal congestion and edema in a horse that is recovering from anesthesia?

(A) Ipratropium
(B) Terbutaline
(C) Albuterol
(D) Phenylephrine
(E) Fluticasone

9. Which one of the following opioids has a strong antitussive effect but is only a mild analgesic?

(A) Fentanyl
(B) Morphine

(C) Codeine
(D) Hydromorphone
(E) Oxymorphone

10. Which one of the following would be the most beneficial in reducing the work of breathing in a preterm foal that was born without endogenous surfactant being produced and exhibiting respiratory distress?

(A) Doxapram injection IV
(B) Saline nebulization
(C) Terbutaline aerosol
(D) Theophylline orally
(E) Beractant injected into the trachea

■ ANSWERS AND EXPLANATIONS

1. The answer is A.
Terbutaline is a rapid acting β_2-selective adrenergic agonist that produces bronchodilation with few side effects. Additionally, terbutaline allows a choice of route of administration because it is available as an injectable, oral, or aerosol preparation. Fluticasone is a glucocorticoid, which may be beneficial, but it is too slow in onset to be used in an emergency situation. Propranolol is a β-adrenergic blocker and, as such, would cause bronchoconstriction rather than dilation. Epinephrine would rapidly cause bronchodilation but has significant side effects because of its mixed α and β effects, that is, tachycardia or bradycardia, vasoconstriction, hypertension, and cardiac arrhythmias. Epinephrine is used for life-threatening anaphylactic reactions to evoke bronchodilation and vasoconstriction to raise blood pressure. However, when treating an "asthmatic" cat, the side effects of epinephrine are too profound and risky. Theophylline is a methylxanthine bronchodilator, but it is slower in onset and less profound in its dilating effect making terbutaline a better choice.

2. The answer is D.
Sildenafil is an inhibitor of phosphodiesterase type V, which inhibits the degradation of cyclic GMP. Cyclic GMP is a potent vascular smooth muscle relaxant that lowers pulmonary blood pressure. Pirbuterol and metaproterenol are selective β_2-adrenergic agonists used for bronchodilation. Nedocromil sodium is a mast cell stabilizer to prevent the release of inflammatory mediators, including histamine. *N*-acetylcysteine is a mucolytic agent, which when nebulized and inhaled breaks the disulfide bonds of mucus, making it less viscous.

3. The answer is B.
Ipratropium is an anticholinergic agent, when inhaled, would induce bronchodilation in a horse with chronic obstructive pulmonary disease. Clenbuterol is a rapid acting selective β_2-adrenergic agonist that will cause bronchodilation in the horse but by a different mechanism. Glycopyrrolate and atropine are anticholinergic agents like ipratropium, but these drugs are not available as an aerosol in a multidose inhaler. Triamcinolone is available as an aerosol but is a glucocorticoid, not an anticholinergic agent.

4. The answer is E.
Epinephrine is a nonselective adrenergic agonist, which activates both α- and β-receptors. All the others are selective β_2-adrenergic agonists.

5. The answer is C.

Theophylline blocks the degradation of cyclic AMP in the smooth muscle, which leads to bronchodilation. Theophylline may block adenosine receptors to increase cyclic AMP as well. β_2-Adrenergic agonists such as clenbuterol block the release of interleuken-1β and tumor necrosis factor as well as dilating bronchi. Cholinergic agonists stimulate the M_3 receptor on the endothelium to increase nitric oxide synthesis. Nitric oxide penetrates into vascular smooth muscle cells to stimulate guanylyl cyclase to produce cyclic GMP, thereby resulting in vasodilation. Doxapram increases the sensitivity of the peripheral chemoreceptors and increases ventilation of the lungs by increasing the tidal volume and rate of breathing.

6. The answer is A.
Doxapram increases ventilatory effort even when the animal is deeply sedated. When the dog breathes with a larger tidal volume, the normal larynx abducts on inspiration to a greater extent while the paralyzed larynx does not move or may even adduct during inspiration. Theophylline is a bronchodilator that can be injected IV, but does not affect laryngeal motion. Sildenafil is a phosphodiesterase inhibitor used to dilate the pulmonary arterioles and reduces hypertension. Zafirlukast is a leukotriene receptor antagonist used to reduce inflammation in the lung.

7. The answer is B.
N-acetylcysteine, when inhaled, breaks the disulfide bonds within the tracheal mucus molecules. Guaifenesin is an oral expectorant that presumably induces a vagal reflex by contact with the gastric mucosa. Potassium iodide is an oral expectorant that stimulates the respiratory tract glands by reflex to evoke a watery secretion. Saline can be nebulized and inhaled to break up mucus by adding more water. Terbutaline can be aerosolized and inhaled. It acts as a bronchodilator that may allow better removal of mucus by coughing, but it does not affect the chemical nature of the mucus.

8. The answer is D.
Phenylephrine is an α-adrenergic agonist, causing vasoconstriction in the mucosa of the nose to induce decongestion. Terbutaline and albuterol are selective β_2-agonists that would not affect the vasculature of the nasal cavity. Ipratropium is an anticholinergic agent and fluticasone is a glucocorticoid. These drugs will not cause acute vasoconstriction in the nasal cavity, but are used to induce bronchodilation. The onset of glucocorticoid-induced bronchodilation is slow, probably would take a few days to see the effect.

9. The answer is C.
Codeine is a potent antitussive drug and is not used as an analgesic. Morphine, fentanyl, hydromorphone, and oxymorphone are strong analgesics, which stimulate the μ-opioid receptor. (See Chapter 4 for detailed information regarding opioids and their receptors.)

10. The answer is E.
Beractant, a bovine lung extract, is used as an exogenous surfactant. It is injected directly into the trachea and distributed to the bronchi and bronchioles by gravity and positive pressure ventilation. Nebulized saline is not a substitute for surfactant. Bronchodilation from terbutaline or theophylline may be slightly beneficial, but is not a substitute for surfactant. Doxapram will increase ventilatory activity, but without surfactant the lungs will not want to stay inflated.

Chapter 11

Drugs Acting on the Gastrointestinal Tract

Albert E. Jergens and Franklin A. Ahrens

I. GENERAL CONSIDERATIONS

A. **Gastrointestinal (GI) disease** is a common clinical problem where signs of vomiting, diarrhea, and anorexia predominate. Rapid diagnosis is essential for symptomatic or specific therapies to be effective. A complete history and physical examination accompanied by appropriate laboratory tests aid in determining the etiology, location, and severity of the disease or disturbance. Endoscopy and mucosal biopsy are frequently required for diagnosis of chronic GI diseases, such as gastritis, malabsorptive syndromes, or idiopathic inflammatory bowel disease (IBD).

B. **Nonspecific therapy**

1. **Correction of fluid and electrolyte balance.** Persistent vomiting or watery small bowel diarrhea produces dehydration, electrolyte loss, and disturbances in acid–base balance that should be corrected by parenteral fluid therapy. With severe vomiting, there is variable loss of sodium, chloride, potassium, hydrogen, and bicarbonate that may cause metabolic acidosis. If the pylorus is obstructed, duodenal bicarbonate is retained while continued loss of gastric chloride, potassium, and hydrogen in the vomitus leads to metabolic alkalosis. Oral fluid and electrolyte replacement may suffice in animals having only mild acute diarrhea or if vomiting is infrequent or absent.

2. **Resting of the GI tract.** Best practice recommendations suggest that withholding food for 24–48 hours in acute GI disturbances is often effective in dogs and cats. Thereafter, feeding a bland diet often and in small amounts is generally indicated for 3–5 days at which time the original diet is gradually introduced. Potential benefits of dietary restriction include decreased gastric secretions, decreased amounts of osmotically active particles in the gut lumen, and the facilitation of mucosal healing (e.g., enterocyte regeneration).

3. **Dietary modification**

    a. **Bland diet.** A bland, easily digested, low-fat diet such as boiled chicken or white fish or low-fat cottage cheese with rice should be offered after withholding food for 24–48 hours. Limiting dietary fat is important because unabsorbed fatty acids are hydroxylated by colonic bacteria into secretagogues which decrease mucosal absorption and promote increased fecal water loss.

    b. **Lactose-free diet.** Milk products should be eliminated from the diet if there is lactose intolerance or a loss of mucosal brush border lactase from GI disturbances.

    c. **Insoluble fiber.** Increased fiber absorbs water and normalizes intestinal transit in constipation and animals with colitis of diverse causes.

    d. **Gluten-free diet.** Gluten-sensitive enteropathy has been reported to occur in Irish setter dogs. Clinical improvement is observed when affected animals are placed on a cereal-free diet.

4. **Provision of nutritional support.** Calories, proteins, and vitamins should be supplied to maintain a positive energy and protein balance. Enteral feeding is preferred over parenteral routes since this is most physiologic and prevents atrophy of the intestinal tract. Initial nutrient deficiencies are gauged by use of body condition scores (BCS), and specific nutrient requirements may be estimated by a variety of methods.

5. **Symptomatic therapies**

    a. **Protectants and adsorbents.** Bismuth-subsalicylate and kaolin-pectin are often administered in acute diarrhea to coat and protect the intestinal mucosa, and because they may reduce intestinal secretions. See more below.

TABLE 11-1. Indications for Antibiotic Use in Gastrointestinal Diseases

Severe Mucosal Injury
- Parvovirus
- hemorrhagic gastroenteritis
- Salmon poisoning disease

Enteropathogenic Bacteria
- *Salmonella, Clostridia*
- *Campylobacter jejuni, E. coli*
- Cocci villus adherence

Antibiotic-responsive diarrhea (± small intestinal bacterial overgrowth)
Inflammatory Bowel Disease

Note: Antibiotics are uncommonly required in most cases of acute or chronic gastroenteritis. Their specific use is indicated in patients with severe mucosal disruption as evidenced by bloody diarrhea, and in animals diagnosed with specific enteropathogenic bacterial infections or other conditions. Indiscriminate use encourages antibiotic drug resistance and may prolong some types of infectious diarrhea (e.g., salmonellosis).

b. **Motility modifying drugs**. Opiates and opioids (loperamide, diphenoxylate) are used to decrease intestinal motility and secretions associated with acute diarrhea. Anticholinergics should be avoided since they can potentiate ileus. See more below.

c. **Antimicrobial therapy**. The routine use of antibiotics for treatment of acute or chronic GI disease is not recommended. Animals having severe mucosal injury (parvoviral enteritis) or infection with specific bacterial pathogens (*Campylobacter jejuni*) of the GI tract should receive antibiotics. Indiscriminate use of antimicrobials promotes bacterial drug resistance (Table 11-1).

d. **Probiotics**. These are live bacterial cultures, which promote beneficial microbial health to the host. The mechanism(s) of action are not fully known and their effects appear to be exquisitely host-specific. Preliminary clinical data supports their use as adjunctive therapy for both acute and chronic diarrhea (see below).

e. **Analgesics**. Indications include alleviation of visceral pain in animals having diverse causes for GI disease (equine colic, pancreatitis in companion animals). **Severe** visceral pain is alleviated by morphine or opioid receptor agonists that inhibit nociceptive reflexes at spinal and supraspinal sites within the CNS.

(1) **Opiates** (see Chapter 4 for more information)
   (a) **Morphine** is used in dogs and cats, IM. Its duration of action is 6 hours in these species. High doses of morphine produce excitement in cats and horses and it is administered at 1/10 of the dose used in dogs (0.05–0.2 mg/kg in cats and horses; 0.5–2 mg/kg in dogs).
   (b) **Butorphanol** is administered IV to horses for the control of colic pain. Butorphanol is a partial agonist for μ-receptors and a full agonist for κ-receptors. Its duration of action is 1–2 hours.

(2) **Nonsteroidal anti-inflammatory drugs (NSAIDs)**. (see Chapter 7 for more information) Flunixin meglumine, or phenylbutazone are given IM or IV to horses for the control of colic pain. They inhibit prostaglandin synthesis by inhibiting the enzyme cyclooxygenase. Duration of action is 1–8 hours, depending on the cause and severity of pain.

(3) **Sedatives**. Xylazine, detomidine, medetomidine, and romifidine are α_2-adrenoreceptor agonists, which produce sedation and analgesia in equine colic. Their duration of action is 1–4 hours following IV or IM administration. (see Chapter 4 for more information).

(4) **Spasmolytics**. *N*-butylscopolammonium bromide (Buscopan®) is an antispasmodic and anticholinergic drug used in horses for control of the abdominal pain of colic.

(a) **Mechanism of action.** Bucospan® competitively inhibits parasympathetic activation of muscarinic receptors on intestinal smooth muscle cells.

(b) **Therapeutic uses.** Bucospan® is administered IV to horses at a dose of 0.3 mg/kg for control of abdominal pain in colic and simple impactions.

(c) **Pharmacokinetics.** The plasma $t_{1/2}$ of Bucospan® is 6 hours. It is eliminated equally via urine and feces.

(d) **Adverse effects.** Transient tachycardia and decreased borborygmal sounds may be present for 30 minutes following administration. Bucospan® should not be used in impaction colics associated with ileus or in horses with glaucoma.

II. APPETITE STIMULANTS

A. **Inappetence or anorexia** is common with GI disease. Insufficient nutrient intake delays clinical recovery and may exacerbate the underlying disease. Note that the use of these drugs should be restricted to animals where nutritional intake is measured because of the inconsistent response to their use. Efficacy studies based on controlled clinical trials for use of any of the appetite stimulants is lacking. Enteral alimentation with liquid supplements is quite practical and very useful in small animals.

B. **Palatable food.** Small amounts of palatable food should be offered at frequent intervals. Warming the food may enhance appetite in carnivores. In general, commercial-derived and nutritionally complete diets should be fed. Homemade diets are quite appropriate for short-term use where the risk of specific deficiencies is minimized by the brief duration of feeding.

C. **Benzodiazepines (see Chapter 4 for more information)**

1. **Mechanism of action.** Benzodiazepines may suppress the satiety center in the hypothalamus via increased γ-aminobutyric acid (GABA) activity.

2. **Therapeutic uses.** Diazepam or oxazepam is used primarily in cats for short-term stimulation of appetite, although the effect is controversial. They are used less frequently in horses, dogs, and goats. Their effectiveness decreases after 2–3 treatments.

3. **Administration**
   a. **Diazepam** is administered orally, IV (0.2 mg/kg), or IM once or twice a day.
   b. **Oxazepam** is administered orally once a day at 2.5 mg/kg in cats.

4. **Adverse effects**
   a. **Sedation and ataxia** are common and may be severe in weak or debilitated animals. Reduced dosage should be employed in these cases. Use cautiously in patients with preexisting renal or hepatic disease.

D. **Cyproheptadine (see Chapter 3 for more information)**

1. **Mechanism of action.** Cyproheptadine is a serotonin antagonist which suppresses the satiety center in the hypothalamus. It is also a histamine-1 (H_1) antagonist and is used as an antiasthmatic in humans.

2. **Therapeutic uses.** Cyproheptadine stimulates appetite in cats and in humans but not in dogs. It has been used experimentally in cats as an appetite stimulant.

3. **Adverse effects.** Sedation and dryness of mucous membranes are the most common side effects. Paradoxically, CNS excitement and marked aggressive behavior may occur in 20% of the cats given cyproheptadine.

E. **Glucocorticoids**

1. Glucocorticoids are frequently employed as appetite stimulants in sick or debilitated animals.

2. **Mechanism of action.** The mechanism by which glucocorticoids stimulate appetite is unknown. It may be due to euphoria—the increased feeling of well-being produced by glucocorticoids. This is, in part, a result of their anti-inflammatory action.
3. **Therapeutic uses.** Glucocorticoids are used as nonspecific, short-term therapy for appetite stimulation.
4. **Administration**
   a. **Small animals.** Prednisolone or prednisone is given once every other day.
   b. **Large animals.** Prednisolone or dexamethasone is given IM once a day.
5. **Adverse effects**
   a. Glucocorticoids are immunosuppressive and may delay recovery from the underlying disease.
   b. Decreased gastric mucus production occurs following glucocorticoid administration. Gastric ulcers may develop with high dose or long-term use or in animals where preexisting gastric mucosal disease is present.

III. ANTIOBESITY DRUGS

A. **General considerations.** Obesity is an important medical condition with serious health implications. Obesity is characterized by the excessive accumulation and storage of fat in the body. Obesity can be defined as exceeding ideal body weight by 20% or more, or BCS of 8 or greater on a 9-point scale. Approximately 20–40% of dogs are considered overweight or obese. The most common cause for obesity is the overconsumption of food combined with inadequate exercise.

B. **Dirlotapide (Slentrol®)**

1. **Mechanism of action.** Dirlotapide is a selective microsomal triglyceride transfer protein (MTP) inhibitor that blocks the assembly and release of lipoprotein particles into the bloodstream (via the lymphatic system) in dogs. Its unique mechanism of action provides for potential weight loss by reducing appetite (which accounts for 90% of its clinical efficacy) and by decreasing fat absorption (accounting for about 10% of dirlotapide's activity).
2. **Therapeutic uses.** To reduce the obesity in dogs that has been associated with increased risk for development of musculoskeletal disease, hypertension, peripheral insulin antagonism, osteoarthritis, and cardiopulmonary diseases.
3. **Pharmacokinetics.** Dirlotapide acts locally in the gut to reduce appetite, increase fecal fat, and produce weight loss. Following oral administration, the mean serum $t_{1/2}$ is 2.8 hours with bioavailability ranging from 20–40%. There is no clinical effect following IV administration. The variable response between animals and decreasing response over time requires that the dose be regularly and individually titrated to effect. The drug undergoes enterohepatic circulation and is primarily excreted in the feces, with small amounts excreted in the bile and urine.
4. **Administration.** Dirlotapide is administered once daily as an oil-based solution formulated at a concentration of 5 mg/mL.
5. **Adverse effects.** The most commonly reported adverse effects include vomiting, diarrhea, anorexia, and lethargy.

IV. DRUGS THAT REDUCE ACID SECRETION AND PROVIDE MUCOSA PROTECTION

A. **General considerations.** Inhibitors of acid secretion and mucosal protectants are used in veterinary medicine to reduce the hydrochloric acid (HCl) content of the stomach and to promote mucosal healing in animals with ulcers and erosions. The parietal cell possesses receptors for histamine, gastrin, and acetylcholine (ACh)—each of which

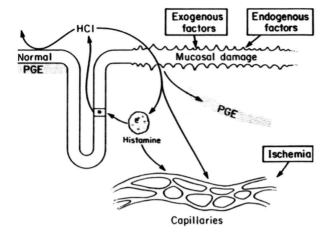

FIGURE 11-1. Overview of the etiopathogenesis of gastric ulceration. A common mechanism of H^+ back diffusion may occur as a consequence of either endogenous (infiltrative mucosal disease, renal or hepatic disease) or exogenous (NSAID use) disorders. Hydrogen ions present within mucosal tissues promote local vasculitis which causes ischemia and subsequent gastric mucosal disruption.

stimulates H^+ secretion into the lumen by the H^+/K^+-ATPase pump located on the apical membrane. Disease conditions which disrupt the gastric mucosal barrier can lead to endoscopic lesions and clinical signs of GI ulceration or erosion. The fundamental lesion in these instances is the presence of an impaired mucosal barrier which permits the back diffusion of hydrogen ions which causes mucosal ischemia and subsequent damage (Figure 11-1).

B. **Gastric secretory inhibitors**

1. H_2-antihistamines (see Chapter 3 for more information)

a. **Mechanism of action.** H_2-antihistamines inactivate H_2-receptors of parietal cells. Histamine-evoked gastric secretions are decreased; some (e.g., ranitidine) also have prokinetic activity mediated by their anticholinesterase activity. Ranitidine or famotidine are first-choice agents since they are safe, effective, and have less hepatic inhibition of microsomal metabolizing enzymes than cimetidine. Ranitidine is 3–13 times more potent as cimetidine. Famotidine has greater gastric inhibitory properties and can be given once daily.

b. **Therapeutic uses**

(1) Ranitidine and famotidine are used to treat gastritis, gastric ulcer/erosions, reflux esophagitis, and gastrinomas (rare) in dogs and cats. Gastric HCl secretion is intermittent in carnivores rather than continuous as in humans; therefore, lower doses are effective. These drugs are also used to treat gastritis and gastric erosions in horses and foals.

(2) H_2-antihistamines are used to prevent acid hydrolysis of replacement pancreatic enzymes in exocrine pancreatic disease in dogs and cats.

(3) Cimetidine or ranitidine are used to treat gastritis and gastric erosions in horses and foals.

(4) **Ranitidine also stimulates gastric and colonic motility by inhibiting acetylcholinesterase activity.** See Section V for additional information

c. **Pharmacokinetics.** Ranitidine and famotidine are well absorbed orally and widely distributed in body tissues. Only 10–20% of drug is bound to plasma proteins. The plasma $t_{1/2}$ is 2–3 hours for ranitidine. Approximately $1/4$ to $1/2$ of the drug is metabolized by the liver. Metabolites and the parent drug are excreted by the kidneys.

d. **Administration**

(1) **Ranitidine** is administered orally, IM, or IV every 12 hours.

(2) **Famotidine** is administered orally or IV once daily.

(3) Ranitidine may stimulate gastric and colonic motility via its prokinetic activity.

e. **Adverse effects.** Side effects are rare in animals at usual dosages. Use ranitidine cautiously in animals with impaired renal function. Liver enzyme alanine

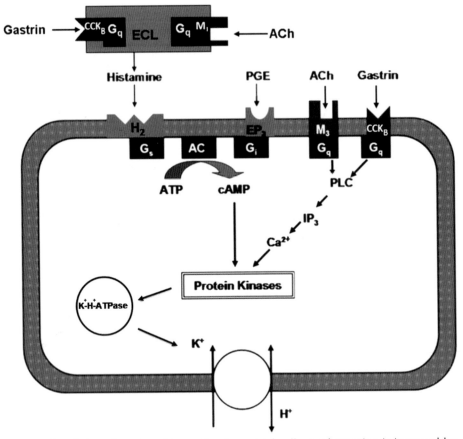

FIGURE 11-2. Regulation of gastric acid secretion in parietal cells. Acid secretion is increased by acetylcholine (ACh) and gastrin, which is mediated by M_3-receptors and cholecystokinin B (CCK_B) receptors, respectively. Stimulation of both receptors increases cytosolic Ca^{2+} levels. Histamine, released from enterochromaffin-like (ECL) cells, increases acid secretion by activating H_2-receptors, which increases cyclic AMP (cAMP) formation. Prostaglandin E decreases acid secretion by activating EP_3 receptors, which inhibits cAMP formation. Ca^{2+} and cAMP activate protein kinases, which translocate H^+, K^+-ATPase to the apical membrane of the cell to pump H^+ into lumen. Also, gastrin and ACh stimulate histamine release from ECL cells by activating CCK_B and M_1-receptors. AC, adenylyl cyclase; PLC, phospholipase C.

aminotransferase (ALT) concentrations should be occasionally monitored in animals receiving ranitidine in high doses for greater than 7 days. Some GI effects (anorexia, vomiting, and diarrhea) noted with famotidine. Famotidine has been associated with intravascular hemolysis when given IV to cats.

2. **Proton pump inhibitors**
   a. **Mechanism of action** (Figure 11-2). Acid pump inhibitors inhibit the H^+/K^+-ATPase on the luminal (secretory) membrane of parietal cells and thus reduce H^+ secretion. Binding to the enzyme is irreversible and restoration of acid secretion requires de novo synthesis of ATPase by the parietal cell. Omeprazole is the protypical agent.
   b. **Therapeutic uses.** Omeprazole is used in the treatment of gastritis, ulcer disease, and esophagitis in dogs, cats, and horses. It is also used in the prevention and treatment of NSAID-induced gastric erosions.
   c. **Pharmacokinetics.** Omeprazole is absorbed orally and enters gastric parietal cells where it is protonated and trapped in the acidic intracellular fluid. The protonated drug is the active form and thus ATPase in nonacid-producing cells is not affected. Since the drug slowly accumulates in parietal cells with repeated

doses, pharmacologic action is not correlated with plasma $t_{1/2}$. Omeprazole is metabolized by hepatic microsomal enzymes and excreted by the kidney.

d. Administration. Omeprazole is administered orally once a day.

e. Adverse effects. Omeprazole, like cimetidine, inhibits hepatic microsomal (cytochrome P-450) metabolism and may prolong the action of concurrently administered drugs that are metabolized by this system (phase 1 reactions) such as phenytoin or phenobarbital. Use cautiously in animals with preexisting hepatopathy.

C. **Mucosal cytoprotectants**

1. **Pharmacologic protection of the gastric mucosa** can be enhanced by administration of a prostaglandin E_1 analog (Misoprostol) or by promoting direct cytoprotection of denuded mucosa (sucralfate).

2. **Misoprostol**

   a. Mechanism of action. Misoprostol has two functions that make it a useful protective agent. It directly inhibits gastric acid secretion by parietal cells and it facilitates PGE-mediated mucosal defenses and healing in response to acid-related injuries.

   b. Therapeutic uses. Misoprostol is used to treat gastric ulceration when caused or aggravated by NSAIDs drugs.

   c. Pharmacokinetics. Approximately 90% of the drug is readily absorbed from the GI tract where a significant amount is metabolized via a first-pass hepatic effect. The presence of food and antacids will delay drug absorption. Metabolites and small amounts of parent drug are excreted in urine. The duration of action is 3–6 hours.

   d. Administration. Misoprostol is given orally three times daily.

   e. Adverse effects. Adverse GI signs include diarrhea, vomiting, and abdominal pain. It should not be given to pregnant animals as it will promote uterine contractions.

3. **Sucralfate**

   a. Mechanism of action. Sucralfate is a sucrose sulfate-aluminum hydroxide complex which polymerizes to a viscous gel at pH < 4 and coats ulcer craters. Sulfate groups bind to proteins in ulcerated tissue and protect ulcers from acid and pepsin.

   b. Therapeutic uses. Sucralfate provides locally acting treatment for GI ulceration. It also provides cytoprotection when used as a slurry in animals having mucosal disruption of the esophagus (esophagitis).

   c. Pharmacokinetics. Only 3–5% of an oral dose of sucralfate is absorbed where it is then excreted in the urine unchanged. The remainder of the drug is converted into sucrose sulfate in the gut by reacting with HCl. The duration of action persists for up to 6 hours after oral dosing.

   d. Route of administration. Sucralfate is given orally 2–3 times daily depending on the severity of mucosal disruption.

   e. Adverse effects. Sucralfate may impair absorption of other oral medications so it is advised to stagger administration with other drugs by 2 hours or more.

V. **PROKINETIC DRUGS**

A. **General considerations.** GI motility disorders result from diseases that, either directly or indirectly, alter normal GI functions (e.g., storage of ingesta, mixing and dispersion of food, and timely propulsion of luminal contents aborally). Briefly, the causes for GI transit disorders are diverse but include both structural (mechanical obstruction) and functional (defective propulsion associated with mucosal inflammation) diseases. Prokinetic drugs act to increase GI motility by stimulating smooth muscle contractions.

B. **Specific drugs**

1. **Cisapride**
   a. **Mechanism of action.** Cisapride enhances the release of acetylcholine at the myenteric plexus, but does not induce nicotinic or muscarinic receptor stimulation. Cisapride blocks dopaminergic receptors to a lesser extent than does metoclopramide. This drug is no longer commercially available and must be obtained from a compounding pharmacy.
   b. **Therapeutic uses.** Cisapride stimulates GI motility from the lower esophageal sphincter (LES) to the descending colon. Proposed uses for cisapride in small animals include gastric/intestinal stasis, reflux esophagitis, and constipation/megacolon in cats.
   c. **Pharmacokinetics.** Information only in humans is available: Cisapride is rapidly absorbed following oral administration with an absolute bioavailability of 35–40%. The drug is highly bound to plasma proteins and is extensively distributed throughout the body. Its elimination $t_{1/2}$ is 8–10 hours.
   d. **Administration.** The drug is administered orally at a range of 0.1–0.5 mg/kg PO q8 hours.
   e. **Adverse effects.** The adverse effect profile is ongoing but the primary adverse effects are GI in origin, including diarrhea and abdominal pain.

2. **Metoclopramide**
   a. Metoclopramide stimulates motility of the proximal GI tract, especially the LES and stomach. See Section IX for more detailed information.
   b. Metoclopramide exerts its effects through antagonism of dopaminergic D_2 receptors and agonism of serotonergic $5\text{-}HT_4$ receptors.
   c. Clinically useful in cases of reflux esophagitis and gastric stasis or hypomotility.

3. **Ranitidine**
   a. In addition to its antisecretory activity, ranitidine stimulates GI motility by inhibiting acetylcholinesterase activity. See gastric antisecretory drugs for more detailed information.
   b. As a parasympathetic potentiating agent, ranitidine stimulates gastric emptying and small intestinal and colonic motility. Its actions appear to be greatest in stimulating gastric motility.

4. **Erythromycin**
   a. The effect of erythromycin on GI motility most closely mimics that of the GI hormone, motilin. It stimulates motility by means of direct motilin-receptor activation (cats) and indirect cholinergic and neurokinin activation (in dogs).
   b. Sub-antimicrobial doses (0.5–1.0 mg/kg) are orally administered to induce prokinetic activity in dogs and cats. GI motility is stimulated most robustly in the proximal GI tract.
   c. Erythromycin is used clinically to increase gastric emptying and for the therapy of reflux esophagitis.

VI. DIGESTANTS

A. **Pancrelipase (Pancreatin)**

1. **Pancrelipase** consists of pancreatic enzymes, including lipase, amylase, and protease, and is derived from porcine pancreas.
2. **Pancrelipase** powder preparations are mixed with food to treat exocrine pancreatic insufficiency in dogs and cats.
3. Enteric coated tablets have limited efficacy and are not recommended because of delayed gastric emptying of these preparations.
4. The maintenance dosage for the powdered preparation is 1 tsp/meal for dogs that weigh 20–30 kg.

An overview of hepatic therapeutic considerations

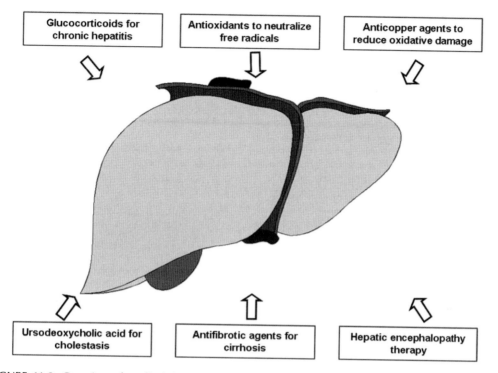

| Glucocorticoids for chronic hepatitis | Antioxidants to neutralize free radicals | Anticopper agents to reduce oxidative damage |

| Ursodeoxycholic acid for cholestasis | Antifibrotic agents for cirrhosis | Hepatic encephalopathy therapy |

FIGURE 11-3. Overview of medical therapy for canine and feline hepatopathy. Therapy may be symptomatic and/or specific as dictated by the histopathologic findings obtained through the performance of hepatic biopsy. Note that both dietary and pharmacotherapy are utilized in dogs and cats to reduce hepatic workload, to treat signs of hepatic encephalopathy, and to facilitate repair of injured liver parenchyma.

VII. DRUGS USED FOR TREATMENT OF LIVER DISEASES

A. **General considerations.** A variety of diverse and clinically useful medications are used to treat dogs and cats with liver diseases. Unfortunately, few controlled clinical trials exist that provide critical evaluation of their effectiveness. Drug therapy is one important arm in treating hepatobiliary diseases along with dietary therapy. Symptomatic and specific therapies for liver disease are diverse but generally include both dietary and pharmacotherapy to induce patient remission (Figure 11-3).

B. **Glucocorticoids (Prednisone and Prednisolone) (see Chapter 12 for more information)**

1. Steroid therapy is the most commonly used therapy for chronic hepatitis in dogs. Prednisone must be metabolized into prednisolone by the liver so it is best to use prednisolone in case of liver disease.
2. Prednisolone is the treatment of first choice for idiopathic chronic hepatitis.
3. Corticosteroids have anti-inflammatory effects but also antifibrotic and choleretic effects. Their principle indication is immunomodulation.
4. Glucocorticoids are contraindicated for infectious diseases of the liver and biliary system.

C. Ursodeoxycholic acid

1. Ursodeoxycholic acid (UDCA), ursodiol, is one of the natural bile acids in the enterohepatic circulation. Ursodiol is an oral medication administered to dogs and cats at a dosage of 15 mg/kg once daily.
2. UCDA has multiple drug actions including protection of hepatic cells from apoptosis, choleresis (induction of bile flow), suppression of hepatic synthesis and secretion of cholesterol, modulation of the immune system to reduce inflammation, and increasing the production of glutathione and metallothionein, which prevent oxidative damage.
3. Although generally well tolerated, UCDA is contraindicated in patients having extrahepatic biliary obstruction.

D. Antioxidants

1. Oxidative stress and damage caused by free oxygen radicals may be a primary or contributory cause of liver disease.
2. The normal host cellular defense mechanisms against oxidative damage include superoxide dismutase (SOD), catalase, and glutathione (GSH) peroxidase.
3. The main antioxidants are vitamins C and E, silymarin, and S-adenosyl-L-methionine (SAMe).
4. SAMe is a normal metabolite in the hepatocytes and is important in the defense against free radicals. Commercially, SAMe is available as a "nutraceutical" and is used as an adjunctive treatment for liver diseases in dogs and cats. Dosage varies as per species and by body weight but it is given once daily.
5. Silymarin (silibinin) is the active component extracted from the fruit of milk thistle. It has several pharmacological actions that may be useful in treating liver disease. It inhibits lipid peroxidase and beta glucuronidase and the cytotoxic actions of tumor necrosis factor (TNF). It is a strong free radical scavenger by induction of cellular SOD and may increase hepatic glutathione content and decrease hepatic collagen formation.

E. Antifibrotic drugs

1. Fibrosis may follow a variety of chronic liver insults and result in cirrhosis and incapacity of the liver to regenerate.
2. Increased lipid peroxidation of hepatocytes (e.g., hepatocellular damage) activates the mesenchymal hepatic stellate cells to produce fibrinogenic substances and extracellular collagen matrix.
3. Colchicine is the only drug used specifically to stop and reduce fibrosis. It is thought to act via stimulation of collagenase activity. Use of this drug is not strongly advocated since clinical studies have not been performed which prove its efficacy.

F. Anticopper medications

1. Chronic copper accumulation may cause oxidative damage to the liver because of the increased intracellular copper concentrations.
2. Hereditary copper toxicosis occurs in Bedlington terriers, and copper accumulation may also occur secondary to diseases in which cholestasis is a prominent feature.
3. Chelating drugs, such as D-penicillamine, can actively bind free extracellular copper and facilitate its excretion in the urine. D-penicillamine is administered orally twice daily with meals.
4. Chelators bind free copper actively and are an effective way to quickly remove increased intracellular copper that causes hepatic damage.
5. Zinc gluconate or acetate is another anti-copper medication for oral use (10 mg elemental zinc/kg twice daily). In the intestinal tract, zinc induces metallothioneine in the enterocytes. This protein binds copper which prevents its absorption, and it is sequestered within senescent enterocytes and shed into the intestinal lumen.

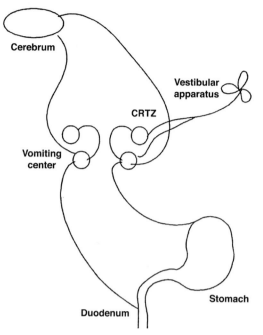

FIGURE 11-4. Simplified schematic showing major input pathways into the vomiting center. While central (CNS disease) and vestibular (motion sickness, vestibular disease) causes for vomiting occur in dogs and cats, they are relatively uncommon. More common causes for vomiting include the stimulation of the CRTZ via blood-borne toxins (uremia, hyperbilirubinemia) or drugs (digitalis, chemotherapy), and abdominal parenchymal disorders that promote irritation, distension, or inflammation of these organs.

G. Drugs to treat hepatic encephalopathy

1. Hepatic encephalopathy (HE) may occur as a consequence of both congenital and acquired hepatic diseases. Ammonia and aromatic amino acids are the two main factors contributing to HE.
2. Portosystemic encephalopathy is the most common cause and is treated with both dietary modification (reduced protein intake of aromatic amino acids) and pharmacologic agents.
3. Lactulose and soluble fibers will reduce ammonia metabolism, and thereby reduce clinical signs. These agents are metabolized by the colonic bacterial flora to produce acids that reduce the pH of the colonic contents. Ammonia is then present in the ionic form that is not absorbed and thus is excreted in the feces.
4. Lactulose is a disaccharide molecule that is metabolized by the resident flora into many osmotically active particles that attract water into the feces. The best guideline for use of lactulose in the management of HE is to give just enough (twice daily) to produce a soft stool.
5. Metronidazole is an antibiotic used as adjuvant therapy in HE. Metronidazole has efficacy against most obligate anaerobes, some of which are urease-producers, which may contribute to ammonia production and exacerbation of HE. Metronidazole is administered orally at 10–20 mg/kg twice daily in dogs and cats.

VIII. EMETICS

A. General considerations

1. The vomiting center in the medulla is activated by vagal and sympathetic afferents from the GI tract, dopaminergic input from the chemoreceptor trigger zone (CRTZ), and cholinergic and histaminergic afferents from the vestibular apparatus (Figure 11-4).
2. The vomiting reflex is developed in carnivores, primates, and swine. Horses, ruminants, rodents, rabbits, and guinea pigs do not possess this protective reflex.

3. Emetics may be used in conscious dogs and cats for elimination of noncorrosive poisons or prior to induction of general anesthesia to minimize gastroesophageal reflux.
4. Emetics generally remove less than 80% of stomach contents.

B. Central acting emetics

1. **Apomorphine HCl**
   a. Apomorphine is a synthetic derivative of morphine which stimulates dopaminergic receptors in the CRTZ to induce vomiting in dogs. It is administered parenterally because oral absorption is slow. It is conjugated in the liver and excreted in urine.
   b. IV administration of a low dose is the preferred route. Onset of vomiting occurs in 1 minute, with a duration of 3–5 minutes. Apomorphine is also effective IM, SQ, or via conjunctival drops. Apomorphine administration should not be repeated because the vomiting center is depressed after the initial CRTZ stimulation.
   c. Apomorphine produces excitement in cats and is not effective in swine.
2. **Xylazine (see Chapter 4 for more information)**
   a. Xylazine is an α_2-adrenoreceptor agonist, which induces vomiting in cats following IV or IM administration.
   b. Onset of vomiting occurs in 2–5 minutes and may be followed by mild sedation for 30–90 minutes.

C. Peripheral acting emetics. Peripheral acting emetics stimulate sympathetic and vagal afferent receptors in pharynx and stomach to induce vomiting. They may be useful as household emetics if the owner has observed ingestion of poison by a pet. They are administered orally as a *single* dose that should not be repeated even if vomiting fails to occur.
   a. **Sodium chloride** is administered as crystals of table salt (1 tsp into pharynx). It is the most effective household emetic in dogs.
   b. **Syrup of Ipecac** contains emetine alkaloid and is the recommended household emetic for children. It is less reliable in dogs and cats but may induce vomiting in 15–30 minutes.
   c. **Copper sulfate** (1%), **zinc sulfate** (1%), or **hydrogen peroxide** (3%) solutions may produce emesis but the response is variable and they are seldomly used now.

IX. ANTIEMETICS

A. General considerations

1. General causes for vomiting include the following:
   a. Stimulation of the vomiting center via vagal and sympathetic afferents from the GI tract in response to irritation, distension, or inflammation. Common clinical examples would include vomiting associated with enteritis, pancreatitis, or intestinal foreign body.
   b. Stimulation of the vomiting center via vestibular afferents from the eighth cranial nerve in response to labyrinthine disease or motion sickness. This is an uncommon cause for vomiting but it might be seen in animals with motion sickness or vestibular diseases.
   c. Stimulation of the vomiting center via inflammation, edema, or tumors of the CNS.
   d. Stimulation of the CRTZ by drugs, bacterial endotoxins, or toxic endogenous metabolites such as urea or bilirubin.
2. Prolonged vomiting may lead to electrolyte and acid-base imbalances and dehydration. Diagnosis and treatment of the primary cause should precede administration of antiemetic drugs.

3. Specific indications for use of antiemetic agents include (1) animals with persistent vomiting in which fluid and electroloyte balance cannot be maintained and (2) abolishing the vomiting "cycle" such that animals can get sufficient rest to recover from their illness.

4. Indiscriminate use of antiemetics in vomiting animals is *not* recommended since this may mask the presence of more serious disease.

B. **Antidopaminergic agents**

1. **Phenothiazines (see Chapter 4 for more information)**
   a. **Mechanism of action.** The phenothiazine tranquilizers exert their antiemetic action by blockade of dopamine (D_2)-receptors in the CRTZ and, at higher doses, the vomiting center. Although they are broad-spectrum antiemetics, they tend to be less effective in vomiting arising from severe inflammation of the GI tract or the inner ear. Blockade of α-adrenoreceptors occurs in addition to dopamine receptor blockade. Phenothiazines also have weak anticholinergic and antihistaminic actions.
   b. **Pharmacokinetics.** Phenothiazines are well absorbed orally although there is significant first-pass metabolism. Distribution is wide. The drugs are metabolized by the liver primarily to glucuronide or sulfate conjugates and excreted by the kidney.
   c. **Administration.** Acepromazine, chlorpromazine, promazine, or prochlorperazine are administered orally or IM every 6 hours to prevent vomiting in dogs and cats.
   d. **Adverse effects.** Hypotension and bradycardia due to α-adrenergic blockade are the most serious side effects of the phenothiazines and are more likely to occur in dehydrated animals. Hypotensive reactions should be treated with α-adrenergic agonists such as phenylephrine. Epinephrine should not be used because of the possibility of epinephrine reversal. Sedation may occur but is usually mild at the doses used for antiemesis.

2. **Metoclopramide**
   a. **Mechanism of action.** Metoclopramide has both central and peripheral antiemetic actions. Its central action is due to blockade of dopamine receptors in the CRTZ and, at higher doses, inhibition of serotonin receptors in the CRTZ. Its peripheral action is due to stimulation of the motility of the stomach and duodenum via increased smooth muscle sensitivity to acetylcholine. This prevents the gastric atony required for the vomiting reflex and ejection of gastric contents.
   b. **Pharmacokinetics.** Oral absorption is rapid with peak plasma levels within two hours. The bioavailability of oral doses is 50–70% due to first pass metabolism. Distribution is wide and includes the CNS. Unchanged drug (25%) and conjugated metabolites (75%) are excreted in the urine. The plasma $t_{1/2}$ is 90 minutes in the dog.
   c. **Administration**. Metoclopramide (Reglan®) is given orally, SC, or IM every 8 hours or by constant rate IV infusion to control severe vomiting in dogs and cats. It is also administered 30 minutes prior to feeding in the treatment of disorders of gastric motility and esophageal reflux in dogs, cats, and foals.
   d. **Adverse effects**. Metoclopramide is contraindicated in animals with gastric outlet obstruction since stimulation of gastric motility may predispose to hemorrhage or perforation. Behavioral changes including excitement or disorientation may be observed in dogs and cats, although the incidence is low.

3. **Butyrophenones**
   a. Droperidol and haloperidol are neuroleptic drugs which are also central-acting antiemetics. They act by blockade of dopaminergic neurons in the CRTZ via their affinity for D_2-receptors. Pharmacokinetic data for animals is lacking. The elimination $t_{1/2}$ in humans is 20–40 hours. They thus have a long duration of action—2–4 days.
   b. Their clinical use in veterinary medicine has been limited but they may be useful in vomiting associated with cancer chemotherapy.

    c. Administration. The butyrophenones are given orally or IM every 2–4 days.
    d. Adverse effects. Butyrophenones may produce mild sedation and tranquilization.

C. **Antihistaminic agents (see Chapter 3 for more information)**

    1. **Mechanism of action.** Antihistaminic agents block histaminergic and cholinergic afferents from the vestibular organs to the vomiting center. They are useful in the prevention of motion sickness in dogs.
    2. **Pharmacokinetics.** Antihistamines are well absorbed orally. Their physiological disposition has not been studied in animals.
    3. **Administration.** Dimenhydrinate, diphenhydramine, or promethazine are administered orally every 8 hours.
    4. **Adverse effects.** Sedation may be observed as a side effect but is much less prominent in animals than in humans.

D. **Anticholinergic agents**

    1. **Mechanism of action.** Anticholinergic drugs block cholinergic afferents from the GI tract to the vomiting center. Although they are generally less active than other antiemetics when used alone, they may be effective when combined with phenothiazines in the control of emesis arising from severe gastroenteritis. An example of this combination is isopropamide + prochlorperazine = Darbazine.® Note that controlled clinical studies attesting to the clinical efficacy of this product have not been performed.
    2. **Administration.** Aminopentamide, propantheline, or isopropamide are administered orally, IM, or SC every 8–12 hours for the symptomatic control of vomiting and diarrhea in dogs and cats.
    3. **Pharmacokinetics. Pharmacokinetics of propantheline are stated in Chapter 2 VI C. Pharmacokinetics of aminopentamide and isopropamide are not available for animals.**
    4. **Adverse effects.** Anticholinergics are contraindicated in patients with glaucoma. Dryness of the mouth (xerostomia) and/or eyes (xerophthalmia), tachycardia, and constipation may occur.

E. **Antiserotonergic agents ondansetron and dolasetron**

    1. **Mechanism of action.** Ondansetron and dolasetron specifically inhibit serotonin type 3 ($5\text{-}HT_3$) receptors located peripherally on vagal nerve terminals and centrally in the CRTZ. Inhibition of $5\text{-}HT_3$ receptors blocks neurotransmission by closing sodium channels. Antineoplastic drugs and radiation therapy damage GI mucosa which results in the release of serotonin and emesis.
    2. **Therapeutic uses.** Ondansetron or dolasetron are used in dogs undergoing cancer chemotherapy or radiation therapy to control emesis.
    3. **Pharmacokinetics.** Animal data are not available. In humans, ondansetron is well absorbed with peak plasma levels in 2 hours and an elimination $t_{1/2}$ of 3–4 hours. Ondansetron is extensively metabolized by the liver. Dolasetron is converted to its active metabolite, hydrolasetron, by plasma carbonyl reductase. Approximately two-third is subsequently metabolized by the liver and one-third is excreted unchanged in the urine. The antiemetic effect of both drugs persists after their disappearance from the circulation suggesting continued binding at the receptor level.
    4. **Administration.** Ondansetron is administered orally or IV once or twice a day. Dolasetron is administered IV once a day.
    5. **Adverse effects.** Side effects are rare. Constipation, extrapyramidal symptoms, hypotension, and cardiac arrhythmias may occur.

F. **Miscellaneous antiemetics**

    1. Alimentary demulcents/adsorbents such as kaolin, pectin, or bismuth salts may reduce vomiting in mild gastritis.

2. Gastric antacids such as magnesium hydroxide, magnesium silicate, aluminum hydroxide, or aluminum silicates may reduce vomiting in cases of gastric hyperacidity.

3. **NK$_1$ receptor antagonist maropitant (Cerenia®)**

   a. A new antiemetic agent for use in dogs with ongoing emesis is a neurokinin (NK) receptor antagonist which serves as a ligand for substance P (NK$_1$) receptors located in the vomiting center. Maropitant blocks neurotransmission of afferent emetic signals from the GI tract and other abdominal organs.

   b. Maropitant is administered to dogs once daily SC at 1 mg/kg/day for up to 5 days for prevention and treatment of acute vomiting. The oral tablets can be used to prevent motion sickness at 8 mg/kg/day for up to 2 days.

   c. Pilot data suggest that maropitant is clinically superior to metoclopramide in the control of general emesis in dogs. Additional studies are needed to confirm these earlier observations.

   d. Pharmacokinetics

   (1) The oral bioavailability of maropitant is 37%. T_{max} is ~2 hours. The plasma protein binding of maropitant in dogs is >99%.

   (2) Maropitant is metabolized by cytochrome P450 enzymes in the liver.

   (3) Renal clearance is a minor route of elimination with <1% of an 8-mg/kg oral dose appearing in the urine as parent drug or metabolite. The data suggest that GI is the major route of elimination for maropitant, when given orally.

   (4) The elimination $t_{1/2}$ is ~4 hours.

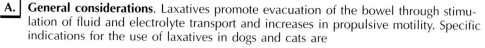

X. LAXATIVES

A. **General considerations**. Laxatives promote evacuation of the bowel through stimulation of fluid and electrolyte transport and increases in propulsive motility. Specific indications for the use of laxatives in dogs and cats are

1. To relieve severe constipation or obstipation which is causing fecal impaction.
2. To enhance intestinal motility that eliminates poisons from the GI tract.
3. To evacuate the large bowel prior to surgery, select radiographic procedures (e.g., excretory urography), or lower GI (e.g., colonoscopy) endoscopic procedures.

B. **Hyperosmotic laxatives**

1. **Mechanism of action.** Hyperosmotic laxatives are nonabsorbable or poorly absorbable salts or polymers which osmotically retain water in the intestinal lumen. They have a rapid onset of action which begins in the small intestine.

2. **Lactulose** is the most effective agent in this group. The organic acids produced from lactulose fermentation stimulate colonic fluid secretion and propulsive motility. Lactulose is administered at a dose of 0.5 mL/kg body weight two or three times daily.

3. **Polyethylene glycol.** Electrolyte solutions (Golytely®., Colyte®.) are isotonic mixtures of polyethylene glycol, sodium sulfate, sodium bicarbonate, sodium chloride, and potassium chloride. They are administered orally prior to colonoscopy in dogs. Anecdotal reports suggest that they are safe to use in cats.

4. **Magnesium sulfate** (Epsom salts) or magnesium hydroxide (Milk of Magnesia®) are administered orally. They should not be used in the presence of renal disease since 20% of the magnesium ions are normally absorbed and are excreted by the kidney. CNS depression may result from elevated levels of plasma magnesium ions.

C. **Bulk laxatives**

1. **Mechanism of action.** Bulk laxatives comprise poorly digestible polysaccharides which absorb water and increase fecal bulk which stimulates large bowel

peristalsis. These products also reduce tenesmus associated with large bowel dysfunction (e.g., colitis, fiber-responsive diarrhea). Most of these products are dietary fiber supplements. Since they act in the large bowel, their onset of action is slow—normally 1–3 days.

2. Methylcellulose, wheat bran, or psyllium are added to the diet. Dietary fiber is preferable because it is well tolerated, more effective, and more physiologic than other laxatives.

3. Their use is indicated in dogs and cats having mild constipation or as adjunctive therapy to reduce clinical signs of colitis.

D. Lubricants and surfactants

1. Mineral oil (liquid petrolatum) and white petrolatum lubricate and soften fecal mass. These agents should only be given via rectal administration to minimize the risk of aspiration if given orally.

2. Docusate is an anionic surfactant which hydrates and softens stools by an emulsifying action.

E. Emollient laxatives

1. Emollient laxatives are anionic detergents that increase the miscibility of water and lipid in digesta, thus enhancing lipid absorption and impairing water absorption. Dioctyl sodium sulfosuccinate and dioctyl calcium sulfosuccinate are two common emollients available in oral formulations.

2. The dosage for both emollient laxatives is 50 mg orally given once daily in the dog and cat.

3. The clinical efficacy of either product in treating canine or feline constipation has not been proven in controlled clinical trials.

F. Irritant laxatives

1. **Mechanism of action.** Irritant cathartics are derived from plants and are activated in the GI tract to release irritant derivatives which activate myenteric neurons and smooth muscle to increase gut motility. They are used primarily in nonruminant large animals.

2. Castor oil is cleaved by pancreatic lipases in the small intestine to yield irritant ricinoleates. These stimulate peristalsis throughout the intestine and reduce fluid absorption. It is used mainly in calves and foals.

3. Anthraquinone (emodin) laxatives include aloe, senna, and cascara sagrada. These contain glycosides which are hydrolyzed in the large intestine to yield irritant anthraquinones which stimulate myenteric plexuses and increase colonic motility. Their onset of action is slow since they act in the large intestine. They are used mainly in horses.

XI. ANTIDIARRHEAL AGENTS

A. General considerations (Figure 11-5)

1. **Diarrhea** is defined as an increase in the frequency, volume, or fluidity of stools. General causes for diarrhea include (1) increased secretion of fluid and electrolytes—example is enterotoxigenic *E. coli* infection; (2) increased intestinal permeability—example is canine protein-losing enteropathy; (3) osmotic diarrhea—example is exocrine pancreatic insufficiency; and (4) alterations in intestinal motility—uncommon. **Acute diarrhea** may respond to symptomatic therapy with antidiarrheal drugs but **chronic diarrhea** requires a definitive diagnosis (often necessitating intestinal mucosal biopsy) and specific therapy.

2. **Oral rehydration** therapy with glucose–electrolyte solutions represents a significant advance in treating secretory diarrheal disease in the absence of vomiting.

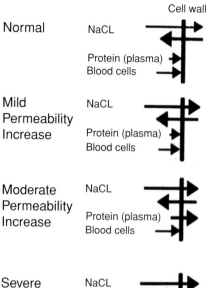

Normal NaCL

Protein (plasma)
Blood cells

Mild Permeability Increase NaCL

Protein (plasma)
Blood cells

Moderate Permeability Increase NaCL

Protein (plasma)
Blood cells

Severe Permeability Increase NaCL

Protein (plasma)
Blood cells

FIGURE 11-5. Altered intestinal permeability can lead to diarrhea. In the healthy intestinal mucosa, selective mucosal permeability leads to minor fluxes of electrolytes and water across the intact epithelial barrier. However, with mucosal inflammation (e.g., infiltrative mucosal diseases or intestinal ulceration with GI bleeding), larger molecular weight substances (albumin, globulins, red blood cells) are progressively lost into the GI lumen as intestinal permeability increases.

Sodium—glucose or fructose and sodium—amino acid-linked absorption by the enterocyte remains intact even in the presence of moderate loss of villus structure. This provides the driving force for water and electrolyte absorption from the lumen to replace fecal losses. In addition to glucose and/or amino acids, solutions contain sodium chloride, potassium chloride, sodium bicarbonate, and potassium phosphate.

B. **Motility-modifying drugs (opiates) (See Chapter 4, V for information on opiates)**

1. **Mechanism of action.** Opiates increase GI rhythmic segmentation and decrease propulsive motility via reduced acetylcholine release. Thus they slow the transit of luminal contents and increase water absorption. In addition, they directly stimulate net absorption of fluid and electrolytes via μ-opiate receptors in the CNS and the intestinal mucosa.

2. **Therapeutic uses.** Opiates are effective in the short-term (5–7 days) symptomatic treatment of acute diarrhea. Opiates are contraindicated in animals with infectious diarrhea because slowing GI transit may increase absorption of bacterial toxins and enhance bacterial growth in the intestinal lumen.

3. **Administration**

   a. **Paregoric** (camphorated tincture of opium) is administered orally two or three times a day to dogs and cats and once a day to calves and foals.
   NOTE: The use of antidiarrheal opiates in cats is controversial because of potential excitatory reactions.

   b. **Diphenoxylate** is a synthetic congener of meperidine. It is combined with atropine as a commercial preparation Lomotil™ and is given orally two to three times a day to dogs. Atropine is added at low concentrations to reduce the abuse potential in humans. Pharmacokinetic data for animals are lacking. In humans, dephenoxylate is well absorbed orally with peak plasma levels in 1–2 hours. It is rapidly deesterified to its active metabolite, difenoxin, which is eliminated with a $t_{1/2}$ of 12 hours.

   c. **Loperamide** is a synthetic piperidine opioid with action limited to the gut. Pharmacokinetic data for animals are not available. In humans, loperamide is absorbed orally with peak plasma levels in 3–5 hours. It undergoes extensive hepatic metabolism with a $t_{1/2}$ of 11 hours. Loperamide (Imodium.™) is given orally once or twice a day to dogs at a dosage of 0.08 mg/kg.

4. **Adverse effects.** Constipation, bloat, and sedation are the most common side effects. Paralytic ileus, toxic megacolon, and pancreatitis are rare but potential adverse effects. Opiates should be used cautiously in cats because of the possibility of excitatory reactions in this species.

C. **Anticholinergic agents**

1. **Mechanism of action.** Anticholinergic agents inhibit GI motility, both propulsive and nonpropulsive. The rationale for their use as antidiarrheals is questionable since hypomotility of the gut is common, especially in diarrheal diseases. Inhibition of cholinergically mediated basal secretions of GI tract may be beneficial but controlled studies are lacking.
2. **Therapeutic uses.** Anticholinergic agents are employed as antidiarrheals and GI antispasmodics.
3. **Administration**
   a. **Isopropamide**—dogs and cats, orally every 12 hours.
   b. **Aminopentamide**—dogs and cats, orally, IM, or SC every 8–12 hours.
   c. **Propantheline**—dogs and cats, orally every 8 hours.
   d. **Methscopolamine**—dogs, orally every 8–12 hours.
4. **Adverse effects.** Xerostomia, tachycardia, loss of accommodation, urinary retention, and paralytic ileus may be observed as side effects of anticholinergic drugs.

D. **Protectants and adsorbents**

1. **Mechanism of action.** Protectants and adsorbents adsorb toxins and provide a protective coating on the inflamed mucosa. They are widely used but their efficacy is questionable. They may decrease fluidity of feces without decreasing fecal water loss.
2. **Therapeutic uses.** Protectants and adsorbents are used for the symptomatic therapy of acute diarrhea.
3. **Administration**
   a. **Kaolin/Pectin**—**Kaolin** (hydrated aluminum silicate) 20% is combined with pectin (polygalacturonic acid carbohydrate polymer) 1% is Kaopectate. It is administered to dogs, cats, birds, horses, cattle, sheep, and swine orally every 4–6 hours.
   b. **Bismuth subsalicylate** has an antiprostaglandin action in addition to its protective/adsorbent properties. It is also used as a component of "triple therapy" for treatment of helicobacteriosis. It is given orally to dogs, horses, cattle, swine, and cats (reduced dosage) every 6–8 hours. Note that cats are sensitive to salicylates.
4. **Adverse effects.** Kaolin/pectin—none; bismuth subsalicylate may produce dark stools which should not be confused with melena. Salicylates should be used cautiously in cats.

XII. DRUGS FOR THERAPY OF INFLAMMATORY BOWEL DISEASE

A. **General considerations.** The IBD represent a diverse group of chronic GI diseases of unknown cause. Both clinical and basic science studies indicate that IBD results from complex interactions between the resident gut flora and the intestinal immune system in a susceptible host. Idiopathic IBD is the most common histologic diagnosis made in dogs and cats having chronic GI signs of vomiting, diarrhea, anorexia, and weight loss. A diagnosis of IBD is one of exclusion and it is only made following rigorous diagnostic evaluation to rule out IBD mimics. Treatment of IBD consists of feeding an elimination (hypoallergenic) diet and the administration of immunomodulatory drugs to reduce intestinal inflammation.

B. **Sulfasalazine**

1. **Chemistry.** Sulfasalazine consists of sulfapyridine plus 5-aminosalicylic acid (5-ASA) linked by a diazo bond.
2. **Mechanism of action.** Sulfasalazine is cleaved by bacteria in the large bowel to release sulfapyridine and salicylate. The anti-inflammatory effects of salicylate (5-ASA) on the bowel mucosa are considered to be primarily responsible for the therapeutic action of sulfasalazine. Salicylates act by inhibiting prostaglandin synthesis and the effects of proinflammatory leukotrienes in the colonic mucosa.
3. **Therapeutic uses and administration.** Sulfasalazine is administered orally two to three times a day for chronic IBD involving the colon (e.g., IBD colitis) in dogs and cats. It is of no therapeutic value to animals having small intestinal IBD.
4. **Pharmacokinetics.** Sulfasalazine is classed as an enteric sulfonamide since oral absorption is generally <30% for sulfapyridine. Salicylate absorption is <10%.
5. **Adverse effects.** Side effects are rare but sulfapyridine toxicity, especially keratoconjunctivitis sicca (KCS), may develop with long-term use. Prophylactic Schirmer tear testing should be performed prior to using this medication. Cats should be monitored for signs of salicylate toxicity if therapy is prolonged.

C. **Olsalazine**

1. **Chemistry.** Olsalazine consists of two molecules of 5-aminosalicylate linked by a diazo bond. Developed for use in humans with IBD where up to 25% may show adverse reactions to sulfasalzine.
2. **Mechanism of action.** After cleavage of the diazo bond by colonic bacteria, salicylates are released to reduce inflammation in the bowel mucosa by inhibition of prostaglandin synthesis.
3. **Therapeutic uses and administration.** Olsalazine is administered orally two to three times a day for chronic IBD in dogs and cats. Controlled studies in the dog attesting to the efficacy of this drug have not been performed.
4. **Pharmacokinetics.** Oral absorption of olsalazine is minimal with over 98% of the dose reaching the colon.
5. **Adverse effects.** Olsalazine is less toxic than sulfasalazine since it lacks the sulfonamide moiety. Cats should be monitored for signs of salicylate toxicity if therapy is prolonged.

D. **Tylosin (see Chapter 15, XI for more information)**

1. **Chemistry.** Tylosin is a macrolide antibiotic structurally related to erythromycin (see Chapter 15). Macrolides are organic bases which form salts with acids such as phosphate or tartrate.
2. **Mechanism of action.** Tylosin inhibits protein synthesis in susceptible bacteria by binding to the 5OS ribosome and blocking long-chain peptide synthesis. Its bacteriostatic action suppresses bacterial overgrowth in chronic intestinal disease. It is thought to possess immunomodulatory actions in IBD patients—possibly related to its antibacterial properties rather than to suppression of the host immune response.
3. **Therapeutic uses and administration.** Tylosin is administered orally with food two or three times a day for chronic colitis in dogs and cats.
4. **Pharmacokinetics.** Tylosin is absorbed from the intestine and widely distributed except to the CNS. It is eliminated unchanged in bile and urine.
5. **Adverse effects.** Mild GI disturbances such as nausea or diarrhea may be observed with tylosin.

E. **Metronidazole**

1. **Mechanism of action.** Metronidazole is an antiprotozoan nitroimidazole (see Chapter 16) and antibacterial, especially against anaerobes (Chapter 15). It may also suppress cell-mediated immune responses which are important in IBD.

2. **Therapeutic uses and administration.** Metronidazole (Flagyl®) is administered orally two to three times a day for the treatment of colitis in dogs.
3. **Pharmacokinetics.** Metronidazole is well absorbed orally, widely distributed to a volume equivalent to total body water. Hepatic metabolites and unchanged drug are excreted in urine and feces. The plasma $t_{1/2}$ in dogs is 4–5 hours
4. **Adverse effects.** Side effects are infrequent in dogs. High or prolonged doses may produce neurotoxicity including tremors and ataxia. Metronidazole should not be used in pregnant animals.

F. FortiFlora®

1. FortiFlora is a specific probiotic (*Enteroccoccus faecium* SF68) which is marketed for dogs and cats with GI disorders. This preparation uses a unique microencapsulated formula which conserves and protects the biologically active *E. faecium* SF68 so it can withstand handling, processing, and storage.
2. **Probiotics** are live bacterial products that affect beneficial health responses to the host. They have diverse ways in which they evoke these changes including exclusion of bacterial pathogens and enhancement of local immunity.
3. Preliminary clinical data suggest that FortiFlora™ is of potential therapeutic benefit in both acute and chronic GI diseases, including IBD. While clinical trials have not been performed in dogs or cats with IBD, evidence-based data in human IBD indicate that probiotics are useful in reducing severity of clinical disease.

XIII. RUMEN PHARMACOLOGY

A. General considerations

1. Development of rumen function starts at 3–6 weeks and is complete at 9–13 weeks.
2. Normal intraruminal pH range is 5.5–7.
3. Extrinsic contractions of the ruminoreticulum are controlled by vagal efferents from the dorsal vagal nucleus in the CNS.
4. Intrinsic contractions are controlled by intramural plexuses.
5. Rumen microflora function depends upon a proper nutrient intake and normal ruminoreticular motor activity.

B. Agents for closure of esophageal groove

1. Closure of the esophageal groove is required for oral medication of calves and lambs in order to bypass the nonfunctioning ruminoreticulum.
2. When stimulated, buccal and pharyngeal receptors activate a vagal reflex to close the groove starting in 2–5 seconds and lasting for 60 seconds.
3. **Administration**
   a. **Milk**—calves and lambs, orally
   b. **Sodium bicarbonate**—10% calves, orally
   c. **Copper sulfate**—5% calves, 2% lambs, orally
   d. **NOTE:** Water is not an effective stimulus for groove closure.

C. Ruminotorics

1. **Bitters** are plant-derived compounds containing alkaloids such as nux vomica, ginger, or capsicum which stimulate salivation. They were components of large animal tonic mixtures for the treatment of inappetence and depressed rumen function. Their efficacy is doubtful and they are seldom used now.
2. **Cholinergics** such as neostigmine or bethanechol (Chapter 2) transiently increase the frequency but not the strength of contractions in rumen atony. Since they do not provide the synchronized contractions and relaxations of the

forestomachs, their value for the movement of ingesta is limited. They are administered SC.

3. **Experimentally, metoclopropamide has been reported to increase ruminoreticular motility and abomasal contractions. Opiate antagonists** such as naloxone stimulate extrinsic contractions in endotoxin-induced ruminal stasis when administered parenterally.

4. **Ruminal fluid transfer.** Oral inoculation of viable rumen bacteria and protozoa is the most effective means of restoring rumen function following correction of the primary cause of stasis.

D. Rumen antacids

1. The principal use of antacids in ruminants is in treating mild cases of lactic acidosis resulting from carbohydrate engorgement.
2. **Administration.** Orally every 8–12 hours
   a. Magnesium oxide (MgO)
   b. Magnesium carbonate
   c. Aluminum hydroxide
3. **Adverse effects.** Systemic alkalosis may occur with overdose, especially with MgO.

E. Rumen acidifiers

1. The principal use of ruminal acidifiers is in treating simple indigestion in which intraruminal pH rises due to the constant inflow of bicarbonate-rich saliva. They are also used in the treatment of acute urea poisoning to decrease ammonia absorption via formation of ammonium ion and to inhibit urease activity of the rumen microflora.
2. **Administration.** Vinegar or dilute acetic acid (4–5%) is administered at a dose of 4–8 liters in cattle via stomach tube every 6–8 hours with several liters of cold water.

F. Bloat therapy

1. Ruminal bloat or tympany is the accumulation of excess gas in the rumen as a result of impaired elimination, *not* excess production. Ruminal gasses may be in the free form or, more commonly, entrapped in froth. Passage of a ruminal tube will alleviate free-gas bloat but viscosity-altering agents are required for the treatment of frothy bloat.
2. **Mechanism of action.** Anti-bloat agents alter the surface tension of froth and break up the bubbles which contain entrapped gases.
3. **Administration.** Anti-bloat agents are administered via drench or stomach tube.
   a. Poloxalene (25–50 g for cattle).
   b. Polymerized methyl silicone (3% emulsion; 30–60 mL in cattle; 7–15 mL in sheep).
   c. Vegetable oils (soybean, peanut, or sunflower oil); 60 mL in cattle; 10–15 mL in sheep.

SUGGESTED READING

Abood SK, McLaughlin MA, Buffington T. 2006. "Enteral nutrition." In *Fluid, Electrolyte, and Acid Base Disorders in Small Animal Practice.* Edited by DiBartola SP. 3rd ed., pp. 584–600. St. Louis, MD: Saunders.

Boothe DM. 2001. "Drugs affecting gastrointestinal function." In *Veterinary Pharmacology and Therapeutics.* Edited by Adams HR. 8th ed., pp. 1041–1063. Ames, IA: Iowa State University Press.

Clarke CR. 2005. "Systemic pharmacotherapeutics of the ruminant digestive system." In *The Merck Veterinary Manual.* Edited by Kahn CM. 9th ed., pp. 1993–1995. Whitehouse Station: Merck & Co. http://www.drugs.com

Plumb DC. 2005. *Veterinary Drug Handbook.* 5th ed. Ames, IA: Blackwell Publishing.

Steiner A. 2003. Modifiers of gastrointestinal motility of cattle. *Vet Clin North Am Food Anim Pract* 19:647–660.

Tams TR. 2003. *Handbook of Small Animal Gastroenterology.* 2nd ed. St. Louis, MD: Saunders.

Washabau RJ. 2003. Gastrointestinal motility disorders and gastrointestinal prokinetic therapy. *Vet Clin North Am Small Anim Pract* 33:1007–1028.

Willard MD. 2003. "Disorders of the stomach." In *Small Animal Internal Medicine.* Edited by Nelson RW, Couto CG. 3rd ed., pp. 418–430. St. Louis, MD: Mosby.

Willard MD. 2003. "Disorders of the intestinal tract." In *Small Animal Internal Medicine.* Edited by Nelson RW, Couto CG. 3rd ed., pp. 431–465. St. Louis, MD: Mosby.

STUDY QUESTIONS

DIRECTIONS: Each of the numbered items or incomplete statements in this section is followed by answers or by completions of the statement. Select the **one** lettered answer or completion that is **best** in each case.

1. You are presented with a 15-year-old cat—depressed, uremic, and dehydrated. Treatment might include *all but one* of the following:

(A) Famotidine, oral
(B) Sucralfate, oral (2 hours prior to or after oral administration of other drugs)
(C) Metoclopramide, oral
(D) Glucose-electrolyte, IV
(E) Polypropylene glycol, enema

2. You have stabilized the above animal but after 3 days in your hospital the cat is still not eating. Increased appetite via depression of the satiety center may result from administration of

(A) terpin hydrate.
(B) scopolamine.
(C) chlorpromazine.
(D) ranitidine.
(E) oxazepam.

3. Appetite has returned to the cat after providing warmed, palatable food, adequate IV fluid therapy, and the correct drug in Question 2. You are about to discharge the cat to its owner when it develops diarrhea. An opiate analog with an action limited to the gut is cautiously administered. The drug is

(A) loperamide.
(B) butorphanol.
(C) domperidone.
(D) meperidine.
(E) propantheline.

4. The cat is sent home. After 2 days, the owner thinks it has a fever and administers two Extra Strength Tylenol® (acetaminophen) tablets. He has second thoughts about this and calls you 15 minutes later. You advise bringing the cat in immediately for induction of emesis with

(A) apomorphine.
(B) ammonium chloride.

(C) nux vomica.
(D) xylazine.
(E) bismuth subsalicylate.

5. The antiemetic actions of metoclopramide (Reglan®) include *all but one* of the following:

(A) Inhibition of H-1 histamine receptors in the vomiting center
(B) Stimulation of gastric motility
(C) Inhibition of dopaminergic receptors in the CRTZ
(D) Increased sensitivity of intestinal smooth muscle to acetylcholine
(E) Relaxation of pylorus

6. Which of the following laxatives act to reduce blood ammonia concentrations and thus is a component of hepatic encephalopathy therapy?

(A) Magnesium sulfate
(B) Lactulose
(C) Castor oil
(D) Bethanechol

7. The primary reason for addition of glucose or fructose to oral rehydration solutions in treating diarrheal disease is

(A) to correct the severe hypoglycemia and weakness.
(B) to stimulate disaccharidase activity in the mucosal brush border
(C) to stimulate sugar-sodium coupled uptake by enterocytes.
(D) to provide a hypertonic gradient for water absorption.

8. Increased segmentation, slowed transit, and stimulation of electrolyte absorption by gut mucosa characterize the antidiarrheal action of *all but one* of the following:

(A) Paregoric
(B) Methscopolamine

(C) Diphenoxylate
(D) Loperamide
(E) Codeine

9. Considering GI antacids, and protectives/adsorbents

(A) Hepatic microsomal inhibition is less likely with cimetidine, than famotidine.
(B) Kaolin is a hydrated aluminum silicate.
(C) Bismuth subsalicylate tends to produce an osmotic laxative effect unless dosage is carefully controlled.
(D) The antidiarrheal action of pectin is due to its rapid breakdown to galactose in the small intestine.

10. Inhibitors of gastric acid secretion are employed in small animals for treatment of gastritis, gastric ulcers, and liver disease. A drug which inhibits the acid (proton) pump in the parietal cell is

(A) famotidine.
(B) ranitidine.
(C) omeprazole.
(D) diazepam.

11. Oral administration of vinegar (acetic acid) in cattle with urea poisoning

(A) reduces the ketonemia by providing acetate as an energy source.
(B) stimulates bacterial urease to increase urea breakdown in the rumen.
(C) slows rumen fermentation to allow regrowth of favorable bacteria.
(D) reduces ammonia absorption into the systemic circulation.

12. Which of the following would be *ineffective* in producing closure of the esophageal (ruminoreticular) groove in a calf?

(A) Water
(B) Milk
(C) Sodium bicarbonate, 10%
(D) Copper sulfate, 5%

13. Synthetic bile acids such as ursodeoxycholic acid

(A) increase fat absorption and bile secretion.
(B) are lipotropic agents useful in preventing fatty liver degeneration.
(C) are used mainly as appetite stimulants in lactose- intolerant patients.
(D) decrease the production of glutamine which promotes oxidative damage to hepatocytes.

14. Vomiting arising from motion sickness or vestibular disease may be reduced by antihistamines such as

(A) propantheline.
(B) metoclopramide.
(C) chlorpromazine.
(D) diphenhydramine.

15. Chelation therapy in dogs with copper toxicosis is best achieved with

(A) colchicines.
(B) D-penicillamine.
(C) S-adenosyl-L-methionine (SAMe).
(D) high protein diets.

16. Anaerobic bacteria serve as microbial antigens which trigger chronic inflammation in canine inflammatory bowel disease (IBD). Bactericidal activity against anaerobes and suppression of mucosal immune reactions characterize the action of which of the following drugs in the treatment of IBD?

(A) Olsalazine
(B) Clindamycin
(C) Metronidazole
(D) Aminopentamide

17. Retention of urine may be observed as an adverse effect of

(A) chlorpromazine.
(B) isopropamide.
(C) droperidol.
(D) diphenoxylate.

18. Antiprostaglandin activity and protective/adsorbent properties characterize the antidiarrheal action of

(A) kaolin.
(B) sucralfate.
(C) magnesium silicate.
(D) bismuth subsalicylate.

19. Poloxalene relieves ruminant bloat by

(A) stimulating the eructation reflex.
(B) inhibiting growth of gas-forming bacteria.
(C) altering the surface tension of froth.
(D) stimulating rumen motility.

20. The elimination of poisons from the GI tract requires administration of a cathartic with a rapid onset of action such as

(A) senna.
(B) methylcellulose.
(C) magnesium sulfate.
(D) docusate.

■ANSWERS AND EXPLANATIONS

1. The answer is E [II C 3].
Polypropylene glycol laxative or enema should not be used in this cat because it will promote fecal water loss and potentiate dehydration. Inhibition of gastric acid secretion with famotidine, protective coating of possible uremia-induced ulcers with sucralfate, prevention of emesis with metoclopramide, and restoration of fluid and electrolyte balance are rational therapeutic measures.

2. The answer is E [II C 3].
Oxazepam may stimulate appetite by suppression of the satiety center in the hypothalamus by increasing GABA and inhibiting serotonin. Terpin hydrate is an antitussive, scopolamine is an anticholinergic, and chlorpromazine is a phenothiazine tranquilizer and central-acting antiemetic. Ranitidine is an H-2 receptor antagonist that inhibits gastric acid secretion.

3. The answer is A [II B 2 c].
Loperamide is a synthetic opiate antidiarrheal with action limited to the gut. Butorphanol and meperidine are opiates that have both central and peripheral actions. Domperidone is a peripheral acting antidopaminergic that stimulates gastric motility. Propantheline is an anticholinergic agent.

4. The answer is D [V B 2].
Xylazine is the central acting emetic of choice in cats. Apomorphine should not be used in cats because of the potential for CNS excitement. Ammonium chloride, nux vomica, or bismuth salts are not emetics.

5. The answer is A [VI B 3].
The central antidopaminergic actions of metoclopramide do not include blockade of histamine H-1 receptors. It inhibits dopamine receptors in the CRTZ and stimulates gastric and intestinal motility and gastric emptying for its antiemetic effects.

6. The answer is B [VI C 2 b].
Lactulose is a disaccharide molecule that is metabolized by luminal bacteria into osmotically active particles that retain water in the intestinal lumen. Bacterial fermentation produces acids that reduce the pH of the colonic contents. Blood ammonia is then converted to the ionic form which is not absorbed and thus is eliminated from the body in the feces.

7. The answer is C [VII A 5].
Glucose or fructose stimulates sodium absorption via a coupled transport mechanism on enterocytes. Sodium uptake then secondarily provides the osmotic force for water absorption. Increased glucose absorption may be beneficial but it is not essential for rehydration. Disaccharidase activity is not altered by monosaccharides.

8. The answer is B [VII B 2; C 1, 2 d].
The actions described characterize the actions of opiates on the gut, and all except **B** are opiates. Methscopolamine is an anticholinergic that does not increase segmentation.

9. The answer is C [VII D 2].
Kaolin is a hydrated, aluminum silicate with protective/adsorbent properties. Cimetidine is more likely to produce hepatic microsomal inhibition than is famotidine . Bismuth subsalicylate has antidiarrheal effects. Pectin is polymerized galacturonic acid that is not readily hydrolyzed in the GI tract.

10. The answer is C [III A 2 b].
Omeprazole decreases gastric acid secretion by inhibiting hydrogen ion generation by parietal cell ATPase. Famotidine and ranitidine are histamine-2 receptor antagonists. Diazepam is a benzodiazepine used for short-term stimulation of appetite.

11. The answer is D [IX E 1, 2].
Acidification of the rumen shifts the equilibrium from ammonia to ammonium ion which slows absorption. Urease activity is also decreased at lower rumen pH, resulting in a slower rate of ammonia formation. Ketonemia or excessive rumen fermentation are not related to urea poisoning.

12. The answer is A [IX B 3 d].
Water is not an effective stimulus for esophageal groove closure. Milk, sodium bicarbonate, or copper sulfates are effective stimuli.

13. The answer is A [IV B 1, 2].
The bile acids emulsify lipids to enhance absorption and stimulate bile flow. Lipotropic agents such as methionine are methyl donors that stimulate hepatic lipoprotein synthesis. Lactose intolerance is treated by eliminating dairy products from the diet. Bile acids increase the production of glutathione which prevents oxidative damage.

14. The answer is D [VI C 1, 2].
Diphenhydramine prevents vomiting via blockade of histaminergic afferents originating in the vestibular organs. Propantheline is an anticholinergic and metoclopramide and chlorpromazine are antidopaminergics with little or no antihistaminic action.

15. The answer is B [I B 4].
Copper toxicosis may occur as a primary disorder in the Bedlington terrier as well as other canine breeds. A variety of hepatic diseases which cause cholestasis may predispose to copper accumulation and subsequent oxidative damage. Colchicine is an antifibrotic agent, while SAMe prevents hepatic oxidative damage but is not a chelation agent. High protein diets should be avoided with hepatopathy since they promote ammonia production. D-penicillamine is the copper chelation agent of first-choice for use in the dog.

16. The answer is C [VIII D 1].
Metronidazole is bactericidal for anaerobes and, in addition, it suppresses cell-mediated immunity. Olsalazine is a salicylate dimer which is cleaved in the large bowel to release two molecules of 5-aminosalicylate which inhibit prostaglandin synthesis. Clindamycin suppresses anaerobic bacterial growth but has no effect on colonic mucosal immune reactions. Aminopentamide is an anticholinergic used in the control of vomiting and diarrhea.

17. The answer is B [VII C 2, 1].
Anticholinergic agents such as isopropamide may produce urinary retention as a side effect by inhibiting bladder contractility and tone. Chlorpromazine and droperidol are dopamine antagonists and diphenoxylate is an opiate agonist.

18. The answer is D [VII D 2 b].
The antidiarrheal action of bismuth subsalicylate is due, in part, to the inhibition of prostaglandins synthesis in gut mucosa. Kaolin, magnesium silicate, and sucralfate are mucosal protectives with no effect on prostaglandin synthesis.

19. The answer is C [IX F 1, 2].
Poloxalene relieves bloat by altering the surface tension of ruminal froth to induce breakup and release of entrapped gases. It does not alter rumen microflora or rumen motility. Breakup of froth permits normal functioning of the eructation reflex.

20. The answer is C [VI B 2, 4].
Osmotic cathartics such as magnesium sulfate act in the small intestine and thus have a rapid onset of action. Senna, methylcellulose, and docusate exert their laxative effect in the large intestine.

Chapter 12

Endocrine Pharmacology

Walter H. Hsu

I. **ENDOCRINE FUNCTION.** Hormones are natural secretions of endocrine glands that can exert powerful effects on other cells/tissues. Compounds that produce hormone-like effects have important therapeutic uses for the treatment of endocrine hypofunction. Compounds that inhibit the hormone synthesis or blocking receptors can be used for the treatment of endocrine hyperfunction.

A. Overview of basic information

1. **Mechanism of action.** Many hormones effect signal transduction through one of four major mechanisms. For detailed information, see Chapter 1, III A 3.
   a. **GTP-binding proteins (G-proteins) in the plasma membrane: G_s, $G_{i/o}$, and G_q.**
   b. **Tyrosine kinase**
      (1) **Receptors with tyrosine kinase activity.**
      (2) **Cystosolic tyrosine kinase.**
   c. **Guanylyl cyclase.**
   d. **Intracellular receptors.**
2. **Pharmacokinetics**
   a. **Polypeptides and proteins**
      (1) **Absorption.** They are destroyed in the GI tract following oral administration, thus they should not be administered via this route. They are well absorbed from the injection sites.
      (2) **Fate**
         (a) **Distribution.** They are evenly distributed in the body. In general, they do not penetrate the blood–brain barrier (BBB).
         (b) **Metabolism.** They are usually rapidly metabolized in the liver and kidney by proteases. Despite their short plasma $t_{1/2}$ (5–20 minutes), their biological actions usually last several hours.
         (c) **Excretion.** Very little is excreted in the urine or feces, if any.
   b. **Glycoproteins**
      (1) **Absorption.** They are destroyed in the GI tract following oral administration. They are well absorbed from the injection sites.
      (2) **Fate**
         (a) **Distribution.** They are evenly distributed in the body. In general, they do not penetrate the BBB.
         (b) **Metabolism.** They are slowly metabolized by the liver and kidneys. In general, the more carbohydrates in the chemical structure, the more resistant the compound is to metabolism. The plasma $t_{1/2}$ ranges from 1 to 24 hours.
         (c) **Excretion.** They are usually not detectable in the urine or feces following parenteral administration.
   c. **Steroids and thyroid hormones**
      (1) **Absorption.** They are well absorbed from the gut following oral administration. However, because the natural steroids are rapidly metabolized by the liver following oral administration, only thyroid hormones and synthetic steroids that are resistant to liver enzymes can be effectively administered orally.
      (2) **Fate.** At least 90% of the circulating steroids and thyroid hormones are bound to plasma-binding proteins (albumin and specific globulins) and are evenly distributed throughout the body, including CNS. Because they are

protected by plasma proteins, they have much longer $t_{1/2}$ (hours to days) than polypeptide and protein hormones.

(3) **Excretion.** When steroids and thyroid hormones are metabolized, they are hydroxylated and then undergo conjugation to form glucuronides and sulfates, which are water-soluble and thus are readily excreted into the urine and feces.

II. COMMON ENDOCRINE DISORDERS

A. Anterior pituitary disorders

1. Hypopituitarism (pituitary dwarfism)
2. Acquired growth hormone (GH) deficiency
3. Neoplasia (functional and nonfunctional)
4. Hypersecretion of pituitary hormones
   a. Acromegaly results from excess of GH.
   b. Cushing's syndrome (hyperadrenocorticism) results from excess of ACTH.
   c. Galactorrhea results from excess of prolactin.

B. Posterior pituitary disorders. Diabetes insipidus results from vasopressin deficiency or vasopressin receptor abnormality.

C. Thyroid disorders

1. Hypothyroidism is usually seen in dogs and horses, which can be treated with thyroid hormones. Overzealous treatment of feline hyperthyroidism can cause this disorder as well.
2. Hyperthyroidism is usually seen in cats. Hyperthyroidism in species other than cats is frequently caused by adenocarcinoma, and the prognosis in these animals is usually poor. Thus, antithyroid agents are only recommended for cats.

D. Parathyroid disorders

1. Hypoparathyroidism leads to hypocalcemia, which is characterized by neuromuscular dysfunction (tetany and paresis), bradycardia, and convulsions.
2. Hyperparathyrodism causes hypercalcemia, which has renal, skeletal, GI, and neurological ramifications.

E. Adrenal dysfunction

1. Hypoadrenocorticism (Addison's disease) is usually the result of primary insufficiency, usually due to autoimmune disorder. Secondary insufficiency, due to a decrease in ACTH secretion, can occur as well.
2. Hyperadrenocorticism (Cushing's syndrome) is usually the result of overproduction of ACTH. The neoplasm of the adrenal cortex can cause this disorder as well.
3. Pheochromocytoma causes excessive production of catecholamines, resulting in hypertension.

F. Disorders of endocrine pancreas

1. Hyperglycemia. Diabetes mellitus is the most common cause.
2. Hypoglycemia (hyperinsulinemia) may be caused by insulin overdose or insulinoma.

G. Gonadal dysfunction results in hypogonadism and ovarian cystic disorders (e.g., follicular cysts and luteal cysts).

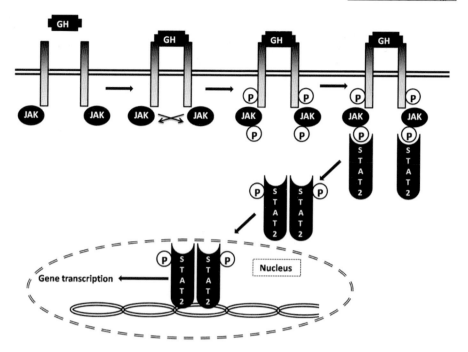

FIGURE 12-1. Mechanism of action of growth hormone (GH). The GH receptor has single subunits that contain both GH-binding and signaling domains. These receptors are associated with Janus kinase (JAK), a cytosolic form of tyrosine kinase. Upon activation and dimerization of GH receptors, 2 JAKs undergo reciprocal phosphorylation, which further attracts signal transduction and activation of transcription-2 (STAT2) proteins. The homodimer of STAT2 binds to DNA and stimulates gene transcription.

III. HORMONES AND AGENTS AFFECTING ENDOCRINE FUNCTION

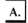 **Growth hormone** is a protein molecule containing 191 amino acids. Because it resembles prolactin and placental lactogen in structure, these three proteins may be evolved from a common ancestral cell. Their function may overlap as well.

1. **Synthesis and secretion.** GH is produced and secreted by somatotrope of the pituitary gland. Production of GH is under hypothalamic control; it is **stimulated by GH-releasing hormone (GHRH) and ghrelin and inhibited by somatostatin.**

2. **Preparations. Sometribove [bovine somatotropin (BST)]** is a prolonged-release injectable formulation of a recombinant DNA-derived BST analog.

3. **Mechanism of action** (Figure 12-1). GH activates **Janus kinase (JAK2)-signal transduction and activation of transcription (STAT) pathway**, which leads to an increase in transcription and protein synthesis. GH also stimulates the secretion of **insulin-like growth factor-1 (IGF-1, somatomedin)** from the liver, which in turn participates in some of the effects of GH (e.g., growth, cartilage, protein metabolism).

4. **Pharmacologic effects.** GH promotes growth of all tissues of body that are capable of growing, including **bone, muscle, and mammary gland.** GH promotes the growth of **epiphyseal** *plate*, which is essential for long bone growth. The following are additional effects of GH:

   a. **It increases uptake of amino acids into cells and promotes lipolysis.**
   b. **It increases milk production, probably due to proliferation of the pituitary gland and prolactin-like activities.**

5. **Therapeutic uses. Sometribove** (Posilac®) is used in cattle to promote milk production.

6. **Administration.** It is injected SC (500 mg) once every 2 weeks, beginning at ninth week after calving and until the end of lactation period.

7. **Pharmacokinetics.** GH is metabolized in the liver and kidney; the unformulated GH has an elimination $t_{1/2}$ of <20 minutes (see I A 2 for general information). However, Sometribove is in the slow release form, which can last >2 weeks.

8. **Adverse effects**
   a. Injection site irritation, swelling, and lameness.
   b. Anorexia and weight loss.
   c. Mastitis and hypogalactia.
   d. Reduced pregnancy rate, due to cystic ovaries and/or uterine disorders, and abortion.
   e. Short gestation periods, decreased birth weights, and increased rates of twinning and placental retention.

B. Corticotropin, corticosteroids, and inhibitors

1. **General considerations**
   a. The adrenal cortex serves as a homeostatic organ, **regulating reactions to stress.**
   b. **Corticosteroid pathway.** The release of adrenal corticosteroids is controlled by a pathway that includes the CNS.
      (1) A number of stimuli, including trauma, chemicals, diurnal rhythms, and stress, can cause the hypothalamus to release corticotrophin-releasing hormone (CRH).
      (2) CRH moves down the hypophyseal portal system and stimulates the anterior pituitary gland to release **ACTH. CRH receptors are coupled to G_q.**
      (3) ACTH stimulates the adrenal cortex to produce corticosteroids.
         (a) Endogenous **glucocorticoids** include **cortisol and corticosterone.**
         (b) Endogenous **mineralocorticoids**
            i. **Deoxycorticosterone is** produced by the adrenal cortex in response to ACTH stimulation.
            ii. **Aldosterone** secretion is stimulated by high plasma angiotensiin, ACTH, or K^+ concentrations.
      (4) **A negative feedback pathway maintains homeostasis.** When the levels of endogenous corticosteroids increase, the hypothalamus–pituitary–adrenal axis is suppressed and the production of CRH and ACTH is decreased.

2. **ACTH** is a polypeptide hormone consisting of 39 amino acids.
   a. **Preparations. Synthetic ACTH [ACTH (1–24)] possesses the biological activity of ACTH and is identical for all species.**
   b. **Mechanism of action.** ACTH receptors are coupled to the **G_s-adenylyl cyclase** system.
   c. **Therapeutic uses.** ACTH is used mainly as a diagnostic tool for distinguishing the two types of adrenal insufficiency.
      (1) **Primary adrenal insufficiency.** IM administration of ACTH produces little or no increase in cortisol secretion because of the underlying adrenal cortical dysfunction.
      (2) **Secondary adrenal insufficiency** (i.e., anterior pituitary dysfunction). ACTH administration may or may not produce large increase in cortisol secretion, depending on the status of the adrenal cortex; if the cortex is atrophied, ACTH would not evoke a pronounced increase in cortisol secretion.
   d. **Pharmacokinetics.** See I A 2 for general information.
   e. **Adverse effects.** ACTH (1–24) is safe when used as directed.

3. **Corticosteroids**
   a. **Chemistry.** The general structure of corticosteroids is shown in Figure 12-2.
   b. **Physiological and pharmacological effects**
      (1) **Glucocorticoids**
         (a) **Effects on intermediary metabolism. Glucocorticoids increase liver glycogen synthesis and storage, gluconeogenesis, and lipolysis and redistribution of lipids.**

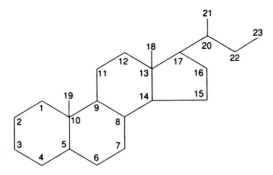

FIGURE 12-2. General structure of corticosteroids. Certain structural features relevant to activity. Positions 1 and 2: The presence of a double bond (delta group) prolongs the activity, especially glucocorticoid activity (most synthetic glucocorticoids have this change). Position 3: The presence of keto group is essential for corticoid function. Positions 4 and 5: The presence of a delta group is essential for corticoid function. Position 6 or 9: Fluorination or methylation potentiates activity, especially glucocorticoid activity. Position 11: The presence of OH increases glucocorticoid activity; the absence of OH increases mineralocorticoid activity. The presence of the 11-keto group abolishes corticoid activity. Examples: cortisone and prednisone; thus, they need to be metabolized to cortisol and prednisolone by having the 11-OH group, respectively. Position 16: The presence of OH or methyl group increases glucocorticoid activity (many synthetic glucocorticoids have this change). Position 17: The presence of OH increases glucocorticoid activity. The presence of acetonide on position 16 or 17 further enhances and prolongs glucocorticoid activity (many synthetic glucocorticoids for topical use have this feature). (From Figure 8-1, *NVMS Pharmacology*.)

  i. The increased gluconeogensis can lead to hyperglycemia and liver glycogen synthesis.
  ii. Hyperglycemia should trigger insulin secretion, which would bring plasma glucose concentrations to the normal range. However, diabetic and diabetes-prone patients would not be able to handle glucocorticoid-induced hyperglycemia.
  iii. Chronic administration of a glucocorticoid may further damage β-cells.
  iv. Glucocorticoids **do not promote glycogenolysis**.
  v. Glucocorticoids **increase protein breakdown**. The amino acids generated can be used for gluconeogenesis and liver protein synthesis.
(b) **CNS effects.** Glucocorticoids may stimulate the CNS, leading to euphoria. CNS depression is associated with the deficiency (hypoadrenocorticism). However, the mechanisms underlying CNS effects of glucocorticoids are not well understood.
(c) **Cardiovascular effects**
  i. **Glucocorticoids increase vasomotor responses and myocardial contractions.**
  ii. Glucocorticoids **increase epinephrine synthesis** by increasing the expression of phenylethanolamine *N*-methyl transferase activity.
  iii. Glucocorticoids increase the **expression of α-adrenergic receptors** in the vascular smooth muscle and β-**adrenergic receptors** in the myocardium.
  iv. Glucocortioids **facilitate the angiotensin system** by increasing expression of angiotensinogen, angiotensin converting enzyme (ACE), and angiotensin II receptors.
  v. Glucocorticoids **promote breakdown of bradykinin** by increasing the expression of ACE and neutral endopeptidase.
  vi. Glucocorticoids **decrease capillary permeability (decongestion).**
(d) **Respiratory effects**
  i. Glucocorticoids cause **bronchodilation** by increasing expression of $β_2$-receptors

    ii. Glucocorticoids **decrease the retention of mast cells** in the respiratory tract and **decrease the expression of autacoids**, for example, histamine and bradykinin.

    iii. Glucocorticoids induce decongestion of the airway (see cardiovascular effects).

(e) Skeletal muscle effects. At physiologic doses, glucocorticoids maintain skeletal muscle function; deficiency causes weakness due to hypoglycemia and poor circulation.

Long-term administration of high doses of glucocorticoids may cause wasting of muscle mass (due to muscle protein breakdown).

(f) Effects on blood cells and lymphoid tissue. Glucocorticoids **increase number of circulatory erythrocytes, neutrophils, monocytes, and platelets**, while **decreasing number of circulatory lymphocytes, eosinophils, and basophils.** Glucocorticoids **decrease the size of lymph nodes and thymus.**

    i. Polycythemia results from decreased phagocytosis of erythrocytes.

    ii. Neutrophilia results from increased entry of neutrophils into the circulation, combined with decreased removal of cells from the circulation. The function of neutrophils, however, is suppressed.

    iii. Eosinopenia, basophilia, and lymphocytopenia result from redistribution of these cells to systems other than blood.

    iv. Apoptosis of lymphocytes may be induced by glucocorticoids.

    v. Production of interleukens (ILs) by macrophages and T-lymphocytes is inhibited; as a result, proliferation of B-lymphocytes and production of immunoglobulins, and activation of T-lymphocytes are suppressed. Phagocytosis activity of macrophages is also suppressed.

(g) Immunological effects

    i. Too little or too much of glucocorticoids can increase susceptibility to infection.

    ii. Glucocorticoids can treat lesions that result from excessive immune reactions; for example, urticaria (humoral immunity) and rejection of transplantation (cellular immunity).

    iii. Glucocorticoid-induced suppression of immunity may be attributable to decreased cytokine production, which can have very serious consequences in animals, particularly exotic birds.

    iv. Involution of the lymph nodes, thymus, and spleen occurs.

(h) Anti-inflammatory and anti-allergic effects occur with pharmacologic doses. Glucocorticoids **suppress inflammatory processes in response to multiple inciting events.** Glucocorticoids **do not address underlying cause of the inflammatory disorders. Anti-inflammatory effects of glucocorticoids are linked to suppression of immune responses. The glucocorticoid-induced anti-inflammation is of enormous clinical utility.**

    i. Leukocyte migration and function are suppressed, which are due to decreased expression of chemoattractive factors (e.g., IL-8) and adhesion factors.

    ii. Plasma and lysosomal membranes are stabilized, resulting in decreased release of proteolytic enzymes and autacoids; the latter effect can lead to decreased capillary permeability. This membrane-stabilizing effect is attributed to a **decrease in phospholipase A_2 (PLA_2) activity**. PLA_2 converts phospholipids into arachidonic acid, which is a precursor of eicosanoids (see Chapter 3 for more information).

    iii. Synthesis of prostaglandins and leukotriene (eicosanoids) is suppressed as a result of inhibition of PLA_2.

    iv. Fibroblast activity, collagen synthesis, and tissue repair are reduced in inflamed areas.

    v. The hair and skin growth is inhibited.

(2) Mineralocorticoids. They **increase reabsorption of sodium and bicarbonate in exchange for excretion of potassium, proton, and chloride in the renal**

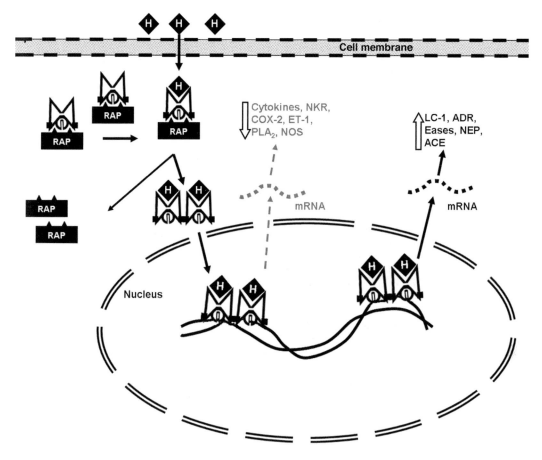

FIGURE 12-3. Mechanism of action of cytosolic corticosteroid receptors. The inactive receptor is surrounded by receptor-associated proteins (RAPs), for example, heat-shock proteins (HSPs). Hormone (H) binding leads to the dissociation of RAPs, and formation of dimers that penetrate into the nucleus and bind to corticosteroid-response element (CRE) of DNA to alter mRNA synthesis. Synthesis of certain mRNAs is increased, while that of others is decreased, particularly in the case of the glucocorticoid receptor. NKR, neurokinin receptor; COX-2, cyclooxygenase 2; ET-1, endothelin-1; PLA$_2$, phospholipase A$_2$; NOS, nitric oxide synthase; LC-1, lipocortin-1; ADR, adrenergic receptor; NEP, neutral endopeptidase; Eases, endonucleases; ACE, angiotensin-converting enzyme.

tubules and, to a lesser extent, in the GI tract (see Figure 9-4). The following events are associated with the changes of these electrolytes:

   (a) Hypernatremia increased blood pressure.

   (b) Hypokalemia decreases excitability of nerves and skeletal muscle and smooth muscle.

   (c) Hypokalemia increases excitability of cardiac muscle. Hypokalemia causes **a poor exchange with intracellular Na$^+$ by Na$^+$, K$^+$-ATPase, resulting in retention of Na$^+$ in myocardium. Increased myocardial Na$^+$ concentration promotes Ca^{2+} influx via Na$^+$–Ca^{2+} antiport.** Increased myocardial Ca^{2+} concentration increases myocardial contractility (see Figure 8-2).

 c. Mechanism of action. Like other steroid hormones, corticosteroids act by altering mRNA synthesis (Figure 12-3). For example, glucocorticoids increase mRNA synthesis of adrenergic receptors; enzymes for breaking down bradykinin, for example, ACE and neutral endopeptidase; enzymes in gluconeogenesis, while decreasing mRNA synthesis of cytokines and their receptors, PLA$_2$, and cyclooxygenase (COX).

TABLE 12-1. Corticosteroids: Anti-Inflammatory and Sodium-Retaining Potencies (Oral Administration)

Corticosteroid	Anti-Inflammatory Potency	Sodium-Retaining Potency
Short-acting (≤12 hours)*		
Hydrocortisone	1	1
Cortisone	0.8	0.8
Fludrocortisone	10	125
Intermediate-acting (12–36 hours)*		
Prednisone	4	0.8
Prednisolone	5	0.8
Methylprednisolone	5	0.5
Triamcinolone	5	0
Long-acting (36–72 hours)*		
Paramethasone	10	0
Betamethasone	25	0
Dexamethasone	25	0
Flumethasone	30	0

* Biologic half-life.

    Aldosterone increases the mRNA synthesis of Na^+ channels, K^+ channels, and H^+-ATPase (in the apical side) and Na^+, K^+-ATPase, and HCO_3^-–Cl^- antiport in the distal renal tubule (see Figure 9-4), and intestine.

  d. Pharmacokinetics.

    (1) Absorption. Corticosteroids are readily absorbed from the GI tract, mucous membranes, and skin.

    (2) Fate. The majority of corticosteroids are bound by plasma proteins (corticosteroid-binding globulin and albumin).

    (3) Metabolism

      (a) The C_3 keto group is reduced to an –OH group, which then undergoes conjugation.

      (b) Reduction of the C_{11} keto group to an –OH group is necessary to convert cortisone to cortisol (hydrocortisone) and prednisone to prednisolone, these are biologically active forms.

    (4) Excretion. The conjugates are excreted by the kidneys.

  e. Preparations

    (1) Depending on duration of action, corticosteroids can be classified as short-acting (biological $t_{1/2}$ of ≤12 hours), intermediate-acting (biological $t_{1/2}$ of 12–36 hours), and long-acting preparations (biological $t_{1/2}$ of 36–72 hours). See Table 12-1.

    (2) For injectable preparations, corticosteroids can be water-soluble or water-insoluble (suspension). Water-soluble injectables are in phosphate or succinate form, or dissolved in polyethylene glycol. These preparations can be administered IV, IM, or SC. Water-insoluble injectables are in acetate, pivalate, or acetonide form. These preparations can be administered IM or SC, but not IV (to avoid embolism). IM or SC administration of suspensions can attain duration of action of the corticosteroid up to 3 weeks.

  f. Therapeutic uses

    (1) Glucocorticoids

      (a) Short-acting drugs (see Table 12-1) are available without prescription for **topical use to treat pruritus and inflammation associated with allergy.**

      (b) Intermediate-acting drugs (see Table 12-1) are used for long-term control of allergy, chronic inflammation (e.g., arthritis), and immunosuppression. They can be used orally in the manner of alternate-day therapy.

      (c) Long-acting drugs (see Table 12-1)

        i. Long-acting drugs are used for the immediate relief of hypersensitivity and shock (particularly hemorrhagic and septic shock) and the long-term control of allergy in cats. They are used topically to treat pruritus and inflammation associated with allergy. In addition to the ones listed in Table 12-1, potent glucocorticoids, for example, mometasone and flucinolone are also used topically.

  ii. They may be used to induce parturition.

  iii. Isoflupredone is used to treat ketosis in cattle.

  (2) Mineralocorticoids

    (a) Aldosterone is not available as a pharmacologic agent because of its short duration of action, particularly when it is administered orally.

    (b) Deoxycorticosterone and fludrocortisone are used in the replacement therapy for hypoadrenocorticism. Deoxycorticosterone pivalate (DOCP, Percorten®-V) is used for mineralocorticoid replacement at 2.2 mg/kg, IM, once every 25 days). **Fludrocortisone has high mineralocorticoid and glucocorticoid potency; thus, it is the preferred drug for the treatment of hypoadrenocorticism.** Fludrocortisone acetate is administered orally at a dose of 0.01 mg/kg, once a day or twice a day as the initial dose. The subsequent doses should be adjusted according to the need.

  g. Administration

    (1) Oral. All synthetic corticosteroids can be administered orally. **Alternate-day oral administration of an intermediate-acting drug helps reduce the inhibition of ACTH secretion. The natural products (hydrocortisone, deoxycorticosterone) should not be administered orally, because they are quickly metabolized by the liver via enterohepatic circulation.**

    (2) IV. Water-soluble drugs (e.g., the succinate, phosphate), and polyethylene glycol form), may be given IV.

    (3) IM administration of steroids, particularly aqueous suspension [e.g., deoxycorticosterone pivalate, methylprednisolone acetate (DepoMedrol®)], may be performed at weekly intervals for chronic use.

    (4) Topical. Water-insoluble drugs are available in water suspension, cream and ointment forms.

 h. Adverse effects

    (1) Iatrogenic hypoadrenocorticism may follow withdrawal from long-term use of high doses due to a decrease in ACTH secretion.

    (2) Toxic effects following continued use of high doses are extensions of the pharmacologic effects and include

      (a) Decreased wound healing.

      (b) Increased susceptibility to infection.

      (c) Fluid and electrolyte imbalance.

      (d) Myopathy.

      (e) Osteoporosis is due to **decreased calcium absorption from the GI tract and reabsorption from the kidneys.** The slight decrease in plasma Ca^{2+} concentration, sends a signal to the parathyroid gland to **increase parathyroid hormone secretion**, which promotes bone resorption. Also, glucocorticoids **inhibit bone formation by decreasing osteoblast activity.**

      (f) Edema (from increased Na^+ retention).

      (g) Congestive heart failure in cats.

      (h) Thrombosis (due to increase in platelets in the blood).

      (i) Hepatotoxicity in dogs, which is manifested by micronodular cirrhosis and hepatomegaly.

      (j) GI ulceration.

      (k) Diabetes mellitus, particularly when used chronically in animals that already have mild diabetes.

      (l) Abortion in late pregnancy.

      (m) Laminitis in horses due to vasoconstriction of venules.

 i. Contraindications include uncontrolled infections, diabetes mellitus, corneal ulcers, cardiac disorders, burns, and pregnancy.

4. Adrenal steroid inhibitors

 a. Mitotane (o,p'-DDD)

    (1) Chemistry. Mitotane is related to DDT, an insecticide. It is a highly lipophilic drug.

(2) **Mechanism of action.** Its mechanism of action is not understood. Mitotane is **cytotoxic to zonae fasciculata and reticularis** of the adrenal cortex, which secrete all endogenous steroids except aldosterone. Zona glomerulosa, which secretes aldosterone, is not affected by mitotane.

(3) **Pharmacokinetics**

(a) Absorption of mitotane through the GI tract is variable, since it is a lipid-soluble drug. The GI absorption can be enhanced by giving the drug with food (especially high in oil/fat content) to increase bile secretion, which will help dissolve mitotane to increase absorption. Distribution of the drug occurs to virtually all tissues in the body. The drug is stored in the fat and does not accumulate in the adrenal glands.

(b) Mitotane has a very long plasma $t_{1/2}$ (in humans), ranging from 18 to 159 days. The drug is metabolized in the liver and is excreted as metabolites in the urine and bile. Approximately 15% of an oral dose is excreted in the bile, and 10% in the urine within 24 hours of dosing.

(4) **Therapeutic uses** include hyperadrenocorticism (Cushing's syndrome) and adrenal adenoma and carcinoma.

(5) **Administration.** Mitotane is administered orally (25 mg/kg, twice daily for 10–14 days, followed by 25–50 mg/kg, once per week).

(6) **Adverse effects**

(a) Animals may show lethargy, ataxia, weakness, anorexia, vomiting, or diarrhea, attributable to lowered corticosteroid secretion.

(b) Hepatotoxicity (i.e., congestion, centrolobular atrophy, and fatty degeneration) may be seen.

(c) Mitotane-induced hypoadrenocorticism may occur.

    i. In ~5% of dogs treated with mitotane, fludrocortisone may be needed as the replacement therapy.

    ii. All animals treated with mitotane should receive glucocorticoid supplementation when undergoing stress.

b. **Ketoconazole inhibits adrenal steroidogenesis** and is used to treat hyperadrenocorticism in dogs that is resistant to mitotane. It is also used as a palliative therapy in dogs with large, malignant, or invasive tumors and in whom surgery is not an option. The recommended dose is 15 mg/kg, twice daily for as long as necessary. The inhibition of steroid synthesis by ketoconazole is reversible.

(1) **Mechanism of action. Ketoconazole inhibits cytochrome P450 enzymes** that are involved in steroid synthesis (see also Chapter 15).

(2) **Pharmacokinetics**

(a) Since ketoconazole has a low pKa of 2.9, oral bioavailability of the drug in dogs is highly variable. Peak serum concentrations occur between 1 and 4 hours after dosing. This wide interpatient variation may have significant clinical implications from both a toxicity and efficacy standpoint. Administration with food may increase GI absorption, since gastric acid will be secreted to increase nonionized form of the drug.

(b) Ketoconazole is >85% bound to plasma proteins. The drug can be found in bitch's milk.

(c) It is metabolized extensively by hepatic cytochrome P450 enzymes into several inactive metabolites. These metabolites are excreted primarily into the feces via the bile. About 13% of a given dose is excreted into the urine and only 2–4% of the drug is excreted unchanged in the urine. $t_{1/2}$ in dogs is 1–6 hours (average 2.7 hours).

(3) **Adverse effects**

(a) Anorexia, vomiting, and/or diarrhea are the most common adverse effects seen with ketoconazole therapy.

(b) Hepatic toxicity consisting of cholangiohepatitis and increased liver enzymes may be seen.

(c) **Reproductive disturbances** may be seen while the dogs are on ketoconazole therapy, since it **inhibits the synthesis of all steroids.**

(d) Ketoconazole can inhibit the metabolism of other drugs that are subjected to cytochrome P450 enzymes. Drug interaction is a very important feature of ketoconazole. For example, ketoconazole and mitotane should not be used concurrently, since the metabolism of mitotane is inhibited by ketoconazole.

(e) Avoid ketoconazole in cats, since they already have deficiency in phase I enzymes.

c. **Trilostane** (Vetoryl®, Desopan®, Modrenal®)
   (1) **Chemistry.** It is a synthetic steroid analog.
   (2) **Mechanism of action.** Trilostane is a competitive inhibitor of 3-β hydroxysteroid dehydrogenase, and thus inhibits corticosteroid synthesis.
   (3) **Therapeutic uses.** Trilostane is used in dogs for treatment of hyperadrenocorticism. Initial therapy is at 2–10 mg/kg, orally once a day. It can be obtained from a compounding pharmacy.
   (4) **Pharmacokinetics**
      (a) In dogs, after oral administration, trilostane is erratically absorbed (because of high lipid solubility) with peak levels occurring within 2 hours. The presence of food in the gut to stimulate bile flow should increase absorption.
      (b) Trilostane is eliminated from the plasma within 18 hours of oral administration (elimination $t_{1/2} = \sim 1$ hour). Inhibition on corticosteroid production apparently last for ≤ 20 hours after dosing.
      (c) Trilostane is metabolized in the liver to several metabolites including ketotrilostane, which is active. The hydroxylated metabolites further undergo conjugation, which will be excreted into urine and feces.
   (5) **Adverse effects.** Lethargy, anorexia, vomiting, electrolyte abnormalities, and diarrhea. Because trilostane **inhibits progesterone synthesis, it should not be used in pregnant animals. Trilostane does not affect the synthesis of estrogens or androgens**.

d. **Selegiline** (Anipryl®)
   (1) **Mechanism of action. Selegiline inhibits ACTH secretion by increasing dopamine concentration** around corticotrope of the anterior pituitary. Selegiline **increases dopamine concentration by inhibiting the metabolism by monoamine oxidase B** (MOA-B) and decreasing the reuptake of dopamine.
   (2) **Therapeutic uses.** Selegiline is labeled for treatment of the pituitary-dependent hyperadrenocorticism in dogs, which is due to excess of ACTH secretion. However, a recent study published in the *Australian Veterinary Journal* (Vol. 82:272, 2004) showed that selegiline was not effective in the treatment of this disease. In addition, it is used to treat **canine cognitive dysfunction syndrome** (see Chapter 5 for more information). It is administered orally at 1–2 mg/kg/day.
   (3) **Pharmacokinetics**
      (a) Selegiline is absorbed rapidly and has an absolute bioavailability of $\sim 10\%$. Elimination $t_{1/2}$ is ~ 1 hour.
      (b) Selegiline is metabolized in the liver into L-desmethylselegiline, **metamphetamine, and L-amphetamine**. Each of these metabolites is active. While l-desmethylselegiline does inhibit MAO-B, the others do not, but are CNS stimulants. The drug is excreted in the urine, primarily as conjugated and unconjugated metabolites.
   (4) **Adverse effects.** Adverse effects include vomiting and diarrhea; CNS disturbances manifested by restlessness, repetitive movements, or lethargy; and salivation and anorexia. Diminished hearing/deafness, pruritus, licking, shivers/trembles/shakes have also been reported. Selegiline has the potential to be abused by humans.

C. | **Gonadotropins are glycoprotein hormones**

1. **Synthesis, secretion, and actions**
   a. **Follicle-stimulating hormone (FSH) and luteinizing hormone (LH)** are produced and secreted by the gonadotrope of the pituitary gland. Production of

FSH and LH is under hypothalamic control; it is **stimulated by gonadotropin-releasing hormone (GnRH). GnRH receptors are coupled to G_q and increases $[Ca^{2+}]_i$.**

(1) **In male animals, FSH increases the diameter of the seminiferous tubules and promotes spermatogenesis. LH increases testosterone synthesis from Leydig cells.** Secretion of FSH and LH is rather consistent in male animals.

(2) **In female animals, FSH stimulates graafian follicle development and estrogen synthesis. LH evokes ovulation and increases luteinization, leading to increased progesterone synthesis.** Secretion in female animals varies with the stage of the estrous cycle.

    (a) **Proestrus (follicular phase).** Rising FSH levels are followed by rising LH levels, which mediate follicular growth and ovulation, respectively. Production of ovarian estrogens increases. The reproductive tract is hypertrophied and hyperemic.

    (b) **Estrus (ovulation) is associated with an LH spike.**

    (c) **Metestrus–diestrus (luteal phase)** is characterized by proliferation of the reproductive tract mucosa as a result of increased progesterone production from the corpus luteum (CL). As CL involutes, ovarian steroid levels decline, causing endometrial degeneration.

b. **Human chorionic gonadotropin (HCG) has LH-like activity.** It is secreted from the placenta and extracted from **the urine of the pregnant women.**

c. **Equine chorionic gonadotropin (ECG, PMSG) has FSH-like activity.** It is secreted from the placenta and extracted from **the serum of pregnant mares.**

d. **Mechanism of action. All gonadotropin receptors are coupled to G_s, which activates adenylyl cylase to increase cyclic AMP formation, which activates protein kinase A. Thus, protein kinase A phosphorylates the cellular constituents for the action.**

2. **Preparations and therapeutic uses**

a. **Gonadorelin** is the drug name for **GnRH; desorelin** is an analog of GnRH. They are administered IM to **induce LH release for treatment of follicular cysts in cows.** They can be used to induce ovulation as well.

b. **LH and HCG**

(1) In female animals, LH and HCG are used to **induce ovulation and to treat persistent infertility.**

(2) In male animals, they can be used to **treat cryptorchidism.** LH increases testosterone production, which causes decent of the testicles into the scrotum.

c. **FSH and ECG**

(1) In females, FSH and ECG are used to **stimulate graafian follicle development**, which leads to estrus and may **increase the incidence of multiple births**.

(2) In males, FSH and ECG are used to **treat infertility**. These hormones may improve libido and spermatozoa counts.

3. **Pharmacokinetics**

a. Plasma $t_{1/2}$ of LH, FSH, HCG, and ECG are ~0.5, ~1, ~8, and ~24 hours, respectively.

b. Gonadotropins are metabolized in the liver and kidney by proteases. However, **gonadotropins as glycoprotein hormones are much more resistant to breakdown than other protein/peptide hormones.** The more carbohydrates are in the structure, the more resistant these glycoproteins are to breakdown. **Carbohydrates account for 13–16% of FSH and LH, 31% of HCG and 47% of ECG.**

4. **Adverse effects. Anaphylactic shock may develop after repeated interspecies administration of a gonadotropin.**

5. **GnRH partial agonist—leuprolide** (Leupron®Depot)

a. **Chemistry and preparation.** Leuprolide is a GnRH analog. The commercial preparation used in animals is a suspension depot form of leuprolide acetate, which should be diluted with saline before use. The diluted form of leuprolide is to negate the muscle necrosis problem and to obtain a more accurate dose than the original form. The diluted form appears to remain active after being stored in the freezer for a year.

   b. Pharmacologic effects. Leuprolide is a partial agonist of GnRH to inhibit the hyperactivity of gonadotropin—sex steroid synthesis.

   c. Therapeutic uses

   (1) Leuprolide is used to **control adrenocortical disease (ACD) in ferrets** that were neutered at 1–3 months of age. ACD is a disease due to overproduction of sex steroids by the adrenal masses. The affected ferrets show aggressive sexual behavior, constant estrus, alopecia, and pruritus. Diluted leuprolide suspension (100 μg) is administered IM once a month for this purpose. It can be used in conjunction with mitotane therapy (see III B 4).

   (2) Leuprolide is used to **inhibit ovulation for the control of inappropriate egg laying in captive cockatiels.** It is administered IM at the dose of 375 μg/bird, once a month.

   d. Pharmacokinetics. See I A 2 a, for general information. No information is available for animals.

   e. Adverse effects. At the recommended doses, leuprolide appears to be safe. The drug should not be used in pregnant animals.

D. **Sex steroids**

1. **Estrogens and anti-estrogens**

   a. Synthesis and secretion of endogenous estrogens. Endogenous estrogens are synthesized and secreted from the **ovaries, testicles (especially in stallions) adrenal cortex, and placenta.**

   b. Preparations

   (1) Steroidal estrogens include estradiol, estrone, and estriol. Estradiol is the most potent endogenous estrogen that is also used therapeutically. Estradiol is available as estradiol cypionate injectable or estradiol and estradiol benzoate ear implants for beef cattle. The estradiol benzoate implant pellets also contain other steroids, for example, progesterone or testosterone propionate/trenbolone acetate (androgen).

   (2) Nonsteroidal estrogens include zeranol (Ralgro®Implants), a mycotoxin which is used as ear implants in cattle and sheep as a growth promotant, and **diethylstilbestrol (DES),** which is used mainly in dogs and cats. DES is difficult to procure.

   c. Pharmacologic effects

   (1) Estrogens stimulate and maintain the reproductive tract and cause hyperemia, hypertrophy, and edema during estrus.

   (2) They cause cervical dilation.

   (3) They stimulate growth of the mammary glands.

   (4) They increase ossification of epiphyseal lines to limit bone growth, particularly in women.

   (5) They increase sexual receptivity.

   (6) They have protein anabolic effects (i.e., they stimulate protein synthesis).

   (7) They antagonize androgen effects by blocking androgenic receptors.

   (8) They can induce growth promotion possibly by increasing GH secretion, expression of GH receptors, insulin-like growth factors secretion.

   d. Mechanism of action. See I A 1 d for general information (also Figure 12-3).

   e. Therapeutic uses

   (1) Treatment of problems associated with **ovariohysterectomy (e.g., urinary incontinence, vaginitis, dermatitis). Phenylpropanolamine, an α-adrenergic agonist, should be used as the primary drug for the treatment of urinary incontinence.**

   (2) To relax the cervix and caudal reproductive tract for parturition induction or abortion.

   (3) It is sometimes effective in **inducing estrus** in anestrous animals.

(4) Treatment of **persistent CL** in cows. Estrogen therapy is occasionally successful.

(5) Treatment of **pyometra and mummified fetus,** however, **prostaglandin F$_{2\alpha}$ is preferred**.

(6) Treatment of **prostatic hyperplasia** or tumors associated with increased androgenic activity. Estrogens can be used as androgen receptor antagonists. However, **finasteride, an androgen inhibitor, is preferred to estrogens for this use (see III C 3 g).**

(7) **Mismating therapy** in dogs. Estrogen preparations decrease implantation and interfere with ovum transport by increasing contraction of the uterotubal sphincter. However, this is a rare practice, because estrogens can cause bone marrow depression in dogs and cats. **Prostaglandin F$_{2\alpha}$ and bromocriptine are preferred drugs for terminating pregnancy in dogs.**

(8) **Growth promotion in ruminants**

(a) **Estradiol is usually combined with progesterone or an androgen** for implantation to promote growth in calves, heifers, and steers. There is no preslaughter withdrawal time indicated for this use.

(b) **Zeranol implantation** is used to promote growth in cattle and sheep. The preslaughter withdrawal period of zeranol is 65 days in cattle and 40 days in sheep.

f. **Pharmacokinetics**

(1) Estradiol cypionate. Following IM administration, estradiol cypionate is absorbed slowly over several days. It is distributed throughout the body and accumulates in adipose tissue. Approximately **90% of estradiol is bound by plasma proteins (i.e., sex steroid-binding globulin and albumin).** Estradiol undergoes hepatic **phase II metabolism** to become estradiol glucuronide and estradiol sulfate. The estradiol metabolites are excreted into the urine and the bile and feces.

(2) Estradiol and estradiol benzoate ear implants. The absorption of estradiol from implants is very slow, taking months before it is completely absorbed.

(3) Zeranol. No information about the pharmacokinetics of zeranol implants is available.

(4) DES is readily absorbed from the GI tract of monogastric animals. It is slowly metabolized (primarily to a glucuronide) by the liver, and then it is excreted into the urine and feces.

g. **Adverse effects.** Estrogens can cause vaginal and rectal prolapse, abortion, follicular cysts, bone fractures (as a result of excessive ossification), **aplastic anemia and leucopenia** (a unique toxic effect of estrogens in dogs and cats caused by bone marrow suppression), and pyometritis.

h. **Contraindications** include pregnancy. High estrogen levels may cause fetal genitourinary malformations and may induce abortion.

i. **Anti-estrogen** (Estrogen receptor antagonist)–**Tamoxifen** (Nolvadex®)

(1) **Therapeutic uses.** Tamoxifen is used to treat **canine mammary gland tumors** at 10–20 mg orally, once every 12 hours.

(2) **Pharmacokinetics.** No information is available for dogs.

(3) **Adverse effects.** Pyometra, nausea, and vomiting.

2. **Progestins**

a. **Synthesis and secretion of progesterone.** Progesterone is synthesized and secreted from the CL and placenta of mares and ewes and from the adrenal cortex.

b. **Pharmacologic effects**

(1) Progestins increase glandular growth after priming with estrogens.

(2) Progestins prolong the luteal phase of the estrous cycle.

(3) Progestins desensitize the myometrium to oxytocin (i.e., it prevents uterine contractions during pregnancy).

(4) Progestins have anabolic effects, probably due to increased appetite and decreased physical activity.

c. **Mechanism of action.** See I A 1 d, for general information (also Figure 12-3).

d. Preparations include progesterone and synthetic progestins, medroxyprogesterone (MPA®), megestrol (Ovaban®), melengestrol (MGA®), and altrenogest (Regu-Mate®, Matrix®).

e. Therapeutic uses

(1) **Altrenogest** is administered orally to mares (0.044 mg/kg, one dose daily for 15 consecutive days) to **synchronize or suppress estrus and extend the luteal phase.** The estrus appears in 4–5 days after last dose of altrenogest. It is also given orally to gilts/sows for 14 days to extend the luteal phase. The estrus appears in 4–9 days after last dose of the drug. When used in pigs, there is a preslaughter withdrawal period of 21 days.

(2) **Melengestrol** is used as a cattle feed additive (0.28–2.2 mg/kg of body weight) for 14 days to suppress estrus and extend the luteal phase. The estrus appears in 2–6 days after the last dose of melengestrol.

(3) Progestins are used (with limited success) to treat **implantation failure and habitual abortion**.

(4) **Megestrol acetate** (2.2 mg/kg/day orally for 32 days starting in anestrus) can be used as a **contraceptive** in bitches.

(5) **Medroxyprogesterone acetate** (IM or SC) and oral **megestrol acetate** are used to **control aggressiveness and inappropriate urination or spraying**. See Chapter 5 for more information.

(6) **Progesterone combined with an estrogen increases sexual receptivity** in bitches and ewes.

(7) **Melengestrol and progesterone** are used as **growth promotants** in cattle.

    (a) Melengestrol is used as a feed additive. A withdrawal period of at least 48 hours should be implemented when using melengestrol in cattle.

    (b) Progesterone is used as an implant. No preslaughter withdrawal time is required.

f. Pharmacokinetics

(1) Progesterone is rapidly inactivated by hepatic enzymes (see below) following GI absorption, thus progesterone should not be administered orally. Synthetic progestins are more resistant to metabolism than progesterone.

(2) **Approximately 90% of progestins are bound by plasma proteins (corticosteroid-binding globulin and albumin).**

(3) The 3-keto group of a progestin is converted to 3-hydroxy group and hydroxyl groups which undergo conjugation with glucuronide or sulfate and thus the metabolites become water soluble and are excreted into urine or feces.

(4) Medroxyprogesterone acetate is an aqueous suspension. No information on the pharmacokinetics is available for animals. However, the duration of action is at least 30 days when used SC or IM to treat behavior problems in cats.

(5) Megestrol acetate is well absorbed from the GI tract of monogastric animals and is metabolized in the liver to conjugates. The $t_{1/2}$ is 8 days in dogs.

(6) Melengestrol and altrenogest. No information about the pharmacokinetics of these agents is available.

g. Adverse effects

(1) Endometrial hyperplasia, endometritis, and pyometra may occur.

(2) The glucocorticoid-like activity of the progestins may induce diabetes mellitus in animals that already have marginal diabetes.

(3) Inhibition of ACTH is also an adverse effect associated with the glucocorticoid-like activity of the progestins, which leads to iatrogenic hypoadrenocorticism after the withdrawal of the progestin.

3. Androgens

a. Synthesis and secretion of testosterone. Testosterone is secreted by the testis and adrenal cortex. In target tissues (e.g., Sertoli cells, prostate gland), testosterone is reduced to 5α-dihydrotestosterone, which has twice the biologic activity of testosterone.

b. Preparations include testosterone esters, **boldenone** (Equipoise®), and **stanozolol** (Winstrol®-V). The latter two are weak androgens and are called **anabolic steroids. Danazol** (Danocrine®) is an **androgen receptor partial agonist.**

c. Pharmacologic effects

(1) Androgens have masculinizing effects.

(a) Testosterone is responsible for the development of the **accessory sex organs, epididymis, vas deferens, prostate, and seminal vesicles,** and the secondary sex characteristics.

(b) Acting in conjunction with FSH, testosterone promotes **spermatogenesis.**

(c) Androgens at the appropriate doses can **increase libido.**

(2) Androgens have **anabolic effects,** leading to increased protein synthesis (particularly in skeletal muscle), retention of potassium and phosphorus, and increased growth of bone cartilage and other tissues.

(3) Androgens increase **erythropoiesis by promoting the secretion of erythropoietin.** This effect of androgens can be used for the **treatment of anemia.**

(4) High doses of androgens can **inhibit gonadotropin secretions** to suppress the estrous cycle, particularly if they are given before the onset of proestrus.

(5) Danazol is a synthetic partial androgen receptor agonist. It can suppress the pituitary–ovarian axis. Danazol may directly inhibit sex steroids synthesis, and binds to sex steroid receptors in cells/tissues, where it may express anabolic, weak androgenic, and antiestrogenic effects. Danazol appears to reduce affinity of antibody with the mononuclear phagocytic system F_c-receptor.

d. Therapeutic uses

(1) Testosterone has been used:

(a) To treat impotency and infertility, with variable success.

(b) To treat urinary incontinence and dermatitis in castrated males.

(c) To produce a teaser animal in cull cows, heifers, and steers.

(2) Stanozolol and boldenone are used for growth promotion, muscle buildup, and reversal of tissue depletion (e.g., cachexia) and to treat anemia, particularly due to chronic renal failure, chronic arthritis, and degenerative myelopathy.

(3) Stanozolol is administered orally on the daily basis, or IM as a suspension at the weekly basis. Boldenone in sesame oil is administered IM once every 3 weeks.

(4) Trenbolone and testosterone are used as implants for growth promotion in cattle. See III C 1 e (8).

(5) Danazol is primarily used as adjunctive therapy with glucocorticoids in the treatment of canine immune-mediated thrombocytopenia and hemolytic anemia, particularly if the patient becomes refractory to glucocorticoids and other immunosuppressants. It is administered orally at 5 mg/kg twice daily; can taper dose once patient is on low dose alternate day prednisone/prednisolone (see III E).

e. Pharmacokinetics

(1) After absorption, androgens are distributed throughout the body and accumulate in adipose tissue. **Approximately 90% of androgens are bound by plasma proteins (i.e., sex steroid-binding globulin and albumin, just like estrogens).** Androgens undergo hepatic metabolism to become glucuronide and sulfate conjugates. The metabolites are excreted into the urine and the bile, further into feces.

(2) Testosterone ester suspensions or in oil are administered IM. The duration of action may persist for 2–4 weeks. The plasma $t_{1/2}$ of testosterone cypionate after IM administration is 8 days.

(3) Boldenone and stanozolol are well absorbed after IM administration; stanozolol may also be administered orally. When administered IM, the effects of boldenone in oil persist up to 8 weeks, while those of stanozolol in suspension persist for >1 week.

(4) Danazol is absorbed from the GI tract, but appears to be a rate-limited process as increasing the dosage does not yield a corresponding increase in plasma concentration. It is metabolized in the liver. Other information is not available.

f. Adverse effects include

(1) Infertility or oligospermia.

(2) Perianal adenomas, perineal hernias, prostatic disorders, and behavioral changes (following long-term androgen administration).

(3) Masculinization of females and female fetuses.

(4) Hepatotoxicity.

g. Antiandrogens–Finasteride (Proscar®)

(1) Pharmacologic effects. Finasteride decreases androgenic activity of the animals by **inhibiting the formation of 5α-dihydrotestosterone**, which is an active and potent testosterone metabolite.

(2) Therapeutic uses. Finasteride can be used orally at 0.1–0.5 mg/kg once a day to treat **benign prostatic hyperplasia** (BPH) in dogs. However, because the drug is expensive, and the long duration of therapy is required to see a response, its usefulness may be limited. **For BPH, the recommended therapy is castration.**

(3) Pharmacokinetics. No information is available for dogs.

(4) Adverse effects. No adverse effects have been seen with recommended doses, except that finasteride is a **teratogen**.

E. **Uterine contractants and drugs to induce luteolysis.** When used to induce labor, these agents are called oxytocic or ecbolic agents. When they are used to induce abortion, they are called abortifacients.

1. General uterine physiology

a. Hormonal influence. Estrogen and progesterone influence uterine activity.

(1) During proestrus and estrus, under the influence of estrogens, the uterus shows large and slow contractions.

(2) During metestrus–diestrus, under the influence of progesterone, the uterus shows weak and rapid contractions.

(3) At parturition, a surge of fetal ACTH and cortisol secretion stimulates synthesis of estrogens and prostaglandins, which lead to luteolysis.

(a) The presence of CL in prepartum animals inhibits the action of an oxytocic agent; therefore, luteolysis may be needed to induce parturition.

(b) Because prepartum mares do not have a functional CL, **an oxytocic agent alone can effectively induce foaling.**

(c) Oxytocin secretion and the density of oxytocin receptors increase, leading to large and effective uterine contractions that expel the fetuses from the reproductive tract. Oxytocin receptors are coupled to G_q.

b. Autonomic influence. Adrenergic and cholinergic activities also influence smooth muscle contraction (see also Chapter 2 for detailed information).

(1) α_1- and α_2-adrenergic receptors mediate excitatory responses, whereas β_2-adrenergic receptors mediate inhibitory responses.

(2) M_3-muscarinic receptors mediate excitatory responses.

2. Preparations

a. Oxytocin is a nonapeptide hypothalamic hormone stored in and released from the posterior pituitary. It is released in response to signals from the genital tract and mammary gland to the hypothalamus.

(1) Actions. Oxytocin increases **uterine contractions and milk ejection and facilitates the transport of sperm in the female genital tract**.

(2) Therapeutic uses

(a) Oxytocin is used to induce labor and reverse uterine inertia. The cervix must be dilated and the fetus must be in normal presentation position. Oxytocin works poorly when CL exists.

(b) It is used to treat agalactia through stimulation of milk ejection. However, oxytocin is not a galactopoietic agent.

(3) Pharmacokinetics. See I A 2 a.

(4) Adverse effects. Oxytocin may cause **uterine dystocia**.

b. Ergonovine is an ergot alkaloid that causes **prolonged contraction of smooth muscle, including the myometrium and blood vessels**.

   (1) Mechanism of action. Its effect on smooth muscle is mainly through activation of **α-adrenergic receptors** and possibly also through modulation of serotonergic and dopaminergic receptors.

   (2) Therapeutic uses

   (a) Induction of uterine involution.

   (b) Postpartum hemorrhage control.

   (c) Expulsion of placenta (particularly in cows and bitches) when oxytocin is ineffective.

   (3) Administration. Ergonovine is administered orally to dogs (0.2 mg) or IM to mares (1–3 mg).

   (4) Pharmacokinetics. Information is not available for animals; however, after administration, the **duration of action is 2–4 hours**.

   (5) Adverse effects. Ergonovine is safe when given as directed; however, overdose may cause **CNS excitation, muscle weakness, hypertension, and vomiting** (in dogs). **It may cause agalactia through inhibition of prolactin release.**

c. Bromocriptine (Parlodel®) and cabergoline (Dostinex®): These drugs are ergot derivatives, having dopaminergic agonistic activity.

   (1) Mechanism of action. The dopaminergic agonistic activity **inhibits prolactin secretion by activating D_2 receptors, resulting in luteolysis. (Prolactin is a luteotropic hormone and it also inhibits gonadotropin release.)** Cabergoline is more potent than bromocriptine in activating D_2 receptors.

   (2) Therapeutic uses

   (a) They are used to **treat galactorrhea.**

   (b) They have been used to **induce luteolysis.**

   i. Bromocriptine is given orally (10–15 μg/kg) twice daily for 3–5 days to terminate pregnancy in dogs or for 10–14 days to **treat pseudopregnancy.**

   ii. Cabergoline is given 5 μg/kg, orally, once daily for 5–10 days to **induce estrus or to treat pseudopregnancy.**

   (3) Pharmacokinetics. The information is not available for animals.

   (a) In humans, after oral administration, both drugs are absorbed from the GI tract. More than 90% of bromocriptine and 50% of cabergoline are bound by albumin.

   (b) Both of them are metabolized by the liver (hydroxylation) to inactive metabolites, which are excreted into urine. Bromocriptine has a biphasic $t_{1/2}$; the α-phase is about 4 hours and the terminal β-phase is about 15 hours. Cabergoline has a $t_{1/2}$ of 60 hours.

   (4) Adverse effects. Both drugs are safe when used as directed. However, they may cause vomiting, sedation, and hypotension (due to α-adrenergic antagonism). They may cause agalactia in lactating animals.

d. Prostaglandin $F_{2\alpha}$ ($PGF_{2\alpha}$, **dinoprost tromethamine**, Lutalyse®) and an analog (cloprostenol, Estrumate®)

   (1) Pharmacologic effects

   (a) $PGF_{2\alpha}$ and analogs cause strong vasoconstriction. The resultant decreased blood supply causes **luteolysis and reduction of progesterone synthesis.**

   (b) $PGF_{2\alpha}$ and analogs have a strong oxytocic effect, especially in mares.

   (2) Therapeutic uses

   (a) Estrous cycle control in cows. $PGF_{2\alpha}$ and analog induce luteolysis of mature corpora. This method is not used in sows, since $PGF_{2\alpha}$ yields inconsistent luteolysis in sows.

   (b) Early abortion usually occurs within 7 days of injection as a result of luteolysis.

   (c) Labor induction. Perform the induction 3–15 days before due. In cows and sows, 1–8 days after administration (average 3 days). In mares, 1–2 days after administration. If milk is present (waxing in mares), labor can be induced in 30 minutes. Because cows and sows have CL in the

prepartum period, $PGF_{2\alpha}$ is used mainly to induce luteolysis. Because mares do not have CL in the prepartum period, $PGF_{2\alpha}$ is mainly to exert an oxytocic effect.

(d) Pyometra. $PGF_{2\alpha}$ can be used to treat pyometra and facilitate the expulsion of mummified fetuses.

(e) Ovarian cysts. Following treatment with GnRH to cause ovulation, $PGF_{2\alpha}$ is administered to induce luteolysis.

(f) The dosage of cloprostenol is 1–5% that of dinoprost because cloprostenol is more resistant to metabolism than dinoprost.

(3) Pharmacokinetics

(a) $PGF_{2\alpha}$ (dinoprost) is distributed rapidly to tissues after IM administration. In cattle, the plasma $t_{1/2}$ is only a few minutes.

(b) Cloprostenol is more resistant to metabolism than dinoprost.

(4) Adverse effects include placental retention, dystocia, and acute systemic toxicity (i.e., salivation, vomiting, colic, defecation, fever, anxiety, tachycardia, tachypnea; sweating and transient decreased rectal temperature are seen in mares).

e. Long-acting glucocorticoids

(1) Mechanism of action. These agents can mimic the action of fetal cortisol surge, thereby inducing parturition. Glucocorticoids increase $PGF_2\alpha$ synthesis in the endometrium.

(2) Therapeutic uses and administration. Dexamethasone has been used to induce parturition in cows and ewes. In prepartum cows, dexamethasone (20 mg IM) may induce parturition within 48 hours. If dexamethasone administration is followed in 40 hours by dinoprost (30 mg IM), calving occurs within 2–5 hours.

(3) Pharmacokinetics. See III B 3 d.

(4) Adverse effects. Placental retention may occur. The adverse effects are usually not a problem when glucocorticoids are used as oxytocic agents.

F. | Antidiabetic agents

1. Introduction. Diabetes mellitus is usually seen in adult animals, particularly dogs and cats >7 years of age. The diabetes mellitus in animals is similar to type 2 diabetes in human; however, it is usually in the very late stage of the disease when it is detected, and thus β-cells have mostly been destroyed by severe hyperglycemia. Therefore, most of diabetic animals need to be on insulin therapy.

2. Insulin remains the most frequently used antidiabetic agent in veterinary medicine.

a. Synthesis, secretion, and actions

(1) Synthesis. Insulin consists of two peptide chains joined by disulfide linkages (Figure 12-4).

(a) Pancreatic β-cells synthesize insulin from a single-chain precursor—proinsulin, which possesses little biologic activity. Inuslin is formed when C-peptide is cleaved from proinsulin.

(b) The amino acid sequence of insulin varies among species.

i. Porcine and canine insulin molecules are identical, and are similar to human insulin (difference in insulin structure: B-30 is alanine in porcine and canine insulin, and is threonine in human insulin).

ii. Feline and bovine insulin are similar in structure.

(2) Secretion. Insulin secretion is controlled mainly by blood glucose levels, GI hormones, and the autonomic nervous system.

(a) Stimulation. Insulin secretion is increased by glucose, amino acids, fatty acids (especially butyric acid in ruminants), Ca^{2+}, and GI hormones [e.g., secretin, gastrin, cholecystokinin, glucagon, glucagon-like polypeptide-1 (GLP-1), gastric inhibitory peptide (GIP), vasoactive intestinal peptide]. GLP-1 and GIP are most potent insulin secretagogues among GI hormones. The receptors of these GI hormones are coupled either to G_s or G_q. Amino acids may stimulate the secretion of GI hormones.

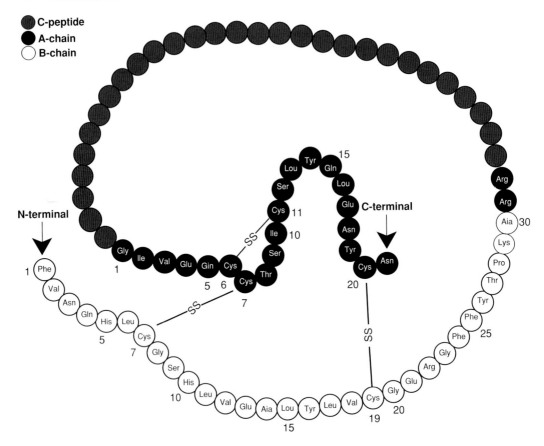

FIGURE 12-4. Structure of porcine (canine) proinsulin. (Modified from Fig. 34.1 of Adams' *Veterinary Pharmacology and Therapeutics*, 8th ed.)

      (b) Inhibition. insulin secretion is inhibited by somatostatin, galanin, epinephrine and norepinephrine. The receptors mediating the inhibition on insulin release are coupled to $G_{i/o}$.

      (c) Autonomic influences

          i. Epinephrine and norepinephrine inhibit insulin secretion by activating α_2-adrenergic receptors (coupled to $G_{i/o}$).

          ii. In the presence of α_2-receptor blockade, epinephrine and norepinephrine stimulate insulin secretion by activating β_2-adrenergic receptors (coupled to G_s).

          iii. Acetylcholine (ACh) stimulates insulin secretion by activating M_3-receptors (coupled to G_q).

    (3) Pharmacologic effects

      (a) Carbohydrate metabolism. Insulin decreases blood glucose concentrations by increasing glycogen synthesis, decreasing hepatic glycogenolysis, decreasing gluconeogenesis, and increasing glucose transport into skeletal muscle cells and adipocytes through activation of type 4 glucose transporters (GLUT4).

      (b) Fat metabolism. Insulin increases lipid synthesis and decreases lipolysis.

      (c) Protein metabolism. Insulin increases the uptake of amino acids and protein synthesis.

      (d) K^+ metabolism. Insulin increases uptake of K^+ into skeletal muscle and fat cells by providing ATP to activate the Na^+, K^+-ATPase (pump). Hyperkalemia may be seen in diabetic patients; after an adequate insulin therapy, hyperkalemia will disappear.

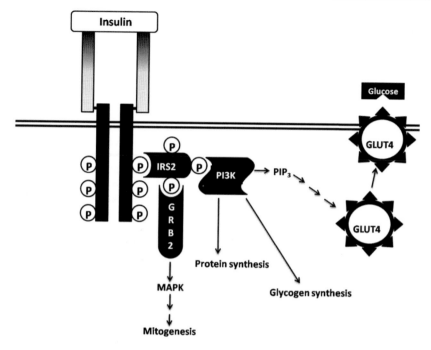

FIGURE 12-5. Mechanism of action of insulin. The insulin receptor is a tetramer; 2α-subunits (ligand binding domain) and 2β-subunits (tyrosine kinase domain). Activation of the receptor by insulin evokes autophosphorylation of tyrosine kinase, which in turn, activates insulin receptor substrates (IRS). Activated IRS binds and activates phosphoinositol 3-kinase (PI3K), which catalyzes the formation of phosphoinositol 3,4,5-triphosphate (PIP$_3$). PIP$_3$ stimulates translocation of glucose transport4 (GLUT4) to plasma membrane, glycogen synthesis, and protein synthesis. Activated IRS can also bind growth factor receptor-binding protein-2 (GRB-2), which stimulates the mitogen-activated protein kinase (MAPK) system to promote mitogenesis.

    b. Mechanism of action. Insulin binds to its receptors and stimulates tyrosine kinase (Figure 12-5).

    c. Pharmacokinetics. Insulin is metabolized by enzymes in the liver and kidney. The plasma $t_{1/2}$ of insulin is 5–10 minutes, but the biologic $t_{1/2}$ is longer (several hours).

    d. Preparations. Commercial insulin preparations are mostly of human origin and are produced using a recombinant DNA technique. **Only two insulin preparations are marketed exclusively for animals: Vetsulin®and PZI Vet®.**

        (1) Crystalline zinc insulin (regular insulin) is a short-acting, soluble human insulin that is prepared in a phosphate buffer with zinc at a pH of 3.5.

            (a) Pharmacokinetics. Onset of effect occurs within 15 minutes of SC injection, peaks within 2–4 hours, and lasts 5–7 hours.

            (b) Administration. It can be administered SC or IV. Injections must be given 4–5 times daily, which can be cumbersome.

            (c) Therapeutic uses. Crystalline zinc insulin is useful for rapidly resolving diabetic ketoacidosis. The frequency with which regular insulin must be administered makes it inconvenient for maintenance of normal plasma glucose concentrations.

        (2) Isophane insulin (NPH) is an intermediate-acting insulin that contains a small amount of protamine (0.3–0.4 mg/100 U insulin), a basic protein that slows down the absorption of insulin. **The onset of action for NPH insulin occurs within 2 hours. Peak effect occurs in 8–12 hours and lasts 24 hours.**

        (3) Lente insulin does not contain protamine. Its insolubility results from the addition of zinc in an acetate buffer, rather than a phosphate buffer. The onset of action for the Lente insulin depends on the physical state, the zinc concentration, and the pH.

  (a) **Semilente insulin** is a microamorphous form of insulin. **Peak effect occurs in 4–8 hours and has duration of action of 12–16 hours.**

  (b) **Ultralente insulin** is a large crystalline form of insulin with high zinc content. **Its onset and duration of action are similar to those of protamine zinc insulin** [see (4)].

  (c) **Lente insulin** consists of seven parts ultralente and three parts semilente. **It is quite similar to isophane insulin in its onset and duration of action. Lente porcine insulin (Vetsulin®)** is available for animal use, particularly in dogs.

(4) **Protamine zinc insulin.** The addition of protamine to crystalline zinc insulin causes the formation of large crystals. **There is a veterinary product consisting of 90% bovine insulin and 10% porcine insulin (PZI Vet®), which is for feline patients.**

  (a) **Pharmacokinetics.** When injected SC, this formulation serves as a tissue depot, producing slow absorption into the blood stream. **The action of protamine zinc insulin begins in 4 hours, peaks in 16–18 hours, and lasts up to 36 hours.**

  (b) **Therapeutic uses.** Fine control of hyperglycemia is difficult with such a long-acting preparation. **However, because of its prolonged action, protamine zinc insulin is convenient for use in veterinary medicine.**

(5) **Insulin glargine (Lantus®).** This is a **recombinant human insulin analog** with a glycine residue at A-chain 21st amino acid residue and 2-arginine residues at B-chain 31st and 32nd amino acid residues. Insulin glargine is soluble at pH 4. **After administration, at pH 7.4, it forms microprecipitates, which slow down the absorption from the injection site.** After SC administration, there is **no pronounced peak levels of insulin detected, but stable antihyperglycemic effect of insulin lasts >24 hours.**

e. **Adverse effects**

(1) **Hypoglycemia.** Early signs of hypoglycemia (e.g., tachycardia, hunger) result from epinephrine release. "Insulin shock," the worst sequela of hypoglycemia, is characterized by CNS disturbances, including convulsions and coma. Severe hypoglycemia is best treated with IV glucose infusion.

(2) **Insulin resistance.** Some diabetic animals may experience insulin resistance.

  (a) **Insulin antibodies** may attenuate responses to exogenous insulin. They are more likely to develop in cats than in dogs given human or porcine insulin preparations.

  (b) **Stress** may induce acute insulin resistance by increasing secretion of epinephrine and corticosteroids.

  (c) **Insulin receptor desensitization/down-regulation** could lead to insulin resistance.

3. **Sulfonylureas (e.g., glipizide, glyburide, and glimepiride)** are rarely used in veterinary medicine, since in most of the diabetic animals by the time the diabetes is diagnosed, they already have lost most, if not all, of the β-cells. Sulfonylureas are lipid soluble drugs.

a. **Mechanism of action.** Sulfonylureas stimulate insulin secretion from β-cells (Figure 12-6).

(1) **They block ATP-sensitive K^+ channels**, which decrease K^+ exit from β-cells.

(2) Retention of intracellular K^+ leads to **depolarization** of the plasma membrane, which activates the **voltage-dependent Ca^{2+} channels** (VDCCs).

(3) **Opening of VDCCs** promotes Ca^{2+} entry to elevate $[Ca^{2+}]_i$. Ca^{2+} evokes exocytosis, resulting in insulin release.

(4) **ATP can block ATP-sensitive K^+ channels** as well. ATP is generated from glucose metabolism. (This also explains how glucose stimulates insulin secretion.)

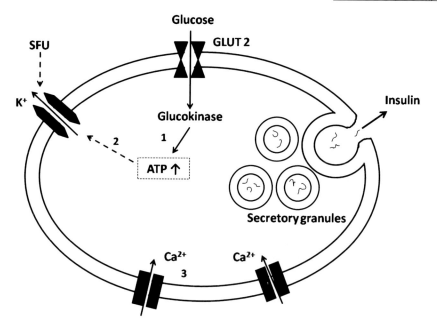

FIGURE 12-6. Mechanism of action of sulfonylurea (SFU) and glucose on insulin release from pancreatic β-cells. 1. Glucose via glucose transporter 2 (GLUT2) enters the cell, which is metabolized by glucokinase to form ATP. 2. ATP blocks ATP-sensitive K^+ channels to stop K^+ efflux, which causes retention of intracellular K^+, leading to depolarization. 3. The depolarization opens L-type Ca^{2+} channels, thereby increasing Ca^{2+} influx. Ca^{2+} promotes insulin exocytosis. SFU also blocks ATP-sensitive K^+ channels to increase insulin exocytosis.

    b. Therapeutic uses. Sulfonylureas have been used with some success to treat diabetes in cats.

    c. Pharmacokinetics

        (1) Glipizide is rapidly and fairly well absorbed after oral administration. Food will enhance absorption because it stimulates bile flow to help dissolve sulfonylureas. Glipizide is very highly bound to plasma proteins. It is primarily biotransformed in the liver by cytochrome P450 enzymes to inactive metabolites that are then excreted by the kidneys. Effects on insulin secretion in cats tend to be short-lived; plasma insulin concentrations peak in ~15 minutes and return to baseline after 60 minutes.

        (2) No information on glyburide and glimpiride is available for animals.

    d. Adverse effects. Sulfonylureas are safe when used as directed. Overdose-induced hypoglycemia is much milder than that induced by insulin and is usually not life-threatening.

  4. Metformin. It is an oral antihyperglycemic, but not hypoglycemic drug.

    a. Mechanism of action. Metformin exerts its antihyperglycemic effect by: **(1) decreasing glucose absorption from GI tract, (2) decreasing glucose output from liver, and (3) increasing insulin receptor sensitivity. Metformin does not stimulate insulin secretion and thus does not cause hypoglycemia.**

    b. Therapeutic uses. Metformin has been used orally (given with food) with some success to treat diabetes in cats, particularly in combination with a sulfonylurea.

    c. Pharmacokinetics. A total of 35–65% of metformin is absorbed after oral administration. In cats, elimination $t_{1/2}$ is ~12 hours. Metformin is primarily eliminated via the kidneys. Metformin's pharmacokinetics in cats are similar to that seen in humans, and that a dosage of 2 mg/kg, twice daily would yield plasma concentrations known to be effective in humans.

    d. Adverse effects. Metformin may cause lethargy, anorexia, vomiting and weight loss in cats. Metformin alone does not cause hypoglycemia.

G. **Thyroid hormones and antithyroid agents**

1. **Thyroid hormones**
   a. **Synthesis**
      (1) Thyroglobulin (TG), a large glycoprotein, is synthesized in the thyroid gland and transported into the follicular lumen (colloid).
      (2) The tyrosine residues on TG are iodinated to form monoiodotyrosine (MIT) and diiodotyrosine (DIT) (Figure 12-7).
         (a) Thyroxine (T_4) is formed by the coupling of DITs.
         (b) Triiodothyronine (T_3) is formed from MIT and DIT.
      (3) Endocytosis and proteolysis of TG from colloid release T_3 and T_4 into follicular cells. The hormones are then transported out of the cells through diffusion into the circulation (Figure 12-8).
   b. **Secretion.** Thyrotropin (TSH) stimulates thyroid hormone secretion by increasing NaI uptake, oxidation to I_2, coupling process, and endocytosis and proteolysis of iodinated TG.
      (1) **Other anions, such as nitrate, thiocyanate, and perchlorate, inhibit NaI uptake** by competing with iodide for active transport.
      (2) **Thioureylene drugs (e.g., methimazole)** inhibit oxidation and coupling processes.
   c. **Pharmacokinetics**
      (1) **Absorption.** T_3 and T_4 are readily absorbed from the GI tract when given orally.
      (2) **Distribution.**
         (a) Both T_3 and T_4 are bound by plasma proteins thyroxine-binding globulin (TBG), transthyretin, and albumin. TBG has much higher affinity for T_3 and T_4 than other plasma proteins. **Humans have four times as much of TBG than dogs.**
         (b) **Cats, rabbits, rodents, and birds do not have detectable TBG level.** High estrogen levels promote synthesis of TBG, leading to increased total T_3 and T_4 concentrations in the plasma.
         (c) Plasma protein-binding activities of thyroid hormones differ among animal species (Figure 12-9), as a result the plasma concentrations of free hormones are also different among species. **Free hormones are the ones that activate receptors, and subject to metabolism and elimination.**
      (3) **Metabolism**
         (a) A total of 30–40% of T_4 is converted to T_3, thereby increasing biologic activity in the liver, kidney, and other peripheral tissues.
         (b) A total of 15–20% of T_4 and ~100% of T_3 form conjugates with glucuronide and sulfate in the liver. These conjugates are then excreted in the bile. Through enterohepatic circulation, some T_3 and T_4 are liberated and reabsorbed from the GI tract.
         (c) Fifty percent of T_4 is converted in peripheral tissues to reverse T_3, which is an inactive metabolite.
      (4) **Plasma $t_{1/2}$ after oral administration**
         (a) **In humans, the plasma $t_{1/2}$ of T_4 and T_3 are 7 days and 1 day, respectively, due to high plasma TBG levels.**
         (b) **In dogs, the plasma $t_{1/2}$ of T_4 and T_3 are 12–24 hours and ~8 hours, respectively.**
         (c) **In cats, the plasma $t_{1/2}$ of T4 is ~11 hours.**
         (d) **Factors affecting plasma $t_{1/2}$**
            i. Conversion rate from T_4 to T_3 is increased during hypothyroidism and is decreased during hyperthyroidism as a compensatory process, attempting to overcome the disorder.
            ii. Increased TBG levels increase plasma $t_{1/2}$.
            iii. Decreased plasma protein levels decrease plasma $t_{1/2}$.
            iv. Other drugs that compete for albumin-binding sites increase free T_3 and T_4 levels, leading to decreased plasma $t_{1/2}$.

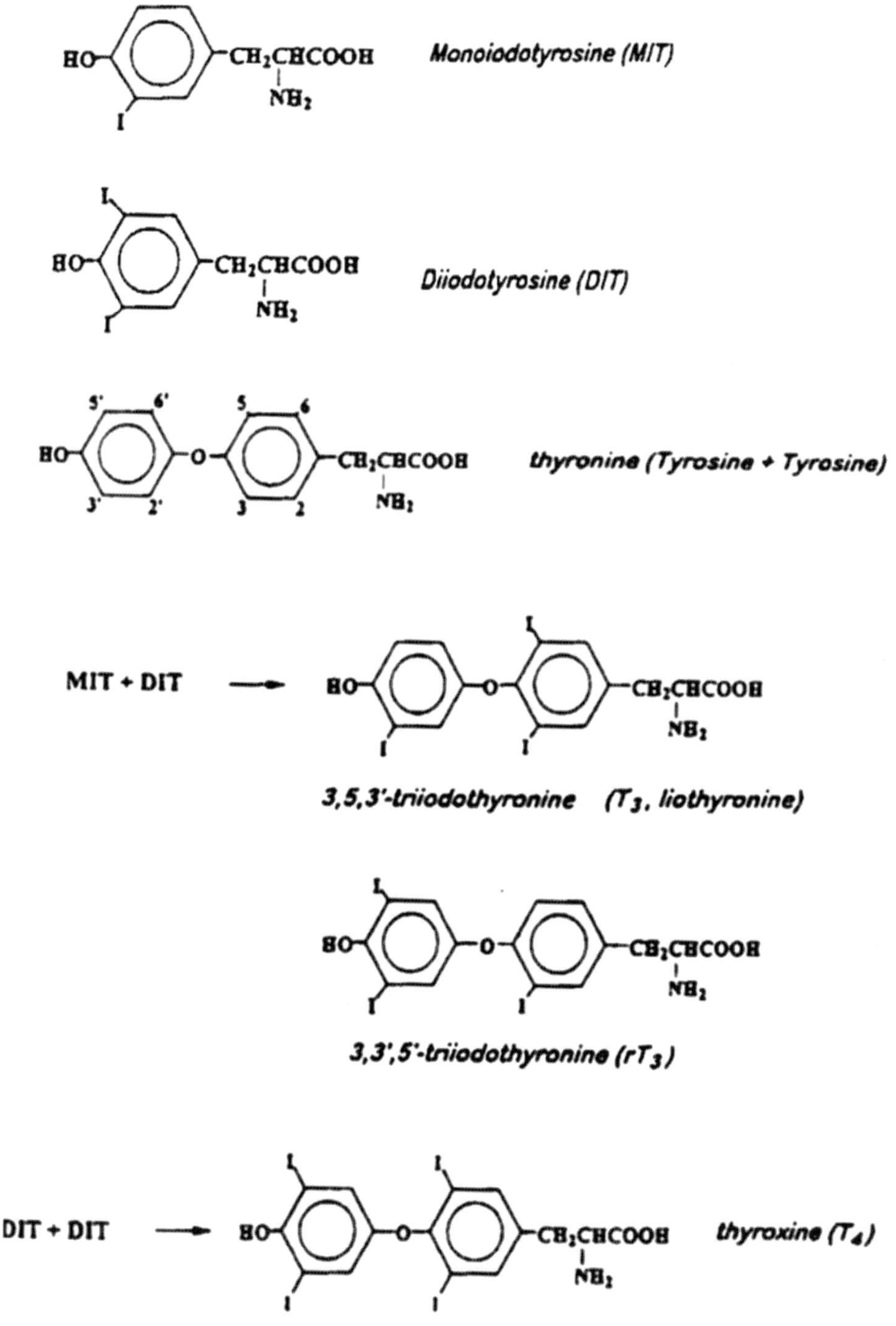

FIGURE 12-7. Structure of iodinated tyrosines and thyroid hormones.

   (6) Excretion. A total of 20–40% of administered T_4 is excreted in the feces.
   d. Physiologic and pharmacologic effects. T_3 is 3–5 times as active as T_4. **T_4 is the prothyroid hormone, and T_3 is the thyroid hormone.**
   (1) T_3 promotes growth and development. These effects of T_3 are attributable in part to the T_3-induced increase in GH secretion and action. T_3 is important for neural growth and maintenance.

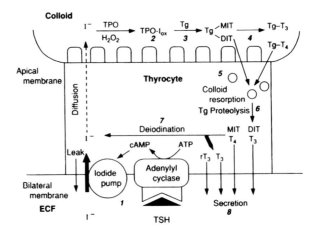

FIGURE 12-8. Thyroid hormone synthesis pathway. 1. Inorganic iodide (I^-) is pumped into the follicular cell from ECF. Activation of TSH receptor stimulates the iodide pump. 2. The iodide is oxidized by thyroid peroxidase (TPO) into iodine (I_{ox}). 3. I_{ox} iodinates tyrosine residues of thyroglobulin (TG) in the colloid to form monoiodotyrosine (MIT) and diiodotyrosine (DIT). 4. The MIT and DIT residues on TG couple to form triiodothyronine (T_3) and reverse T_3. Two DIT residues couple to form thyroxine (T_4). 5. The TG containing T_3, rT_3, and T_4 returns to follicular cells. 6. The TG complex undergoes proteolysis to release T_3, rT_3, T_4, MIT, and DIT. 7. MIT and DIT are deiodinated, allowing recycling of I^-. 8. The newly synthesized T_3, rT_3, and T_4 diffuse into the circulation. (Reprinted From S. J. Ettinger. *Textbook of Veterinary Internal Medicine*, W. B. Saunders, 1990.)

(2) T_3 increases the basal metabolic rate; therefore, it is calorigenic. In addition, T_3 increases heat production by activating uncoupling oxidative phosphorylation in brown fat cells. T_3 exerts this effect by increasing the synthesis of uncoupling proteins in the mitochondria, and thus inhibits ATP formation and produces heat.

(3) T_3 is a cardiovascular stimulant, since it increases cardiac output and enhances the sensitivity of the myocardium to catecholamines. T_3 increases the expression of α- and β-adrenergic receptors, α-myosin light chain, Na^+,

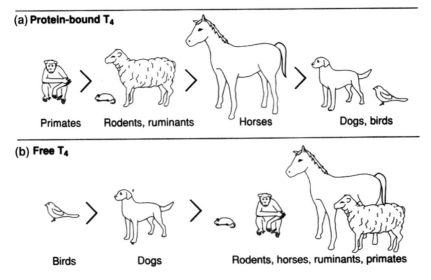

FIGURE 12-9. Thyroxine (T_4)-binding activity of plasma proteins by species. (From Figure 8-3, *NVMS Pharmacology*, page 166.)

K^+-ATPase, and Na^+ and Ca^{2+} channels in both myocardial muscle and vascular smooth muscle (all of these proteins may have contributed to cardiovascular effects of thyroid hormones).

(4) T_3 enhances carbohydrate utilization and lipolysis. T_3 decreases plasma concentrations of low-density lipoprotein (LDL) by increasing the expression of LDL transport receptors in the liver, thereby increasing utilization of LDL by the liver.

(5) T_3 can promote milk production. Many years ago, iodinated casein was used as a feed additive for dairy cattle to promote milk production. However, it was not a profitable practice, since the cattle consumed large amount of feed and produced large amount of waste after becoming hyperthyroid.

e. Mechanism of action

(1) T_3 increases mRNA synthesis for a number of proteins that are important for thyroid hormone functions.

(2) T_3 activates its mitochondrial receptors to increase mRNA synthesis in this organelle.

(3) Thyroid hormone metabolites may activate G protein-coupled receptors (e.g., G_q) to mediate its acute and nongenomic effects.

f. Preparations

(1) Levothyroxine is T_4.

(2) Liothyronine is the drug name for T_3.

g. Administration. Because of different plasma protein-binding activities of the thyroid hormones in humans and dogs, human dosages should not be used in dogs. T_4 is preferred to T_3 in the replacement therapy due to the fact that T_4 can maintain higher thyroid hormone activity in brain than T_3.

(1) Levothyroxine. The initial dose in dogs is 20 μg/kg/day, orally.

(2) Liothyronine. The initial dose in dogs is 5 μg/kg orally, 2–3 times daily.

(3) Doses may need to be adjusted following the initial dose.

h. Adverse effects. Overdose with thyroid hormones will produce signs of hyperthyroidism.

2. Antithyroid agents

a. Thioureylenes (methimazole). Methimazole is a preferred antithyroid medication for hyperthyroid cats.

(1) Mechanism of action. Methimazole inhibits the synthesis of T_3 and T_4 (see G 1 b).

(2) Pharmacokinetics

(a) GI absorption after oral administration in cats is rapid and complete with bioavailability of near 80%.

(b) Methimazole is widely distributed in the body with no significant protein-binding activity.

(c) It is metabolized by hepatic cytochrome P450 enzymes, followed by conjugation with glucuronide in other species than cats. Since cats tend to have drug metabolism problems, this might explain the wide range of elimination $t_{1/2}$ of methimazole in cats (see below).

(d) No information is available for cats. In humans, only 10% of methimazole is excreted in urine.

(e) The elimination $t_{1/2}$ of methimazole in cats is 2–10 hours (average 6.6 hours).

(f) Because of the high plasma-binding activity of thyroid hormones, plasma levels of T_3 and T_4 decline slowly. Significant reduction of signs of hyperthyroidism is usually seen in 1–3 weeks.

(3) Adverse effects. Anorexia, vomiting, lethargy, pruritus, hepatopathy, hemorrhage, thrombocytopenia, agranulocytosis, leukopenia, eosinophilia, and lymphocytosis may occur.

b. Ipodate can be used in cats that cannot tolerate methimazole. It can be obtained from a compounding pharmacy.

(1) Mechanism of action. Ipodate is an iodine-containing compound that inhibits the conversion of T_4 into T_3 by binding to iodinases. It might also block T_3 receptors and actions of TSH.

(2) Therapeutic uses. Ipodate is useful in feline hyperthyroidism, who cannot tolerate the adverse effects of methimazole.

(3) Pharmacokinetics. Ipodate is well absorbed from the GI tract after oral administration (100–200 mg/cat/day). The other information is not available for animals.

(4) Adverse effects. Cats may become refractory to ipodate treatment after a relatively short time. GI distress (nausea, vomiting, diarrhea, cramping, inappetence) may be seen in cats dosed with ipodate. Skin rashes, itching, dizziness, and headache have been reported by human patients.

c. Radioactive iodide (Na^{131} I)

(1) Mechanism of action. Na^{131}I destroys thyroid follicles. Therefore, it is an alternative to surgical thyroidectomy, which runs a risk for damaging parathyroid glands.

(2) Pharmacokinetics. Na^{131}I is rapidly incorporated into the thyroid follicles. It has a $t_{1/2}$ of 8 days and emits β-particles and X-ray. Serum T_4 and T_3 concentrations will normalize within 1–2 weeks of administration.

(3) Therapeutic uses. Na^{131}I is used to treat hyperthyroidism in cats and thyroid adenocarcinoma in both cats and dogs.

(4) Administration. Na^{131}I is administered SC at 1–5 mCi in cats; 5% patients need a second dose.

The treated animals should be hospitalized for 1–4 weeks. The use of Na^{131}I is under strict federal regulation. The treated animals and excreta need to be handled carefully to avoid contamination; the excreta need to be safely stored until radioactivity is gone.

(5) Adverse effects. Hypothyroidism may result.

(6) Contraindications. Na^{131}I is contraindicated in pregnant and nursing queens.

H. **Agents for the treatment of hypocalcemia**

1. Regulation of serum calcium levels

a. Secretion and actions of parathyroid hormone (PTH). PTH is secreted from the parathyroid gland. Its secretion is increased in response to hypocalcemia and decreased in response to hypercalcemia. PTH increases calcium and decreases phosphate levels in the extracellular fluid (ECF).

(1) PTH acts on the bone, small intestine, and kidneys to transfer calcium to the ECF.

(2) PTH increases the absorption of calcium from the small intestine. (This is a vitamin D-dependent process.)

(3) PTH increases the rate of resorption of calcium and phosphate from bone.

(4) PTH increases renal tubular reabsorption of calcium and the excretion of phosphate.

b. Secretion and actions of calcitonin. Calcitonin (CT) is secreted from the parafollicular cells of the thyroid gland. Its secretion is increased in response to hypercalcemia and decreased in response to hypocalcemia. CT decreases calcium and phosphate levels in the ECF.

(1) CT acts on the bone and kidneys to decrease the transfer of calcium and phosphate to the ECF.

(2) CT decreases the rate of resorption of calcium and phosphate from the bone.

(3) CT decreases distal tubular reabsorption of calcium and phosphate.

c. Synthesis, metabolism, and actions of vitamin D$_3$

(1) Vitamin D$_3$ is synthesized in the skin from 7-dehydrocholesterol by sunlight.

(2) Vitamin D$_3$ is metabolized in the liver to 25(OH)D$_3$, which is then metabolized in the kidney to 1,25(OH)$_2$D$_3$. 1,25(OH)$_2$D$_3$ is the most potent vitamin D metabolite.

(3) Vitamin D$_3$ and its metabolites increase serum concentrations of calcium and phosphate by:

(a) increasing calcium and phosphate absorption from the gut.

(b) increasing calcium and phosphate reabsorption from the renal tubules.

(c) increasing bone resorption.

2. Preparations used to treat hypocalcemia
    a. Calcium gluconate, calcium borogluconate, and so forth.
        (1) Pharmacokinetics
            (a) Absorption. Calcium is absorbed from the small intestine.
                i. Vitamin D_3, PTH, and an acidic pH facilitate absorption.
                ii. Dietary fiber, phytates, fatty acids, steatorrhea, and uremia interfere with absorption.
            (b) Fate. After absorption, calcium enters ECF and then is readily incorporated into bone. Nearly 99% of total body calcium is found in bone. Of circulating calcium, ~50% is bound to serum proteins or complexes with anions and the other 50% is in free Ca^{2+}, which is distributed to all tissues.
            (c) Excretion. Both unabsorbed calcium and calcium secreted into the bile and pancreatic juice are eliminated primarily into the feces. Only a small amount of calcium is excreted into the urine because most of it is reabsorbed from the renal tubules.
        (2) Therapeutic uses include hypocalcemia and cardiac dysrhythmias induced by hyperkalemia.
        (3) Administration
            (a) Calcium gluconate is usually administered to effect by slow IV infusion.
            (b) IP route may be used as well.
            (c) Oral route is rarely used because of limited absorption from the gut.
            (d) Long-term therapy can be accomplished by increasing dietary calcium and administering vitamin D.
        (4) Adverse effects
            (a) Hypercalcemia may occur, which is particularly detrimental to animals with cardiac or renal disease.
            (b) Rapid IV injection of calcium gluconate can cause cardiac arrhythmias and arrest. Treatment should be discontinued in the presence of elevated ST segments, shortened QT intervals in ECG, or arrhythmias.
        (5) Contraindications include ventricular fibrillation, hypercalcemia, renal or cardiac disease, and concurrent treatment with digitalis.
    b. Dihydrotachysterol (DHT)
        (1) Chemistry. DHT is a vitamin D_2 analog.
        (2) Therapeutic uses. DHT is used in small animals to treat hypocalcemia secondary to hypoparathyroidism or severe renal disease.
        (3) Pharmacologic effects. See H 1 c (3).
        (4) Mechanism of action
            (a) Vitamin D and its analogs increase the synthesis of calcium-binding proteins through promoting mRNA synthesis. These calcium-binding proteins facilitate the transport of calcium from the gut mucosa to ECF, thereby promoting calcium absorption from the gut and reabsorption in the renal tubules.
            (b) Vitamin D metabolites rapidly increase Ca^{2+} influx by activating the G_q-protein coupled receptors.
        (5) Pharmacokinetics
            (a) After oral administration, in the presence of food, the GI absorption is good; food stimulates bile flow, which helps dissolve DHT.
            (b) Like other vitamin D analogs, DHT is bound tightly by vitamin D-binding globulin.
            (c) DHT is hydroxylated in the liver to 25-hydroxy-DHT, which is the active form of the drug. The drug is not hdyroxylated in the kidney to form 1,25-dihydroxy metabolite.
            (d) The $t_{1/2}$ of DHT is 8 days (in humans); as a result, overdose can be a problem with DHT. The $t_{1/2}$ in patients with renal disease is not known; it is likely to be shorter than healthy subjects, since plasma concentration of vitamin D-binding globulin should be low in patients with renal disease.
            (e) DHT is excreted mostly in the feces.

      (6) Adverse effects. Hypercalcemia, nephrocalcinosis, and hyperphosphatemia are potential complications of DHT therapy. Because of its long $t_{1/2}$, DHT toxicity lasts 17–30 days.

    c. Calcitriol (1,25-$(OH)_2D_3$). It is the most potent vitamin D_3 metabolite that increases plasma calcium and phosphorus concentrations.

      (1) Therapeutic uses. Calcitriol is used in small animals to treat hypocalcemia secondary to hypoparathyroidism or severe renal disease. It may also be of benefit in treating primary idiopathic seborrhea, since it serves as a growth factor to promote differentiation of skin cells.

      (2) Pharmacokinetics

        (a) The GI absorption after oral administration is similar to that of DHT.

        (b) Calcitriol is bound by vitamin D-binding globulin.

        (c) Unlike DHT, calcitriol has a more rapid onset and much shorter $t_{1/2}$ of 4–6 hours. The $t_{1/2}$ in patients with renal disease could be shorter than healthy subjects, since plasma concentration of vitamin D-binding globulin may be low in patients with renal disease. The duration of action is 1–3 days.

        (d) Like other vitamin D analogs, calcitriol is excreted mostly into the feces.

      (3) Adverse effects. Hypercalcemia, nephrocalcinosis and hyperphosphatemia are potential complications of calcitriol therapy, but the duration of these adverse effects of calcitriol is shorter than that of DHT. If the hypercalcemia is severe, furosemide, calcium-free IV fluids (e.g., normal saline), urine acidifiers, and glucocorticoids may be employed to lower serum calcium levels.

I. **Human recombinant erythropoietin (EPO, Epoetin Alfa, Epogen®).** EPO, a naturally occurring hormone, is produced in the kidney. EPO promotes erythropoiesis.

    1. Chemistry. As a recombinant EPO, Epoetin Alfa® has a molecular weight of ~30 kDa.

    2. Pharmacologic effects. It promotes erythrocyte production by stimulating the differentiation and proliferation of committed red cell precursors. EPO also stimulates the release of reticulocytes. Recombinant human EPO alfa (r-HuEPO-alpha) serves as a substitute for endogenous EPO, primarily in patients with renal disease. Various uremic toxins may be responsible for the decreased production of EPO by the kidney.

    3. Mechanism of action. EPO activates EPO receptors and stimulates the Janus kinase cascade, which is similar to GH (see Figure 12-1 for GH signaling).

    4. Therapeutic uses. EPO has been used in dogs and cats for anemia associated with chronic renal failure.

    5. Pharmacokinetics. No information is available for animals. Depending on initial hematocrit and dose, correction of hematocrit may require 2–8 weeks to occur.

    6. Adverse effects. In dogs and cats, EPO therapy may induce antibodies with resultant resistance to further treatment. EPO should be withdrawn if PCV starts to drop while on therapy. Recombinant canine and feline EPOs are under development to treat anemia more effectively and safely in these species. There is a great need for the development of recombinant feline and canine EPOs in veterinary medicine.

SUGGESTED READING

Behrend EN. 2006. Update on drugs used to treat endocrine diseases in small animals. *Vet Clin North Am Small Anim Pract* 36:1087–1105.

Braddock JA, Church DB, Robertson ID, Watson AD. 2004. Inefficacy of selegiline in treatment of canine pituitary-dependent hyperadrenocorticism. *Aust Vet J* 82:272–277.

Ferguson DC. 2001. "Thyroid hormones and antithyroid drugs." In *Veterinary Pharmacology and Therapeutics.* Edited by Adams HR. 8th ed., pp. 626–648. Ames, IA: Iowa State University Press.

http://www.drugs.com

Plumb DC. 2005. *Veterinary Drug Handbook.* 5th ed. Ames, IA: Blackwell Publishing.

STUDY QUESTIONS

DIRECTIONS: Each of the numbered items or incomplete statements in this section is followed by answers or by completions of the statement. Select the **one** lettered answer or completion that is **best** in each case.

1. Oxytocin without a preceding prostaglandin $F_{2\alpha}$ treatment can consistently induce parturition in

(A) mares.
(B) sows.
(C) cows.
(D) bitches.

2. Which of the following is a preferred drug for the treatment of postpartum hemorrhage and uterine involution?

(A) Oxytocin
(B) Bromocriptine
(C) Cloprostenol
(D) Dexamethasone
(E) Ergonovine

3. Chronic administration of a glucocorticoid may

(A) induce anemia.
(B) increase the amount of adipose tissue in the body by decreasing lipolysis.
(C) induce osteoporosis.
(D) induce lymphocytosis.

4. Frequent administration of which one of the following sex steroids in animals would most likely inhibit growth of the adrenal cortex and adrenocorticotropic hormone (ACTH) secretion?

(A) Boldenone
(B) Estradiol
(C) Megestrol
(D) Stanozolol

5. Which of the following steroids is used to treat anemia?

(A) Deoxycorticosterone
(B) Estradiol
(C) Medroxyprogesterone
(D) Boldenone

6. Administration of megestrol acetate in queens as an oral contraceptive may cause

(A) masculinization.
(B) diabetes mellitus
(C) aplastic anemia.
(D) hepatopathy.

7. All of the following statements concerning agents for treatment of hypocalcemia are true except

(A) only a small amount of calcium administered is excreted in the urine.
(B) calcium gluconate is also used for the treatment of cardiac arrhythmias induced by hyperkalemia.
(C) dihydrotachysterol (DHT), like parathyroid hormone (PTH), elevates serum calcium concentrations and lowers serum phosphate concentrations.
(D) DHT is metabolized in the liver to a 25(OH)-metabolite, which is the active form of the drug.

8. Use of a glucocorticoid is contraindicated in all of the following conditions except

(A) diabetes mellitus.
(B) corneal ulceration.
(C) anaphylactic shock.
(D) infection uncontrolled by antibiotics.
(E) burns.

9. All of the following statements concerning antidiabetic agents are true except

(A) commercial insulin preparations are mostly of human origin.
(B) hepatocytes, erythrocytes, leukocytes, adrenal medullary chromaffin cells, and brain cells do not require insulin to transport glucose.
(C) dogs are more likely than cats to develop insulin antibodies to porcine or human insulin preparations.
(D) glipizide, a sulfonylurea, has been used with some success in treating cats with moderate diabetes.

10. All of the following progestins are effective when administered orally to an animal except

(A) progesterone.
(B) megestrol.
(C) melengestrol.
(D) altrenogest.

11. Which of the following drug is the preferred drug for the treatment of the adrenal cortical disease in ferrets?

(A) Ketoconazole
(B) Trilostane
(C) Leuprolide
(D) Mitotane

ANSWERS AND EXPLANATIONS

1. The answer is A.
The presence of CL may inhibit the action of an oxytocic agent. Because prepartum mares do not have a functional CL, oxytocin can effectively induce foaling. All prepartum sows, cows, and bitches have corpora lutea; therefore, luteolysis must occur [or be induced, for example, with prostaglandin $F_{2\alpha}$ ($PGF_{2\alpha}$)] before an oxytocic agent can work effectively.

2. The answer is E.
Ergonovine causes prolonged contraction of myometrium and uterine blood vessels; therefore, it is a preferred drug for the treatment of postpartum hemorrhage and uterine involution. Oxytocin is a peptide hormone that evokes short-term uterine contractions. Bromocriptine at therapeutic doses has an insignificant effect on smooth muscle contraction. Cloprostenol is a prostaglandin $F_{2\alpha}$ ($PGF_{2\alpha}$) analog that is used to induce parturition and abortion, to treat pyometra, and to expel mummified fetuses. Dexamethasone is used to induce parturition.

3. The answer is C.
Glucocorticoids may create a negative calcium balance by inhibiting calcium absorption from the gastrointestinal tract and reabsorption from the kidney. Glucocorticoids induce polycythemia, lipolysis, and lymphocytopenia.

4. The answer is C.
Progestins, such as megestrol, have glucocorticoid-like activities that can inhibit adrenocorticotropic hormone (ACTH) secretion, inducing iatrogenic hypoadrenocorticism. Estrogens (e.g., estradiol) and androgens (e.g., stanozolol, boldenone) do not have significant glucocorticoid activities.

5. The answer is D.
Androgens increase erythropoiesis by promoting erythropoietin synthesis. Therefore, androgens such as boldenone can be used to treat anemia. Deoxycorticosterone, estradiol, and medroxyprogesterone are not androgens, and thus do not promote erythropoiesis.

6. The answer is B.
Megestrol, a progestin, may cause diabetes mellitus, particularly in a diabetes-prone animal; this is due to progestin's glucocorticoid activity. Megestrol is not an androgen, so it does not cause masculinization or hepatopathy. It is not an estrogen, so it does not cause aplastic anemia.

7. The answer is C.
Dihydrotachysterol (DHT) elevates both serum calcium and phosphate concentrations. Like parathyroid hormone (PTH), DHT increases serum calcium concentrations by promoting calcium and phosphorus absorption from the GI tract and by deceasing calcium excretion from the kidney. However, unlike PTH, DHT decreases phosphorus excretion from the kidney.

8. The answer is C.
Glucocorticoids are not contraindicated in anaphylactic shock. They should not be used in animals with corneal ulceration, diabetes mellitus, infections uncontrolled by antibiotics, or burns.

9. The answer is C.
Following administration of a human or porcine insulin preparation, cats are more likely than dogs to develop insulin antibodies. Most commercial products are developed using recombinant DNA techniques and are of human origin. Hepatocytes, erythrocytes, leukocytes, adrenal medullary chromaffin cells, and brain cells do not require insulin for glucose transport. Glipizide, a sulfonylurea, has been used with some success to treat feline diabetes.

10. The answer is A.
Progesterone is a natural steroid that is rapidly inactivated by liver enzymes following absorption from the GI tract. Synthetic progestins (e.g., megestrol, melengestrol, altrenogest) are more resistant to liver enzymes.

11. The answer is C.
Leuprolide is a partial agonist of GnRH. The adrenal cortical disease (ACD) of ferrets is due to an increase in GnRH secretion from the hypothalamus in neutered ferrets. GnRH evokes hyperadrenocorticism in these animals with a great increase in sex steroids. Other inhibitors of the corticosteroid synthesis may be used in conjunction with leuprolide treatment.

Chapter 13

Topical Dermatology Therapy

James O. Noxon

I. **INTRODUCTION.** Drugs applied to the surface of the skin have four possible outcomes. (1) They may remain on the surface, where they may exert their medicinal qualities. (2) They may have local effects on the stratum corneum. (3) They may be absorbed by the skin and exert deeper effects on the epidermis and dermis. (4) They may be absorbed and exert systemic effects.

A. **Structure and function of the skin**

1. **Functions of the skin.** The skin is considered the largest organ of the body. It has several key functions in normal and diseased states, including maintenance of hydration; protection from chemical/mechanical damage, radiation, and infectious agents; sensation; aiding in motion and shape; metabolism; and communication. These functions are accomplished in part by the anatomical structure of the skin and in part by the physiological actions of the skin, especially the epidermis. These same physiological processes are responsible for the behavior of drugs applied to or on the skin. For example, desquamation is an important part of the physiologic renewal of the epidermis. Any substances, including drugs, placed on the skin will naturally be removed by this normal turnover of epithelial cells, thus limiting the residual effects of topical medication.

2. **Structure of the skin.** The skin consists of three basic layers, from outside to inside: the epidermis, the dermis, and the hypodermis.
   a. **The epidermis.** The epidermis is the most crucial layer affecting drug absorption and pharmacokinetics. There are four anatomic layers in the skin. From the deepest layer to the most superficial, these are the stratum basale (basal cell layer), the stratum spinosum (prickle cell layer), the stratum granulosum (granular cell layer), and the stratum corneum (horny layer). The germinal layer is the stratum granulosum and keratinocytes move outward through these layers and undergo several important physiologic alterations, in a process called cornification. This process includes production of various proteins that contribute to the development of a thick cell envelope and production of intercellular lipids that contribute to the lipid layer found between keratinocytes. The epidermis is constantly regenerating in the basal cell layer and sloughing from the stratum corneum. The epidermal turnover time in the dog is approximately 21–25 days
      (1) Keratinocytes. Keratinocytes undergo several physiologic changes as they move from the stratum basale to the stratum corneum. The cell envelope becomes thick and insoluble; however, the keratinocyte is very hygroscopic and may absorb large amounts of water or hydrophilic substances. Keratinocytes may act as reservoirs of hydrophilic substances, which then diffuse long after the topical agent has been applied.
      (2) Epidermal lipids. The keratinocytes are surrounded by lipids produced in lamellar granules of keratinocytes and sebaceous glands. These lipids include ceramides, fatty acids, cholesterol, squalene, sterol/wax esters, and sphingolipids. These lipids form a bipolar layer between the keratinocytes and play a key role in the barrier functions of the skin and in keratinocyte cohesion within the epidermis. Obviously, hydrophobic, the lipids retard passage of hydrophilic substances, such as water through the layer.

B. **Factors affecting cutaneous pharmacokinetics**

1. **Routes of drug passage.** Drugs may move through the skin by movement through the epidermis, through the hair follicles, or through apocrine or sebaceous glands.

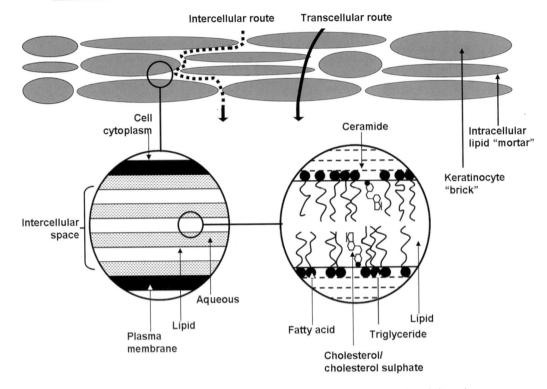

FIGURE 13-1. Two-compartment model of the skin. Intercellular lipids allow lipophilic substances to pass through the skin more readily than hydrophilic substances. (Modified from Fig. 53.4. of *Adams's Veterinary Pharmacology and Therapeutics*, 8th ed. 2001).

The vast majority of drug movement occurs through the epidermis; however, the movement through other structures could alter the pharmacokinetics required for good drug absorption.

2. **Two-compartment system (Figure 13-1).** The structure of the epidermis consisting of keratinocytes surrounded by a lipid layer has been compared to a brick and mortar wall, where the keratinocytes are the "bricks" and the lipids produced by the keratinocytes and sebaceous glands surround the keratinocytes like mortar in a brick wall. This results in a lipophobic (or hydrophilic) structure, the keratinocytes, that are surrounded by a lipohilic (or hydrophobic) layer, the bipolar lipids. In order for drugs to pass through the epidermis, they must pass through the lipid layer. Logically, lipid soluble drugs are generally able to accomplish this more readily than water-soluble drugs.

3. **Reservoir actions of the epidermis.** Many drugs, especially hydrophilic drugs, may be concentrated within the keratinocytes or bound to epidermal sites providing a high concentration and an osmotic gradient for drugs to move passively into the deeper layers of the epidermis and dermis, even after the drug has been removed from the surface of the skin. This principle is used in topical application of systemically active medications, such as patches for pain or motion sickness.

C. Factors affecting drug disposition

1. **Properties of the topical agent**
   a. **Properties of the active agent.** Because of the lipid layer between the keratinocytes, lipid soluble drugs penetrate the epidermis more efficiently. Water-soluble drugs are more likely to be absorbed by keratinocytes, but have a difficult time penetrating the epidermis.
      (1) **Solubility of the drug.** The solubility of the drug has a major effect on the absorption of the drug into the skin. The drug must be soluble enough to be

carried in high concentrations in the vehicle, but it must not be too soluble, which would tend to hold the drug in the vehicle and not allow it to diffuse into the keratinocytes or lipid layer of the epidermis.

    (a) Partition coefficient. The partition coefficient is the term that describes the affinity of a drug for the lipid phase of the skin. A higher partition coefficient suggests better movement of a drug into the lipid components of the skin, and thus better topical absorption.

  (2) Concentration of the drug. Since drug movement into and through the stratum corneum is a passive process (i.e., diffusion), higher concentrations of the drug within the vehicle will promote greater movement of the drug into the keratinocytes or lipid layer.

  (3) Molecular weight. Smaller molecular weight compounds will pass through the lipid barrier more readily than larger molecular weight compounds. This remains the case even with hydrophilic compounds, which in general, do not pass through the lipid layer readily.

 b. Vehicle. The vehicle carries the active drug, in which it is suspended or dissolved, and provides a delivery mechanism for active agents. An oil-based vehicle allows for better movement of the drug into the lipid barrier. Vehicles may, in some cases, have therapeutic effects by themselves, for example, by functioning as occlusive dressings which increase cutaneous hydration.

 c. Occlusive dressings. Occlusive dressings may include a physical dressing or a layer of the vehicle that prevents loss of the drug from the surface of the skin. Bandages, even band-aids, act as occlusive dressing by preventing removal of the drug by mechanical means or evaporation. An oil preparation may also act as an occlusive dressing when applied after other medications. Bath oil applied after bathing is an example of the use of an occlusive dressing. The oil slows down water loss through the skin and from keratinocytes that have absorbed water in the bathing process.

2. Cutaneous factors affecting drug disposition

 a. Thickness of the stratum corneum. Movement of a drug through the skin involves movement through the lipid layer surrounding the stratum corneum, and in some cases, movement through the keratinocytes. Drug movement is more difficult as the stratum corneum becomes thicker and is enhanced by application on areas of the skin, such as the axillary, inguinal, and abdominal regions, where the epidermis is thinner.

 b. Integrity of the stratum corneum. Damage to the stratum corneum, from excoriations or abrasions, will reduce the effectiveness of the barrier function and increase the drug absorption.

 c. Alterations in physiological behavior. Desquamation is an important factor in epithelial turnover. Inflammatory diseases, metabolic disorders, and familial conditions, such as familial seborrhea, may alter the desquamation of keratinocytes by increasing or decreasing the turnover of keratinocytes. Loss of keratinocytes would definitely change disposition of any drugs using the stratum corneum as a reservoir and would increase the loss of any drug remaining on the surface of the skin.

 d. Temperature. Increased temperature of the skin will allow for enhance absorption of most drugs by increasing solubility of the drug and increasing vascular flow to the area.

 e. Hydration status of the epidermis. As the epidermis becomes dehydrated, keratinocytes become shrunken and the cell envelope tougher, resulting in less drug absorption.

D. **Indications for topical therapy.** Topical therapy using any of the agents or formulations described in this chapter may be used for a wide range of dermatological problems. **The most common uses in veterinary dermatology are (1) for control of ectoparasites, (2) for control of pruritus, (3) for treatment of cutaneous infections by bacteria, yeast, and dermatophytes, and (4) as an aid for the management of seborrhea and other scaling disorders.**

II. PHARMACOLOGICAL AGENTS

A. Antimicrobial agents

1. **Topical antibacterial agents**
   a. **Preparations and chemistry.** Topical antibacterial agents fall into one of two main categories, antibiotics or antiseptic agents. However, keratolytic agents and other compounds may also exhibit antibacterial properties. Glycotechnology is the use of simple mono- or polysaccharide sugar moieties to competitively inhibit binding of microbes to the skin surface.
      (1) **Various antibiotics** have been used topically, including neomycin, gentamicin, chloramphenicol, bacitracin, polymyxin B sulfates, nitrofurazone, and others. Mupirocin is a highly effective topical antibiotic in an ointment formulation. It is highly effective against staphylococci and many gram-negative bacteria.
      (2) **Antiseptics** used on the skin include alcohol, acetic acid, propylene glycol, chlorhexidine, iodophors, phenols (e.g., resorcinol, hexylresorcinol), potassium permanganate, triclosan, and sodium hypochlorite.
      (3) **Many of the topical keratolytic agents** found in shampoos used for anti-seborrheic therapy also demonstrate potent antimicrobial properties. These include sulfur, salicylic acid, selenium disulfide, ethyl lactate, and benzoyl peroxide. Benzoyl peroxide is highly effective as a topical antibacterial agent used in a shampoo formulation.
      (4) **Glycotechnology.** It is recognized that some monosaccharides or polysaccharides will bind to lectins found on microbes. These lectins, or binding sites, are used by the bacteria to attach to keratinocytes which contain other sugars on their surface. This competitive inhibition is incorporated in some shampoos available commercially, such as Keratolux® (containing salicylic acid) and KetoChlor® (containing chlorhexidine and ketoconazole), and will likely be found in other topical agents in the future.
   b. **Mechanism of action.** The mechanism of action of antibiotic varies with the class of drug. Antiseptics work through various mechanisms, including denaturing proteins that damage cell walls or membranes, lowering surface tension, inhibition of essential enzymes, or by acting as reactive oxidating or alkylating agents. Mono- and polysaccharides bind to lectins on microbes, preventing their adherence to keratinocytes.
   c. **Therapeutic uses.** Topical antibacterial therapy in the form of ointments, creams, and sprays is indicated for focal bacterial infections, such as acute moist dermatitis and wounds. Generalized bacterial dermatitis, such as folliculitis, is best managed with shampoos or rinses containing antibacterial agents such as benzoyl peroxide.
   d. **Administration.** Topical antibacterial agents are used once or twice daily on affected areas. Shampoos containing residual agents, such as benzoyl peroxide, are administered once or twice weekly in most cases.
   e. **Adverse effects.** Any topical antibacterial agent may potentially induce irritation or result in a contact allergic reaction. Such problems are infrequently reported.

2. **Topical antifungal therapy**
   a. **Topical therapy for yeast (*Malassezia pachydermatis*)**
      (1) **Preparations and chemistry.** Several antibiotics and antiseptics have efficacy against yeast including azoles (miconazole, clotrimazole, enilconazole, and ketoconazole), nystatin, iodine, chlorhexidine, selenium sulfide, and lime sulfur.
      (2) **Mechanism of action.** Antiseptics, such as chlorhexidine and iodine, work through various mechanisms. The azole compounds inhibit ergosterol synthesis, which disrupts fungal cell membranes.
      (3) **Therapeutic uses.** Anti-yeast medications are indicated to treat localized or generalized yeast infections. Their primary use is to manage infections caused by *M. pachydermatis*.

(4) Administration

(a) Localized infections. *Malassezia* are found in areas of higher humidity and temperature, such as lip folds, interdigital areas (both dorsally and ventrally), axillary and inguinal regions, or any intertriginous area.

i. The goal is to clean and dry the affected area. This may be done using detergents or commercial products designed with astringents included in the formulation.

ii. Excellent products for "spot" treatment of focal lesions include towelettes containing miconazole and chlorhexidine (Malaseb Toweletts®) or acetic acid plus boric acid (Malcetic Wipes®). The latter product is safe around the eyes, making it ideal for treating periocular infections.

(b) Generalized *Malassezia* infections. Generalized or multifocal yeast infections require wider distribution of medication. Shampoos or rinses are best suited for this purpose.

i. Active ingredients found in shampoo or rinse formulations that are effective in controlling *Malassezia* infections include selenium sulfide, miconazole, ketoconazole, enilconazole, lime sulfur, acetic acid-boric acid, and chlorhexidine.

ii. Shampoos must be applied 2–3 times weekly to effectively control yeast infections of the skin. Contact time of 10 minutes is important to achieve the best results from these agents.

(5) Adverse effects. Patients may rarely develop irritation or hypersensitivity to the active agent or other ingredients of the products. Clinical signs may include redness or pruritus following topical application. A patient may rarely develop urticarial reactions to topical medications.

b. Topical therapy for dermatophytosis

(1) Preparations and chemistry. Agents found in commercial veterinary formulations with activity against dermatophytes include (in decreasing order of effectiveness) lime sulfur, enilconazole, chlorhexidine, povidone iodine, and ketoconazole. The combination of miconazole and chlorhexidine appears to have superior activity over the use of either agent alone. Antiseptics, including sodium hypochlorite, also have some activity against dermatophytes.

(2) Mechanism of action. The agents work in various manners. The azoles inhibit ergosterol synthesis in fungal cell walls (see Chapter 15 for detailed information).

(3) Therapeutic uses. Topical antifungal agents are used as adjunctive therapy for dermatophytes infections in companion animals. They are often used as the sole treatment in large animals.

(4) Administration.

(a) Formulations. Antifungal agents may be administered in lotions (e.g., Conofite®), sprays or rinses (e.g., Malaseb Rinse®), and shampoos (e.g., Malaseb® shampoo, Miconazole® shampoo, KetoChlor®).

(b) Application. Products are generally applied once or twice weekly as adjunctive therapy to systemic antifungal therapy.

(5) Adverse effects. Possible adverse effects include irritation or hypersensitivity reactions to ingredients of these formulations. Products should be used with caution around eyes to avoid irritation.

B. Antipruritic agents

1. Preparation and chemistry. Substances present for topical application that reduce pruritus include glucocorticoids (e.g., hydrocortisone), antihistamines (e.g., diphenhydramine), hydrating agents, sulfur, tar, topical anesthetics (e.g., lidocaine, pramoxine), and cooling agents (e.g., methol, camphor). Any topical therapy that moisturizes the skin tends to reduce pruritus, since dry or dehydrated skin exacerbates pruritus. This may include bathing and/or the use of occlusive dressings.

2. Mechanism of action. There are many mechanisms for induction of pruritus, which is thought primarily in dermatology conditions to arise from irritation of unmyelinated nerves by various cytokines (e.g., leukotriene B_4, kallikreins, prostaglandins), external enzymes (e.g., proteases), and other inflammatory mediators (e.g., kinins, opioids, acetylcholine). As might be expected, there are many mechanisms of action to disrupt that sensation. Glucocorticoids work by reducing the inflammation and the production of various cytokines that induce pruritus. Topical anesthetics are presumed to desensitize the peripheral nerves or receptors that trigger pruritus. The cooling agents will substitute a cool sensation that functionally may displace the sensation of itch. Cool soaks or dressings work to reduce the pruritic threshold thorough several mechanisms including desensitizing nerve receptors.

3. **Therapeutic uses and administration.** Topical antipruritic agents may reduce pruritus in allergic, parasitic, seborrheic, neoplastic, and other skin conditions where inflammation or dry skin is present. **Topical therapy is rarely effective as the sole treatment for moderate or severe pruritus.** It is best used as adjunctive therapy or for spot treatment of focally pruritic lesions. Hydrating agents works best in allergy skin diseases and conditions where the skin is dehydrated (i.e., dry). Spot treatment of focal lesions may be applied once or more daily to affected areas in lotions, creams, ointments, or sprays. Generalized pruritus is best managed with agents formulation in shampoos.

4. **Adverse effects.** In general, these topical antipruritic agents are safe. Rarely, a patient may show focal cutaneous irritation at the site of application. Repeated applications of topical anesthetics may result in a contact allergic reaction, although is not considered a problem for products containing pramoxine.

C. **Anti-inflammatory and immunomodulating agents**

1. **Preparations.** Various substances may have anti-inflammatory effects, including cool water applications, glucocorticoids, dimethyl sulfoxide (DMSO), aloe vera, and others.
   a. Glucocorticoids vary greatly in their topical potency. The more common topical glucocorticoids for skin and ear use are, in order of increasing potency, hydrocortisone, prednisone and prednisolone, triamcinolone, dexamethasone, betamethasone, mometasone, and flucinolone. The salt used to formulate the glucocorticoid will affect the pharmacokinetics, especially $t_{1/2}$. For example, triamcinolone generally has a stronger anti-inflammatory effect on the skin and ears than dexamethasone, despite their opposite potencies in vivo.
   b. **Tacrolimus.** Tacrolimus is a macrolide produced by *Streptomyces tsukubaensis*. It is available for topical administration as a 0.03% and 0.1% ointment (Protopic®), although the higher concentration is primarily used in veterinary dermatology. Pimecrolimus (Elidel Cream®) is a similar drug that is also available commercially but is not used extensively in veterinary medicine.
   c. **Imiquimod.** Imiquimod is an immune response modifier sold as a 5% cream (Aldara®).

2. **Mechanism of action.** The mechanisms of action vary in this group.
   a. Glucocorticoids, the most commonly used anti-inflammatory drugs, exert their anti-inflammatory properties by decreasing migration of and phagocytosis by inflammatory cells, decreased elaboration of C-reactive protein, suppression of cytokine production and release from inflammatory cells, and prevention of the release of lysosomal enzymes that cause tissue damage and generation of leukotactic substances.
   b. Tacrolimus has anti-inflammatory and immunomodulating effects through calcineurin inhibition, which results in inhibition of various cytokines (interleukin-2, 3, and 4; TNF-α, and interferon) and down-regulation of cytokine expression in inflammatory cells. Tacrolimus has similar properties as cyclosporine but is reportedly 10–100 times more potent when applied topically.
   c. Imiquimod actives immune cells by ligating toll-like receptors (TLR7, TLR8), resulting in cytokine production and release (interferon-α), interleukin-6, and tumor necrosis factor-α. In addition, imiqimod may activate Langerhans cells to activate additional immunoregulatory responses.

3. **Therapeutic uses and administration.**
   a. Topical anti-inflammatory agents are used to reduce the inflammation caused by various skin disorders. They are used most often for their antipruritic activities.
   b. Tacrolimus has been shown to be effective in the management of perianal fistula, effective in reducing the severity of clinical lesions in atopic dermatitis, and for management of various autoimmune skin conditions, such as discoid lupus erythematosus.
   c. Imiquimod has been used in human medicine to manage various cutaneous neoplasms (e.g., basal cell carcinoma), precancerous lesions (e.g., Bowen's disease), genital warts, and actinic (i.e., solar) keratosis. In veterinary medicine, the drug has been shown in limited studies to be effective in managing sarcoids in horses. Other potential uses, that need additional investigation, include Bowen's disease in cats and cutaneous herpes virus infections.

4. **Adverse effects**
   a. All topical glucocorticoids are absorbed and may exert systemic effects, though the degree to which they are absorbed varies from agent to agent with the formulation and salt used. For example, mometasone has significantly more potency than betamethasone, but is absorbed much less and therefore is safer for prolonged topical application. Specific adverse effects may be iatrogenic hyperadrenocorticism, suppression of the hypothalamic-pituitary-adrenal axis, and cutaneous manifestations of hyperadrenocorticism (e.g., comedone formation, cutaneous atrophy, alopecia).
   b. Tacrolimus is very safe when applied topically, though gloves should be worn by humans applying the medication. Rarely, mild erythema may be seen at the site of application.
   c. Imiquimod does induce inflammation, so cutaneous erythema, edema, and pruritus may be seen following topical application. Gloves should be worn by humans applying this compound.

D. **Astringents**

1. **Preparations and chemistry.** The principal astringents are salts of aluminum, zinc, iron, and bismuth or salts that contain these metals (e.g., permanganates). Tannins and other polyphenolic compounds also act as astringents. Commonly used astringents in veterinary medicine include zinc sulfate and aluminum acetate (Domeboro® solution).
2. **Mechanism of action.** Astringents are substances that precipitate protein, reduce permeability of the cell membrane, and reduce transcapillary movement of plasma proteins, and thus inflammation, edema, and exudation.
3. **Therapeutic uses.** Astringents are used to dry the skin, toughen the skin, and promote healing. They are also used to coagulate blood (i.e., styptic actions).
4. **Administration.** These agents are applied topically to dry moist areas. They are helpful in the topical management of acute moist dermatitis and other moist pyoderma, for irritant dermatitis (e.g., urine scald), and for drying the ear canal in suppurative otitis externa and yeast infections of the ears.
5. **Adverse effects.** Astringents may cause mild irritation following topical application. Overuse may cause excessive drying of the skin, which can result in secondary infections.

E. **Demulcents**

1. **Preparation and chemistry.** Demulcents may be applied as sticky lotions that adhere to the skin or as powders that mix with fluids excreted from the affected area. Substances that have demulcent properties include alginates, mucilages, starches, dextrins, gums, sugars, and polymeric polyhydric glycols. The most common demulcents used for skin and ear application in veterinary dermatologic formulations are propylene glycol, polyethylene glycol, and glycerin.
2. **Mechanisms of action.** Demulcents adhere to the skin to provide physical protection and to allow prolonged topical exposure of any drug that might be suspended in the preparation used. Some demulcents, such as propylene glycol, have

bacteriostatic and fungistatic properties. Most demulcents have hydrophilic colloidal properties that allow them to serve as emulsifiers and suspending agents for water-soluble agents.

3. **Therapeutic uses and administration.** Demulcents are protective agents that are used to relieve irritation and irritation, especially of abraded tissues or mucous membranes. They are applied topically to irritated areas. Propylene glycol is commonly used because of its antimicrobial actions and physical properties: nongreasy, nonstaining, and the ability to spread easily over the surface.

4. **Adverse effects.** Topical irritation may be seen in some animals following repeated application of propylene glycol on the skin or in the ear canal.

F. Adsorbents

1. **Preparations and chemistry.** Adsorbents are inert and insoluble substances, generally fine powders, that may consist of starch, calcium carbonate, boric acid, zinc oxide, titanium dioxide, or talc.

2. **Mechanism of action.** Adsorbents generally absorb moisture on the skin and act as dessicants.

3. **Therapeutic uses and administration.**
   a. Adsorbents may be used as a vehicle for parasiticides or antimicrobial agents.
   b. Powders may be used to absorb moisture on the skin as long as they are not allowed to form adherent crusts.

4. **Adverse effects.** If applied to wet surfaces, adsorbents may form crusts of powder and liquid. Powders may promote granulation tissue, especially if used within body cavities.

G. Protectives

1. **Preparations and chemistry.** Mechanical protectives may form an adherent film that may be flexible or inflexible. Ingredients considered as protectives include lanolin, mineral oil, olive oil, zinc stearate, petrolatum, silicones, and various polymers. Several products recently introduced into veterinary dermatology contain sugars that may serve as protectives against microbes.

2. **Mechanism of action.** A protective may provide a physical and/or occlusive layer on the skin. In addition, these materials may also serve as a vehicle for medications. These agents may protect from physical (e.g., radiation) or chemical insult to the skin. The most recent agents released in veterinary medicine in this class are shampoos containing monosaccharides.

3. **Therapeutic uses and administration.**
   a. Protectives may be applied to wounds or nonhealing ulcers.
   b. Petrolatum or other protectives may be applied daily around inguinal region to protect the skin from irritation from urinary or fecal incontinence.

4. **Adverse effects.** Protectives may be occlusive and may therefore allow infections to spread. They should not be used without the appropriate antimicrobial therapy in infected skin.

H. Humectants and moisturizing agents

1. **Preparations.** Many substances have hygroscopic qualities and will attract water, including α-hydroxy acids (lactic acid, malic acid, glycolic acid, and others), urea, colloidal oatmeal, propylene glycol, glycerin, and DMSO.

2. **Mechanism of action.** These agents generally attract water molecules, which are chemically bound to the agent. They are often used in conjunction with an emollient to retain water that has been attracted or bound to the skin.

3. **Therapeutic uses and administration.** Humectants are indicated whenever the skin is dry or dehydrated.

4. **Adverse effects.** Adverse effects are uncommon. Overuse could potentially lead to excessive maceration of the skin.

I. Emollients

1. **Preparations and chemistry.** Emollients are bland fatty substances that are applied locally to the skin. Numerous animal fats and oils may act as emollients, including

lanolin and lard. Sources found in vegetable oils include olive oil, castor oil, cottonseed oil, corn oil, coconut oil, peanut oil, persic oil, sesame oil, and cocoa butter. Waxes and other hydrocarbons, such as glycerin, isopropyl myristate, beeswax, paraffin, and petrolatum also serve as emollients. Products containing fatty acids and phytosphingosines will also act as emollients when applied topically.

2. **Mechanism of action.** Emollients act to increase the tissue moisture content by (1) preventing moisture loss by acting as an occlusive dressing or protective, (2) increasing the water holding capabilities through the use of humectants, and (3) altering the desquamation of the stratum corneum.

3. **Therapeutic uses and administration.** Emollients are indicated in patients with dry and scaly skin to increase cutaneous hydration and soften the skin. Their chief use is as a vehicle for many lipid-soluble topical medications. Emollients used after shampoo therapy will increase or reduce evaporative water loss from the skin by forming an occlusive dressing.

4. **Adverse effects.** Emollients may result in retention of moisture that may trap bacteria and possibly favor growth of some organisms, including anaerobic bacteria. Some emollients, such as lanolin, may promote formation of comedones.

J. **Keratolytic and keratoplastic agents (antiseborrheic agents)**

1. **Preparations.** Benzoyl peroxide, urea, salicylic acid, sulfur, selenium disulfide, resorcinol, coal tar, various phenols, and sulfur all have keratolytic actions. Tar (from coal or pine distillation), sulfur, salicylic acid, and sulfur have keratoplastic properties.

2. **Mechanism of action.**
   a. Phenols and sulfhydryl compounds may loosen the keratin to promote desquamation.
   b. Keratolytic agents also increase hydration of keratinocytes. Maceration of the epidermis results from this increased hydration, which also enhances the desquamation process. Sulfur, salicylic acid, benzoyl peroxide, colloidal oatmeal, urea, and coal tar are all used with frequency in veterinary dermatology to hydrate the skin and promote desquamation.
   c. The term keratoplastic implies normalization of the cornification process by slowing epithelial turnover. It is presumed that this process occurs due to alterations in DNA synthesis. **Coal tar is the most widely used keratoplastic agent in veterinary medicine.** Salicylic acid and selenium sulfide may also have mild keratoplastic properties.

3. **Therapeutic uses and administration**
   a. Keratolytic agents are used primarily in shampoo therapy for the management of scaling skin conditions, including familial seborrhea and ichthyosis, and for softening and removal of crusts in parasitic or infectious dermatologic conditions. Topical gels or ointments containing salicylic acid (e.g., KeraSolv®) are an excellent adjunctive therapy for nasal hyperkeratosis.
   b. Coal tar and other keratoplastic agents are indicated as part of shampoo therapy for the management of familial seborrhea and other scaling disorders.

4. **Adverse effects.** Mild irritation may ensue following topical application of keratolytic or keratoplastic agents. **Coal tar may be photosensitizing, irritating, carcinogenic, and it may stain hair coats and clothing. Coal tar is not recommended for use on cats because of its irritant nature in that species.**

K. **Caustic and escharotics**

1. **Preparations and chemistry.** Active ingredients include potassium hydroxide, silver nitrate, gentian violet, aluminum chloride, alum, glacial acetic acid, trichloroacetic acid, and salicylic acid.

2. **Mechanism of action.** These agents are used to induce desquamation of cornified epithelium, and thus cause destruction of tissue at the site of application. Agents that also precipitate protein to form a crust, and eventually a scar, are called an escharotic.

3. **Therapeutic uses and administration.** These agents may be applied topically to proliferative lesions. They are not used with much frequency in veterinary medicine.

4. **Adverse effects.** Cutaneous irritation, crust formation, scar formation, and discomfort are the primary adverse effects of topical application of caustic agents.

L. **Rubefacients, irritants, and vesicants**

1. **Preparations.** Rubefacients include volatile aromatic irritants, such as camphor and menthol. Locally applied heat, from hot packs, heating pads, or heat lamps, also serves as a rubefacient. Capsicum, coal tar, creosote, iodine, turpentine, alcohols, and pine tar are some of the better-known irritants used in veterinary medicine.
2. **Mechanism of action.** These agents work on the skin to induce hyperemia (rubefacients), inflammation and hyperemia (irritants), and vesicles (vesicants) caused by leakage of fluid from damaged capillaries. Rubefacients may act by increasing circulation to the area.
3. **Therapeutic uses and administration.** Rubefacients are often used to increase the absorption of topical medications, to increase the circulation to an area of the body, and to induce the feeling of warmth. Some irritants have medicinal qualities that support their use. For example, menthol will induce the sensation of coolness and has some antipruritic activity.
4. **Adverse effects.** Inflammation, hyperemia, vesicles, irritation, discomfort, or pain are likely adverse effects of topical application, since that is the classification of these agents.

III. VEHICLES AND DELIVERY SYSTEMS

A. **Vehicles (Figure 13-2).** Substances used to carry active ingredients in pharmacological preparations are called vehicles. These substances do not generally have therapeutic properties, but they may provide some support for the management of skin diseases by acting as occlusive dressings or protectives.

1. Solubility of the active drug is a key in selection of the vehicle. Insufficient solubility results in poor movement of a drug into the skin and excessive solubility may result in a drug that fails to move from the vehicle into the skin.

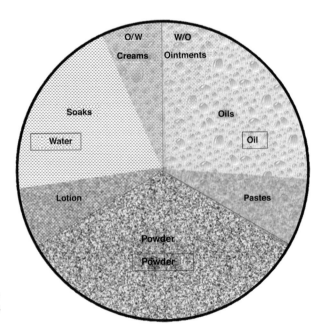

FIGURE 13-2. Representation of the formulations of topical medications. Topical preparations consist of oil, solids (powders), or water and various mixtures of these substances.

2. **Emulsifiers.** Emulsifying agents are used to allow mixing of a lipid (or oil) soluble substance with a water-soluble substance. Emulsifying agents may be classified as natural agents (e.g., hydrophilic colloids), synthetic agents (e.g., soaps, sulfates, sulfonates), or as finely divided solids (e.g., colloidal clays, metallic hydroxides). Common emulsifying agents include cetyl alcohol, glyceryl monosterate, methycellulose, stearic acid, stearyl alcohol, DMSO, lanolin, polyethylene glycol, benzalkonium chloride, and many others.

3. **Liposomes.** When phospholipids disperse in liquids, they swell, hydrate, and form multilamellar, concentric layers of aqueous materials separated by the lipid bilayers. These aggregates, called liposomes, are used as carriers of water, various drugs, and macromolecules that can be trapped between these layers for dispersal in or on the skin.

   a. **Novosomes®.** Liposome technology was used to incorporate moisturizing agents into lipid microvesicles that have been incorporated into various veterinary shampoos (e.g., HydraPearls®) and cream rinses. These novosomes bind to hair and keratinocytes and slowly disperse their contents (moisturizing agents) as the liposomes break down. Studies have shown that these provide superior moisturizing effects on the skin of dogs.

   b. **Spherulites®.** These are liposomes that also contain active agents, such as moisturizers, stabilizers, fatty acids, chlorhexidine, and more. Spherulites may be nonionic to allow for deeper penetration into the skin or cationic, which facilitates binding to the surface of the skin. These structures release their contents as the liposome degrades over time.

B. **Dispersants and penetration enhancers**

1. **Preparations and chemistry.** These agents tend to fall into four categories: (1) azone and its derivatives, (2) terpenes, (3) urea and derivatives, and (4) aparotic solvents. DMSO belongs to the latter class and is a common agent used to enhance the penetration of water, antibiotics, glucocorticoids, and other commonly used medications in veterinary medicine. Dispersants, such as transcutol (i.e., diethyleneglycol monoethyl ether), are becoming more extensively used in veterinary medicine to facilitate absorption and diffusion of agents throughout the lipid layer of the skin. Limited data are available on many because of their proprietary nature.

2. **Mechanisms of action.** Penetration enhancers, such as DMSO, may alter lipids in the stratum corneum or induction of a more porous intercellular matrix of the epidermis. Dispersants act to facilitate the movement of the active chemical throughout the lipid layer of the skin. These are commonly employed in veterinary medicine in pour-on products to rapidly disperse the active ingredients. These agents may also affect (increase or decrease) drug solubility and affect the depot effects of some drugs.

3. **Therapeutic uses and administration.**

   a. Dispersants are key ingredients in several "pour-on" flea control products, including Frontline® and Advantage®. These agents allow the active ingredients, fipronil and imidacloprid, respectively, to dispense throughout the lipid layers of the epidermis and provide antiparasitic concentrations of insecticides.

   b. Newer commercial products containing sphingolipids also contain dispersants to facilitate the distribution of the lipids when applied to only one area of the body.

4. **Adverse effects.** DMSO has a strong odor associated with topical application and is reported to induce the taste of garlic when applied topically to the skin. Gloves should be worn when applying products containing DMSO. No adverse effects attributed to dispersants have been reported.

C. **Liquid preparations**

1. **Wet dressings**

   a. **Definition.** Wet dressings consist of cloth or bandage material soaked in solutions, generally astringents or antimicrobial agents, and applied to localized areas for treatment.

     b. Mechanism of action. Dressings act to physically protect the lesion while delivering high concentrations of the therapeutic agent directly to the area.

     c. Therapeutic uses and administration. Wet dressings are helpful to debride wounds and decubital ulcers.

     d. Adverse effects and limitations. Dressings should be changed frequently to avoid overhydration (maceration) and trapping microbes in the treated area. Many animals will not tolerate a physical dressing and will bite or chew at the application to remove it.

2. Soaks

     a. Definition. Soaks are a form of hydrotherapy containing medications, usually keratolytic agents. Animals are either allowed to sit in the medicated solution or the solution is applied with sponges, cotton balls, or other dressings and allowed to remain for several minutes before drying.

     b. Mechanism of action. The soaking process will increase water absorption by keratinocytes, thus promoting desquamation. Keratolytic agents, such as colloidal oatmeal, are often added to enhance the process.

     c. Therapeutic uses and administration. Soaks are rarely used in veterinary medicine. However, colloidal oatmeal is available as veterinary products and over-the-counter (OTC) as fine powders for soaks. Oatmeal soaks may be used to reduce pruritus in dogs or cats with allergic skin disease. Retention of the water in the keratinocytes is increased when an emollient is used as an occlusive dressing after the soak.

     d. Adverse effects and limitations. Overhydration of the skin is a potential adverse effect. Soaking the entire body is difficult since many patients will not sit still in a soak for 10 minutes.

3. Shampoo therapy

     a. Definition. Shampoos are the most common topical formulation used in veterinary dermatology. Medicated shampoos are used to kill or control ectoparasites, reduce inflammation or control pruritus, facilitate the removal of scale or "normalize" epidermal kinetics, or aid in the control of microbes. Shampoos may contain detergents or be free of soaps, using various bases and emulsifying agents to facilitate distribution of the active ingredients.

     b. Mechanism of action. Shampoos provide topical application of various active ingredients over a large surface of the body. In most cases, the active ingredient is largely removed as the shampoo is rinsed off the patient.

     c. Therapeutic uses and administration.

       (1) Rules of shampoo administration.

         (a) Shampoos should be applied using water that is of room temperature or slightly cool, especially when used for the reduction of pruritus. Heat exacerbates pruritus, and animals bathed with hot water, even if an antipruritic shampoo was used, will be more pruritic after bathing.

         (b) Medicated shampoos should have a contact time of 10 minutes. This allows the active ingredients to work and may allow some absorption of active agents into the stratum corneum.

         (c) Shampoos should be thoroughly rinsed from the hair coat.

         (d) Patients treated for pruritus should be towel dried only. Hair drying, even with those blowing cool air, tends to dry the skin or exacerbate pruritus.

       (2) Frequency of bathing. Shampoos may be administered as often as every other day, depending on the dermatologic condition in the patient. The frequency of shampoo therapy of most dermatologic conditions may be reduced as the condition is controlled.

     d. Adverse effects and limitations. Shampoo therapy may be difficult in some animals, such as cats. In addition, it is very difficult to get sufficient contact on lesions of the head and face. It is best to avoid distributing the shampoo above the neck area for that reason. Other delivery systems (e.g., lotions) are more effective in those areas. Some medications and inactive substances found in the shampoo may be irritating to the eyes or mucous membranes.

4. Sprays
  a. Definition. Sprays are water-based formulations that often contain an emulsifier to aid in distribution of the active agent. Humectants and emollients are common ingredients to facilitate moisturizing the treated area.
  b. Mechanism of action. Sprays deliver the active agent directly to the skin in a mist using a pump spray bottle or aerosol delivery system.
  c. Therapeutic use and administration. Sprays are used to deliver medications for parasite control, control of infectious agents, medications to reduce pruritus, hydrating agents and emollients to condition the skin, and medications for the management of seborrheic conditions. Sprays are excellent for focal treatment of dermatologic conditions, as in treatment of pruritus on the feet or perianal region. They are easy to apply and can be used for spot treatment or generalized application.
  d. Adverse effects and limitations. Sprays of all types (hand pumps or aerosol) may startle or frighten some patients, such as cats or horses. A dense hair coat will reduce the effectiveness of sprays, unless the area is thoroughly soaked.

5. Rinses/dips
  a. Definition. Rinses consist of soluble powders or concentrated liquids mixed with water applied by spraying, rinsing, sponging, or pouring on the diluted medication and allowing it to sit for a prescribed period of time. Most rinses are allowed to dry, or in some cases, they may be rinsed off with more water. The primary advantage of this delivery system is that the medication is left on the patient providing significant residual action.
  b. Mechanism of action. Rinses are used to directly apply the medication on the skin. The therapeutic agent has direct topical effects, and in many cases, will be absorbed and provide some systemic effects.
  c. Therapeutic use and administration.
    (1) Indications. Rinses are an excellent treatment method for generalized disease requiring aggressive therapy. They are usually used to manage ectoparasitic infestations, for example, mange, lice, and fleas.
    (2) Administration. Hair of long- or medium-coated dogs and cats should be removed by clipping to facilitate the contact of the active agent on the skin. Patients should generally be bathed to remove excess dirt or debris, if it is sufficient to block access of the rinse to the skin. The rinse is applied by either pouring the medication onto the animal, by using some type of spray system, or by using a sponge to wet the animal. The rinse solution is generally left on the patient to dry.
  d. Adverse effects and limitations. Adverse effects are largely dependent upon the therapeutic agent found in the rinse or dip. The application of medication as a rinse is more tedious than as a shampoo. In addition, active ingredients of many rinses (e.g., amitraz, lime sulfur) are more odiferous and pose a higher risk to those applying these agents. Most rinses are best performed by trained personnel wearing appropriate protective gear (e.g., gloves, respirator) on well-ventilated areas.

6. Lotions
  a. Definition. Lotions are powders dissolved in water. Some veterinary products use the term "residuals" for these formulations.
  b. Mechanism of action. Lotions are generally liquid to semisolid. The water-based lotions evaporate leaving the active ingredient and emulsifiers and/or emollients on the surface of the skin.
  c. Therapeutic use and administration. Lotions are used for localized treatment of skin conditions. They are useful for the management of parasitic conditions, for focal control of inflammation, for control of pruritus, and for focal scaling or hyperplastic skin conditions.
  d. Adverse effects and limitations. Lotions may be messy to apply where there is hair over the lesion. Hair may also reduce the effectiveness by blocking penetration or coverage of the medication on the skin.

D. **Solids or semisolid preparations**

1. Powders

a. **Definition.** Powders are pulverized solids.

b. **Mechanism of action.** Powders may contain active medications (e.g., parasiticides), be used as dessicants (substances that absorb moisture), or intended to be mixed with liquids to form other formulations (e.g, a paste).

c. **Therapeutic use and administration.** Powder formulations in veterinary medicine may contain antiparasitic agents, antimicrobials, or anti-inflammatory agents. There are intended for spot treatment of localized skin conditions.

d. **Adverse effects and limitations.** Powders tend to be messy and may cause a "cloud" of medication during the application process. As such, care should be taken by those applying powders not to inhale any of the material. Powders tend to form a crust when mixed with water or serum on skin lesions.

2. Ointments

a. **Definition.** An ointment is a semisolid preparation intended for external application. The properties of ointments vary with their intended use, ease of application, and extent of application. Ointments consist of oil-based products, emulsions of water and oil, and water-soluble bases. The emulsions may be considered water-in-oil (W/O), meaning a water-soluble agent emulsified into an oil base, or oil-in-water (O/W), meaning a lipid soluble agent or medication emulsified into a water-soluble base. The latter is more esthetically acceptable, as it tends not to leave as noticeable oily residue at the site of application.

b. **Mechanism of action.** Ointments provide delivery of medication that is dissolved in the best vehicle for the medication. For example, lipid-soluble medications may be dissolved in lipid vehicle and then formulated as an emulsion to allow for better esthetics and distribution of the active agent. Water-soluble medications may be emulsified into an oil base to allow for better penetration into and through the skin.

c. **Therapeutic use and administration.** Ointments are applied locally to skin lesions. They provide the best delivery system to enhance penetration through the two-compartment barrier of the skin. Ointments are generally applied to affected areas once or twice daily.

d. **Adverse effects and limitations.** Most adverse effects of ointments are related to effects from the active medications contained within. However, the oil base or emulsfiers used in ointments may cause irritation or hypersensitivity reactions in some animals. The products are limited by the hair coat of animals. Many pet owners do not like the greasy medications and residue that may be left on the skin (to potentially stain carpets or clothing).

3. Creams

a. **Definition.** A cream is a type of ointment with a water-soluble base. Creams are emulsions of either a water-soluble medication or a lipid-soluble medication in an aqueous base. Creams have an oil phase typically containing petrolatum with higher molecular weight alcohols (e.g., stearyl or cetyl alcohol) as emulsifiers. The aqueous phase, which is generally the largest component of the cream, contains preservatives, emulsifiers, and humectants, such as propylene glycol, glycerin, or polyethylene glycol.

b. **Mechanism of action.** Active medications may be dissolved in the oil phase or aqueous phase of a cream.

c. **Therapeutic use and administration.** Creams provide topical delivery of medications in high concentrations to focal area. In addition, they may hydrate focal areas, since they often contain humectants.

d. **Adverse effects and limitations.** Most adverse effects are due to the active ingredients of specific medications. Like ointments, creams are less effective in patients with a thick hair coat. Likewise, they are not logistically suitable for treating large surface areas.

4. Pastes

a. **Definition.** A paste is an ointment or cream containing a large amount of powder.

b. Mechanism of action. Pastes allow for topical medications to be delivered in high concentrations to the surface of the skin. They may also act as a protective and an occlusive dressing, and as such, enhance absorption of medications into the skin.

c. Therapeutic use and administration. Pastes may be used in veterinary medicine to protect the skin from ultraviolet exposure (e.g., zinc oxide on the nasal planum) or from caustic effects of topical substances (e.g., for urinary incontinence), to facilitate hydration of localized lesions (e.g., hydration of nasal hyperkeratosis), or to deliver medication in high concentrations to focal lesions.

d. Adverse effects and limitations. Adverse effects and limitations are similar to those seen with application of ointments.

5. Gels

a. Definition. Gels are semisolid preparations that form a clear, greaseless, and water-soluble base. There are various types of gels based on their composition, but they may contain polyvinyl alcohol, methycellulose and similar compounds, gelatins, or propylene glycol.

b. Mechanism of action. Gels contain active ingredients in solution. After a gel is distributed onto the skin, the base rapidly evaporates leaving the active agent with no oily or greasy residue.

c. Therapeutic use and administration. Gels are widely accepted by pet owners because they are cosmetically acceptable. Veterinary and medical formulations are available that contain, hydrating agents (e.g., salicylic acid, KeraSolv®), antibacterial agents (e.g., benzoyl peroxide, BPO Gel®), glucocorticoids, and antifungal agents. These are applied to affected skin once or twice daily.

d. Adverse effects and limitations. Adverse affects from topical application of gels are due to active ingredients or topical sensitization to humectants (e.g., propylene glycol) or other components of the gel. Gels have similar limitations as ointments and creams by the nature of the hair coat of animals.

IV. CLINICAL APPLICATION OF TOPICAL THERAPY

A. Antimicrobial therapy

1. Topical antibacterial therapy

a. Indications. Topical antimicrobial therapy is indicated for focal bacterial skin lesions and as adjunctive therapy for superficial pyoderma (e.g., folliculitis).

b. Therapeutic options

(1) Topical antibiotics are generally not highly effective because of their limited ability to penetrate deep into the skin and provide high concentrations of the active ingredient. **One antibiotic, known for its ability to penetrate into granulation tissue, is mupirocin.** Mupirocin is available as an ointment and may be useful for draining tracts or focal granulomas caused by bacteria when applied to the affected area once or twice daily. **Mupirocin is highly effective against staphylococci and many gram-negative bacteria.**

(2) Shampoo therapy is widely used as adjunctive therapy for generalized pyoderma. Ingredients with efficacy against staphylococci are preferred and include benzoyl peroxide, chlorhexidine, ethyl lactate, iodifors, triclosan, salicylic acid, and sulfur.

(a) Benzoyl peroxide has been shown to be the most effective topical antibacterial agent, providing up to 48 hours of bactericidal activity. It is found in several veterinary products, sometimes in combination with salicylic acid and/or sulfur.

(b) Ethyl lactate is available in a veterinary shampoo formulation (EtiDerm®). This agent penetrates the hair follicle and sebaceous glands where it dissociates into ethyl alcohol and lactic acid, which provide comdolytic and antibacterial activities, respectively.

c. Administration and clinical use

(1) Antibacterial shampoos are generally administered as baths every 3–7 days as adjunctive therapy for surface and superficial pyoderma. Disease conditions where shampoo therapy is beneficial includes puppy pyoderma, acute moist dermatitis, and folliculitis.

(2) Good principles of bathing should be followed.

(3) Antibacterial shampoos are not effective for management of deep pyodermas.

2. Topical antifungal therapy

a. Topical therapy for yeast (*M. pachydermatis*)

(1) Indications. Topical therapy is often effective as the sole therapy for localized or generalized *Malassezia* dermatitis. It is also useful as adjunctive therapy when systemic management of yeast infections is utilized. Topical therapy is highly effective as the sole treatment of *Malassezia* infections in otitis externa.

(2) Therapeutic options. Topical agents that have some activity against *Malassezia* spp. yeast include nystatin, azoles (miconazole, clotrimazole, ketoconazole, enilconazole), chlorhexidine, lime sulfur, iodifors, and acetic acid/boric acid. The combination of miconazole with chlorhexidine (Malaseb® Shampoo) has shown superior efficacy as a shampoo for yeast dermatitis. Other similar combination products (e.g., ketoconazole and chlorhexidine, KetoChlor®) may have similar efficacy.

(3) Clinical use.

(a) For sole therapy, shampoos should be administered three times weekly for 2–3 weeks, then twice weekly for 2–3 weeks, then every 7–10 days as maintenance therapy.

(b) As adjunctive therapy, shampoos should be administered every 7–10 days.

(c) Good principles of bathing should be followed (e.g., contact time).

(d) Several areas of the body are difficult to treat using shampoos. These include the lip folds, facial folds on brachcephalic breeds, and even the ventral and dorsal interdigital areas. Topical therapy against yeast can be greatly enhanced using moist towelettes or pledgets containing miconazole and chlorhexidine (e.g., Malaseb® towelettes) or boric acid and acetic acid (e.g., Malcetic Wipes) to clean the affected areas once daily.

b. Topical therapy for dermatophytosis

(1) Indications. Topical therapy is not recommended as the sole treatment for dermatophytosis in companion animals. It may be more effective in large animals. However, topical therapy is not recommended for the sole therapy of any animal that is in frequent contact with humans.

(2) Therapeutic options.

(a) Agents with antifungal activity against dermatophytes include the azoles (miconazole, clotrimazole, ketoconazole, and enilconazole), nystatin, lime sulfur, terbinafine, and sodium hypochlorite.

(b) These active ingredients may be found in lotions, creams and ointments, powders, and shampoos, and as concentrates that may be diluted down and used as a rinse or spray.

(c) Several commercially available veterinary products contain combinations of active ingredients, such as miconazole and chlorhexidine.

(3) Administration and clinical use.

(a) Lotions or creams may be applied to lesions once or twice daily. These products must be used with care to avoid dispersal of infective components. Therefore, if used, it is recommended that they should be applied from the periphery of the lesion and then distributed toward the center of the lesion.

(b) Shampoo therapy is a highly effective as an adjunct therapy for dermatophytosis. While it is not recommended as the sole therapy, routine bathing with antifungal shampoos has been shown to speed clinical recovery and may reduce the time period in which the animal is contagious.

    i. As adjunctive therapy, animals should be bathed once weekly following good principles of bathing.

   ii. Topical application of products as sprays may also be helpful. One spray that contains both miconazole and chlorhexidine (Malaseb® spray) is commercially available and can be very effective as an adjunctive therapy for dermatophytosis.

B. **Topical management of pruritus**

1. **Indications.** Topical agents are very useful to manage generalized pruritic skin conditions, especially atopic dermatitis. They may also be helpful, though often not as effective, in the management of contact allergy, food allergy, and many other skin disorders that induce pruritus. Topical therapy can be very useful to facilitate withdrawal for systemic antipruritic medications in preparation for allergy testing. In addition, topical therapy may provide the additional therapy required for "trouble areas," such as the interdigital areas or the perianal region, in animals with atopic dermatitis. However, topical therapy is generally not highly effective as the sole treatment of pruritic skin conditions, especially for extended time periods.

2. **Therapeutic options**

   a. Shampoos containing keratolytic agents or topical antipruritic agents, such as colloidal oatmeal or sulfur, will hydrate the skin and reduce the pruritus. The duration of activity of these products is generally ~24 hours.

   b. A shampoo containing diphenhydramine in a colloidal oatmeal base is available for adjunctive management of allergic pruritus.

   c. A topical anesthetic, pramoxine, is available in shampoos (combined with colloidal oatmeal). This agent provides enhanced antipruritic activity over colloidal oatmeal alone and is available as a spray or shampoo (Dermal Soothe®; Relief®).

   d. Ointments, creams, and lotions (i.e., residuals) containing glucocorticoids may be useful for focal pruritic skin lesions. Topical glucocorticoids are also considered a key element in topical management of otitis externa. For generalized pruritus, shampoos, rinses, or sprays provide dispersion to a greater surface area. Glucocorticoids, available for topical use in increasing order of potency, include hydrocortisone, prednisolone, triamcinolone, dexamethasone, betamethasone, flucinolone, and mometasone. Hydrocortisone is the most commonly used topical glucocorticoid and is available in lotions, shampoos, and sprays. Triamcinolone is also available in lotions, creams, ointments, and sprays (e.g., Genesis® Spray).

     (1) Glucocorticoids applied topically will be absorbed and may induce systemic effects, including suppression of the hypothalamic–pituitary–adrenal axis, hyperglycemia, polyuria/polydipsia, and other signs of hyperadrenocorticism. Hydrocortisone is a mild glucocorticoid and is the least likely to result in these adverse effects.

     (2) Prolonged application of any glucocorticoid, and even short-term application of potent glucocorticoids, may result in cutaneous atrophy, comedone formation, and scarring of the skin. The glucocorticoid selected for topical use should be based on the potency required for the problem. Use of more potent topical glucocorticoids will likely increase the incidence of adverse effects.

     (3) Topical tacrolimus (Protopic-Fujisawa) has been shown to provide some anti-inflammatory and antipruritic effects in dogs with atopic dermatitis.

3. **Administration and clinical use**

   a. For adjunctive management of generalized pruritus accompanying atopic dermatitis, shampoos containing hydrocortisone, diphenhydramine, or pramoxine may be administered once weekly or as needed.

     (1) These agents may be effective as the sole therapy of pruritus in mild atopy cases.

     (2) Good principles of shampoo therapy should be followed, especially contact time and the use of neutral temperature or cool water for bathing.

b. For managing trouble spots, such as the perianal or interdigital regions, lotions (residuals), sprays, or creams/ointments may be applied to the affected areas.

(1) Prolonged use of products containing glucocorticoids, other than hydrocortisone, should be avoided.

(2) Products containing pramoxine or diphenhydramine may be used daily or as needed.

(3) Pentoxyfylline ointment may be applied twice weekly for adjunctive management of pruritus associated with atopic dermatitis. Humans should wear gloves when applying this product.

C. **Topical antiseborrheic therapy**

1. Indications. Topical antiseborrheic therapy is indicated to reduce scaling associated with primary seborrhea and to reduce scaling and pruritus associated with other scaling disorders. These products may be helpful in the management of familial seborrhea, ichthyosis (i.e., ichthyosis of the golden retriever), sebaceous adenitis, or any other parasitic or infectious skin disorder that is characterized by excessive scale formation. Familial seborrhea is the classical disease condition for which these products are used.

2. Therapeutic options

a. Shampoos are the most commonly employed delivery system for antiseborrheic agents, although rinses, sprays, and lotions may also be used.

b. Active ingredients provide some reduction in scale formation (keratoplastic agents) or facilitate removal of scale (keratolytic agents).

(1) Tar is the most effective keratoplastic ingredient used in topical veterinary formulations. It also has keratolytic, degreasing, and antipruritic properties. Tars have been refined to remove many of the more irritating hydrocarbons; however, they may still cause irritation and photosensitization in some animals. Tars have historically been combined with sulfur to antagonize this irritant effect.

(2) Sulfur is keratolytic, mildly keratoplastic, antipruritic, antibacterial, antifungal, and antiparasitic, depending on the formulation and concentration. It is considered to be mild and is often combined with tar or salicylic acid.

(3) Salicylic acid is an active ingredient that may be found as the primary ingredient (e.g., Keratolux®) or combined with sulfur, where there may be synergistic effects. Salicylic acid is keratoplastic, keratolytic, mildly antipruritic, and antibacterial. It is considered a mild product making it safe for use on cats.

(4) Selenium disulfide is a potent degreasing agent that is also keratolytic, antibacterial, and has some anti-yeast activity. It may stain some hair coats and clothing. Overuse will result is dry skin and pruritus. However, this is an excellent agent for greasy skin conditions.

(5) Benzoyl peroxide is antibacterial, degreasing, keratolytic, antipruritic, and is often reported to have the ability to penetrate into the follicles, often call follicular flushing activity. It has been shown to dry the skin and allow for increased transepidermal water loss and decrease surface skin lipid concentrations. It is the best topical antibacterial agent for dogs and is also effective to remove excessive oils in greasy skin conditions. Benzoyl peroxide may be irritating, especially in cats and when concentrations exceed 5%. Benzoyl peroxide may bleach clothing.

(6) **Recently, a line of topical veterinary products containing phytosphingosines has been introduced in North America. These lipid-containing products may act as emollients and keratoplastic agents and have some antibacterial and antifungal properties.**

3. Administration and clinical use

a. For familial seborrhea, shampoo therapy may be a very effective method to manage the disease.

(1) Two shampoos are selected for initial use on the basis of clinical features. For animals with a bacterial component, benzoyl peroxide would be recommended. Sulfur would be recommended for patients with pruritus and no clinical infections. Animals with yeast dermatitis and greasy skin would benefit more with initial application of shampoos containing selenium disulfide. Clinical judgment is used to select the best two initial shampoos.

(2) Animals are bathed three times weekly for 3 weeks following good principles of shampoo therapy.

(3) After 3 weeks, the shampoo perceived by the client to work the best is combined with a 1% salicylic acid shampoo or tar shampoo. These are utilized for their superior keratoplastic properties. Patients are then bathed twice weekly, alternating use of the one shampoo from the first round that worked the best and the shampoo added during the recheck examination.

(4) The frequency of shampoos is slowly reduced to allow the best clinical control of the condition. In general, owners are very capable to determine the best long-term schedule for shampoos. A tar or 1% salicylic acid shampoo is recommended as part of the long-term management.

b. For sebaceous adentitis or other scaling conditions, shampoos containing sulfur-salicylic acid, 1% salicylic acid, or tar will generally provide the best reduction of scale formation. The frequency of bathing required varies greatly with the patient and disease condition.

c. Scaling may also be reduced for familial seborrhea and other scaling disorders through the topical application of products containing phytosphingosines. These products are available in various formulations, including shampoos, pour-ons, sprays, and otic formulations. Combinations of shampoos, sprays, and the pour-on formulation appear to facilitate the reduction of scale in these disease conditions.

D. Antiparasitic therapy

1. Indications. Topical therapy is an effective method to control parasitic infestations caused by mites, lice, fleas, and other ectoparasites. However, the development of several excellent systemic parasiticides has reduced the use of topical antiparasitic agents over the past several years.

2. Therapeutic options

a. Topical antiparasitic agents

(1) **Delivery systems.** Antiparasitic agents are commercially available as powders, sprays, shampoos, foaming agents, pour-ons, and rinses. Some of the agents are absorbed and have systemic effects, including distribution to the skin through lipid secretions (e.g., selamectin).

(a) Microencapsulation suspends insecticides in microscopic spherules made of various substances. This technology has been used for pyrethrin-containing products. The insecticide is inactive while contain within the microspheres, but when released onto the parasite, through diffusion or breakdown of the sphere, the insecticide is active. Microencapsulation reduces the toxicity, since the insecticide is inactive in these suspensions. The ability to rapidly kill insects upon exposure, known as knockdown, may be reduced through this process while the residual activity of the product is extended.

(2) **Active ingredients**

(a) **Sulfur** remains an excellent parasiticide. It is available in two veterinary formulations (LymDyp®; Sulfurated Lime Dip®) and is effective against various mites, lice, and chiggers. The most effective application is through weekly rinses. The product is very safe for dogs and cats, as well as puppies and kittens, and may be used on horses. The primary adverse effects are the foul, rotten-egg odor, and staining of hair coat and clothing.

(b) **Pyrethrins** are volatile oil extracts of the chrysanthemum flower. They act as neurotoxins to kill fleas, mites, lice, and flies and may be used on dogs, and in low concentrations, on cats. Products containing pyrethrins are very common in OTC products. They have excellent knockdown ability but are rapidly inactivated by UV light. Most products containing pyrethrins also contain piperonyl butoxide, a microsomal enzyme inhibitor, to prevent insects from rapidly inactivating the insecticide.

(c) **Pyrethroids** are synthetic insecticides based on the pyrethrin molecule. In general, these agents have less knockdown ability than pyrethrin, but more residual activity. Permethrin and other pyrethroids also exhibit some repellent activity and have been labeled as repellents for mosquitoes (K9 Advantix®). Pyrethroids are, in general, significantly safer than the natural pyrethrins. Permethrin is the most commonly found pyrethroid in prescription and OTC veterinary formulations, but there are many pyrethroids available for common use, including etofenprox, d-trans allethrin, resmethrin, and others. Pyrethroids are toxic to cats and should not be used in that species.

(d) **Two types of cholinesterase inhibitors** remain available for use, though their use has declined greatly due to the availability of less toxic, effective antiparasitic agents.

    i. Carbamates, such as carbaryl, remain available in powders, sprays, and rinses.

    ii. Organophosphates, once a mainstay in insecticidal products, are infrequently used due to the development of safer, more effective agents. In general, these are highly toxic substances, and with the exception of malathion, should never be used on cats. Examples of organophosphates include malathion, dichlorvos, diazinon, phosmet, and coumaphous. Organophosphates are used more often for environmental control than for direct application on pets.

(e) **Amitraz** (Mitaban®), an octopamine receptor agonist, is available as a rinse for the treatment of canine demodicosis. It has been shown to be effective and is licensed in other countries for the treatment of sarcoptic mange. Side effects of amitraz include sedation, bradycardia, hypotension, pruritus, and hyperglycemia. Most of these side effects are due to activation of α_2-adrenergic receptors and hence are reversible with yohimbine.

(f) **Fipronil** is a neurotoxin of the phenylprazole class and is available as a pour-on product (Frontline®) for the treatment of fleas, ticks, and lice in dogs and cats. This drug distributes throughout the body in the lipid layer of the skin. It is not significantly absorbed. It is reported to be rapidly effective (within 24 hours) and persist in therapeutic concentrations for 1 month.

(g) **Neonicotinoids** are insecticides that act as neurotoxins by serving as agonists at the insect nicotinic acetylcholine receptor.

    i. Imidacloprid is available as a pour-on product (Advantage®, Advantage Multi®) for the treatment of fleas. Imidacloprid is not systemically absorbed. It is distributed through the lipid layers of the epidermis. Like fipronil, imidacloprid is reported to kill greater than 95% of fleas on an animal within the first 24 hours and duration of activity for 1 month in dogs and 3 weeks in cats. It is also effective against some lice.

    ii. Nitenpyram (Capstar®) is an orally effective neonicotinoid insecticide related to imidacloprid. It kills fleas within a few hours of oral dosing in dogs and cats, but has little to no residual activity. It is very safe and ideal for treating flea-infested pets before admission to hospitals or boarding facilities.

    iii. Dinotefuran (Vectra 3D®) is a third-generation neonicotinoid with slightly faster knockdown than imidocloprid while retaining residual activity against fleas for at least 30 days. It is available in combination with permethrin and pyriproxifen for use on dogs and in combination with pyriproxifen for use on cats.

(h) Macrocyclic lactones. See Chapter 16 for detailed information on these drugs.

i. Selamectin (Revolution®) is an avermectin compound that stimulates glutamate-gated chloride channels to cause hyperpolarization of neurons and muscle, resulting in paralysis and death in susceptible parasites. It is safe in puppies and kittens greater than 6 weeks of age, in lactating and pregnant bitches, and is safe in ivermectin-sensitive dogs. Selamectin is systemically absorbed following topical application as a pour-on product. The active agent is then redistributed through lipids secreted by sebaceous glands of the skin. Selamectin is effective for the treatment of flea infestations and a wide range of mite infestations, including sarcoptic mange, otoacariasis, and notoedric mange. It is also an effective heartworm preventative, kills some internal parasites (e.g., *Ancylostoma tubaeforme*, *Toxocara cati*) and kills some ticks (*Dermacentor* spp.)

ii. Moxidectin is a pentacyclic lactone of the milbemycin class, and is closely related to avermectins. It is available as a pour-on product for cattle and in combination with imidacloprid (Advantage®) for use on dogs and cats. Moxidectin may be effective against a wide range of mites; however, detailed studies are currently underway to evaluate its safety and efficacy.

iii. Doramectin is another avermectin that has been used to manage canine demodicosis outside the United States. Doramectin has shown efficacy and safety in treating sarcoptic mange in rabbits. At this time, it is not recommended for use in dogs or cats.

iv. Milbemycin oxime (Interceptor® Flavor Tabs) is closely related to avermectins and is administered orally for heartworm control. It is also effective against *Sarcoptes canis* when administered daily in high doses (0.5–1.0 mg/kg) for 30–120 days. It is not available as a topical product but is included in this chapter because it is related to several topical antiparasitic agents.

(i) Metaflumizone (ProMeris®) is a neurotoxin that works by blocking sodium influx in nerves of fleas, causing paralysis and death. It is available as a pour-on product for cat (older than 8 weeks of age) and dogs and labeled for monthly application. Field efficacy of this new product is not clear at this time. (See Chapter 16 for detailed information on metaflumizone.)

b. Insect growth regulators

(1) Juvenile hormone analogs. These agents interfere with the metabolism, development, and reproductions of the various life stages of fleas by mimicking chemicals that act as growth hormones in the flea. (See Chapter 16 for detailed information on juvenile hormone analogs.)

(a) Methoprene is a juvenile hormone analogue that is available in sprays (Frontline® Spray Treatment), rinses, flea collars, and in combination with fipronil as a pour-on product (Frontline® Plus). It is degraded by exposure to UV light. Methoprene is very safe and may be used on puppies and kittens with a high degree of safety.

(b) Pyriproxifen is available in sprays and has the advantage of being UV-stabile. It is widely available in products found OTC in combination with insecticides.

(2) Chitin inhibitors, such as lufenuron (Program®), are given orally to disrupt the synthesis and deposition of chitin in the exoskeleton of fleas. It is an oral product that works through systemic activity. (See Chapter 16 for detailed information on lufenuron.)

3. Administration and clinical use

a. Flea control

(1) For knockdown (i.e., rapid kill of adult fleas), pyrethrin sprays, rinses, or shampoos are effective. Orally administered nitenpyram is an excellent knockdown product and provides the fastest kill of adult fleas available. It is labeled for use in animals over 4 weeks of age and 2 pounds body weight.

(2) For rapid kill (less than 24 hours) of adult fleas with excellent residual effects, monthly application of fipronil, imidacloprid, or selamectin in dogs and cats or metaflumizome in cats.

(3) Integrated flea control is the principle of applying multiple flea control products that work in different manners (e.g., insecticide vs. insect growth regulator) to provide better flea control. Several veterinary products are combinations of insecticides and growth regulators. Frontline® Plus (fipronil and methoprene) and Knockout® (permethrin and pyriproxifen) are good examples of these products.

(a) Combinations of various flea control products can accomplish the same task. For example, nitenpyram could be administered orally once weekly while a patient is receiving monthly lufenuron as an insect growth regulator.

(b) Products that have different mechanisms of action may be used in combination therapy. To avoid toxicity drugs of the same class should not be used together.

b. **Control of mite infestations**

(1) The selection of a miticidal agent should be based on the safety and toxicity studies in the species to be treated and efficacy studies for the various mites.

(2) For sarcoptic mange of dogs, highly effective products labeled for treating this condition include selamectin and lime sulfur. Other products showing efficacy, but not labeled for this infestation include ivermectin, amitraz, moxidectin, fipronil sprays, and milbemycin oxime.

(3) For generalized demodicosis of dogs caused by *Demodex canis*, amitraz is the only labeled product available in the United States. Other products showing efficacy include ivermectin (give orally in high doses), moxidectin, and milbemycin oxime. The extra-label use of these agents in high doses may result in drug toxicity.

(4) For generalized demodicosis in cats caused by *Demodex gatoi*, lime sulfur rinses are the treatment of choice.

(5) For the treatment of notoderic mange in cats caused by *Notoedres cati*, effective products include ivermectin (orally), selamectin, and lime sulfur rinses. Other macrocyclic lactones may also be effective.

c. **Pediculosis (lice infestations).** For pediculosis of dogs and cats, topical application of lime sulfur, pyrethrin, pyrethroids (for dogs only), imidacloprid, fipronil sprays, and cholinesterase inhibitors (both organophosphates and carbamates for dogs only) have been shown to be effective. The efficacy of newer pour-on products containing selamectin, moxidectin, or metaflumizone is unclear. In addition, there may be some variability between species of lice.

d. **Tick control.** For tick control, several products may be used to kill or remove ticks in various life stages from the animals. Powders, rinses, sprays, pour-on products, and systemic parasiticides may all exhibit some efficacy. Products with a proven record for prevention of tick infestation and/or removal of ticks from animals include fipronil pour-on or sprays, permethrin pour-on products (dogs only), and flea collars containing amitraz (Preventic® Plus Tick and Flea IGR Collar for Dogs). Selamectin has efficacy against *Dermacentor* spp. ticks but poor activity against other canine ticks.

V. SYSTEMIC THERAPY OF DERMATOLOGIC CONDITIONS

A. **Therapeutic uses.** Systemic therapy is indicated for the management of most dermatology conditions, including allergy, autoimmune disorders, infectious diseases, metabolic and endocrine conditions, genetic and congenital skin disorders, and many others. Systemic therapy is necessary for generalized conditions, conditions manifested below the epidermis (e.g., deep pyoderma), when clients are unable to apply topical medications (e.g., due to physical limitations of the owners), when animals are not cooperative in the topical application process, or in some cases, for financial reasons.

B. **Preparations.** The most common systemic medications used in dermatology include antimicrobial agents, anti-inflammatory agents (e.g., glucocorticoids), antihistamines, nutraceuticals (e.g., fatty acid supplements), cytotoxic agents, hormones (e.g., thyroid supplements), vitamins (e.g., vitamin A), and antiparasitic compounds.

C. **Administration.** These systemic medications are administered orally, parenterally, or by absorption of topically applied medications.

D. **Adverse effects.** Naturally, the administration of pharmacological agents orally or parenterally is more likely to be associated with systemic side effects. Allergic reactions and other adverse effects, such as retinal damage in cats receiving some fluoroquinolone antibiotics in high doses, are a potential problem with any antimicrobial. Glucocorticoids are well recognized for creating iatrogenic hyperadrenocorticism (both cutaneous and systemic) and for suppressing the hypothalamic-pituitary-adrenal axis. Antiparasitic compounds may lead to adverse effects directly due to the neurotoxic activities. In addition, some animals have increased sensitivity to some antiparasitic agents, such as macrocyclic lactones, due to mutations in the multiple drug resistance-1 gene.

VI. SAFETY

A. **Application of medications.** Care should always be taken when applying topical medications since direct application of most of these agents can have effects on human skin or be absorbed systemically in humans. Gloves should be worn by those applying rinse, creams, ointments, or when rubbing in sprays or lotions. Medications should be applied in well-ventilated areas, especially for medications applied as topical sprays, to avoid inhalation of aerosolized drugs. Clients with small children should be instructed to keep animals with recent applications of topical agents away from the children, at least until the medicine is dry or dissipated. Caution and warning labels should always be consulted and followed. We generally recommend that topical applications are not applied by children, people with debilitating or immunosuppressive diseases, or the elderly.

B. **Storage of medication.** All medications should be stored in a secure location, safe from small children and from animals that might accidentally ingest or come into inappropriate contact with the agents. Products should be stored according to label instructions.

SUGGESTED READING

Block LH. 2000. "Medicated topicals." In *Remington: The Science and Practice of Pharmacy.* Edited by Gennaro AR. 20th ed., pp. 837–857. Baltimore, MD: Lippincott Williams & Wilkins.
Brunner SR. 2006. Updates in therapeutics in veterinary dermatology. *Vet Clin North Am Small Anim Pract* 36:39–58.
Gortel K. 2006. Update on canine demodicosis. *Vet Clin North Am Small Anim Pract* 36:229–241.
Knutson K, Pershing LK. 2000. "Topical drugs." In *Remington: The Science and Practice of Pharmacy.* Edited by Gennaro AR. 20th ed., pp. 1200–1218. Baltimore, MD: Lippincott Williams & Wilkins.
Marsella R. 2006. Atopy: New targets and new therapies. *Vet Clin North Am Small Anim Pract* 36:161–174.
Plumb DC. 2005. *Veterinary Drug Handbook.* 5th ed. Ames, IA: Blackwell Publishing.

Riviere JE, Spoo JW. 2001. "Dermatopharmacology: Drugs acting locally on the skin." In *Veterinary Pharmacology and Therapeutics*. Edited by Adams HR. 8th ed., pp. 1084–1104. Ames, IA: Iowa State University Press.

Scott DW, MIller WH, Griffin CE. 2001. "Dermatologic therapy." In *Muller and Kirk's Small Animal Dermatology*. Edited by Scott DW, Miller WH, Griffin CE. 6th ed., pp. 207–273. Philadelphia, PA: Saunders.

STUDY QUESTIONS

DIRECTIONS: Each of the numbered items or incomplete statements in this section is followed by answers or by completions of the statement. Select the **one** lettered answer or completion that is **best** in each case.

1. Which one of the following shampoo ingredients would be most suitable for the treatment of a dog with *Malassezia* dermatitis, where the dog is severely greasy and has 4+ yeasts on the skin?

(A) Benzoyl peroxide
(B) Sulfur/salicylic acid
(C) Tar/sulfur
(D) Selenium disulfide
(E) Salicylic acid alone

2. What is the main objective of using an emollient after shampooing?

(A) To prevent secondary bacterial infection
(B) To act as an occlusive dressing to trap water and hydrate the skin
(C) To activate the active ingredient of the shampoo
(D) To remove the active ingredient to prevent irritation
(E) To suppress pruritus

3. Which shampoo ingredient is used primarily for its keratoplastic property?

(A) Tar
(B) Sulfur
(C) Salicylic acid
(D) Selenium disulfide
(E) Benzoyl peroxide

4. Which of the following *delivery vehicles* would be the most occlusive? In other words, which would be best used on a dry lesion in an attempt to treat the lesion and hydrate the area?

(A) Powder
(B) Rinse
(C) Lotion
(D) Ointment
(E) Gel

5. Which of the following is used to allow mixture of an oil (or lipid) material with an aqueous (or water) material?

(A) A gel
(B) An emulsifier
(C) A humectant

(D) An emollient
(E) An alcohol

6. In general, shampoos should be applied and allowed to sit for what period of time?

(A) A few moments
(B) 2–3 minutes
(C) 10 minutes
(D) 30 minutes
(E) The time to sit prior to rinsing is not important.

7. The term used to describe the pharmacological behavior of the skin is

(A) hydrophilic.
(B) lipophilic.
(C) two-compartment system.
(D) complete barrier.
(E) completely soluble system.

8. Keratolytic agents work primarily by

(A) lysing keratinocytes by destroying sulfur bonds.
(B) acting as softening agents by hydrating keratinocytes.
(C) slowing epidermal turnover.
(D) dissolving the keratinocytes.
(E) stopping the production of keratin within keratinocytes.

9. Which of the following delivery systems would most likely be the most esthetically acceptable to pet owners?

(A) Paste
(B) Water-in-oil ointment
(C) Poultice
(D) Oil-in-water ointment
(E) Gel

10. Phytosphingosines are

(A) plant extracts used for dermatology therapy.
(B) oils derived from marine mammals.
(C) lipids produced by keratinocytes.
(D) emulsions of lipids and aqueous sweat.
(E) structures found on keratinocytes that act as drug receptors.

ANSWERS AND EXPLANATIONS

1. The answer is D.
Selenium disulfide is the best and most powerful degreasing agent listed as an option. It also appears to have some direct anti-yeast activity. Benzoyl peroxide is also an excellent degreasing agent, but has no activity on yeast. If the patient was greasy and had a bacterial infection, the answer would have been benzoyl peroxide.

2. The answer is B.
An emollient is used to act as an occlusive dressing. This will trap water to enhance water absorption by keratinocytes and slow the evaporation process that is inevitable. Emollients allow the skin to stay hydrated for a longer time period.

3. The answer is A.
Tar has many pharmacological properties, but its keratoplastic properties are their main indication for use. Tar is also mildly antipruritic, mildly degreasing, and has keratolytic properties, but we use it in dermatology for the keratoplastic effects. Other agents listed also have mild keratoplastic properties, but they are primarily used for other qualities.

4. The answer is D.
Ointments contain lipids that act as a barrier or occlusive dressing. This will trap medications and water on the skin to facilitate hydraton. This barrier also serves to slow transepidermal water loss through the epidermis.

5. The answer is B.
Emulsifiers are the agents that allow for oil and water-based materials to effective disperse and mix. Emulsifiers include sodium lauryl sulfate, soaps, quaternary ammonium salts, and polyoxyethylene glycols, fatty acids, and alcohols.

6. The answer is C.
In general, 10 minutes is the ideal time to allow a shampoo to sit on a patient. Shorter times will not allow the active ingredients to be effective topically or diffuse into the epidermis. Longer times become tedious for pet owners and could result in overhydration of the skin.

7. The answer is C.
The skin is considered a two-compartment system because it has lipophobic (hydrophilic) keratinocytes that are surrounded by lipohilic (hydrophobic) lipids. Any topical agent must be able to transverse these structures, and to be active topically, must be able to be compatible with areas.

8. The answer is B.
The term keratolytic is somewhat confusing. While these agents do cause some changes in the keratinocytes and desmosomes, they primarily allow increased hydration and softening of the keratinocytes. These softer cells are then more easily desquamated or removed.

9. The answer is E.
Gels evaporate leaving little to no residue behind. Even the oil-in-water ointments leave some residue after absorption. Most pet owners prefer topical medications that do not leave such a residue that could stain clothing, carpets, and furniture, or be detected by handling the pet.

10. The answer is C.
Phytosphingosines are produced naturally by keratinocytes in lamellar bodies. These lipids then are released into the intercellular spaces where the help from the lipid layer found between epithelial cells. They are a key part of the barrier produced by the epidermis.

Chapter 14

Ocular Pharmacology

Daniel M. Betts

I. **GENERAL CONSIDERATIONS.** Many drugs that are used for other organs or systems, for example, the nervous, cardiovascular, immune, and endocrine systems, are used orally or parenterally for ocular disease conditions. **With few exceptions, the content of this chapter is limited to the topically administered drugs for the eye.**

A. Considerations for drug delivery in topical administration

1. **The blood–ocular barriers** to drug penetration are complex, protective mechanisms that complicate drug delivery to the interior of the uninflamed eye. In corneal and conjunctival diseases where the epithelium is compromised or removed, resistance to drug absorption/corneal penetration is reduced or eliminated.
2. **Vascular supply of the eye. The eye is a complex organ with an intricate vascular supply** to nourish highly specialized neuroreceptors and unique tissues that must remain transparent to focus light on the photo receptors deep within the organ, and a system for secretion, circulation, and absorption of a fluid to nourish and maintain intraocular pressure compatible with the primary function of vision.

B. Mechanism of action. Drugs used in ophthalmic practice are generally the same as those targeted for other systems in regard to their mechanism of action. **The uniqueness of ocular pharmacology is in the vehicle or formulation appropriate for delivery of these drugs for absorption and distribution to the targeted tissues or compartments of the eye at a sufficiently high concentration without creating toxic or physical damage to other ocular tissues.**

C. Pharmacokinetics. In contrast to the abundance of pharmacokinetic data for systemic drugs, few data are available for ophthalmic drugs. In many analyses, the effects of the drug (change in pupil size, lowered intraocular pressure, change in corneal thickness, changes in optical transparency, or electrophysiologic or imaging recordings) are the basis for determining absorption, distribution, and metabolism. Drug concentrations in tissues or compartments of the eye cannot be done without disturbing and impairing the "system."

II. **OPHTHALMIC DRUG DELIVERY**

A. Treatment of precorneal tissues and tearfilm, cornea, iris, and ciliary body

1. **Topical preparations** are preferred as they achieve relatively high local concentrations with only marginal drug exposure of the rest of the body.
   a. Preparations are solutions, suspensions, emulsions, and lipid- or oil-based ointments for periodic application to the surface of the eye.
   b. Ocular (conjunctival) inserts and impregnated soft contact lenses for slow release facilitate convenient uniform drug delivery.
   c. Subconjunctival and subtenon's injections may provide a long-lasting slow release depot of drug for the anterior segment.
   d. Systemic delivery of some agents is limited by poor penetration due to the blood–ocular barriers or the paucity or absence of blood supply (cornea, sclera, lens).

B. **Other local forms of delivery** to other tissues or compartments

1. **Intracameral injections** into the vitreous or aqueous humor.
2. **Retrobulbar injections**
3. **Implantion of various drug impregnated**, slow-release polymers intravitreally or suprachoroidally.

C. **When a drop is instilled into the conjunctival sac**

1. Absorption of an ocular medication from the cul-de-sac begins with mixing of the drug with tears to give some unknown dilution that is exposed to the entire conjunctival and corneal surface.
2. Tear volume (in canine) is 8–12 μL; conjunctival sac is about 3–6 μL; delivery volume is about 50 μL; at most 20 μL can be retained.
3. Excess spills over the lid margin or goes down the nasolacrimal duct.
4. Tear turnover rate is 0.5–1.0 μL/min, so the $t_{1/2}$ of the initial drug concentration is 3–6 minutes.
5. Slower elimination is achieved with ointments.
6. Washout times are shortened with increased lacrimation due to irritation/discomfort or increased drainage induced by blinking. (Restraint of the dog increases the blink rate.)
7. The spillover or drained portion may be absorbed by the mucous membranes in the nose or digestive tract and can lead to systemic side effects.
8. The principal route into the eye is through the cornea.
   a. Epithelial and endothelial cell membrane and intercellular tight junctions limit penetration to the lipophilic agents; the stroma is hydrophilic and water-soluble agents diffuse most readily.
   b. Ideally, one should couple lipophilic component to a more hydrophilic drug that would cleave or dissociate after passage through the cornea.
9. **Drug binding to protein in tears** or to conjunctival pigment may reduce bioavailability. Degradation by enzymes within the cornea may destroy the drug enroute, and binding to protein in aqueous humor may inactivate and hasten elimination from the anterior chamber.
10. **Drug molecules** pass between compartments by diffusion and active transport processes.
    a. Diffusion follows concentration gradient. Related inversely to molecular size and directly to temperature.
    b. Related to chemical structure and stearic configuration.
    c. Active transport is affected by competition of other substrates for the transport system.
11. Binding, diffusion, and transport processes are quite variable between individuals and species, and are affected by pathologic conditions such as inflammation.
12. Penetration into the eye through the conjunctiva is generally not relevant. Conjunctival epithelium is similar to corneal epithelium. The subconjunctiva, episclera, sclera, and choroid are not significant barriers to diffusion.
13. Drugs crossing the conjunctiva and sclera are eliminated by the blood circulation in the choroid.
14. Once through the cornea, drugs diffuse in the aqueous humor and are taken up in the iris, base of the ciliary body and the lens. There is little to no flow into the posterior segment. **Posterior segment diseases cannot be treated effectively with topical medications.**
15. Cornea and lens can absorb drugs, then retain and release them over a prolonged time, such as corticosteroids in the lens.
16. Drugs are eliminated from the eye in the aqueous humor outflow into the aqueous veins or by diffusion through the uveal tissues, and washout by the venous blood circulation. (There are no lymphatics in the eye.)
17. Breakdown and metabolism of drugs applied to the eye may begin in the tears and the conjunctival and corneal epithelium as well as other ocular tissues, although these processes in the eye are somewhat limited. **Enzymes for**

oxidizing, reducing, and conjugating are present in ocular tissues (esterases, oxidases, reductases, lysosomal enzymes, peptidases, transferases, catechol-*O*-methyl transferase, monoamine oxidase, corticosteroid hydroxylase).

18. Many of the topically applied drugs, particularly antibiotics and corticosteroids, are not broken down in the eye, but leave the eye unchanged and enter the general circulation.

19. Eyelids and orbital tissue are best treated with systemically administered drugs as ophthalmic preparations applied to the surface of the eye do not reach these areas.

III. PRACTICAL TOPICAL DRUG THERAPY

A. Eye drops

1. **Delivery volume** should not exceed 50 μL; 20 μL is ideal for small animals.
2. **Repeat or continuous dosing** increases the pharmacologic effect. Frequent dosing can be facilitated with subpalpebral lavage or reverse nasolacrimal lavage, especially in horses.
3. **A 5-minute interval between drops** reduces irritation and is consistent with the average washout period of 3–6 minutes.
4. **Punctal occlusion** prolongs clearance time from tears and reduces systemic side effects.

B. Ointments. Prolonged contact time due to delayed melting, dilution, and breakdown, and punctual occlusion.

C. Suspensions have no advantages; only result from poorly soluble drugs.

D. Inactive ingredients

1. They are added to adjust pH, prevent oxidation, and increase absorption. Increased lipid solubility results from pH buffering with acetic acid, boric acid, hydrochloric acid or bicarbonate, phosphates, citrates, or borates.
2. Controlling the pH (7.2–7.4) and tonicity (0.9%) of the preparation to match the tears increases the comfort of the patient.
3. Methyl, hydroxyl, and hydoxypropyl methylcellulose polyvinyl alcohol, polyvinylpyrrolidone, Dextran 70, polysorbate 80, and PEG400 are viscous substances used as tear substitutes as well as drug delivery vehicles to increase corneal contact time (see XV Tear Substitutes).

IV. AUTONOMIC DRUGS

A. Introduction (see Chapter 2 for detailed information)

1. These are drugs that act primarily on the smooth muscles of the iris (sphincter and dilator) and the ciliary body (muscles of accommodation) and the smooth muscles of the arteriolar vessels.
2. Miotic agents constrict the pupil.
3. Mydriatic agents dilate the pupil.

B. Miotics: Cholinergic stimulants (parasympathomimetics). There are direct and indirect acting cholinergic stimulants to constrict the pupil and contract ciliary muscles to facilitate outflow of aqueous humor.

1. **Direct acting cholinergic stimulants**
   a. **Mechanism of action.** These drugs have the muscarinic effects of acetylcholine (ACh). In the eye they activate the muscarinic receptors of the iris sphincter and

ciliary muscles at the postganglionic parasympathetic neuroeffector junction. They can act on denervated structures.

b. Agents

(1) Pilocarpine (1–8% solution, 4% ointment)

    (a) Chemistry. Pilocarpine is a naturally occurring lipid-soluble alkaloid.

    (b) Ocular effects

        i. Topical pilocarpine induces slowly increasing contraction of the iris sphincter and ciliary muscles. Miosis begins within 10 minutes, peaks in 30 minutes, and slowly decreases over 6 hours.

        ii. The effect of ciliary muscle contraction on decreasing outflow resistance in the ciliary cleft is unclear, but intraocular pressure (IOP) decreases with decreased outflow resistance in the conventional trabecular meshwork pathway.

        iii. The iris sphincter contraction pulls the peripheral iris from the drainage angle to minimize obstruction to outflow if the angle is narrow or closed, but the state of contraction or relaxation of the iris does not necessarily affect outflow facility.

        iv. IOP is reduced 30–40% for up to 6 hours in the beagle dog. This drug is most useful in open angle glaucoma, but is usually not effective when used alone. The high IOP and structural changes in closed angle glaucoma limit the effectiveness of miotic drugs in lowering IOP in dogs.

        v. Other drugs, β-blockers, carbonic anhydrase inhibitors, and prostaglandin analogs are more effective in lowering IOP than pilocarpine.

    (c) Pharmacokinetics. Pilocarpine is absorbed readily into the eye primarily through the cornea after topical administration. It is degraded in the cornea but the small portion of the administered dose that reaches the anterior chamber is taken up by uveal tissue. The drug does not enter the posterior segment of the eye in significant quantities.

    (d) Therapeutic uses. The principal uses for pilocarpine are the treatment of primary glaucoma, and to stimulate lacrimation through activation of muscarinic receptors in the lacrimal gland when administered orally for neurogenic keratoconjunctivitis sicea. It is also useful for closing the pupil to keep a luxated lens from obstructing the pupil, to facilitate resolution of hyphema by increasing outflow, and in localization of parasympathetic denervation of the iris sphincter (along with physostigmine).

    (e) Administration. Usually, 1–2% solution four times a day.

    (f) Adverse effects include local irritation, salivation, lacrimation, nausea, vomiting, and diarrhea. Transient breakdown of blood–aqueous barrier and aqueous flare may occur. Miosis will decrease vision in low light. Cholinergic agents decrease uveoscleral outflow (most significant in the horse), so these agents are less effective in lowering IOP. Pilocarpine alone is not effective for reducing high IOP.

(2) Carbachol (0.75–3% solution)

    (a) Chemistry. Carbachol is a carbamyl ester of choline that is a combination of the molecules of ACh and physostigmine, thus it also has some indirect action by inhibition of cholinesterase. It is not lipid soluble, but is stable in water solution.

    (b) Mechanism of action. Carbachol enhances outflow facility and reduces IOP the same as pilocarpine. Miosis is maximal in 5 minutes and may last up to 2 days in a normal canine eye. Carbachol is more potent and has longer duration of action than pilocarpine.

    (c) Pharmacokinetics. This drug is not lipid soluble so it penetrates the corneal epithelium poorly unless combined with a wetting agent such as benzylalkonium chloride.

    (d) Therapeutic uses. When administered intraocularly at the conclusion of cataract surgery, the induced miosis can prevent postsurgical elevation of IOP, and may remove iris from the area of the corneal incision and decrease the potential for peripheral anterior synechia. By constricting the pupil an implanted prosthetic lens is stabilized.

(e) **Administration.** It is applied topically 2–4 times a day, or one time in the anterior chamber at the conclusion of cataract surgery.

(f) **Adverse effects** are similar to pilocarpine. There is no systemic toxicity from topical application.

(3) **ACh.** Topical application is of no value as cholinesterase destroys the drug before it can penetrate the cornea. The drug is used intraocularly during surgery to briefly but rapidly constrict the pupil (10 minutes).

2. Indirect acting cholinergic stimulants

a. Introduction. Cholinesterase inhibitors allow ACh to persist at the nerve ending by inhibiting the enzymatic hydrolysis of the neurotransmitter. Therefore, there will not be any effect on denervated tissues where there is no production of ACh.

b. Agents

(1) **Demecarium bromide** (0.125 and 0.25% solutions)

(a) **Chemistry.** It is synthesized by connecting two neostigmine molecules. It is water soluble and stable in aqueous solution.

(b) **Mechanism of action.** It reversibly inhibits cholinesterase. It is potent and long-acting. Miosis occurs within 2–4 hours and may persist for several days.

(c) **Therapeutic uses.** It is used in the management of primary glaucoma. It is administered prophylactically in the unaffected eye after an acute primary glaucoma attack in the first eye.

(d) **Pharmacokinetics.** It is readily absorbed through the cornea and taken up in the anterior uveal tissues.

(e) **Administration.** Apply topically once or twice daily.

(f) **Adverse effects/contraindications.**

i. Do not use a miotic in secondary glaucoma (usually due to uveitis) as it may increase pupillary block. As with other miotics, it is not effective for high IOP—first reduce IOP with IV mannitol.

ii. Salivation, vomiting, and diarrhea are common when the drug is first administered.

iii. Do not use on animals concurrently treated with antiparasitic products containing cholinesterase inhibitors.

(2) **Echothiophate** (0.03, 0.125, and 0.25% solution)

(a) **Chemistry.** It is phospholine iodide, a hygroscopic powder that is stable indefinitely but must be tightly capped. It has a short shelf-life in solution and must be refrigerated. It loses potency within a month; discard after 2 months.

(b) **Mechanism of action.** It irreversibly binds cholinesterase permitting ACh to persist at neuroeffector junction for prolonged action.

(c) **Pharmacokinetics.** It readily penetrates the eye through the intact cornea and the conjunctiva–sclera. Echothiophate has prolonged action with maximum effect in 4–6 hours and maintained for 24 hours.

(d) **Therapeutic uses.** It is for control of primary glaucoma. It is seldom used due to the inconveniences in handling: powder to be dissolved, need to refrigerate, short shelf-life, and toxicity to people handling it.

(e) **Administration.** It is applied topically once or twice daily.

(f) **Adverse effects.** It is very toxic when ingested. With prolonged topical use, corneal clouding, iritis, and iris cysts may occur; cataracts not reported for dogs as in humans.

(3) **Physostigmine**

(a) It is short acting and reversible.

(b) It may be used as a diagnostic agent in a normotensive eye with unexplained mydriasis and normal retinas. See pilocarpine.

(c) There are no proprietary preparations, but USP powder is available for generic compounding.

(d) **Adverse effects** are similar to demecarium.

Note: Pralidoxime (Protopam®) can reverse the effects of toxic doses of anticholinesterase drugs. (See Chapter 2 for more information.)

C. **Mydriatics** dilate the pupil (parasympatholytics and sympathomimetics)

1. **Parasympatholytics (Cholinergic antagonists)**
   a. **Introduction.** These drugs compete with ACh to reversibly block cholinergic receptors of iris sphincter muscle and ciliary muscles (cycloplegia). The pupil dilates due to tone in the unopposed iris dilator muscle. They also paralyze accommodation but that is of little significance in animals.
   b. **Agents**
      (1) **Atropine** (0.5–2% solution)
         (a) This mydriatic agent has slow onset, but prolonged action. Maximum dilation occurs in the dog in 60 minutes and may last for 4–5 days; and 10–48 hours to maximum in horse and last up to 14 days.
         (b) **Therapeutic uses**
            i. Atropine is used in acute inflammatory conditions of the iris or uveal tract to relieve the pain of sphincter muscle and ciliary muscle spasms.
            ii. Dilating the pupil will minimize the possibilities of posterior synechia, pupillary block, and secondary glaucoma.
            iii. Pupil dilation facilitates surgery of the lens and posterior segment, and may improve vision when opacities of the lens or cornea partially obstruct vision.
            iv. Because of the large alternative uveoscleral outflow of aqueous humor in the horse, atropine is beneficial in treating primary glaucoma.
         (c) **Administration.** Topically as needed to achieve effect, up to hourly.
         (d) **Adverse effects** include salivation due to bitter taste, predisposition to glaucoma if there is a preexisting narrow angle or inflammatory infiltrates in the angle. GI stasis and colic may be induced in horses. Systemic toxicity with behavior changes may occur in small animals. Less commonly, diminished tear production may predispose to dry eyes and keratoconjunctivitis. Luxated lens may fall into anterior chamber.
      (2) **Tropicamide** (0.5–1% solution)
         (a) **Pharmacokinetics.** It has a rapid onset, short duration of action. Maximum dilation in 20 minutes, lasts for 3 hours.
         (b) **Therapeutic uses.** Mostly to dilate pupil to facilitate examination of lens and posterior segment of the eye. Also, because it reduces blood–aqueous barrier permeability it is a good choice for intraocular surgery.
      (3) **Other parasympatholytics** that are seldom used include homatropine, scopolamine, and cyclopentolate.
2. **Adrenergic agents.** Drugs with α_2-agonistic activity or β_2-blocking activity to decrease cAMP levels, which decrease aqueous humor formation.
   a. **Adrenergic agonists** stimulate adrenergic receptors (α_1, α_2, β_1, β_2).
      (1) **Epinephrine** (1–2% sol) decreases aqueous production through vasoconstriction in the ciliary body. Increased facility of aqueous outflow is mediated by α_2-receptors and is correlated with increased cAMP production by the trabecular meshwork.
      (2) **Dipivalyl epinephrine** (0.1% solution). It is a lipophilic prodrug that is metabolized by corneal esterases to two epinephrine molecules.
      (3) **Phenylephrine** (2–10% solution). A direct acting α_1-agonist with little effect on β-adrenergic receptors that is used diagnostically for Horner's syndrome and therapeutically as an adjunct to atropine. Ten percent phenylephrine will dilate the dog's pupil in 2 hours and it persists for 12–18 hours. Because of the time to complete mydriasis, this drug is not useful as a mydriatic when used alone. It does not dilate the pupil of the cat, horse, or cow. It is used topically for its local vasoconstrictive effect.
   b. **Selective α_2-agonists**
      (1) **Preparations.** Apraclonidine (1% solution) and brimonidine (0.2% solution).

(2) Therapeutic uses. It is used to treat complications related to postoperative IOP spikes and augment other glaucoma medications. These agents are not an important group for veterinary medicine due to their limited effectiveness and significant side effects of vomiting and bradycardia.

(3) Mechanism of action. Aqueous humor secretion is decreased by:

(a) Activation of presynaptic α_2-receptors, which inhibits norepinephrine (NE) release, thereby blocking the tonic adrenergic stimulation of the secretory ciliary epithelium by endogenous NE.

(b) Stimulation of postsynaptic α_2-receptor in the ciliary body suppresses adenylyl cyclase and thus decreases cAMP synthesis, which results in decreased aqueous humor formation.

(c) Constriction of the afferent arterioles of the ciliary body reduces ciliary body blood flow that may also account for reduced aqueous secretion.

(d) Enhanced uveoscleral outflow may also contribute to lowered IOP.

(e) In the dog, apraclonidine causes mydriasis through interaction with inhibitory prejunctional α_2-receptors on adrenergic nerves to the iris sphincter. In the cat, apraclonidine produces miosis, but the mechanism is uncertain.

(4) Adverse effects. Apraclonidine may reduce heart rate and blood pressure so systemic β-blockers should be used with caution.

c. **Indirect-acting adrenergic stimulants** stimulate the release of NE. Hydroxyamphetamine is used for diagnosis of first-order Horner's syndrome. It causes pupillary dilation in eyes with preganglionic sympathetic disruption but not in eyes with a postganglionic lesion.

d. **β-Adrenergic blockers**

(1) Mechanism of action

(a) Nonspecific agents block both β_1- and β_2-receptors in the epithelium of the ciliary processes. The subsequent inhibition of cAMP production leads to diminished aqueous humor production. The major receptor in the anterior segment is β_2.

(b) β-Blockers do not affect carbonic anhydrase (CA) nor aqueous humor outflow.

(2) Therapeutic uses. These agents are useful in combination with other ocular hypotensive drugs such as CA inhibitors or parasympathomimetics for treating glaucoma and prophylactically in preglaucomatous eyes in the dog and cat. β-Agonists used with CA inhibitors or parasympathomimetics can achieve 50–60% reduction in IOP.

(3) Nonselective β-blockers. Timolol (0.25–0.5% solution), levobunolol (0.25–0.5% solution), carteolol (1% solution), metipranolol (0.3% solution):

These drugs have significant hypotensive effect for cats at 0.5%, but 4–8% solution is required for dogs. They have variable hypotensive effects in different animals possibly due to variations in β-receptors. Betaxol (0.25–0.5% sol) is a selective β_1-blocker.

(4) Administration. They are used topically, twice daily.

(5) Adverse effects. Bradycardia is the most significant side effect.

V. **ANTIMICROBIALS** (for chemistry, mechanism of action, and spectrum of activity refer to Chapter 15). **Intraocular inflammation accompanying infections reduces or eliminates blood–ocular barriers to drug penetration so choices of antibiotics are similar to selection of antimicrobials for treatment of soft tissue infections.**

A. **Antibacterial agents**

1. General considerations

a. Topical preparations are intended for ocular surface infections or prophylaxis, but there are a limited number of commercially available preparations.

Alternative topical formulations may be prepared with injectable antibiotic solutions if indicated.

b. Systemically administered antibiotics are generally ineffective in treating corneal and conjunctival infections.

c. Culture and sensitivity testing are advised but selection of an antibiotic for initial treatment is often an empirical decision or based on cytology.

d. Concern for penetration of the corneal epithelium (to the stroma or intraocularly) is not relevant in ulcerative keratitis as the epithelial barrier has been lost. For a stromal abscess in the deep cornea where the surface epithelium is intact, penetration is a concern. Intraocular inflammation breaks down blood–ocular barriers so transport of systemically administered antibiotics to intraocular structures is usually not an issue.

e. Topical antibiotics should be administered frequently as the preparation will not remain on the ocular surface more than a few minutes. Dilution and washout in the tears may be overcome with fortified solutions created with injectable solutions added to proprietary preparations or to methylcellulose (artificial tears) especially for horses. Increased frequency of medication may be preferable as high concentrations may be toxic to regenerating epithelium.

f. Topical antibiotics are combined, that is, neomycin, polymyxin, and gramicidin, to increase the spectrum of activity of the preparation. Synergy is sometimes achieved such as with an aminoglycoside and a cephalosporin. Antagonism between drugs in combination is uncommon.

g. Topical antibiotics are typically those not used systemically. Bactericidal and bacteriostatic antibiotics should not be used concurrently.

h. Adverse effects vary among the different topical antibiotic preparations, but all have the potential to be irritating leading to tearing, blepharospasm, conjunctival hyperemia, or chemosis. Tonicity, pH, and preservatives, or the drug itself may be the cause (Table 14-1).

2. Antibacterial classes

a. Penicillins. These antibiotics are rarely used topically in veterinary medicine. Preparations for intramammary infusion in bovine mastitis are often used topically for infectious keratitis (pink eye), and subconjunctival injections of systemic injectables may be efficacious for bovine or equine infectious keratitis.

Agents. Any of the natural or synthetic injectable penicillin preparations may be compounded for topical use or administered subconjunctivally. They include natural penicillins G, V, and K; penicillinase-resistant oxacillin, cloxacillin, dicloxacillin, nafcillin; and the aminopenicillins and carboxycillins including ampicillin, amoxicillin, carbenicillin, piperacillin, and ticarcillin.

b. Cephalosporins. There are no topical ophthalmic preparations available. Agents for systemic use are compounded for topical treatment of infected corneal ulcers. First-generation drugs: cefazolin, cefadroxyl, cephalexin, and cephalothin are active against most Gram-positive organisms. Second-generation and third-generation drugs in this category are rarely used in ophthalmic preparations except when sensitivity testing dictates. Compounded fortified cephazolin solution for infected corneal ulcers in horses is commonly used in combination with fortified amikacin.

c. Aminoglycosides. Neomycin, gentamicin, and tobramycin are widely available as topical solutions and ointments. Neomycin is commonly combined with bacitracin or gramicidin and polymyxin B (referred to as "**triple antibiotic**") to increase the spectrum of activity. Topically these drugs do not penetrate the intact cornea. Amikacin is compounded and used to complement cephazolin for treatment of infected equine corneal ulcers.

(1) Subconjunctival injections of gentamicin and tobramycin readily enter the corneal stroma and aqueous humor, and pass through the sclera into vitreous of inflamed eyes.

(2) The low pH of gentamicin parenteral solution is locally irritating and may be painful. Neomycin and kanamycin do not penetrate eye from the subconjunctival injection site.

TABLE 14-1. Antibiotic Choices for Ocular Infections

Drug	Topical Propriety Prep Sol/Ointment	Topical Compounded Fortified Solutions	Subconjunctiva 1 Injection Dose	Systemic Oral/ Parenteral
Amoxicillin	–	–	–	G
Amikacin	–	10 mg/mL P	25 mg G	G
Ampicillin	–	50 mg/mL P	50–250 mg G	P
Bacitracin	500 units/g	–	–	–
Carbamicillin		5 mg/mL P	100 mg G	P
Cephaloridine	–	32–35 mg/mL P	100 mg G	P
Cephalothin	–	–	50–100 mg G	P
Cefazolin	–	30–50 mg/mL	100 mg G	P
Clindamycin	–	50 mg/mL	15–50 mg	P
Chloramphenicol	5–10 mg/mL G	50–100 mg/mL G	50–100 mg G	P
Chlortetracycline	10 mg/g G	–	3–5 mg G	G
Ciprofloxacin	3.5 mg/mL P	10–12 mg/mL P	–	G
Colistin	5 mg/mL P	10 mg/mL P	15–35 mg G	P
Enrofloxacin	–	7 mg/mL P	–	G
Erythromycin	5 mg/gm G	10–50 mg/mL G	50–100 mg G	P
Gentamicin	3 mg/mL or gm P	8–15 mg/mL P	10–20 mg G	P
Kanamycin	–	30–50 mg/mL P	30 mg P	P
Lincomycin	–	–	150 mg G	G
Methicillin	–	50 mg/mL P	50–100 mg G	P
Moxalactam	–	100 mg/mL P	50 mg G	P
Neomycin	3.5–8 mg/mL P	35 mg/mL P	125–25 mg P	–
Penicillin G	–	100–300,000 units P	0.5–1 million units G	F
Norfloxacin	3 mg/mL	–	–	G
Ofloxacin	3 mg/mL	–	–	G
Oxacillin	–	65 mg/mL	–	–
Polymyxin B	10,000 units/mL P	–	100,000 units P	–
Streptomycin	–	–	50–100 mg	–
Tetracycline	10 mg/g G	–	2.5–5 mg G	P
Ticarcillin	–	6 mg/mL	100 mg	P
Tobramycin	3 mg/mL or gm P	5–15 mg/mL P	10–20 mg G	P

Intraocular penetration: good (G), fair (F), poor (P), no information (–).

(3) Parenteral (or oral) administration results in low concentrations in the anterior segment.

(4) Except for neomycin, aminoglycosides should be reserved for use in established infections. **Allergic and hypersensitivity reactions are more common in this group, especially to neomycin.**

(5) **All aminoglycosides are toxic to intraocular structures.** Amikacin is safer for intravitreal injections than gentamicin. Gentamicin is used for chemical ablation of the ciliary body in blind, chronically glaucomatous eyes.

d. Tetracyclines

(1) Topical proprietary preparations are either ointments or suspensions of topical tetracycline or oxytetracycline combined with polymyxin B.

(2) Doxycycline and minocycline are lipophilic and penetrate the eye well when given systemically to dogs for rickettsia and cats for chlamydial infections, but do not penetrate aqueous or vitreous of horse to be sufficiently effective against *Leptospira*.

(3) Oral doxycycline is more beneficial for chlamydial infection in cats than topical preparations. Subconjunctival oxytetracycline gives therapeutic concentrations in tears for treatment of *Moraxella*, but not when administered IM.

(4) Adverse effects. Oxytetracycline is painful when given subconjunctivally, and causes chemosis and hyperemia.

e. Polypeptides. Polymyxin B, bacitracin, and ointments are used. Vancomycin is rarely indicated parenterally, but is the drug of choice for intravitreal injection for Gram-positive bacteria. There are no topical forms. Polypeptides do not penetrate the intact cornea or conjunctiva.

f. Fluoroquinolones. Norfloxacin and ofloxacin solutions, and ciprofloxacin solution and ointment are the common topical preparations. They are well tolerated and not toxic topically. Ofloxacin and norfloxacin penetrate the intact cornea readily; ciprofloxacin does poorly. Levofloxacin, pefloxacin, marbofloxacin, and enrofloxacin parenterally penetrate to therapeutic levels in aqueous and vitreous humor in the dog and cat; however, they may cause retinal degeneration in cats even at recommended doses. Toxicity is dose-related and aged cats are more susceptible.

g. Chloramphenicol. Readily diffuses through the cornea into anterior chamber, especially if ointment form is used. Through systemic administration, it crosses the blood–ocular barriers and enters the aqueous at the same rate that it enters the cerebrospinal fluid. Topical dosing in the cat leads to systemic absorption. Chloramphenicol is antagonistic to erythromycin.

h. Lincosamides and macrolides. Erythromycin ointment is the only topical preparation in this class. Clindamycin orally is the drug of choice for toxoplasmosis endophthalmitis. Azithromycin orally is used for *Borrelia* and *Bartonella* infections.

i. Sulfonamides. Sulfacetamide and sulfisoxazole topicals are rarely used in veterinary medicine. Trimethoprim-sulfadiazine orally penetrates the aqueous and vitreous humor readily. Systemic sulfonamides may be toxic to the lacrimal gland leading to keratoconjunctivitis sicca.

B. **Antivirals**

1. Pyrimidine nucleoside analogs
   a. idoxuridine (2.5% ointment, 0.1% solution compounded) and triflurothymidine (1% solution) for topical use.
   b. Mechanism of action. These compounds substitute for thymidine in DNA synthesis and interfere with viral replication. They are virostatic, and thus competent mucosal surface immunity is required for efficacy.
   c. Pharmacokinetics. Idoxuridine is not absorbed by the conjunctiva nor cornea unless there is an erosion. Trifluorothymidine is better absorbed.
   d. Therapeutic uses. They are for the treatment of feline herpesvirus-1 conjunctivitis and keratitis, and punctate keratitis in horses due to equine herpesvirus-2. Triflurothymidine is the drug of choice. However, latent infections are resistant.
   e. Adverse effects. Local irritation and hypersensitivity are occasional problems especially in cats. Trifluorothymidine is the least toxic of nucleic acid analogs.

2. Purine nucleoside analogs
   a. Preparations. Adenine arabinoside (or vidarabine 3% ointment, 1% suspension compounded) for topical use.
   b. Mechanism of action. Vidarabine is a structural analog for adenosine that interferes with viral DNA synthesis. It is virastatic.
   c. Pharmacokinetics. They are not absorbed by the conjunctiva nor cornea unless there is an epithelial defect due to viral replication in the epithelium.
   d. Therapeutic uses. They are used to treat feline herpesvirus-1 conjunctivitis and keratitis and punctate keratitis in horses due to equine herpesvirus-2.
   e. Adverse effects. Local irritation and hypersensitivity are occasional problems for cats.

3. Acyclovir is a guanidine derivative of vidarabine. It is not available commercially as a topical.
   a. Preparation. Five percent ointment; oral and parenteral preparations are not effective for FHV-1.

    b. Mechanism of action. Acyclovir is an analog of guanosine with selective affinity for substitution in viral DNA, but not in normal uninfected cells. It acts by selectively inhibiting viral thymidine kinase but not cellular thymidine kinase.

    c. Therapeutic uses. Antiherpetic treatment for cats with chronic conjunctivokeratitis.

    d. Administration. Use topically as oral administration does not achieve plasma concentrations sufficient to inhibit FHV-1.

    e. Adverse effects. There is renal, liver, and bone marrow toxicity potential at therapeutic levels. It is reserved for severe, unresponsive cases.

  4. Gangciclovir, cidofovir, and penciclovir are new compounds. Gangciclovir is related to acyclovir, cidofovir is cytotoxic and less potent.

  5. Betadine 1:20 dilution of disinfectant in artificial tear solution is administered one drop twice daily on the eye.

  6. Interferons (IFNs)

    a. Preparations. Human recombinant IFN-α and feline recombinant IFN-ω.

    b. Mechanism of action. These are cytokines component of natural defense mechanism.

      (1) They are released by host cells in response to viral infection. Attached to the receptors on adjacent cells, IFNs increase the transcription of host cell DNA and activate endonuclease in the cell, increasing the resistance of the cell to virus infection.

      (2) They stimulate cell-mediated lysis of virus-infected cells.

      (3) Interferons are synergistic with acyclovir.

    c. Therapeutic uses. They are for the treatment of FHV-1 conjunctivitis and keratitis. Topical administration is effective only for active infection that is in the conjunctival and corneal epithelium. Combinations of IFN and topical antiviral drugs are synergistic. Parenteral administration prior to exposure does not prevent infection but the symptoms are less severe. Oral dosing within 48 hours postexposure diminishes the severity of the clinical disease. It is less effective for established infections and has no effect on latent infection or the carrier state.

    d. Administration. It is used topically, one drop, 30 IU/mL (diluted in artificial tear solution) and orally, 30 IU/day.

    e. Pharmacokinetics. Direct contact with the epithelial surface is sufficient for benefit of topical administration. Oral administration has been demonstrated to be beneficial even though the large protein molecule is degraded in the GI tract. Benefit is presumed from unknown immunologic mechanisms.

    f. Adverse effects. None reported at recommended doses.

  7. L-lysine

    a. Preparations. USP, tablets or powder, OTC; commercially in flavored vehicle.

    b. Mechanism of action. L-lysine interferes with viral replication.

    c. Therapeutic uses. It prevents or suppresses feline herpesvirus-1 conjunctivitis and keratitis.

    e. Administration. It is given orally, 500 mg in food twice daily.

    f. Pharmacokinetics. It is readily absorbed from GI tract and secreted in tears.

    g. Adverse effects. None reported at recommended doses.

C. Antifungals

  1. General considerations. Keratomycoses are most common in horses, especially in warmer climates, and dogs and cats less frequently. Deep puncture wounds in the cornea may lead to stromal abscesses beneath an intact surface epithelium. Intraocular infection with systemic mycotic organisms occurs mostly in dogs.

  2. Agents. Polyenes, azoles, 5-fluorocytosine, and iodides

    a. Betadine and tincture of iodine

      (1) Therapeutic uses. Betadine is an iodine antiseptic and is effective at 1:10–1:20 dilution in saline or ocular irrigation solution. It is more effective in an electrolyte solution. Betadine is effective for mycotic and bacterial infection in stromal ulcers, but not for deep stromal abscesses as it does not penetrate intact epithelium. Tincture of iodine is absorbed into the corneal stroma better than betadine. Each is antibacterial and antifungal at the same dilutions. As a presurgical disinfectant for the conjunctiva and cornea, betadine is used at 1:50 dilution to minimize chemosis.

   (2) **Administration.** Repeat topical betadine application every 2–3 hours for 24–48 hours. Tincture (2 or 7%) is used only once at the time of initial debridement of the wound.

   (3) **Adverse effects.** Betadine causes a local irritation, and chemosis in some individuals. Tincture of iodine is very irritating and should be preceded with a topical anesthetic.

b. **Silver sulfadiazine.** This is a broad spectrum antibacterial and antifungal dermatologic cream that is compatible with the cornea and conjunctiva. It is used for topical application for equine keratomycosis.

c. **Azoles** (Imidazoles) (see Chapter 15 for detailed information).

   (1) **Preparations.** Itraconazole, miconazole, clotrimazole, ketoconazole, and fluconazole.

   (2) **Mechanism of action.** They inhibit mitochondrial oxidative enzymes resulting in cell death. Damage to the cell wall by interaction with phospholipids leads to increased permeability.

   (3) **Pharmacokinetics.** Miconazole and ketoconazole penetrate the cornea moderately well; fluconazole penetrates well due to minimal protein binding. Itraconazole penetrates the blood–ocular barriers well.

   (4) **Therapeutic uses**

      (a) Imidazoles have a broad spectrum of activity against filamentous and dimorphic fungi and yeasts.

      (b) Intraocular infections by systemic fungi are treated with oral or IV preparations; **itraconazole is preferred.**

      (c) Keratomycoses are treated using IV preparations topically. Oral forms of miconazole and itraconazole are compounded as ointments for topical use. Itraconazole and fluconazole systemically are effective against filamentous organisms infecting the deep cornea.

      (d) **Clotrimazole and miconazole vaginal and dermatologic creams have been used topically on the eye, but the alcohols in these preparations are harmful to the corneal epithelium and should not be used on the eye.**

   (5) **Administration.** They can be mixed to a 1% ointment in 30% dimethyl sulfoxide (DMSO) for topical use for superior penetration deep into the cornea. Fluconazole solution can be given subconjunctivally and intracamerally. Topical treatment of keratomycosis requires hourly or every other hour application for 2–3 days then tapering to four times a day for at least 4–6 weeks.

   (6) **Adverse effects.** Except for vaginal and dermatologic creams, oral and injectable preparations are well tolerated topically. DMSO preparations should be handled with gloves to minimize skin absorption that is enhanced by the DMSO solvent.

d. **Polyene macrolide antibiotics**

   (1) **Preparations**

      (a) **Natamycin** (5% suspension) is the only topical antifungal commercially available.

      (b) **Amphotericin B** is compounded in 0.3–0.5% colloidal suspension for topical use.

      (c) **Nystatin** is compounded in isohydric phosphate buffer solution for topical use.

   (2) **Mechanism of action.** They bind to a sterol moiety in the fungal cell membrane and form a polyene–sterol complex that alters the selective permeability of the membrane and results in K^+ efflux and oxidative damage, cytoplasmic organelle destruction. It is fungicidal or fungistatic depending on the concentration and the susceptibility of the organism.

   (3) **Therapeutic uses**

      (a) Amphotericin B has a broad spectrum of activity against systemic fungal infections. It may be formulated for topical use on fungal keratitis.

(b) Natamycin has a broad spectrum of activity against filamentous fungi and yeasts.

(c) Nystatin is effective on some filamentous fungi and yeast (*Candida*).

(4) Administration. They are applied topically for keratomycosis. Parenteral amphotericin B is rarely used due to nephrotoxicity and availability of azole agents.

(5) Pharmacokinetics

(a) Amphotericin B penetrates the cornea poorly unless the epithelium debrided. Amphotericin B penetrates the blood–ocular barrier poorly when given parenterally.

(b) Natamycin will penetrate in effective concentrations in the corneal stroma if the epithelium is debrided.

(6) Adverse effects

(a) **Amphotericin B.** At >0.3%, applied topically causes conjunctival hyperemia, chemosis, and iritis. Corneal epithelial toxicity interferes with healing of ulcers. It is too irritating to administer subconjunctivally.

Amphotericin B is toxic to retina if injected into the vitreous. Renal toxicity if B given parenterally in small animals.

(b) Natamycin is not toxic topically but is too irritating to use subconjunctivally or intracamerally.

(c) Nystatin is well tolerated.

VI. ANTI-INFLAMMATORY DRUGS

A. **Glucocorticoids** (see Chapter 12 for more information)

1. **General considerations.** Scarring may be inconsequential to healing in most other tissues, but the need to control and prevent the sequelae of ocular inflammation to preserve transparency for vision is essential in treating ocular diseases. Anti-inflammatory and immunosuppressive effects of glucocorticoids reduce resistance to infectious organisms. **Infectious or allergic causes of inflammation are not eliminated even if signs are reduced.** Impaired keratocyte and fibroblast activity is dose-related.

2. **Chemistry/agents/preparations selection**

   a. Phosphate solutions are water soluble. Acetates and alcohols preparations are aqueous suspensions of lipophilic glucocorticoids, and are biphasic, facilitating absorption through the cornea. They deliver higher concentrations than solutions. Lipophilic acetate and alcohol preparations penetrate the cornea up to 20 times greater than water-soluble phosphate preparations.

   b. **Agents.** Hydrocortisone, dexamethasone alcohol and sodium phosphate, betamethasone, triamcinolone, prednisone, prednisolone acetate, and sodium phosphate. Progestins (having glucocorticoid activity): fluorometholone, medrysone, megestrol acetate.

   c. **Selection of a preparation for topical use**

      (1) Consider relative potency, corneal penetration, duration of action, retention of vehicle, and adverse effects of the drug and the vehicle in selecting a product.

      (2) Dexamethasone and betamethasone are 5–10 times more potent than prednisolone and 20 times more potent than hydrocortisone (see Chapter 12, Table 12-1). The higher concentration of prednisolone negates the difference in potency.

      (3) An acetate suspension penetrates into the anterior chamber through the intact corneal epithelium making it the preparation of choice for treating anterior uveitis.

      (4) Hydrocortisone is commonly combined with the "triple antibiotic" mixture, but it does not penetrate the cornea and is inappropriate for intraocular inflammation.

(5) Dexamethasone sodium phosphate is more potent, but prednisolone acetate suspension is better absorbed into the anterior segment of the eye. Penetration into the eyelids and posterior segment is poor.

d. **Selection of a glucocorticoid preparation for systemic use** is not significantly affected by its ability to cross the blood–ocular barriers as those barriers are broken in inflammation. Relative potency and duration of action are more important considerations.

3. **Effects on the eye.** Glucocorticoids have anti-inflammatory effects. At high doses, they exert immunosuppressive effects.

4. **Therapeutic uses** of topical preparations. They suppress vascular and cellular aspects of inflammation of the conjunctiva, cornea, sclera, iris, and ciliary body.

5. **Administration.** Apply topically solutions, suspensions, or ointments. Suspensions must be shaken gently to assure consistent dosing. Subconjunctival injection of par enteral injectable solutions or suspensions.

6. **Pharmacokinetics.** Potency and penetration of different glucocorticoid preparations is important in the management of an ocular disease.

7. **Adverse effects and contraindications**
   a. Do not use for conjunctivitis in cats unless herpesvirus infection is controlled or ruled out.
   b. Do not use on ulcerated corneas as steroids inhibit healing (mitosis and epithelial cell migration, keratocyte proliferation and collagen deposition), potentiate matrix metalloproteinases that lead to corneal necrosis.
   c. Host immune defenses are impaired by reducing neutrophil and macrophage migration, and suppression of cytokine activity.
   d. Subconjunctival granuloma from injection of repository preparations.
   e. Superficial calcification of the cornea with prolonged use of phosphate preparations; lipid keratopathy.
   f. Rarely, cataracts or glaucoma.
   g. Iatrogenic Cushing's syndrome.

B. **Nonsteroidal anti-inflammatory drugs (NSAIDs)** (see Chapter 7 for detailed information).

1. **Preparations**
   a. **Topical NSAIDs**: flurbiprofen, diclofenac, suprofen, ketorolac
   b. **Systemic NSAIDs**: flunixin meglumine, carprofen, deracoxib, phenylbutazone

2. **Mechanism of action.**
   a. Topical preparations, like the systemic drugs, are predominately COX-2 inhibitors but have anti-COX-1 activity as well.
   b. NSAIDs prevent prostaglandin production that causes blood–aqueous barrier breakdown, lowered pain threshold, miosis, photophobia, and decreased aqueous humor formation.
   c. They also suppress PMN motility and chemotaxis, decrease mast cell degranulation and expression of inflammatory cytokines, and may act as free radical scavengers.

3. **Therapeutic uses.** NSAIDs suppress ocular inflammation. They depress pain and photophobia of uveitis of all causes including postoperative inflammation. Used preoperatively they prevent intraoperative miosis. Control symptoms of allergic conjunctivitis. NSAIDs avoid the undesirable side effects of glucocorticoids. Systemic NSAIDs are used for posterior segment inflammation.

4. **Administration.** Topicals are applied 2–4 times a day.
   Systemic products, oral or injectable should not be given more than twice daily due to adverse GI effects.

5. **Pharmacokinetics.** Oral drugs are readily absorbed by the gastric mucosa (see Chapter 7 for detailed pharmacokinetics information). Topical drugs are absorbed by the cornea and into the anterior chamber of the eye. Corneal epithelial compromise or loss leads to much enhanced absorption.

6. **Adverse effects.** Local irritation and corneal epithelial toxicity, infiltrates, and punctate keratopathy are reported. A modest decrease in aqueous humor outflow may

occur. Systemic products commonly predispose to gastrointestinal damages due to breakdown of prostaglandin-dependent mucosal protective mechanisms by COX-1 inhibition. Signs include anorexia, vomiting, diarrhea, hematemesis, and gastric ulcers. Horses are most vulnerable. Hepatic and renal toxicity occur in the dog and cat (see Chapter 7 for more information). Absorption of topical products rarely causes systemic effects.

VII. **IMMUNOMODULATING DRUGS.** Miscellaneous immunosuppressive agents have been introduced to veterinary medicine to manage chronic ocular inflammatory diseases where long-term glucocorticoids and NSAIDs are inadequate or inappropriate.

A. **Azathioprine** (see Chapter 17 for more information)

1. **Mechanism of action.** Interferes with the synthesis of purine bases, nucleic acid synthesis. Effect is limited to helper T lymphocytes.
2. **Therapeutic uses.** The most common alternative treatment of steroid-resistant uveitis and nodular granulomatous episclerokeratitis.
3. **Administration.** It is given orally; there are no topical formulations.
4. **Pharmacokinetics.** See Chapter 17 for information.
5. **Adverse effects** include vomiting, diarrhea, bone marrow suppression, hepatic necrosis.

B. **Other cytotoxic immunomodulating agents** for inflammatory ocular diseases that are resistant to conventional doses of glucocorticoids (see Chapter 17 for detailed information).

1. **Cytosine arabinoside**, an antimetabolite, and **Procarbazine**, an MAO inhibitor, are used for optic neuritis associated with granulomatous meningioencephalitis.
2. **Chlorambucil**, an alkalating agent, is used for refractory immune-mediated uveitis in dogs.
3. **Mitoxantrone**, an antitumor antibiotic, is an alternative for treatment of optic neuritis.
4. **Tetracylcine and niacinamide combined** have immunomodulatory and anti-inflammatory effects used for pyogranulomatous blepharitis and episcleritis.

C. **T-lymphocyte Inhibitors (calcineurin inhibitors)**

1. **Preparations**
   a. **Cyclosporine** is available commercially as a 0.2% ointment and an oral solution that is diluted to 1 or 2% in olive or corn oil. Intravitreal or suprachoroidal cyclosporine implants for control of equine recurrent uveitis.
   b. **Tacrolimus** is compounded to 0.03% in olive or corn oil.
2. **Mechanism of action.** These compounds inhibit T-lymphocytes by inhibiting cytokine production (IL-2, IFN-γ) so helper T cell activation is blocked, inhibiting the initiation of specific T-cell responses. Rapamycin blocks signal transduction pathways of cytokine (IL-2) receptors and inhibits proliferation of T cells.
3. **Therapeutic uses**
   a. In treatment of keratoconjunctivitis sicca, corneal and conjunctival inflammatory changes are reversed. They are lacromimetic by inhibiting immune-mediated inflammation in the lacrimal gland, and has an independent lacrimogenic effect.
   b. Control superficial keratitis (pannus) by inhibiting neovascularization.
   c. Control eosinophilic keratitis, episcleritis, and superficial punctate keratitis.
   d. Prevent corneal graft rejection.
4. **Administration.** Apply topically twice daily on the surface of the eye.

5. Pharmacokinetics
   a. They readily penetrate corneal epithelium, but not endothelium, so they accumulate in the corneal stroma.
   b. They penetrate conjunctival epithelium and are taken up into the lacrimal gland.
   c. There is minimal penetration into the aqueous humor; but systemic absorption is sufficient for measurable cellular immunity suppression.
6. Adverse effects. Ocular and periocular irritation may occur. Local and systemic immunosuppression may result from systemic absorption.

VIII. ANTIALLERGIC, ANTIHISTAMINIC, AND DECONGESTANT DRUGS (see Chapters 2 and 3 for detailed information).

A. **General considerations.** Upon repeated exposure to an antigen, sensitized mast cells in the conjunctiva rupture and release granules, which contain inflammatory mediators, including histamine, prostaglandins, leukotrienes, and eosinophil chemotactic factors, for example, IL-8. Histamine activates H_1-receptors on blood vessels causing vasodilation, increased capillary permeability, chemosis and pruritis. Intraocular (iris) inflammation may occur.

B. **Mechanism of action.** These drugs inhibit degranulation of mast cells and release of histamine, leukotrienes, and so forth, by stabilizing cell membranes, inhibiting the pathophysiologic effects, or competing for receptor sites of the mediators.

C. **Therapeutic uses.** For control of allergic conjunctivitis and blepharitis. These agents are used in place of glucocorticoids with variable results. Their efficacy in animals is unsubstantiated.

D. **Pharmacokinetics.** These agents are all active on the surface of the mucous membrane (palpebral and bulbar conjunctiva), but **do not penetrate the intact corneal epithelium**.

E. **Agents**
   1. H_1-antihistamines: levocabastine, emedastine
   2. Mast cell stabilizers: cromolyn sodium, lodoxamide
   3. Both mast cell stabilizers and H_1-antihistamines: olopatidine, ketotifen, azelastine, nedocromil
   4. Vasoconstrictors (decongestants): in topical preparations include naphazoline, tetrahydrozoline, and phenylephrine (see Chapter 2 for more information).
   5. Antihistamine/decongestant combinations are used in small animals with negligible or variable results which are often due to inaccurate diagnosis: pyrilamine/phenylephrine, pheneramine/naphazoline, antazoline/naphazoline.

F. **Adverse effects/contraindications.** Most first-generation antihistamines have a sedative effect. Topical application may cause local irritation.

IX. PROSTAGLANDIN ANALOGS

A. **Agents.** Latanoprost (0.005% solution), bimatoprost (0.03% solution), travoprost (0.004% solution).

   1. Chemistry. These are esters of prostaglandin $F_{2\alpha}$ analogs that increase lipid solubility to facilitate uptake through cornea. Hydrolysis during passage through epithelium releases the active form for distribution to the interior of the eye.

2. **Mechanism of action.** They activate G_q-coupled prostanoid FP receptors in dogs. **They do not work in cats or horses**, probably due to FP receptor problems in these species.
   a. The increased uveoscleral outflow is the primary mechanism for lowering IOP with $PGF_{2\alpha}$ in the dog. There is evidence of the pressure-dependent conventional outflow increasing due to alterations in the trabecular meshwork.
   b. Matrix metalloproteinases are increased and collagen is decreased with evidence of lysis of extracellular matrix, widening of intermuscular spaces concurrent with reduced outflow resistance. Blood vessels dilate in the optic nerve head and the increased perfusion spares the inner retina.
3. **Therapeutic uses.** $PGF_{2\alpha}$ analogs lower IOP in primary glaucoma in dogs, but not in cats or horses.
4. **Administration.** Apply topically once or twice daily.
5. **Pharmacokinetics.** Esterified drugs are readily absorbed through the cornea and taken up in the ciliary body and trabecular meshwork.
6. **Adverse effects.** Miosis; conjunctival irritation, melanogenesis in the iris.
7. **Contraindications**
   a. Luxated lens where pupil block could result from vitreous entrapment.
   b. Ocular inflammation is exacerbated by prostaglandin analogs.

X. ANTIFIBRIN AGENTS

A. Tissue plasminogen activator (TPA)

1. **Preparations/mechanism of action.** Human recombinant TPA; a protease that converts plasminogen to plasmin which lyses fibrin; it does not contribute to intraocular hemorrhage. It is reconstituted from human product, alteplase (Activase®), to 25 µg/100 µL and frozen at $-70°C$ in 100 µL aliquots.
2. **Therapeutic uses.** It is injected into the anterior chamber to lyse intraocular fibrin or blood clot formed from inflammatory disease, intraocular surgery, or ocular trauma. It prevents posterior synechia, secondary glaucoma, cyclitic membranes, and corneal blood staining.
3. **Administration.** Intracameral injection of 25 µg, most commonly into anterior chamber but may be used intravitreally.
4. **Pharmacokinetics.** It is not absorbed through the cornea after topical administration.
5. **Adverse effects.** The TPA doses that are higher than the recommended ones may damage corneal endothelium. TPA may be retinotoxic when injected in deep vitreous.

B. Heparin

1. **Mechanism of action.** It impairs thrombin-mediated formation of fibrin.
2. **Therapeutic uses.** Heparin is added to intraocular irrigating solutions for use in intraocular surgery to minimize the formation of fibrin clots.
3. **Adverse effects.** It may predispose to intraoperative or postoperative hemorrhage. It does not lyse fibrin or blood clots already formed (see fibrinolytics, TPA).

C. Hirudin

1. **Mechanism of action.** Hirudin is the direct acting antithrombin agent that blocks formation of fibrin from fibrinogen without affecting platelets.
2. **Therapeutic uses.** It is used intraoperatively to block formation of fibrin.
3. **Administration.** Hirudin is added to intraocular irrigating solutions for use during surgery.
4. **Adverse effects.** None reported.

XI. **TOPICAL ANESTHETICS** (see Chapter 6 for detailed information).

A. **General considerations.** The cornea has a dense sensory innervation, most dense in the superficial stromal and notably intraepithelial.

B. **Chemistry.** These agents consist of a lipid soluble aromatic ring with a linked hydrophilic amino group, giving the molecule biphasic solubility.

C. **Preparations.** Proparacaine, 0.5% solution (best tolerated, fewest adverse effects), also tetracaine, 0.5–2% ointment or solution, piperocaine, dibucaine, benoxinate.

D. **Mechanism of action.** These agents block Na^+ channels, preventing axon depolarization, progressively decreasing the nerve action potential leading to reversible block of conduction through nerve fibers.

E. **Therapeutic uses**
1. **Topical anesthesia of the conjunctiva and cornea** facilitate diagnostic, manipulative and minor treatment procedures including tonometry, nasolacrimal duct irrigation, corneal debridement, subconjunctival injections, and elevating and everting the membrana nictitans to search for foreign bodies. It is sufficient for anterior chamber centesis with small needle. **These agents are useful preoperatively in cataract surgery to maintain mydriasis and stabilize the blood–aqueous barrier. They are not a treatment for painful conditions.**
2. **Regional (infiltrative) anesthesia** (see Chapter 6 for more information) by palpebral, auriculopalpebral, supraorbital nerve blocks and eyelid infiltration for the horse and deep orbital injections (Peterson eye block) for cattle are often employed using injectable agents such as lidocaine, but general anesthesia is preferred for the dog and cat.

F. **Administration.** One to two drops on the surface of the eye 15 seconds prior to tonometry, longer for more extensive procedures. One minute is usually satisfactory for debriding corneal epithelium or anterior chamber centesis. The duration of anesthesia is up to 45 minutes in the dog, 25 minutes in the cat.

G. **Pharmacokinetics.** These drugs traverse the cornea and nerve membrane readily due to equilibrium of ionized and nonionized forms that is pH dependent. Bicarbonate buffering to increase pH facilitates penetration; inflammation lowers the pH of tissue and diminishes effectiveness. It does not penetrate into aqueous humor.

H. **Adverse effects**
1. Tetracaine causes burning sensation, hyperemia, and chemosis.
2. All agents induce minor surface irregularities in the corneal epithelium that may interfere with examination of the posterior segment.
3. Faint fluorescein uptake may be seen after anesthetic instillation.
4. Repeated application may lead to ulceration of an edematous cornea.
5. Topical anesthesia reduces tear production.
6. These agents are bactericidal so cultures must be procured prior to instillation.
7. Topical anesthesia will permit an animal to rub at an eye with clouded vision or deep pain and damage the cornea without awareness of pain.

XII. **CARBONIC ANHYDRASE INHIBITORS (CAIS)**

A. **Preparations**
1. **Systemic preparations.** Acetazolamide, dichlorphenamide, methazolamide, ethoxzolamide (see Chapter 9 for more information).
2. **Topical preparations.** Dorzolamide, brinzolamide.

B. **Chemistry.** All clinically active CAIs have the same active configuration.

C. **Mechanism of action.** CA catalyzes the formation of bicarbonate (HCO_3^-) in nonpigmented ciliary epithelium. Aqueous humor is created as sodium accompanies and water follows the transport of bicarbonate into the posterior chamber of the eye due to the created osmotic gradient. CAIs obstruct the enzyme surface and block the catalyst availability for the formation of bicarbonate.

   Given systemically, a CAI must block >99% of CA to achieve significant decrease in IOP. Aqueous humor production is decreased 30–60%. Uncatalyzed hydration of CO_2 is sufficient to maintain at least 40% of normal aqueous production.

D. **Ocular therapeutic uses.** These agents are to reduce IOP. **They are the only systemic agents for long-term medical management of glaucoma.** Topical CAIs are less effective (<50%) than systemic agents, but lack of side effects makes topical agents preferable. IOP reduction in dogs is ~20%. Topical CAIs are used prophylactically and therapeutically. **Both topical and systemic preparations are inadequate for acute high-pressure, closed-angle glaucoma without first administering an osmotic diuretic (mannitol). The effects of concomitant use of a topical and a systemic CAI are not additive and therefore not warranted in glaucoma therapy.**

E. **Pharmacokinetics.** Absorption through cornea is sufficient for topical preparations to reach concentrations comparable to systemic administration.

F. **Administration.** Injectable acetazolamide is for IV administration. Other systemic preparations are given orally. Topicals are used twice daily for cat and three times daily for dog and horse.

G. **Adverse effects.** Systemic CAIs create systemic acidosis and compensatory hyperpnea, GI disturbances, diuresis, and depression. Hypokalemia is rarely seen.

XIII. **OSMOTIC DIURETICS** (see Chapter 9 for more information). IV Mannitol and oral glycerol are osmotic diuretics that lower IOP by reducing the volume of the vitreous.

XIV. **MATRIX METALLOPROTEINASE (MMP) INHIBITORS**

A. **Introduction.** MMPs are zinc-dependent endopeptidases categorized according to their structure and matrix specificity: **collagenases (MMP1,8,13)**, **gelatinases (MMP2,9)**, **stromelysins (MMP 3,10)**, elastase, and serine proteases of plasmin and tissue plasminogen activator (TPA).

1. MMPs are present in normal tissue and are important to maintenance and remodeling of damaged corneal epithelial cells and stromal collagen, but upregulated in inflammation.
2. MMPs are present in various cells: invading leukocytes, phagocytes, keratocytes, and bacteria (*Pseudomonas*).
3. In the cornea, small amounts of proteinases are liberated in response to trauma to liquefy and remove damaged collagen, facilitating epithelialization. In excess the proteinases cleave the stromal collagen and create a rapidly progressive, expanding ulcer.

B. **Agents for inhibiting MMPs.** Topical sodium EDTA, calcium EDTA; acetylcysteine; sodium citrate and sodium ascorbate; doxycycline and tetracycline administered systemically accumulate in the cornea; betadine, serum.

C. **Mechanism of action.** Most inhibitors act by chelating calcium and/or zinc, which prevents the activation of the latent MMP. α-2 macroglobulins in serum bind collagenase and have been shown to promote corneal healing.

D. **Therapeutic uses.** They are topically applied to inhibit rapidly progressive corneal stromal necrosis secondary to bacterial or fungal infection of an ulcer.

E. **Adverse effects.** None documented; use of these agents is empirical and benefits are inconsistent.

XV. TEAR SUBSTITUTES

A. **Introduction.** The natural tearfilm is a three-layered mucin, water, lipid film that has not been duplicated. The most common defect in the tearfilm is lack of the aqueous portion but there may be a mucin deficiency as well. A chronic tearfilm deficiency results in metaplastic changes in the corneal and conjunctival epithelium, leading to scarring and vision loss. Tear replacement products are not pharmacologically active.

B. **Agents.** Numerous products of varying viscosity and wetting qualities are available.

1. **Methylcellulose, hydroxypropylmethlycellulose, carboxymethylcellulose.**
2. **Polyvinyl alcohol, polyvinyl pyrrolidone (mucomimetic).**
3. **Hyaluronic acid (hyaluronate) for prolonged retention, improved tearfilm stability.**
4. **Mineral oil, white petrolatum, lanolin for maximum retention.**

C. **Therapeutic advantages**

1. Lubricate the surface of the eye for comfort.
2. Duplicate the optical characteristics of the tears.
3. Better agents are hypotonic as tear tonicity increases with decreased aqueous tear production.

D. **Adverse effects.** None except for the inability to duplicate the trilaminar structure of the natural tears. Preservatives may be irritating and many products are available without preservatives.

SUGGESTED READING

Bentley E, Murphy CJ. 2004. Topical therapeutic agents that modulate corneal wound healing. *Vet Clin North Am Small Anim Pract* 34:623–638.

Brooks DE, Ollivier FJ. 2004. Matrix metalloproteinase inhibition in corneal ulceration. *Vet Clin North Am Small Anim Pract* 34:611–622.

Ford MM. 2004. Antifungals and their use in veterinary ophthalmology. *Vet Clin North Am Small Anim Pract* 34:669–691.

Galle LE. 2004. Antiviral therapy for ocular viral disease. *Vet Clin North Am Small Anim Pract* 34:639–653.

Giuliano EA. 2004. Nonsteroidal anti-inflammatory drugs in veterinary ophthalmology. *Vet Clin North Am Small Anim Pract* 34:707–723.

Grahn BH, Storey ES. 2004. Lacrimostimulants and lacrimomimetics. *Vet Clin North Am Small Anim Pract* 34:739–753.

Holmberg BJ, Maggs DJ. 2004. The use of corticosteroids to treat ocular inflammation. *Vet Clin North Am Small Anim Pract* 34:693–705.

http://www.drugs.com

Kern TJ. 2004. Antibacterial agents for ocular therapeutics. *Vet Clin North Am Small Anim Pract* 34:655–668.

Mauger TF, Craig EL. 1994. *Havener's Ocular Pharmacology.* 6th ed. St. Louis, MD: Mosby.

Moore CP. 2004. Immunomodulating agents. *Vet Clin North Am Small Anim Pract* 34:725–737.

Plumb DC. 2005. *Veterinary Drug Handbook.* 5th ed. Ames, IA: Blackwell Publishing.

Regnier A, Herring I. 2007. "Clinical pharmacology and therapeutics." In *Veterinary Ophthalmology.* Edited by Gelatt KN. 4th ed., pp. 271–354. Ames, IA: Blackwell Publishing.

Wilkie DA, Gemensky-Metzler AJ. 2004. Agents for intraocular surgery. *Vet Clin North Am Small Anim Pract* 34:801–823.

Willis AM. 2004. Ocular hypotensive drugs. *Vet Clin North Am Small Anim Pract* 34:755–776.

STUDY QUESTIONS

DIRECTIONS: Each of the numbered items or incomplete statements in this section is followed by answers or by completions of the statement. Select the **one** lettered answer or completion that is **best** in each case.

1. For a through examination of the lens, retina, and optic nerve of a dog, which drug is most appropriate for dilating the pupil?

(A) Atropine
(B) Pilocarpine
(C) Tropicamide
(D) Acetylcholine

2. A dog has presented with classic signs of glaucoma including a very high intraocular pressure (IOP) of 65 mm Hg. You administer IV mannitol to lower the IOP and now must select medications to attempt to keep the pressure in a more normal range. Which of these drugs would decrease the secretion of aqueous humor?

(A) Atropine
(B) Pilocarpine
(C) Demecarium
(D) Dorzolamide

3. Which of these drugs would be most effective in facilitating aqueous humor outflow?

(A) Latanoprost
(B) Flurbiprofen
(C) Pilocarpine
(D) Demecarium

4. With signs of keratoconjunctivitis and a low Schirmer tear test bilaterally (2 mm in each eye, where 15–25 mm is normal), what medication would you choose as your primary agent to reverse the signs and symptoms of this problem?

(A) Cyclosporine ointment
(B) Pilocarpine
(C) Prednisolone acetate
(D) A lubricating ointment tear substitute

5. You have adopted a cat from a humane shelter and they have given you a small bottle of idoxuridine to continue treating the eyes. They do not know what the problem is, but you know that this drug is used to treat

(A) glaucoma.
(B) herpesvirus infection of the conjunctiva.
(C) a fungal keratitis.
(D) a chlamydial conjunctivitis.

6. A small terrier dog has presented with a posterior lens luxation and you have arranged for referral to an ophthalmologist for removal of the lens next week. If you can keep the lens in the posterior of the eye, there is less chance that it will obstruct the pupil and cause glaucoma. Which of these drugs will accomplish this?

(A) Atropine
(B) Dorzolamide
(C) Pilocarpine
(D) Timolol

7. A horse is presented with a very painful eye with a 1 cm diameter deep stromal corneal ulcer with necrotic margins. Examination of a scraping from the ulcer reveals numerous septate hyphae so you submit a sample for culture. A logical initial topical treatment until culture results are available would include

(A) Nystatin, calcium EDTA, and atropine.
(B) Neomycin, bacitracin, gramicidin ointment, and atropine.
(C) Natamycin, acetylcysteine, and atropine.
(D) Itraconazole in DMSO, atropine, and betadine.

8. You apply a 2% solution of phenylephrine to each eye of a dog with unilateral Horner's syndrome (miosis, ptosis, enophthalmos, and elevated nictitating membrane) and no other neurologic or oculars signs. The Horner's signs diminish significantly within 10 minutes. You correctly conclude that

(A) this is a postganglionic Horner's.
(B) this is a preganglionic Horner's.
(C) this is a central Horner's.
(D) this is not Horner's syndrome.

9. A horse with severe recurring anterior uveitis should be given a systemic nonsteroidal anti-inflammatory drug such as flunixin meglumine but other medications are equally important to use concurrently to suppress the intraocular inflammation and related signs and symptoms. In addition to atropine, which of the following is most appropriate?

(A) Prednisolone acetate drops and subconjunctival triamcinolone.
(B) Hydrocortisone acetate and triple antibiotic drops, and dexamethasone subconjunctivally.
(C) Flurbiprofen drops and dexamethasone drops.
(D) Dexamethasone drops and subconjunctival gentamicin.

10. A dog with a shallow, epithelial erosion of the cornea is to be treated with a topical triple antibiotic solution but the owner is distressed about relieving pain in the cornea. She inquires about using a topical anesthetic on the eye for a few days. Your response should be:

(A) Yes, of course, proparacaine will provide good anesthesia rapidly and for several hours a day.
(B) Yes, but the proparacaine will anesthetize the cornea for only 20–30 minutes so it will have to be repeated frequently.
(C) We should not use a topical anesthetic on a corneal ulcer because the dog may rub at it and not feel the pain of further trauma to the eye and cause a worse wound.
(D) Topical anesthetics will stop mitosis of epithelial cells and greatly delay the healing of the wound.

ANSWERS AND EXPLANATIONS

1. The answer is C.
Tropicamide causes rapid mydriasis that returns to normal in 2–3 hours. Atropine takes too long to dilate a pupil and the mydriasis may last for 2–3 days. Acetylcholine is much too short acting and is neutralized by esterases in the cornea. Pilocarpine is a miotic.

2. The answer is D.
Dorzolamide is the topical carbonic anhydrase inhibitor. Demecarium and pilocarpine facilitate outflow of aqueous humor. Atropine would predispose to obstruction of outflow when the pupil is dilated.

3. The answer is A.
Latanoprost is the most effective agent for facilitating outflow through increased uveal scleral outflow that is not altered by a narrow or closed angle. It only needs once a day dosing. Pilocarpine and demecarium facilitate outflow but pilocarpine must be used 3–4 times a day and often is irritating to the eye. Demecarium is potent and long acting, but is toxic (a cholinesterase inhibitor) and can only be procured from one compounding pharmacy.

4. The answer is A.
Cyclosporine ointment will reverse inflammatory changes of the immune-mediated lacrimal adenitis, the most likely cause for the loss of tear secretion; it will help reverse the corneal changes resulting from the lack of tears, and it is lacrimomimetic.
Pilocarpine topically is a poor lacrimomimetic but does not affect inflammation on the cornea, conjunctiva, or in the lacrimal gland. Prednisolone will help to diminish inflammatory changes on the cornea but will not affect tear production. In the absence of normal tears there are no antibacterial components such as lysozyme that are normally present and there may be opportunistic bacterial overgrowth. A lubricating ointment alone is inadequate for all aspects of the problem. It would need to be applied several times a day.

5. The answer is B.
Conjunctivitis and keratitis caused by herpesvirus. None of the other conditions are treatable with idoxuridine.

6. Pilocarpine is a direct acting cholinergic that will constrict the pupil to a diameter smaller than the lens thereby keeping it behind the iris where it is less likely to obstruct the circulation of aqueous until the time of surgery. It will "wear off" rapidly when withdrawn so that the pupil can be dilated at the time of surgery so that the lens can be retrieved from the posterior chamber. Atropine dilates the pupil and the lens may wedge in the pupil, obstructing aqueous humor circulation or permit the lens to enter the anterior chamber where it can rub on the interior of the cornea. Timolol, a nonselective β-blocker, lowers IOP by reducing aqueous production. It does cause some miosis though not reliably enough to keep the lens behind the iris. The hypotensive effect may cause the IOP to go too low as the inflammation secondary to the loose lens may already have decreased aqueous production. Dorzolamide is a CAI that reduces aqueous production more than timolol.

7. The answer is C.
Natamycin, acetylcysteine, and atropine. Natamycin is the only antifungal drug approved for use on the eye and the only one commercially available, although azoles can be compounded for topical use. This ulcer has characteristics strongly suggestive of matrix metalloproteinase overactivity that is causing corneal "melting" (necrosis). Acetylcysteine may be helpful, although betadine is MMP inhibiting as well as fungicidal. Atropine will benefit the secondary iritis (sphincter spasm) that accompanies corneal trauma. Itraconazole is a good choice but DMSO is an unnecessary irritant on the open ulcer.

8. The answer is A.
This is a postganglionic Horner's syndrome with obvious improvement of signs within a short time—10 minutes—indicating denervation supersensitivity at the terminal ending of the adrenergic nerve(s).

9. The answer is A.
Prednisolone acetate drops topically will penetrate the intact cornea effectively and the subconjunctival triamcinolone (a

suspension) will provide a slow release steroid that will be absorbed into the eye for as much as 7–10 days. Dexamethasone is equal to prednisolone topically but the subconjunctival depot lasts only 24 hours. Hydrocortisone is insufficiently potent. Antibiotics are not indicated. Flurbiprofen, a topical NSAID, is good but very expensive and must be applied at least 4 times a day. With horses owner compliance with treatment schedules more than 2–3 times a day is seldom achieved, even with lavage tubes.

10. The answer is D.
Topical anesthetics must not be used on corneal wounds as they are toxic to epithelial cells and will inhibit mitosis. It is true that a dog may rub at an anesthetized cornea and further damage the cornea without realizing the damage being done. Topical anesthetics are for diagnostic purposes, not treatment.

Chapter 15

Antimicrobial Drugs

Franklin A. Ahrens and Richard J. Martin

I. INTRODUCTION

A. **Selection of an antimicrobial drug.** Antimicrobial therapy is based upon the selective toxicity of the drug for invading organisms rather than mammalian cells. It is important to select an agent to which the organism is sensitive and to maintain the effective tissue concentrations (above the minimal inhibitory concentration or MIC) until the infection is eliminated. A practical approach is to select an antimicrobial agent where the measured MIC is less than the concentration known as the breakpoint concentration. Sensitivity tests using either sensitivity disks or sensititer micro-well plates can be used to estimate the MIC of specific bacteria and then tables are consulted to see if the MIC is below the breakpoint. If the MIC is below the breakpoint, it is predicted that the microbe will be Susceptible (S) to therapy; if it is equal to the breakpoint, it is predicted that the microbe will be Intermediate (I)—where high therapeutic doses may work; if the MIC is above the breakpoint, it is predicted that the microbe will be Resistant (R). The breakpoint concentrations have been determined by groups like the Clinical and Laboratory Standards Institute (CLSI) following review of clinical and laboratory data. The pharmacokinetic data on data labels of more recently introduced antimicrobials contain breakpoint information. It is pointed out that the sensitivity tests and breakpoints are useful indicators for the clinical outcome, but in the whole animal, additional factors like drug binding, drug distribution, and an active immune system affect the outcome so that clinical experience is still essential.

Extra-label use of specific antimicrobial drugs in food animals is prohibited for reasons of safety or limitation of resistance spread. These drugs include the fluoroquinolones, chloramphenicol, nitroimidazoles, furazolidone, nitrofurazone and other nitrofurans, and sulfonamide drugs in lactating dairy cattle (except approved use of sufadimethoxine, glycopeptides, and vancomycin).

There are six selection questions that are helpful to use routinely to aid selection:

1. **Is an antimicrobial agent required—is there an infection that will respond to your treatment?** Avoid: "Just in case."
2. **Where is the infection (which organ/tissue)—what are the access problems to be overcome?**
3. **Which pathogen(s) are usually found at the location of the infection?**
4. **Which antimicrobial agent has the necessary pharmacokinetic properties to get to the location and also will get there at a concentration above the MIC so that the MIC is below the breakpoint?**
5. **What dose and route is necessary to achieve the desired effect?**
6. **How long should the treatment be for?**

There are 4 additional factors to help the selection:

1. **A bactericidal compound is preferable to a bacteriostatic compound.**
2. **Toxicity and cost limit the selection of an antimicrobial drug.**
3. **In food-producing animals, residues in milk and meat requiring the need for withdrawal times before slaughter (preslaughter withdrawal times) are very important and limit the use of specific antimicrobial drugs. Animals must not be slaughtered for meat or their milk used within the preslaughter period (see appendix for the withdrawal period for each drug).**
4. **It should be appreciated that the plasma concentration governs the dose intervals on a treatment regimen but it is the tissue residence times that govern the preslaughter withdrawal times in production animals.**

B. **Resistance to antimicrobials**

1. **Mechanisms by which bacteria manifest resistance:**
   a. **Organisms may produce enzymes**, constitutive or inducible, which inactivate the drug.
   b. **The permeability to or uptake of the drug by organisms** may be decreased or transport out of the cell may be increased.
   c. **Alteration of the drug receptor or binding site** may result in reduced drug affinity at target loci.
   d. **The organism may develop alternate metabolic or synthetic pathways** to bypass or repair the effects of the antimicrobial.

2. **Mechanisms by which bacteria develop resistance**
   a. **Mutation.** Within a large population of bacteria, chromosomal mutations may occur, which confer resistance either slowly, in a step-wise fashion with each succeeding generation of the mutant more resistant or rapidly, in a single step in which the bacterium is resistant after the initial mutation. Mutation is a random event. Antimicrobials do not induce mutations but may exert a selecting out of resistant strains by suppression of susceptible bacteria.
   b. **Conjugation.** Certain Gram(–) bacteria undergo conjugation, a type of reproduction in which genetic material is transferred from cell to cell via a pilus that is encoded by a resistance transfer factor (RTF) on a plasmid. Resistance factors (R-factors) from plasmid DNA and/or chromosomal DNA may encode for resistance to multiple drugs and may be rapidly transferred to the bacterial population. This is termed **infectious drug resistance or transferable drug resistance** and has been observed clinically in enteric infections with *Salmonella* spp., *Shigella* spp., and *Escherichia coli*.
   c. **Transduction.** The process of transference of drug resistant genes by bacteriophage is termed transduction. It may be important in the development of resistant strains of *Staphylococcus aureus*.
   d. **Transformation.** Bacteria may incorporate DNA encoding for drug resistance from their environment after its secretion or release by resistant organisms. Acquisition of resistance by this mechanism is relatively infrequent.

II. SULFONAMIDES

A. **Chemistry.** The sulfonamides are derivatives of *p*-aminobenzene sulfonic acid (Figure 15-1) and are structurally similar to *p*-aminobenzoic acid (PABA), an intermediate in bacterial synthesis of folic acid. They behave as weak organic acids which are poorly water soluble unless prepared as sodium salts. Concentrated solutions of the sodium salts of most sulfonamides are very alkaline and may be corrosive. The solubility of a sulfonamide is not influenced by the presence of other sulfonamides in the solution. This is termed the law of independent solubility and is the primary reason for the use of sulfonamide mixtures in order to increase the combined total sulfonamide concentration to prevent renal precipitation and thus reduce toxicity.

B. **Mechanism of action.** Sulfonamides competitively inhibit dihydropteroate synthase, the enzyme which catalyzes the incorporation of PABA into dihydrofolic acid (Figure 15-2). Folic acid is required for purine and DNA synthesis and thus bacterial growth is inhibited. Mammalian cells and bacteria that use preformed folic acid are not affected. Sulfonamides are broad spectrum (including protozoa) and bacteriostatic.

C. **Therapeutic uses.** Sulfonamides were widely used in the prevention and treatment of local and systemic infections in all species but now resistance is common. Examples of sulfonamides used in veterinary medicine include the following:

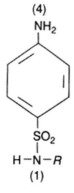

(4)
NH₂

SO₂
H−N−R
(1)

FIGURE 15-1. General structure of the sulfonamides. The *p*-amino group at position 4 must be free for antimicrobial activity to occur. Substitution with a heterocyclic ring (e.g., thiazole, pyrimidine, pyridine) at the *R* position on position 1 distinguishes the various sulfonamides. Replacement of the hydrogen with sodium at position 1 greatly increases the water solubility of the sulfonamide. (Adapted from Figure 11-1, *NVMS Pharmacology*, by Ahrens, F. A. 1996.)

1. **Sulfamethazine is used in cattle, sheep, and swine.** It is slowly excreted and therapeutic levels are maintained in plasma for 24 hours with a single dose.
2. **Sulfadimethoxine is a long-acting sulfonamide.** It is more soluble and less toxic than sulfamethazine. The plasma $t_{1/2}$ is 10–15 hours.
3. **Sulfachlorpyridazine is a rapidly absorbed and rapidly excreted sulfonamide used orally in calves under 1 month of age and in swine for the treatment of respiratory and enteric infections,** especially colibacillosis. Peak levels occur in 1–2 hours in nonruminants and in preruminant calves. The plasma $t_{1/2}$ is 1.2 hours.
4. **Sulfamethoxazole is used to treat urinary tract infections in small animals.** It is rapidly excreted and very soluble. Thus high concentrations may be attained in urine with minimal danger of renal crystalluria.
5. **Sulfacetamide is the only sulfonamide that can be prepared as the sodium salt at neutral pH and thus can be used in ophthalmic preparations.**
6. **Sulfasalazine is an "enteric" sulfonamide employed in the therapy of colitis and inflammatory bowel disease in dogs and cats.** It consists of a molecule of sulfapyridine linked to a molecule of 5-aminosalicylic acid (5-ASA) by a diazo bond. This prevents absorption in the small intestine and allows drug transit to the large bowel where it is cleaved by gut bacteria to sulfapyridine and 5-ASA. These have antibacterial and anti-inflammatory actions, respectively.
7. **Other sulfonamides used in veterinary medicine are** sulfathiazole and sulfaquinoxaline.

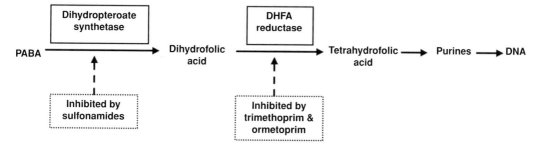

FIGURE 15-2. Mechanism of action of sulfonamides. Sulfonamides block dihydrofolic acid synthesis by competing with *p*-aminobenzoic acid (PABA) for binding sites on dihydropteroate synthetase. Dihydrofolic acid is necessary for the synthesis of tetrahydrofolic acid, and ultimately, purines and DNA. Trimethoprim and ormetoprim inhibit dihydrofolic acid (DHFA) reductase, which is necessary for tetrahydrofolic acid synthesis. Therefore, potentiated sulfonamides (i.e., those combined with trimethoprim or ormetoprim) block the second step of protein synthesis.

8. **Potentiated sulfonamides are fixed combinations of a sulfonamide with trimethoprim or ormetoprim.** This results in a synergistic action via sequential blockade of folate synthesis (Figure 15-2).

   a. Trimethoprim and ormetoprim inhibit dihydrofolate reductase in bacteria (but not mammalian cells) and thus block the formation of tetrahydrofolic acid essential for purine and DNA synthesis.

   b. Potentiated sulfonamides have a broader spectrum of action and a reduced rate of development of bacterial resistance.

   c. Preparations include sulfadiazine plus trimethoprim, sulfamethoxazole plus trimethoprim, and sulfadimethoxine plus ormetoprim. They are used in the treatment of susceptible infections in all species.

   d. Trimethoprim and ormetoprim are organic bases in contrast to the organic acid nature of the sulfonamides. They accumulate by ion-trapping in acidic environments and will concentrate differently in the tissues to the sulfonamides. Trimethoprim plasma $t_{1/2}$ is 2–3 hours in most species.

D. **Pharmacokinetics**

1. Sulfonamides are well absorbed orally and widely distributed to tissues. Transcellular fluid concentrations are 80% of plasma concentration. Binding to plasma albumin varies with each sulfonamide but is generally 50–75%.

2. Metabolism by acetylation at N_4 and glucuronide conjugation occurs in most species. Acetylation does not occur in the dog. Oxidation of the benzene and heterocyclic rings to quinone derivatives also occurs, especially in dogs. The type and extent of metabolism varies with the sulfonamide and the animal species.

3. Renal excretion of unchanged drug and metabolites is via glomerular filtration, active secretion, and passive tubular reabsorption. Reabsorption is pH–pKa dependent.

E. **Administration.** Sulfonamides and potentiated sulfonamides can be administered orally or by injection, depending on species. Frequency of dosing varies with the individual sulfonamides.

F. **Bacterial resistance.** Bacteria develop resistance by mechanisms, which include increased PABA production, decreased binding of sulfonamide to dihydropteroate synthase, and bacterial metabolism of sulfonamide. Bacteria which are resistant to one sulfonamide are resistant to all. Resistance to the potentiated sulfonamide does occur but is less common than to the sulfonamide. The spectrum of action of the potentiated sulfonamides is broader and the combination is considered bactericidal rather than bacteriostatic.

G. **Adverse effects**

1. **Renal crystalluria** due to precipitation of sulfonamides in neutral or acidic urine may occur with large or prolonged doses or inadequate water intake, especially with the older, less soluble sulfonamides such as sulfathiazole. Therapeutic regimens generally do not extend beyond 5 days and renal crystalluria is rare.

2. **Keratoconjunctivitis sicca (KCS) may be observed in dogs treated with sulfonamides**, such as sulfadiazine, which contain the pyrimidine nucleus. The mechanism of the toxic effect on lacrimal acinar cells is unknown.

3. **Hypoprothrombinemia, thrombocytopenia, and anemia occur rarely** and are probably immune-mediated reactions. Sulfonamides should not be used in animals with preexisting bleeding disorders.

III. FLUOROQUINOLONES

A. **Chemistry.** The fluoroquinolones consist of a quinoline ring to which is attached a carboxyl group, fluorine atom, and piperazine ring. They are weak acids and are lipophilic. Water-soluble salts are used in parenteral preparations.

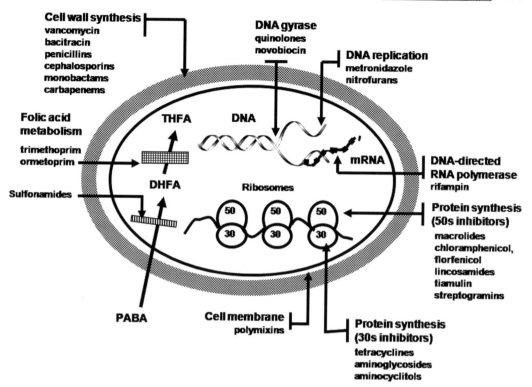

FIGURE 15-3. Mechanisms of action of antibacterial drugs. The five general mechanisms are (1) inhibit synthesis of cell wall, (2) damage outer membrane, (3) modify nucleic acid/DNA synthesis, (4) modify protein synthesis, and (5) modify energy metabolism in the cytoplasm (at folate cycle). (Modified from Figure 46.2, *Human Pharmacology*, 2nd ed., by Brody, T. M., Larner, J., Minneman, K. P., and Neu, H. C. 1994.)

B. **Mechanism of action.** The fluoroquinolones inhibit bacterial DNA gyrase, an enzyme which controls DNA supercoiling as the replicating strands separate. Inhibition of gyrase results in degradation of chromosomal DNA at the replicating fork. Fluoroquinolones are broad spectrum and bactericidal. Anaerobes tend to be resistant (Figure 15-3).

C. **Therapeutic uses**

1. **Enrofloxacin** is used in the treatment of dermal, respiratory, and urinary tract infections (including prostatitis) in dogs, cats, and birds and in respiratory infections in cattle.
2. **Danofloxacin** is used for the treatment of bovine respiratory infections including *Mannheimia* species.
3. **Difloxacin** is used for treatment of dermal, respiratory, and urinary tract infections in dogs.
4. **Orbifloxacin** and Marbofloxacin are used for the treatment of dermal, respiratory, and urinary tract infections of dogs and cats. Orbifloxacin is used for susceptible Gram(–) infections in horses.
5. **Extralabel use of fluoroquinolones in food animals is prohibited.**

D. **Pharmacokinetics.** Oral absorption of the fluoroquinolones is rapid with peak plasma concentrations at 1 hour in dogs. Distribution is wide and includes the CNS, bone, and prostate. Some hepatic metabolism occurs and both parent drug (15–50%) and metabolites are excreted in urine and bile. Renal tubular active secretion results in high urinary concentrations. The plasma $t_{1/2}$ for enrofloxacin is 3–5 hours in dogs and

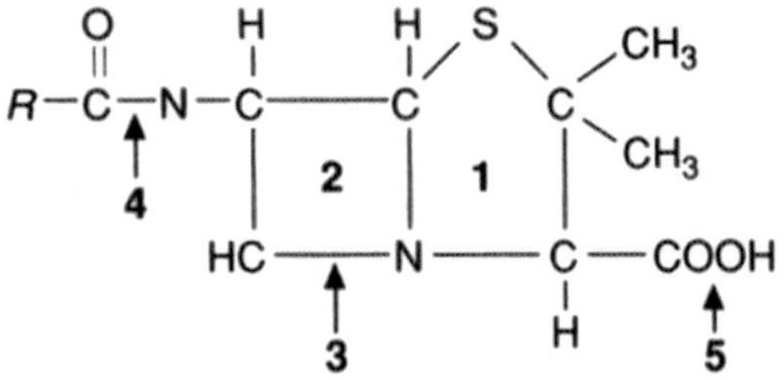

FIGURE 15-4. General structure of penicillins. Substituents at *R* distinguish the various penicillins. (1) Thiazolidone ring. (2) β-Lactam ring. (3) Site of action of β-lactamases (penicillinases). (4) Site of amidase cleavage to yield 6-aminopenicillanic acid (6-APA) nucleus for semisynthetic penicillins. (5) site of salt formation (e.g., sodium, procaine). (Adapted from Figure 11-3, *NVMS Pharmacology*, by Ahrens, F. A. 1996).

6 hours in cats and horses. The elimination $t_{1/2}$ for difloxacin and marbofloxacin is 9–12 hours in dog and cats and for orbifloxacin is 6 hours in dogs and cats and 9 hours in horses.

E. **Administration.** Fluoroquinolines are administered orally or parenterally once or twice a day in all species. Enrofloxacin is administered SC once a day for treatment of respiratory infections in cattle.

F. **Resistance.** Development of bacterial resistance is relatively rare. Long periods of subtherapeutic levels may allow the growth of mutants in which fluoroquinolones are not bound to DNA gyrase.

G. **Adverse effects.** Toxicity associated with fluoroquinolones is **erosion of articular cartilage** in young dogs and foals, particularly, if they are used at high doses for longer than 14 days in rapid growth phase. Enrofloxacin has also been reported to produce **seizures** in dogs on phenobarbital for epilepsy; other quinolones evoke headaches in humans. **Retinal degeneration** has been reported due to acute and diffuse retinal damage in cats.

IV. PENICILLINS

A. **Chemistry.** The structure of penicillins includes a β-lactam ring and a thiazolidone ring (Figure 15-4). Cleavage of the β-lactam ring destroys antibiotic activity. Amidase cleavage of the amide bond side chain yields the 6-amino-penicillanic acid (6-APA) nucleus used in producing semisynthetic penicillins. The carboxyl group attached to the thiazolidone ring is the site of salt formation (sodium, potassium, procaine, etc.) which stabilizes the penicillins and affects solubility and absorption rates.

B. **Mechanism of action.** Penicillins bind to and inhibit the transpeptidase involved in the cross-linking of the bacterial cell wall, the third and final step in cell-wall synthesis (Figure 15-3). The weakened cell wall ruptures, resulting in lysis and cell death. Penicillins also inhibit other peptidases (penicillin-binding proteins) involved in cell wall synthesis and block the inhibition of autolysins. Rapidly growing bacteria are most susceptible to the bactericidal effect of penicillin. The penicillins are primarily effective against Gram(+) aerobes and anaerobes. The broad-spectrum, semisynthetic penicillins are also effective against some Gram(–) pathogens.

C. **Therapeutic uses**

1. **Natural penicillins**
   a. **Penicillin G (benzylpenicillin)** is used in all species for the treatment of infections caused by Gram(+), nonpenicillinase producing pathogens. It is the most potent penicillin for these organisms.
   b. **Penicillin V** now used infrequently for long-term oral therapy of Gram(+) bacterial infections in dogs, cats, and horses.
2. **Penicillinase-resistant penicillins** include methicillin, oxacillin, and cloxacillin. Their use is suited for severe staphylococcal infections caused by β-lactamase-producing

organisms (some bovine mastitis) but they are less effective against *Streptococcus* than the natural penicillins.

3. **Broad-spectrum penicillins**
    a. **Aminopenicillins.** Ampicillin and amoxicillin are active against many Gram(–) aerobes (*E. coli, Proteus, Haemophilus* spp.) as well as Gram(+) pathogens. They are used in all species for the treatment of susceptible infections. They are acid-stable but are not penicillinase stable. GI absorption of amoxicillin is better than ampicillin.
    b. **Carbenicillin and ticarcillin** are carboxypenicillins that have antipseudomonal actions when used alone or in combination with or gentamicin or tobramycin. They are useful for ear and skin infections in dogs caused by *Pseudomonas* spp.
    c. **Piperacillin** is an ureidopenicillin that has an extended Gram(–) spectrum including *Pseudomonas, Enterobacter,* and *Klebsiella* spp. Cost limits its use to the treatment of severe Gram(–) bacterial infections in dogs and cats.
4. **Potentiated penicillins.** Clavulanic acid has minimal antibacterial action but it inhibits many of the β-lactamases produced by penicillin-resistant organisms. It is combined with amoxicillin or ticarcillin in commercial preparations. Sulbactam has an action similar to clavulanic acid and is combined with ampicillin. The potentiated penicillins are used in small animals for extended spectrum antimicrobial action. Tazobactam is another β-lactamase inhibitor.

D. **Pharmacokinetics.** Many penicillins are broken down by gastric HCl and are thus poorly absorbed orally. These include penicillin G, methicillin, and ticarcillin. Acid stable penicillins are well absorbed orally. These include penicillin V, ampicillin, amoxicillin, oxacillin, cloxacillin, and the indanyl salt of carbenicillin. The distributions of penicillins are confined mostly to the extracellular spaces occur, but clinically effective concentrations in most tissues except for the CNS, bones, prostate, and eye. More than 90% of an administered dose is excreted unchanged in the urine by glomerular filtration and active tubular secretion. The remainder is metabolized by the liver to penicilloic acid derivatives, which may act as antigenic determinants in penicillin hypersensitivity.

E. **Administration.** Penicillins are generally administered IM. The acid-stable penicillins are administered orally 2–3 times a day. Procaine penicillin G is slowly absorbed from IM sites and may provide therapeutic levels for 24 hours with a single dose. Benzathine penicillin G is even more slowly absorbed over 48–72 hours but blood levels attained are relatively low. Sodium or potassium salts of penicillin G may be administered IV or IM every 4–6 hours.

F. **Resistance.** Inactivation of penicillins by bacteria-producing penicillinases (β-lactamases) is the most common mechanisms of resistance. Failure of the drug to bind to penicillin-binding proteins (PBPs) may also occur.

G. **Adverse effects.** Allergic reactions to penicillin may occur in animals, especially cattle. Signs include skin eruptions, angioedema, and anaphylaxis. Procaine salts of penicillin should not be used in birds, snakes, turtles, guinea pigs, or chinchillas because these species are sensitive to procaine. Procaine penicillin G should not be used in race horses 30 days before racing. Release of procaine due to high levels of plasma esterases in horses may produce CNS effects. Hyperkalemia and cardiac arrhythmias may result from IV administration of potassium penicillin in all species.

V. CEPHALOSPORINS

A. **Chemistry.** Cephalosporins are β-lactam antibiotics, which have a 7-amino-cephalosporanic acid nucleus analogous to the 6-APA nucleus of penicillins. They are weak acids and are administered as the sodium salt, monohydrate, or free base.

B. **Mechanism of action.** Cephalosporins inhibit the third stage of bacterial cell wall synthesis—the cross-linking of the peptidoglycan chain, by the same mechanism as the penicillins (Figure 15-3). Cephalosporins are bactericidal.

C. **Therapeutic uses.** Cephalosporins may be used in penicillin-intolerant patients, but this should be done with caution since cross-reactivity can occur.

1. **First generation cephalosporins** include cephalexin (oral), cefadroxil (oral), cephapirin (parenteral), and cephalothin (parenteral). They are effective against Gram(+) aerobes. **Cephalosporins are frequently employed for antibiotic prophylaxis because of their ability to penetrate tissues. They are a first alternate to penicillins in the treatment of many infections caused by Gram(+) pathogens.**

2. **Second-generation cephalosporins** include cefaclor (oral) and cefoxitin (parenteral). Their antibacterial spectrum is broader than that of first-generation cephalosporins and includes some Gram(–) pathogens. They are not widely used in veterinary medicine.

3. **Third-generation cephalosporins** include ceftiofur, cefoperazone, cefotaxime, cefixime, and cefpodoxime (Simplicef®). They have an extended spectrum of action against Gram(–) organisms, are resistant to β-lactamases cephalosporinases), and penetrate the blood–brain barrier. Ceftiofur is used in the treatment of respiratory disease in cattle, horses, sheep, and swine following IM injection and for intramammary treatment of mastitis in cattle. It is also used for treating urinary tract infections and soft tissue infections in dogs and cats. Cefoperazone is used in dogs to treat soft tissue infections and Gram(–) bacteremia. Cefotaxime is used in dogs, cats, and foals to treat Gram(–) sepsis, soft tissue infections meningitis, and CNS infections. Cefpodoxime proxetil is the prodrug marketed for use in the treatment of skin infections in dogs and cats. Cefixime is used in the treatment of urinary tract infections and respiratory infections in dogs and cats and for bacterial endocarditis in dogs.

4. **Fourth-Generation cephalosporins** include cefepime and cefquinone and have more activity against bacteria, particularly *Pseudomonas*, showing resistance to other cephalosporins. Some manufacturers have implied incorrectly that their third-generation cephalosporins are fourth generation.

D. **Pharmacokinetics.** Most cephalosporins are unstable in gastric acid and must be given parenterally. Cephalexin and cefadroxil, cefachlor, and cefixime are acid stable and are well absorbed orally. Cephalosporins are distributed in the extracellular fluid and penetrate body tissues except the CSF. Metabolism is minimal except for a few cephalosporins such as cephalothin, which is deacetylated by the liver. The plasma $t_{1/2}$ for most cephalosporins is 1–2 hours. The $t_{1/2}$ for cefixime in dogs is 7 hours. The elimination $t_{1/2}$ for ceftiofur in cattle is 8–12 hours following IM administration. Ceftiofur tissue concentration fall in food animals below tolerance levels in liver and kidney after 4 days. Renal excretion is by glomerular filtration and active tubular secretion like penicillins.

E. **Administration.** The acid-stable cephalosporins (cephalexin, cefadroxil, cefachlor, and cefixime) are administered orally every 8–12 hours in dogs and cats. Parental cephalosporins are administered IM, IV, or SC every 8–12 hours in all species. An exception is ceftiofur, which is administered once a day in cattle, horses, sheep, dogs, and cats.

F. **Resistance.** Bacterial β-lactamase production may confer resistance, although cephalosporins tend to retain efficacy in contrast to the penicillins.

G. **Adverse effects.** Side effects are rare and **cephaolsporins are considered to be among the safest antimicrobials in use.** Prolonged treatment or high doses may produce **hemopoietic effects with anemia and bone marrow depression. Hypersensitivity and allergic reactions** may occur.

VI. CARBAPENEMS

A. **Chemistry.** Carbapenems are β-lactams with a structure similar to penicillin but the –S– in the thiazolidine is replaced by a methyl group.

B. **Mechanism of action** is similar to other β-lactam antimicrobial drugs but the carbapenems bind to more penicillin-binding proteins so that **they have a very broad spectrum of action, one of the widest spectrum antimicrobials** (Figure 15-3).

C. **Therapeutic uses.** The carbapenems are used to treat very serious infections like peritonitis associated with ruptured GI tract or intestinal spillage during surgery. They are effective against Gram(+) and Gram(–) aerobic and anaerobic bacteria including *Pseudomonas* and *Enterobacteriaciae.*

D. **Pharmacokinetics. Oral administration is not possible because of acid hydrolysis and poor absorption.** Imipenem is given IV over a period of 15–30 minutes and elimination in humans is governed by a $t_{1/2}$ of 2 hours where 75% is eliminated by renal filtration and metabolism in the renal tubules. No information on $t_{1/2}$ is available for animals. Imipenem undergoes extensive metabolism by the kidney dehydropeptidase (DHP-1) in the brush border of the proximal tubule. The metabolite is nephrotoxic and exhibits antimicrobial action in the urine. Imepenem is used with a DHP-1 inhibitor, cilastatin, to decrease toxicity and increase elimination $t_{1/2}$. Meropenem is a more recent derivative that is more DHP-1 stable that does not need cilastatin to inhibit kidney metabolism.

E. **Adverse effects.** Side effects may include anorexia, vomiting, and diarrhea; CNS toxicity including seizures and tremors; and hypersensitivity reactions including pruritis, fever, and rarely, anaphylaxis.

VII. MONOBACTAMS

A. **Chemistry.** Monobactams have a β-lactam ring but the adjacent thiazolidine ring has been replaced.

B. **Mechanism of action.** Aztreonem binds to penicillin binding proteins present in Gram(–) aerobic bacteria and disrupt cell wall synthesis (Figure 15-3). **It is stable to most β-lactamases**.

C. **Therapeutic uses.** Aztreonem is used in humans to replace aminoglycosides, which are more toxic when used with macrolides and lincosamides. **It may be used as a reserve antibiotic in veterinary medicine to treat severe Gram(–) infections.**

D. **Pharmacokinetics.** When given parenterally, aztreonem has a similar distribution to penicillin G. Penetration of CSF is good. It is excreted by the kidneys with an elimination $t_{1/2}$ of 1.2 hours in humans. No other information is available for animals.

E. **Adverse effects.** Hypersensitivity reactions may occur but cross-allergy with penicillins or cephalosporins has not been observed.

VIII. AMINOGLYCOSIDES

A. **Chemistry.** Aminoglycosides consist of two or three amino sugars joined to a hexose (aminocyclitol) by glycosidic bonds. Numerous amino groups contribute to their very polar and basic character. Sulfate salts are water soluble.

B. **Mechanism of action.** The aminoglycosides bind to the 30S ribosomal fragment and inhibit the rate of protein synthesis and the fidelity of mRNA translation which results in the synthesis of abnormal proteins (Figure 15-3). Their uptake by bacteria includes an energy-dependent step (EDP_1), which is oxygen linked and is inhibited by an anaerobic or acidic environment and by Ca^{2+} or Mg^{2+}. They are bactericidal against Gram(–) aerobes and are synergistic with β-lactams against many Gram(+) pathogens.

C. **Therapeutic uses.** The aminoglycosides are used in the treatment of Gram(–) infections in all species.

1. **Streptomycin and dihydrostreptomycin** are the oldest members of this class of antibiotics. Their use has declined with the advent of broader spectrum aminoglycosides such as gentamicin and amikacin.
2. **Neomycin** is used orally for the treatment of enteric infections and topically for treating skin, ear, and eye infections.
3. **Gentamicin and amikacin** are expanded spectrum aminoglycosides with activity against *Pseudomonas*, *Proteus*, *Staphylococcus*, and *Corynebacterium* spp., as well as Gram(–) aerobes. They are used in all species for the treatment of susceptible infections of the skin, respiratory tract, ear, eye, urinary tract, and septicemia. Tobramycin is similar to gentamicin but has more potent antipseudomonal activity and reduced nephrotoxicity.
4. **Kanamycin** has an antimicrobial spectrum similar to gentamicin except it is not effective against *Pseudomonas* spp. It is currently used in veterinary medicine only as an oral preparation combined with bismuth subcarbonate and aluminum magnesium silicate for the treatment of bacterial enteritis in dogs and for symptomatic relief of the associated diarrhea.

D. **Pharmacokinetics. Aminoglycosides are not absorbed from the GI tract because of their high polar nature.** They are distributed to the extracellular fluid and to transcellular fluids such as pleural and peritoneal fluids. Distribution is limited with penetration of the CNS or ocular tissue being minimal. **Aminoglycosides tend to accumulate in the renal cortex and otic endolymph, which predisposes these tissues to their toxicity.** They are excreted unchanged in the urine by glomerular filtration. The plasma $t_{1/2}$ is 1–3 hours for most species. **The prolonged residues values in kidney severely limits the use of aminoglycosides in production animals to label use only.**

E. **Administration.** Aminoglycosides are administered IM or SC for systemic infections. Because the bactericidal effects of aminoglycosides are concentration-dependent for systemic infections, some clinicians advocate a high dose once daily (pulse therapy, rather than twice daily) to allow full clearance to reduce renal and cochlear toxicity. For enteric infections, an oral dose twice a day may be used.

F. **Resistance.** Inactivation of aminoglycosides by bacterial enzymes is the most common form of resistance. **The numerous amino and hydroxyl side groups are sites of attack by acetylases, phosphorylases, and adenylases.** Resistance may be plasmid-mediated and develop quickly. Amikacin is more resistant to enzymatic degradation than other members of this class.

G. **Adverse effects**

1. **The aminoglycosides are relatively more toxic than other classes of antimicrobials.** Toxicity is reversible if the treatment is stopped early. Dosage regimens must be adjusted in animals with decreased renal function and they should not be used with other ototoxic or nephrotoxic drugs such as furosemide or amphotericin B.
2. **Ototoxicity** is due to progressive damage to cochlear sensory cells and/or vestibular cells of the inner ear resulting in deafness and ataxia, respectively.
3. **Nephrotoxicity** is due to the damage of the membranes of proximal tubular cells resulting in a loss of brush border enzymes, impaired absorption, proteinuria, and decreased glomerular filtration rate.

4. Neuromuscular blockade is a relatively rare adverse effect of aminoglycosides. It is caused by prejunctional blockade of acetylcholine (ACh) release and decreased postsynaptic sensitivity to ACh. Muscle paralysis and apnea are treated with calcium gluconate.

IX. TETRACYCLINES

A. **Chemistry.** The tetracyclines are polycyclic compounds that are amphoteric and that fluoresce when exposed to ultraviolet light. Most are prepared as the hydrochloride salt. They form insoluble chelates with cations such as Ca^{2+}, Mg^{2+}, Fe^{3+}, and Al^{3+}. They accumulate in growing teeth and bones.

B. **Mechanism of action.** Tetracyclines reversibly inhibit bacterial protein synthesis by binding to the 30S ribosome and preventing attachment of aminoacyl tRNA to the mRNA-ribosome complex (Figure 15-3). They block the addition of amino acids to the growing peptide chain. They are bacteriostatic and broad spectrum. Their antimicrobial spectrum includes Gram(+) and Gram(−) aerobes and anaerobes, *Rickettsiae*, *Spirochetes*, *Chlamydiae*, *Mycoplasma*, and some protozoans such as *Anaplasma* spp. and *Haemobartonella* spp.

C. **Therapeutic uses**

1. **Large animals.** Tetracycline, chlortetracycline, and oxytetracycline are used in the treatment of local and systemic bacterial, chlamydial, rickettsial, and protozoal infections in cattle, sheep, horses, and swine and as feed additive/growth promoters in cattle and swine.
2. **Small animals.** Doxycycline, minocycline, and tetracycline are used in the treatment of respiratory and urinary tract infections in dogs and cats and as specific therapy for *Borrelia* (Lyme disease), *Brucella*, *Haemobartonella*, and *Ehrlichia* spp. infections. They are also effective in the treatment of psittacosis in birds.

D. **Pharmacokinetics.** Oral absorption of tetracyclines ranges from 60–90% of the administered dose except for chlortetracycline, which is only 35% absorbed. Divalent or trivalent cations impair absorption and thus milk, antacids, or iron salts should be avoided 3 hours before and after oral administration. Distribution is wide and includes all tissues except those of the CNS. **Doxycycline and minocycline are more lipid soluble than tetracycline, chlortetracycline, or oxytetracycline and penetrate the CNS, eye, and prostate at therapeutic concentrations.** Metabolism is minimal in domestic animals, except for minocycline, which is extensively metabolized by the liver. Renal excretion by glomerular filtration is the major route of elimination for most tetracyclines, but small amounts are excreted into feces via bile and/or diffusion from the blood into the intestine. **Doxycycline is unique in that intestinal excretion is the major route of elimination (75%).** The plasma $t_{1/2}$ ranges from 6–12 hours for most tetracyclines. A recent derivative of the glycylcyclines, **tigecycline**, has been developed that has an effect against methicillin-resistant *S. aureus* (MRSA).

E. **Administration.** Tetracyclines are administered orally or IV every 8–12 hours. IM injections produce pain, irritation, and sterile abscesses unless special buffered solutions are used. **Oral therapeutic doses should be avoided in adult ruminants and used with caution in horses because of the danger of disrupting ruminal or colonic microflora, respectively.**

F. **Resistance** is now common because of widespread use. Resistance may be plasmid-mediated and is usually due to decreased drug uptake or active transport of the tetracycline out of the bacterial cell.

G. **Preslaughter withdrawal of oxytetracycline in food animals**

1. The Food Animal Residue Avoidance Databank (FARAD) recommends, in cattle, an extralabel withdrawal of 28 days for intrauterine treatment. It also recommends testing milk after intrauterine treatment, as there is inter-cow variability in the residue elimination profiles in milk.
2. FARAD recommends an extralabel preslaughter withdrawal of 28 days in sheep and goats after IM or SC oxytetracycline administration. A milk withdrawal of 96 hours is recommended for sheep and goats.
3. For swine, FARAD recommends an extralabel preslaughter period of 14 days following administration of tetracycline product in feed or water to swine.

H. **Adverse effects**

1. **The tetracyclines (except doxycycline and minocycline) are potentially nephrotoxic** and should be avoided if renal function is impaired.
2. **Permanent staining of unerupted teeth may occur in young animals** due to the formation of a tetracycline-calcium phosphate complex in enamel and dentine.
3. **Suprainfections of fungi, yeast, or resistant bacteria** may occur in the GI tract with prolonged administration of broad-spectrum antibiotics such as the tetracyclines. GI adverse effects are seen frequently in cats. **Oral tetracyclines should not be used with herbivores because of serious effects on ruminant digestion.**
4. **Antianabolic effects are seen at high doses** because of binding to mitochondrial ribosomes. This may result in an elevated blood urea nitrogen (BUN) especially with preexisting renal disease.
5. **Photosensitivity and hepatotoxicity are rare side effects in animals.**

X. CHLORAMPHENICOL GROUP

A. **Chemistry.** Chloramphenicol is an unusual natural compound because it contains dichloracetate and nitrobenzene moieties as part of its structure. Palmitate salts are water insoluble and are administered orally. Chloramphenicol sodium succinate is water soluble for parenteral use. Florfenicol is a fluorinated derivative where the $-NO_2$ group has been replaced by $-SO_2CH_3$ to treat respiratory infections in beef cattle. It does not leave the toxic residues in meat that chloramphenicol does.

B. **Mechanism of action.** Chloramphenicol and florfenicol bind to the bacterial 50S ribosome unit to inhibit peptide bond formation and protein synthesis (Figure 15-3). They are bacteriostatic and broad spectrum and are effective against most anaerobic bacteria.

C. **Therapeutic uses.** Chloramphenicol is not allowed for use in food-producing animals because the potential danger of residue-induced toxicity in humans (see below). It is used in dogs, cats, horses, and birds for local and systemic infections, inducing respiratory, CNS, and ocular infections, and infections caused by anaerobes and *Salmonella* spp. Florfenicol is approved for use only in cattle for the treatment of bovine respiratory disease (BRD) caused by *Pasteurella* spp. and *Haemophilus somnus*. It is used in dogs and cats for treating susceptible infections when the myelotoxic potential of chloramphenicol must be avoided.

D. **Pharmacokinetics**

1. **Chloramphenicol** is rapidly absorbed from the GI tract and widely distributed to all tissues including the CNS and eye. Hepatic metabolism by glucuronide conjugation occurs slowly for 75% of the administered drug in cats, but faster to 90% in dogs. The elimination $t_{1/2}$ is 1–1.5 hours for dogs and horses and 4–5 hours in cats.

2. Florfenicol is absorbed orally in dogs and cats and from IM sites in cattle. It is widely distributed, including the CNS, similar to chloramphenicol. The serum $t_{1/2}$ is 18 hours in cattle and 4–6 hours in dogs and cats. In cattle, two-thirds of a dose is excreted as the parent drug in the urine and one-third is metabolized by the liver.

E. **Administration.** Chloramphenicol is administered orally, IM, IV, or SC every 6–8 hours to dogs, birds, or horses and every 12 hours to cats. Florfenicol is administered IM in cattle and repeated 48 hours later for a total of two doses of the slow-release preparation. It is administered IM or SC every 8 hours in dogs and every 12 hours in cats.

F. **Resistance.** Resistant bacteria inactivate chloramphenicol by production of an acetyl-transferase and other metabolizing enzymes. Similar inactivation is expected with florfenicol.

G. **Adverse effects**

1. **Anemia,** which is dose-related, may occur in animals and humans. Chloramphenicol may inhibit the uptake of iron by erythrocytes and their rate of maturation in bone marrow. A second type of anemia may occur in humans treated with chloramphenicol. **It is non-dose-related and rare but the resulting aplastic anemia is often fatal and this is the reason for the drug's ban in food-producing animals.**
2. **Anorexia and diarrhea** may occur especially in cats with high or prolonged dosage.
3. **Florfenicol is not known to produce aplastic anemia** and its use is permitted in beef cattle.

XI. MACROLIDES

A. **Chemistry.** The macrolide antibiotics include erythromycin, azithromycin, clarithromycin, tulathromycin, tylosin, and tilmicosin. They are basic, lipid-soluble compounds consisting of a lactone ring to which are attached deoxy sugars. They are prepared as sulfate salts or as esterified salts of stearate, tartrate, estolate, or lactobionate.

B. **Mechanism of action.** Macrolides are bacteriostatic by inhibiting bacterial protein synthesis (Figure 15-3). They bind to the 50S ribosome to prevent translocation of amino acids to the growing peptide chain. Binding sites on the 50S ribosome overlap with binding sites of chloramphenicol and the lincosamides (especially clindamycin) and combination therapy should be avoided. Their antimicrobial activity is primarily against Gram(+) aerobes and anaerobes and *Mycoplasma* spp. Tylosin and tiamulin are effective against some Gram(–) pathogens, including *Pasteurella* and *Haemophilus* spp.

C. **Therapeutic uses**

1. **Erythromycin** is an alternate to penicillin for infections caused by Gram(+) aerobes and anaerobes in dogs, cats, and horses. It is a drug often chosen for the treatment of enteritis caused by *Campylobacter jejuni* in dogs and foals and for *Rhodococcus equi* pneumonia in foals.
2. **Tylosin** is used in cattle, sheep, and swine for the treatment of local and systemic infections caused by *Mycoplasma* and Gram(+) bacteria. It is also added to feed as a growth promotant in these species. Tylosin is used in dogs and cats for the treatment of chronic colitis.
3. **Tilmicosin** is used in cattle for the treatment of respiratory disease caused by *Pasteurella* spp. It has potentially fatal toxic effects in horses and humans.
4. **Azithromycin** is used in dogs, cats, and horses and is effective against *Staphylococcus, Streptococcus,* and *Mycoplasma*. It is used as an alternative for erythromycin for *R. equi* pneumonia in foals

5. **Tulathromycin** is used for the treatment of bovine and swine respiratory diseases. It is effective against *Mannheimia*, *Mycoplasma*, and *Haemophilus*; it is concentrated in leucocytes and lung tissue.

6. **Clarithromycin** is used in dogs and cats for the treatment of mycobacterial infections including canine leproid granuloma, feline leprosy, and for *Helicobacter* spp. in cats and ferrets, and for *R. equi* in foals.

D. **Pharmacokinetics.** Macrolides are absorbed orally if protected from gastric acid destruction by enteric coated preparations or administration of the stable, esterified salts. They are weak organic bases that are widely distributed to all tissues except those of the CNS. They are concentrated in acidic environments like the respiratory secretions, milk, and leukocytes. Tilmicosin concentrates in lung tissue at levels 60-fold higher than serum. Erythromycin is mainly excreted unchanged in bile but a fraction is metabolized by N-demethylation in the liver. Tylosin, tilmicosin, and azithromycin are excreted unchanged in bile and urine. The plasma $t_{1/2}$ for the macrolides are erythromycin—1–3 hours in most species; azithromycin—20 hours in cats and 35 hours in foals; tilmicosin—1 hour in cattle and 25 hours in pigs; tylosin—1 hour in dogs and cattle and 4 hours in sheep, pigs, and goats; tulathromycin—90 hours in cattle and pigs. Information is not available for the $t_{1/2}$ of clarithromycin.

E. **Administration**

1. **Erythromycin** is administered orally or IM three times a day to dogs, cats, and foals, and IM once a day in cattle, sheep, and swine.

2. **Tylosin** is administered IM or orally once or twice a day to swine, calves, lambs, dogs, and cats.

3. **Tilmicosin** is administered SC to cattle every 72 hours.

4. **Tulathromycin.** A single IM injection is claimed to be effective against bovine and swine respiratory infections.

5. **Azithromycin** is administered orally once a day to dogs, cats, and foals.

6. **Clarithromycin** is administered orally twice a day to dogs, cats, ferrets, and foals.

F. **Resistance.** Bacterial resistance to macrolide antibiotics may be chromosomal or plasmid mediated and is due to decreased drug binding by the 50S ribosome. Less frequently, active efflux, or enzymatic inactivation by resistant bacteria may occur.

G. **Adverse effects.** Erythromycin, tylosin, azithromycin, clarithromycin, and tulathromycin have relatively few side effects. Mild GI upset with oral doses and pain and irritation at IM injection sites may occur. Erythromycin is recognized to be an agonist of the motilin (a peptide that stimulates contraction of GI smooth muscle) receptor and acts on the stomach, ileum, cecum, and pelvic flexure and can produce abdominal pain and diarrhea. Edema of the rectal mucosa with mild anal prolapse may be seen in swine following IM administration of tylosin. Erythromycin should not be administered orally to adult ruminants or tylosin, orally or parenterally, to adult horses because of the danger of severe diarrhea. Tilmicosin produces cardiovascular toxicity in species other than cattle by increasing myocardial Ca^{2+} concentrations. Side effects are rare for others in the group.

XII. LINCOSAMIDES

A. **Chemistry.** Lincomycin, clindamycin, and pirlimycin are derivatives of a sulfur-containing octose with an amino acid-like side chain and are highly lipid soluble. They are prepared as HCl or phosphate salts, which are water soluble, or clindamycin palmitate for oral administration.

B. **Mechanism of action.** The lincosamides bind to the bacterial 50S ribosome to inhibit protein synthesis (Figure 15-3). Since this is the same binding site of chloramphenicol and the macrolides, combined therapy should be avoided. Lincomycin and clindamycin are bacteriostatic and are active against Gram(+) aerobes and obligate anaerobes, *Toxoplasma* spp. *Neospora canis,* and *Mycoplasma* spp. The antibacterial activity of clindamycin is greater than that of lincomycin, especially against anaerobes.

C. **Therapeutic uses.** Lincomycin is used in swine for the control and treatment of swine dysentery, and the treatment of staphylococcal, streptococcal, and mycoplasmal infections. Clindamycin is used in dogs and cats for periodontal disease, osteomyelitis, dermatitis, and deep soft tissue infections caused by Gram(+) organisms. It is used for treating toxoplasmosis in dogs and cats and neosporosis in dogs. Pirlimycin is prepared and used for the treatment of bovine mastitis.

D. **Pharmacokinetics.** Oral absorption is 50% for lincomycin and 90% for clindamycin. Distribution is wide with excellent penetration of bone and soft tissues, including tendon sheaths. CNS levels are low unless the meninges are inflamed. Lincosamides are metabolized by the hepatic microsomal enzymes into sulfoxide and other metabolites (60%, lincomycin; 90%, clindamycin). Parent drug and metabolites are excreted in urine, bile, and feces. The elimination $t_{1/2}$ is 3–5 hours in dogs and cats. No information is available for other species.

E. **Administration.** Lincomycin is administered IM to swine once a day or added to the drinking water. Clindamycin is administered orally or IM twice a day to dogs and cats. Pirlimycin is given by intramammary infusion.

F. **Resistance.** Altered drug binding by bacterial ribosomes is the usual form of resistance. **Cross-resistance between lincosamides and macrolides is common.**

G. **Adverse effects. Lincosamides are contraindicated in horses, rabbits, hamsters, and guinea pigs because they may produce a severe, often fatal, diarrhea due to altered GI flora.** Side effects are rare in dogs, cats, cattle, and swine except for neuromuscular blockade at high doses or when used with anesthetics.

XIII. MISCELLANEOUS ANTIBACTERIAL DRUGS

A. **Aminocyclitols**

1. **Mechanism of action.** Spectinomycin and apramycin are **chemically related to the aminoglycosides but are bacteriostatic, not bactericidal.** They bind to the 30S ribosome and inhibit protein synthesis (Figure 15-3). They are active primarily against Gram(–) aerobes and *Mycoplasma* infections.

2. **Therapeutic uses.** Spectinomycin is used in dogs, cats, horses, swine, calves, and poultry for the treatment of enteric and respiratory infectious disease. Apramycin is used to treat enteric infections, especially colibacillosis in swine and calves.

3. **Pharmacokinetics.** The pharmacokinetics of aminocyclitols is similar to that of the aminoglycosides. Less than 10% is absorbed orally. Parenterally administered spectinomycin distributes to the ECF and is excreted unchanged by the kidney. Other information is not available for animals.

4. **Administration.** Spectinomycin is administered orally or parenterally twice a day in all species. Apramycin is administered to swine and cattle in the drinking water once a day.

5. **Adverse effects.** No significant toxicity is associated with clinical use of spectinomycin.

B. **Metronidazole**

1. **Chemistry.** The nitroimidazoles include metronidazole, ipronidazole, dimetridazole, and ronidazole. They are heterocyclic compounds containing a five-membered ring similar to the nitrofurans. Only metronidazole is used in veterinary medicine.

2. **Mechanism of action.** Metronidazole is taken up by anaerobic bacteria and protozoa and reduced to a cytotoxic metabolite, which disrupts DNA (Figure 15-3). It is bactericidal against most obligate anaerobes and is active against protozoa, including *Giardia* and *Trichomonas* spp.

3. **Therapeutic uses.** Nitroimidazoles have demonstrated carcinogenicity in laboratory animals and their use is banned in food-producing animals. Metronidazole is used in dogs, cats, and horses for the treatment of severe infections caused by anaerobic pathogens, especially brain abscesses and pelvic, genitourinary tract, and respiratory infections. Metronidazole is also used to treat protozoal infections such as giardiasis and trichomoniasis in dogs and cats.

4. **Pharmacokinetics.** Metronidazole is well absorbed orally and widely distributed, including the CNS. Hepatic metabolism by oxidation and conjugation occurs for one-third to one-half of administered drug. Metabolites and unchanged drug are excreted in urine and feces. The elimination $t_{1/2}$ in dogs and horses are 3–5 hours.

5. **Administration.** Metronidazole is administered orally twice a day in dogs, cats, and horses.

6. **Adverse effects.** High or prolonged dosage may produce neurotoxicity with signs that include nystagmus, ataxia, and seizures.

C. **Rifampin**

1. **Mechanism of action.** Rifampin inhibits DNA-dependent RNA polymerase, which prevents initiation of RNA synthesis (Figure 15-3). It is bactericidal for mycobacteria and Gram(+) pathogens. It is effective against intracellular infections.

2. **Therapeutic uses.** Rifampin is combined with erythromycin in the treatment of *R. equi* infections in foals. Rifampin is also used in combination with other antifungal agents to treat fungal infections such as aspergillosis or histoplasmosis in dogs and cats when infection involves the CNS.

3. **Pharmacokinetics.** Rifampin is absorbed orally and rapidly distributed to cells and tissues. Rifampin is metabolized in the liver to a deacetylated form that also has antibacterial activity. Both this metabolite and parent drug are excreted primarily in the bile, but up to 30% may be excreted in the urine. The parent drug is substantially reabsorbed in the gut, but the metabolite is not. Reported elimination $t_{1/2}$ for various species are 6–8 hours in horses, 8 hours in dogs, and 3–5 hours in sheep. Because rifampin can induce hepatic microsomal enzymes, elimination rates may increase with repeated doses.

4. **Administration.** Rifampin is administered orally three times a day in foals, dogs, and cats.

5. **Adverse effects.** Side effects are rare. **Hepatotoxicity** may occur in animals with preexisting liver disease. Rifampin may produce red-orange colored urine, sweat, and saliva but this is not harmful.

D. **Tiamulin**

1. **Mechanism of action.** Tiamulin binds to the 50S bacterial ribosome to inhibit protein synthesis (Figure 15-3). Its mechanism of action and antibacterial spectrum are similar to macrolides such as tylosin. It is active against Gram(+) cocci, *Mycoplasma*, *spirochetes*, and some Gram(−) pathogens such as *Haemophilus* spp.

2. **Therapeutic uses.** Tiamulin is administered in medicated feed or water in swine for the control and treatment of *Haemophilus* pneumonia and swine dysentery.

3. **Pharmacokinetics.** Tiamulin is well absorbed orally, widely distributed, and metabolized by the liver. Elimination of metabolites occurs in feces (70%) and urine (30%). The $t_{1/2}$ is 4–12 hours in pigs.

4. **Adverse effects.** Dermatitis with erythema and pruritus may be observed if pigs are overcrowded and is due to the irritant metabolites in urine.

E. **Vancomycin**

1. **Mechanism of action.** Vancomycin blocks the second step of bacterial cell wall synthesis by inhibiting polymer release from the cell membrane (Figure 15-3). It is bactericidal for Gram(+) organisms.

2. **Therapeutic uses.** Vancomycin is a reserve antibiotic administered IV over 30–60 minutes every 6–8 hours for methicillin-resistant staphylococcal infections of bone and soft tissue in dogs and cats. It is administered orally every 6–8 hours in dogs for the treatment of multidrug-resistant enteric infection.

3. **Pharmacokinetics.** Vancomycin is not absorbed orally. It distributes to the ECF and transcellular fluids and is excreted unchanged by glomerular filtration. It has a plasma $t_{1/2}$ of 2 hours.

4. **Adverse effects.** Ototoxicity and nephrotoxicity occur with large or prolonged dosage.

F. Bacitracin

1. **Mechanism of action.** Bacitracin inhibits the second step of cell wall synthesis (Figure 15-3). It is bactericidal for Gram(+) bacteria and *Spirochetes*.

2. **Therapeutic uses.** Bacitracin is used in topical ointments and solutions and is frequently combined with polymixin B and/or neomycin in these preparations. It is also added to swine and poultry rations for the prevention and treatment of clostridial enteritis and as a growth promotant.

3. **Pharmacokinetics.** Bacitracin is not absorbed orally. It is too nephrotoxic for systemic use.

4. **Adverse effects.** Systemic toxicity does not occur with topical or oral administration of bacitracin.

G. Polymyxin B

1. **Mechanism of action.** Polymyxin B interacts with phospholipids in the bacterial cell membrane to produce a detergent-like effect and membrane disruption (Figure 15-3). It is rapidly bactericidal to Gram(–) organisms.

2. **Therapeutic uses.** Polymyxin B is used topically to treat Gram(–) bacterial infections of the skin, eye, and ear in all species. It is usually combined with bacitracin for broad-spectrum antibacterial effects. Polymyxin B is administered orally to cattle and swine for the treatment of Gram(–) enteric infections.

3. **Pharmacokinetics.** Polymyxin B is not absorbed orally. **It is too nephrotoxic for parenteral use.**

4. **Adverse effects.** Polymyxin B does not produce systemic toxicity when administered topically or orally, since it is not absorbed systemically using these routes of administration.

H. Nitrofurans

1. **Mechanism of action.** The nitrofurans are reduced by bacteria to reactive intermediates that inhibit nucleic acid synthesis (Figure 15-3). They produce DNA fragmentation and may also block mRNA translation. They are broad spectrum and bacteriostatic.

2. **Therapeutic uses.** Nitrofurantoin is occasionally used in the treatment of lower urinary tract infections in dogs and cats. It is administered orally every 6–8 hours and is most effective in acid urine. Nitrofurazone is used topically as an antibacterial ointment, powder, and water-soluble wound dressings in all species.

3. **Pharmacokinetics.** Nitrofurantoin is absorbed orally and rapidly excreted by glomerular filtration and active secretion. Peak urine levels are achieved less than 1 hour after administration. The plasma $t_{1/2}$ is 20 minutes in humans; no information is available for animals.

4. **Adverse effects.** Side effects are rare. Nausea, vomiting, and diarrhea may occur in dogs and cats following oral administration. Nitrofurans may not be used in food-producing animals (include topically) because they have been shown to be potential carcinogens in laboratory animals.

I. Novobiocin

1. **Chemistry.** Novobiocin is a coumarin antibiotic and is acidic.

2. **Mechanism of action.** It blocks binding of ATP to DNA gyrase to inhibit super-coiling of bacterial DNA (Figure 15-3). It is bacteriostatic for Gram(+) cocci, especially *S. aureus*.

3. **Therapeutic uses. Novobiocin** is used for wound treatment and the treatment of mastitis particularly *Staphylococcus* infections. It is less potent against *Streptococcus* infections.

4. **Pharmacokinetics.** Novobiocin is absorbed orally with peak levels in 2–4 hours. Tissue penetration is relatively poor. It is excreted primarily into bile and feces. The plasma $t_{1/2}$ after oral administration in humans is ~6 hours; no information is available for animals.

5. **Administration.** Novobiocin is given by intramammary infusion usually combined with procaine penicillin to limit the development of resistance. Novobiocin is combined with tetracycline in a proprietary preparation (AlbaPlex®) for oral administration twice a day in dogs for susceptible infections.

6. **Adverse effects.** Novobiocin does not produce systemic toxicity when administered topically or orally

J. **Streptogramins**

1. **Chemistry.** Virginiamycin is used for poultry and is a mixture of streptogramin B, a macrolide (virginiamycin M), and streptogramin A, a cyclic hexadepsipeptide (virginiamycin S). The human preparation Synercid® is a mixture of the macrolide, dalfopristin, and the cyclic hexadepsipeptide, quinupristin.

2. **Mechanism of action.** Streptogramins bind to the 50S ribosome to inhibit protein synthesis (Figure 15-3). Virginiamycin is bactericidal against Gram(+) aerobic and anaerobic bacteria.

3. **Therapeutic uses.** Virginiamycin is administered as a medicated feed additive in broiler chickens and swine as a growth promotant and for the prevention of necrotic enteritis in broiler chickens and for the control of swine dysentery in pigs weighing up to 120 lbs. It is also used as a feed additive in cattle to increase feed efficiency and to reduce the incidence of liver abscesses. Synercid® is used in humans for the treatment of vancomycin-resistant enterococcal infection and methicillin-resistant *S. aureus*.

   There is concern that the use of virginiamycin in poultry may lead to transferable resistance to humans and limit the value of Synercid®.

4. **Pharmacokinetics.** Virginiamycin is administered orally. Since it is not absorbed, its antibacterial effects are limited to the GI tract.

K. **Ionophore antibiotics**

1. **Chemistry.** Ionophores are polyether antibiotics derived from *Streptomyces* used primarily in poultry and swine for feed efficiency and anticoccidial activity. They include monensin, lasalocid, laidlomycin, salinomycin, and narasin.

2. **Mechanism of action.** Ionophores act as alkali metal ionophores. They complex with Na^+ in the cell membrane to produce passive extracellular transport of K^+ and intracellular influx of H^+, which kills bacteria and coccidian by lowering intracellular pH. In the rumen, ionophores selectively affect Gram(+) organisms resulting in a shift to Gram(–) populations in the rumen microflora. This increases the production of propionic acid and decreases the production of acetic and butyric acids by rumen bacteria. This change in volatile acids (VFA) increases feed efficiency by reducing bacterial energy losses to CO_2 and methane, thereby increasing the energy content per unit of feed.

3. **Therapeutic uses.** Monensin, lasalocid, and laidlomycin are administered as premixes or medicated feed for growth promotion, feed efficiency, and control of coccidiosis in cattle and broiler chickens. Salinomycin and narasin are administered as medicated feed to broiler chickens for prevention of coccidiosis.

4. **Pharmacokinetics.** Ionophores are absorbed orally. Monensin absorption is 50% in ruminants. They are rapidly and extensively metabolized by the liver and the numerous metabolites are excreted by bile and eliminated in the feces. Absorption

is more complete and metabolism is slower in monogastric animals, especially horses, which may explain the greater toxicity in this species.

5. **Adverse effects.** Toxicity of ionophores when used in species for which they are approved is uncommon, unless mixing errors occur. Ionophore toxicity is due to cellular electrolyte imbalances, increased extracellular K^+, and intracellular Na^+ and Ca^{2+} concentrations, resulting in cellular damage and death. The increased intracellular Ca^{2+} concentration is due to the exchange of Na^+ for Ca^{2+} by $Na^+–Ca^{2+}$ exchanger; this exchange is particularly prominent in cardiac and skeletal muscles and these are usually the most severely affected. Horses are the most susceptible species to toxic effects when accidentally exposed to ionophore-containing feeds.

XIV. ANTIFUNGAL AGENTS

A. Griseofulvin

1. **Chemistry.** Griseofulvin is a cyclohexane benzofuran antibiotic derived from Penicillium griseofulvin. It is insoluble in water.
2. **Mechanism of action.** Griseofulvin is actively taken up by growing dermatophytes (ringworm). It binds to microtubules to inhibit spindle formation and mitosis. It is fungistatic for dermatophytes such as *Microsporum* spp. and *Trichophyton* spp. Its action is slow as infected cells are shed and replaced with uninfected cells.
3. **Therapeutic uses.** Griseofulvin is used in dogs, cats, and horses for multifocal dermatophyte infections.
4. **Pharmacokinetics.** The GI absorption rate varies from 25–70%. The absorption is increased by high-fat foods and by preparations consisting of micronized particles. It distributes to keratin precursor cells of skin, hair shafts, and nails. It is metabolized by the liver by demethylation and glucuronide conjugation and excreted in urine. Griseofulvin's plasma $t_{1/2}$ in dogs is less than 6 hours, but is stored in the growing keratin cell producing skin, hair, and horn.
5. **Administration.** Griseofulvin is administered orally twice a day to dogs and cats and once daily to horses for 4–6 weeks.
6. **Adverse effects.** Untoward effects are rare. Leucopenia and anemia may occur as an idiosyncratic reaction in kittens.

B. Nystatin and Natamycin

1. **Chemistry.** Nystatin and natamycin are polyene antibiotics derived from *Streptomyces* spp.
2. **Mechanism of action.** Nystatin and natamycin are fungicidal to yeast infections caused by *Candida* spp. and *Malassezia* spp. They act by binding to erogsterol of the protoplast membrane of fungi to alter permeability and allow leakage of cell contents.
3. **Therapeutic uses.** Nystatin and natamycin are too toxic for parenteral use. They are administered topically for yeast infections of the eye, ear, and skin, and administered orally for treating mucosal yeast infections of the mouth and GI tract. Nystatin is used as a feed additive in poultry to prevent crop mycosis and mycotic diarrhea. Nystatin is a component of topical proprietary preparations such as Panalog®, which also include thiostrepton, a polypeptide antibiotic, and triamcinolone, a glucocorticoid.
4. **Pharmacokinetics. Nystatin is** not absorbed orally and is excreted in the feces.
5. **Administration.** Nystatin is administered orally every 6–8 hours for Candidal infections in dogs and cats. Natamycin is used topically primarily for ocular mycotic infections and is the drug of choice for treating fungal keratitis in horses.
6. **Adverse effects.** Adverse effects are rare since the drugs are not supposed to enter the systemic circulation. Occasional GI upset may be observed with high dose.

C. Azoles

1. **Chemistry.** Ketoconazole, itraconazole, and fluconazole are imidazole antifungals for systemic use. Other imidazoles used only topically for dermatophyte, *Aspergillus* or yeast infections include miconazole and clotrimazole.

2. **Mechanism of action.** The azoles inhibit the synthesis of ergosterol in fungal cytoplasmic membranes by blocking cytochrome P450 enzymes and increasing cellular permeability. At high doses, mammalian steroid synthesis (corticosteroids and sex steroids) is inhibited. Azoles are fungistatic for most pathogenic fungi causing systemic infections such as *Blastomyces*, *Coccidioides*, *Cryptococcus*, and *Histoplasma* spp. They are also effective against candidiasis and griseofulvin-resistant dermatophytes.

3. **Therapeutic uses.** Ketoconazole is used in dogs, cats, horses, and birds for systemic mycoses and for severe yeast infections. It is also used in dogs and cats at high dosage for the treatment of hyperadrenocorticism (see Chapter 12, III E 4 b). Fluconazole and itraconazole have replaced ketoconazole in most treatment regimens for the systemic mycoses because of their longer $t_{1/2}$, greater activity, and lower toxicity. Clotrimazole and miconazole are used topically in the treatment of *Candida*, *Aspergillus*, and dermatophyte infections.

4. **Pharmacokinetics**
   a. Following oral administration, azoles are well absorbed in the presence of food that stimulates bile flow.
   b. They are widely distributed, particularly in tissues high in lipid content; however, minimal amounts are found in cerebrospinal fluid (~10% of other tissue levels).
   c. They are metabolized by microsomal enzymes of the liver and excreted in bile.
   d. The $t_{1/2}$ of ketoconazole in dogs is 1–6 hours. In humans, fluconazole's plasma $t_{1/2}$ is ~30 hours and itraconazole's $t_{1/2}$ is 20–60 hours. Because of their long $t_{1/2}$, these two azoles do not reach steady state plasma levels for 6–14 days after beginning therapy, unless loading doses are given. **Patients with impaired renal function may have $t_{1/2}$ extended significantly and dosage adjustment may be required.**

5. **Administration.** Ketoconazole is administered orally twice a day for 3–6 months for systemic mycotic infections. Fluconazole and itraconazole are administered orally or IV once a day to dogs and cats for systemic mycoses for periods of 1–3 months, depending on the type of pathogenic fungi being treated. Clotrimazole and miconazole are applied topically for the treatment of yeast or dermatophyte infections or via nasal infusion for treating nasal aspergillosis.

6. **Adverse effects.** Anorexia, vomiting, and diarrhea may occur, especially in cats, treated with ketoconazole. Suppression of adrenal or gonadal steroids may also occur but the effects are transient at doses employed in antifungal therapy. Adverse effects are rare with fluconazole or itraconazole therapy, unless in patients with impaired renal function.

D. Amphotericin B

1. **Chemistry.** Amphotericin B is a polyene macrolide that is stabilized with sodium desoxycholate as a colloidal suspension.

2. **Mechanism of action.** Amphotericin B binds to ergosterol of fungal cell membranes to form pores or channels, which result in leakage of cell contents. It is fungicidal against most organisms causing systemic mycoses, including *Aspergillus*, *Blastomyces*, *Coccidioides*, *Cryptococcus*, and *Histoplasma* spp.

3. **Therapeutic uses.** Amphotericin B is used to treat systemic fungal infections in dogs, cats, horses, and birds. Combined therapy with ketoconazole, fluconazole, itraconazole (to reduce toxicity), or flucytosine (for CNS, bone, or ocular infections) is common.

4. **Pharmacokinetics.** Amphotericin B is not absorbed from the GI tract. After IV administration, it slowly distributes to most tissues except the CNS, eye, and bone. Elimination is biphasic with plasma $t_{1/2}$ of 24–48 hours and 1–2 weeks.

Approximately 65% of amphotericin B is excreted unchanged into urine (20%) and feces (45%).

5. **Administration.** Amphotericin B is diluted in 5% dextrose and administered IV. Treatment frequency and duration vary with the type of infection.

6. **Adverse effects.** Renal toxicity is a serious side effect. Amphotericin B produces renal vasoconstriction, decreased GFR, and damage to tubular epithelium. BUN must be monitored weekly during therapy.

E. **Flucytosine**

1. **Chemistry.** Flucytosine (5-FC) is a fluorinated pyrimidinethat is deaminated by fungi (not mammalian cells) to 5-fluorouracil, a potent antimetabolite.

2. **Mechanism of action.** Flucytosine inhibits thymidylate synthase and DNA and RNA synthesis in susceptible fungi. It is fungicidal against *Cryptococcus, Candida,* and *Aspergillus* spp.

3. **Therapeutic uses.** Flucytosine is combined with amphotericin B for synergistic action in the treatment of cryptococcosis (especially meningeal cryptococcosis) in dogs and cats. It is used alone in treating aspergillosis and candidiasis in psittacine birds.

4. **Pharmacokinetics.** Flucytosine is well absorbed orally and widely distributed, including the CNS. It is excreted unchanged in urine. The plasma $t_{1/2}$ in humans is 3–6 hours. No information is available for animals. The $t_{1/2}$ may be prolonged in patients with compromised renal function.

5. **Administration.** Flucytosine is administered orally 3–4 times a day for a minimum of 4 weeks.

6. **Adverse effects.** Toxicity is low. Mild GI disturbances and, more rarely, bone marrow suppression have been reported.

F. **Terbinafine**

1. **Chemistry.** Terbinafine is an allylamine derivative.

2. **Mechanism of action.** Terbinafine inhibits the synthesis of ergosterol—a component of fungal cell membranes. By blocking the enzyme squalene monooxygenase (squalene 2,3-epoxidase), terbinafine inhibits the conversion of squalene to sterols (especially ergosterol) and causes accumulation of squalene. Both these effects are thought to contribute to its antifungal action. Unlike azoles, **terbinafine does not block cytochrome P450 enzymes. It is fungicidal against dermatophytes and fungistatic against yeast.**

3. **Therapeutic uses.** When administered orally (30 mg/kg/day) or topically, terbinafine is useful for treating dermatophytic infections in dogs and cats. It is also useful for treating birds for systemic mycotic infections such as aspergillosis.

4. **Pharmacokinetics.** No information is available for animals. In humans, it is readily absorbed (>70%) when given orally. Since terbinafine is lipophilic, food may enhance GI absorption of the drug by increasing bile secretion. Terbinafine is distributed to skin and into the sebum. Over 99% of drug in the plasma is bound to albumin. Drug in the circulation is metabolized in the liver into demethylated, deaminated, and dealkylated conjugates, which are excreted into urine. The elimination $t_{1/2}$ is ~36 hours. The drug may persist in adipose tissue and skin for more than 30 days.

5. **Adverse effects.** Terbinafine appears to be well tolerated by animals.

XV. **ANTIVIRAL AGENTS**

A. **Amantadine**

1. **Chemistry.** Amantadine is 1-aminoadamantane.

2. **Mechanism of action.** When influenza viruses replicate within the host cell, a viral membrane protein known as M_2 forms an ion-channel for H^+ influx from the

endosome into the virion prior to fusion of the viral membrane with the endosomal membrane. Amantadine binds to M_2 protein and blocks its ion channel activity and thus inhibits viral uncoating and replication.

In addition to its antiviral activity, amantadine antagonizes the N-methyl-D-aspartate (NMDA) receptor in the CNS. NMDA receptors are important in pain sensation, especially chronic pain. Amantadine combined with other analgesics such as opiates or NSAIDs alleviates chronic pain.

3. **Therapeutic uses.** The primary use of amantadine in veterinary medicine is as an adjunct to NSAIDs for the treatment of chronic pain in dogs and cats. It is effective for treating some, but not all, influenza viruses. Because oral absorption in horses is variable, it has been used IV to treat equine-2 influenza but its potential for inducing seizures when administered by this route limits its use.

4. **Pharmacokinetics.** Given orally, ~50% of the dose of amantadine is absorbed in horses and high levels are attained in secretions. It is excreted unchanged by the kidneys. The elimination $t_{1/2}$ in horses is ~3.5 hours. The information for dogs and cats is not available.

5. **Administration.** As an adjunct to chronic pain therapy, amantadine is administered orally once a day to dogs and cats.

6. **Resistance.** Develops quite rapidly.

7. **Adverse effects.** Infrequently, the following signs are seen: agitation, loose stools, flatulence, or diarrhea, particularly early in therapy.

B. **Acyclovir**

1. **Chemistry.** Acyclovir is a guanosine derivative with selectivity for particular herpes viruses.

2. **Mechanism of action.** Acyclovir is metabolized to the monophosphate by thymidine kinase, which is more active in the virus than in the host cell. The host cell then converts the monophosphate to the triphosphate that inhibits the viral DNA polymerase, ending the nucleotide chain prematurely.

3. **Therapeutic uses.** Acyclovir is used to treat ocular and respiratory infections of herpes virus 1 of cats. Although acyclovir is active against equine herpes virus type-l in vitro, oral absorption is poor in horses and therapeutic levels are not attained

4. **Pharmacokinetics.** Acyclovir is poorly absorbed (~20%) after oral administration. It is widely distributed throughout body tissues and fluids, including the brain, semen, and CSF. It has low protein binding and crosses the placenta. Acyclovir is primarily metabolized by the liver and has a $t_{1/2}$ of ~3 hours in humans. No information is available for animals.

5. **Administration.** Acyclovir is administered orally twice a day to cats.

6. **Adverse effects.** Leucopenia and anemia may occur. These are reversible if therapy is discontinued.

C. **Zidovudine (AZT)**

1. **Chemistry.** Zidovudine is an analog of thymidine.

2. **Mechanism of action.** Zidovudine is phosphorylated by host cell enzymes to AZT 5'-triphosphate, which competes with host 5'-thymidine, which is essential for proviral DNA formation by reverse transcriptase of the virus. The incorporation of the 5'-triphosphate zidovudine into the viral DNA chain produces the termination of viral DNA synthesis. Mammalian α-DNA polymerase does not incorporate the zidovudine.

3. **Therapeutic uses.** Zidovudine may be used in cats to treat FIV infection where it produces temporary alleviation of the clinical signs and increase in quality of life and survival time in most cats, particularly when clinical signs of immunodeficiency are evident. It does not inhibit the viremia. Clinical improvement occurs 14 days after the start of treatment. Zidovudine is not effective against feline leukemia virus at nontoxic doses

4. **Pharmacokinetics.** Zidovudine is well absorbed orally and has a $t_{1/2}$ of ~2 hours in cats. It is metabolized in the liver by glucuronide conjugation and excreted in urine. $t_{1/2}$ may be extended in cats that have low levels of glucuronyl transferase.

TABLE 15-1. Websites for Antimicrobial Information

VIN	http://www.vin.com/
FDA—human	http://www.accessdata.fda.gov/scripts/cder/drugsatfda
Compendium veterinary product	http://www.bayerdvm.com/ Resources/cvp_main.cfm?CFID=307632&CFTOKEN=61494892
Merck veterinary manual	http://www.merckvetmanual.com/ mvm/index.jsp?cfile=htm/bc/toc_191200.htm

5. **Administration.** Zidovudine is administered orally 2–3 times a day for a minimum of 4 weeks.
6. **Resistance.** Mutation of virus target sites may result rapidly and resistance to zidovudine is expected with long-term use.
7. **Adverse effects.** Anemia and reduction in hemoglobin are the most common side effects observed in cats. Diarrhea and weakness may also occur. Reduced dosage should be employed in cats with renal or hepatic insufficiency.

D. **Cat omega interferon**

1. **Chemistry. Interferons are cytokines**, proteins produced by host cells when they are attacked by viruses. Cat omega interferon is produced by genetic engineering and is a type 1 interferon closely related to alpha interferon. **It has a $t_{1/2}$ of 1–2 hours in dogs and cats.**
2. **Mechanism of action.** Interferon's mechanism of action is not a direct attack on the virus but by altering host cell metabolism to induce proteins that protect against viral invasion by several methods including destruction of mRNA and blockade of translational proteins resulting in the inhibition of viral replication.
3. **Therapeutic uses.** Feline omega interferon can be used to treat cat viral infections, including calci virus, FeLF, FIV, and other feline viral infections as well as canine parvovirus.
4. **Administration.** Interferons may be given SC or by other parenteral routes (depending on the virus to be treated) once a day.
5. **Adverse effects.** Transient anorexia and weight loss may occur in cats. Fever, myelotoxicity, and myalgia may develop with parenteral administration at higher dosages (Tables 15-1 and 15-2).

TABLE 15-2. Generic and Trade Names for Antimicrobial Drugs

Class	Generic Name	Trade Name
Penicillins		
Old penicillins		
	Penicillin G—benzylpenicillin	Many
	Penicillin V—Phenoxymenthyl Penicillin	Many
	Benzathine penicillin G	Many
	Procaine penicillin G	Many
	Penicillin G potassium	Many
Penicillinase resistant		
	Methicillin	Staphcillin®
	Nafcillin	Nafcillin®
	Oxacillin	Oxacillin®
	Cloxacillin	Orbenin®, Dry-Clox®
Aminopenicillins		
	Ampicillin	Polyflex®
	Amoxicillin	Amoxi-Tab®, Biomax®
Carboxypencillins		
	Carbenicillin	Geopen®, Geocillin®
	Ticarcillin	Ticar®
Ureidopenicillins		
	Piperacillin	Pipercil®
Potentiated penicillins		
	Amoxicillin-clavulanate	Clavamox®
	Ticarcillin-clavulanate	Timentin®
	Ampicillin-sulbactam	
Cephalosporins		
First generation		
Oral	Cefadroxil	Cefa-Drops®
Oral	Cephalexin	Keflex®
Parenteral	Cephaparin	
	Cefazolin	Ancef®, Kefzol®
Second generation		
Oral	Cefachlor	Ceclor®
Parenteral	Cefoxitin	
Third generation		
Parenteral	Ceftiofur	Naxcel®
Fourth generation		
Parenteral	Cefapime	Maxipime®
Carbapenems		
	Imipenem	Primaxin®
	Meropenem	Merrem®
Monobactams		
	Azetreonem	Azactam®
Polypeptids		
	Bacitracin	Many
Aminoglycosides		
	Streptomycin	Streptomycin Bulk®
	Neomycin	Neomix, Biosol®
	Kanamycin	Kantrim® Amforal®
	Amikacin	Amiglyde-V®
	Gentamicin	Gentavet®, Gentocin®

(continued)

TABLE 15-2. (*Continued*)

Class	Generic Name	Trade Name
Aminocyclitols		
	Spectinomycin	Adspec®
	Apramycin	Apralan®
Tetracyclines		
	Chlortetracycline	Aureomycin®
	Oxytetracycline	Terramycin®
	Tetracycline	Panmycin®
	Doxycycline	Doxyrobe®
	Minocycline	Minocin®
Macrolides		
14-molecule ring	Erythromycin	Galimycin®, Ery-Tab®
15-molecule ring	Azithromycin	Zithromax®
	Tulathromycin	Draxxin®
16-molecule ring	Tylosin	Tylan®
	Tilmicosin	Micotil®
Lincosamides		
	Lincosamides	Lincosin®
	Clindamycin	Antirobe®, Clinsol®
	Pirlimycin	Pirsue®
Amphenicols		
	Chloramphenicol	Chloromycetin®
	Florfenicol	Nuflor®
Streptogramins		
	Streptogramin A and B	
	Virginiamycin M and A	Stafac®
	Dalfopristin and quinupristin	
Polymixins		
	Polymixin B	Aerosporin®
	Polymixin E	Colistin®
Mupirocins		
	Mupirocin	Bactroban®
Sulfonamides		
	Sulfamethoxazole + trimethoprim	Bactrim®, Septra®
	Sulfadiazine	
	Sulfadimethoxine	Albon®
Diaminopyridazines		
	Trimethoprim + sulfadiazine	Tribrissen®
	Ormethoprim + sulfadimethoxine	
Methenamine		
	Methenamine	Hiprex®, Mandelamine®
Fluoroguinolones	Enrofloxacin	Baytril®
	Sarafloxacin	Saraflox®
	Difloxacin	Dicural®
	Orbifloxacin	Orbax®
	Marbofloxacin	Zeniquin®
Novobiocins		
	Novobiocin	Albamycin®
	Novobiocin + tetracycline	Albaplex®

(*continued*)

TABLE 15-2. (*Continued*)

Class	Generic Name	Trade Name
Nitroimidazoles		
	Metronidazole	Flagyl®
Nitrofurans		
	Nitrofurantoin	Furadantin®
	Furazolidone	Topazone®
	Nitrofurazone	NFZ Puffer®
Isoniazid		
	Isoniazid	Nidrazid®
Rifampin		
	Rifampin	RiFadin®
Pleuromutilins		
	Tiamulin	Denagard®
Glycopeptides		
	Vancomycin	Vancocin®
Ionophores		
	Monensin	Rumensin®
	Lasalocid	Bovatec®
	Narasin	Monteban®
	Salinomycin	Biocox®
	Laidlomycin	Cattlyst®
Antifungals		
	Griseofulvin	Fulcin®
	Flucytosine	5-FC®, Ancoban®
	amphotericin	Amphocin®, Fungizone®
	Terbinafine	Lamisil®
Azoles	Clotrimazole	Lotrimin®, Mycelex®
	Fluconazole	Diflucan®
	Itraconazole	Sporanox®
	Ketoconazole	Nizoral®
	Miconazole	Many
Topical Antifungals	Nystatin natamycin	Natacyn®, Mycostatin®

SUGGESTED READING

Booth DM. 2000. "Do's and don'ts of antimicrobial therapy." In *Kirk's Current Veterinary Therapy*. Edited by Bonagura JD. 13th ed., pp. 33–40. Philadelphia, PA: Saunders.
  http://www.drugs.com
Plumb DC. 2005. *Veterinary Drug Handbook*. 5th ed. Ames, IA: Blackwell Publishing.
Giguers S, Prescott, JF, Baggot, JD, Walker RD, Dowling PM. 2006. *Antimicrobial Therapy in Veterinary Medicine*. 4th ed. Ames, IA: Blackwell Publishing.

STUDY QUESTIONS

DIRECTIONS: Each of the numbered items or incomplete statements in this section is followed by answers or by completions of the statement. Select the **one** lettered answer or completion that is **best** in each case.

1. Bacterial resistance due to drug-inactivating enzymes is important for all of the following antibiotics except:

(A) Penicillin G
(B) Ampicillin
(C) Gentamicin
(D) Tetracycline
(E) Cephalexin

2. Infectious or transferable drug resistance, which involves transfer of multiple-drug resistant genes via pili, has been observed clinically in Gram(–) infections of the

(A) urinary tract.
(B) intestinal tract.
(C) respiratory tract.
(D) skin.

3. The primary reason for using mixtures of sulfonamides in cattle is

(A) to decrease the likelihood of bacterial resistance since most organisms would be sensitive to one of the sulfonamides in the mixture even if resistant to the others.
(B) to decrease the rate of acetylation since each sulfonamide competes for enzyme.
(C) to provide a broader spectrum of antimicrobial action.
(D) to reduce renal toxicity based on the law of independent solubility.
(E) to allow the formulation of neutral solutions.

4. Trimethoprim or ormetoprim combined with a sulfonamide results in all of the following EXCEPT

(A) a sequential blockade of folate synthesis in susceptible bacteria.
(B) a decreased ability of sulfonamides to produce keratoconjunctivitis sicca (KCS).
(C) a decrease in the rate of development of resistant bacteria.
(D) an extended antibacterial spectrum.

(E) an increased inhibition of purine and DNA synthesis in susceptible bacteria.

5. The fluoroquinolones, enrofloxacin, and marbofloxacin

(A) have an antibacterial spectrum, which is limited to Gram(–) pathogens, especially anaerobes.
(B) are used primarily for enteric infections since they are not absorbed from the gut.
(C) are useful for respiratory, skin, and urinary tract infections in puppies.
(D) are bactericidal via inhibition of DNA gyrase.

6. Considering the pharmacology of the penicillin G and the first-generation cephalosporins, all of the following are true EXCEPT:

(A) They inhibit peptidoglycan cross-linking in the third stage of bacterial cell wall synthesis.
(B) Bacterial resistance is most commonly due to β-lactamase production.
(C) Tissue penetration of cephalosporins is superior to penicillin G and thus they are preferred for antibiotic prophylaxis in surgery.
(D) They are eliminated primarily by hepatic metabolism and biliary excretion of conjugated drug.
(E) Nephrotoxicity is more likely to occur with high or prolonged dosage of cephalosporins.

7. The antibacterial activity of amoxicillin may include penicillinase-producing organisms if it is combined with

(A) phenethicillin.
(B) enrofloxacin.
(C) penicilloic acid.
(D) ampicillin.
(E) clavulanic acid.

8. Two semisynthetic penicillins that are effective against *Pseudomonas* spp. are

(A) methicillin and ampicillin.
(B) ampicillin and amoxicillin.
(C) amoxicillin and ticarcillin.
(D) ticarcillin and piperacillin.
(E) ticarcillin and oxacillin.

9. The aminoglycoside antibiotics such as amikacin and gentamicin

(A) are lipid soluble and distribute widely to tissues including the CNS.
(B) are not effective against Gram(–) anaerobes because their uptake by bacteria is oxygen linked.
(C) are bacteriostatic at therapeutic concentrations.
(D) are well absorbed orally if they are enteric coated to protect them from gastric acid.

10. Adverse reactions to the aminoglycoside antibiotics include all of the following EXCEPT:

(A) neuromuscular blockade.
(B) myelosuppression and anemia.
(C) nephrotoxicity.
(D) ototoxicity—auditory.
(E) ototoxicity—vestibular

11. Tetracyclines are broad spectrum and bacteriostatic by a mechanism of action that involves

(A) binding to the 30S ribosome to inhibit the addition of amino acids to the growing peptide chain.
(B) binding to phospholipids in bacterial cell membranes to increase permeability.
(C) binding to the 50S ribosome to inhibit peptidyl transferase.
(D) Inhibition of DNA gyrase.

12. Tylosin

(A) inhibits the first step of cell wall synthesis and thus is bactericidal in growing bacteria.
(B) may produce anemia by blocking iron uptake in erythroblasts.
(C) antibacterial spectrum includes mycoplasma.
(D) is usually effective in organisms resistant to erythromycin.

13. Clindamycin

(A) is primarily active against Gram(–) pathogens.

(B) is used in equine enteric infections since it is a poorly absorbed "enteric" macrolide.
(C) distribution is generally limited to the ECF.
(D) is frequently effective in staphylococcal osteomyelitis.

14. You are presented with an aged cat with *Haemobartonella* infection but also with impaired renal function. A tetracycline that may be safely administered is

(A) chlortetracycline.
(B) doxycycline.
(C) oxytetracycline.
(D) tetracycline.

15. An antibiotic that is combined with erythromycin for treating *Rhodococcus equi* infections in foals is

(A) spectinomycin.
(B) vancomycin.
(C) rifampin.
(D) tylosin.

16. Which of the following therapies is not correct?

(A) Metronidazole—anaerobic infection of the pelvis in cats
(B) Lincomycin—swine dysentery
(C) Florfenicol—bovine respiratory disease
(D) Tetracycline—psittacosis in birds
(E) Chloramphenicol—mycoplasmal pneumonia in swine

17. Three antibiotic used topically or orally but not parenterally (primarily because of nephrotoxicity) are

(A) streptomycin, kanamycin, bacitracin.
(B) polymixin B, bacitracin, neomycin.
(C) bacitracin, tiamulin, polymixin B.
(D) neomycin, gentamicin, rifampin.

18. Weekly monitoring of renal function (e.g. BUN) is necessary in antifungal therapy with

(A) amphotericin B.
(B) ketoconazole.
(C) flucytosine.
(D) griseofulvin.

19. All of the following statements concerning griseofulvin are true EXCEPT:

(A) oral absorption is increased by dietary fats.
(B) distribution is to keratin precursor cells.
(C) its action is rapid and fungicidal.

(D) it inhibits mitosis in dermatophytes (ringworm).

20. All of the following statements concerning ketoconazole are true EXCEPT:

(A) it is more effective than flucytosine for meningeal cryptococcosis since it penetrates the CNS more completely.

(B) it inhibits ergosterol synthesis in both systemic mycotic infections and candidiasis (yeast infections).

(C) cortisol and testosterone synthesis in mammals is inhibited at high doses.

(D) it must be administered for 3–6 months in therapy for systemic mycoses.

ANSWERS AND EXPLANATIONS

1. The answer is D.
Bacterial resistance to tetracyclines is usually due to decreased uptake or active transport of drug out of the bacterial cell. Resistance to penicillin G, ampicillin, and cephalexin is due to β-lactamase production. Gentamicin is enzymatically inactivated by resistant bacteria, which acetylate, phosphorylate, or adenylate the drug.

2. The answer is B.
Infectious or transferable drug resistance may occur in Gram(–) bacteria, which reproduce by conjugation and has been observed clinically in enteric infections caused by Salmonella, *Shigella*, or *E. coli*.

3. The answer is D.
The renal toxicity of sulfonamides is due to their precipitation in neutral or acid urine. Because of their independent solubility, mixtures of sulfonamides provide greater solubility for a given concentration. Bacterial resistance, metabolism, spectrum of activity, or neutrality of solutions are minimally affected by mixtures.

4. The answer is B.
The ocular toxicity of sulfonamides, especially the sulfapyrimidines, is not reduced by combination with trimethoprim or ormetoprim. Potentiated sulfonamides have an extended spectrum and reduced rate of development of bacterial resistance via a sequential blockade of folate, purine, and DNA synthesis.

5. The answer is D.
The fluoroquinolones are bactericidal by inhibiting bacterial DNA gyrase, which results in degradation of replicating DNA. They are broad spectrum but anaerobes tend to be resistant. They are absorbed orally. They should not be administered to puppies because they may produce erosion of articular cartilage in growing dogs.

6. The answer is D.
Penicillins and cephalosporins are eliminated by renal mechanisms of glomerular filtration and active tubular secretion. Their mechanism of action and inactivation by resistant bacteria are similar. Tissue penetration and nephrotoxicity are greater for the cephalosporins.

7. The answer is E.
Clavulanic acid inhibits β-lactamases and prevents inactivation of amoxicillin by otherwise resistant organisms. Phenethicillin, enrofloxacin, or ampicillin do not inhibit penicillinases. Penicilloic acid is a degradation product of penicillinase action, which acts as an antigenic determinant in penicillin allergy.

8. The answer is D.
Piperacillin and ticarcillin are antipseudomonal penicillins used alone or in combination with gentamicin, tobramycin, or clavulanate in severe infections caused by this organism. Methicillin and oxacillin are penicillinase stable and ampicillin and amoxicillin are broad spectrum but are not effective against *Pseudomonas* spp.

9. The answer is B.
The uptake of aminoglycosides by bacteria includes an energy-dependent step (EDP_1), which is oxygen-linked. Since anaerobes do not use oxygen, the uptake of aminoglycosides is minimal. Aminoglycosides are highly polar and poorly lipid soluble. They are bactericidal and are not absorbed orally.

10. The answer is B.
Aminoglycosides do not produce myelosuppression. Nephrotoxicity and ototoxicity are most likely in patients with impaired renal function. Neuromuscular blockade occurs rarely and is reversed by calcium.

11. The answer is A.
Tetracyclines inhibit bacterial protein synthesis by binding to the 30S ribosome of bacteria and preventing attachment of aminoacyl tRNA to the ribosome and thus block the addition of amino acids to protein synthesis. Polymyxin B disrupts bacterial cell membranes and fluoroquinolones inhibit DNA gyrase. Chloramphenicol binds to the 50S ribosome and inhibits peptidyl transferase.

12. The answer is C.

Tylosin is a macrolide antibiotic effective against Gram(+) pathogens and mycoplasmal infections. It is also active against some Gram(–) bacteria, including *Pasteurella* and *Haemophilus* spp. It inhibits protein synthesis by binding to the 50S ribosome like other macrolides including erythromycin and thus cross-resistance would be expected.

13. The answer is D.

Clindamycin is active against Gram(+) aerobes and anaerobes and has excellent penetration of soft tissues and bones, which renders it effective in staphylococcal osteomyelitis. It is contraindicated in horses because it suppresses colonic flora and produces a severe, often fatal, diarrhea.

14. The answer is B.

Tetracyclines are effective in treating *Haemobartonella* infection, but are excreted by the kidney and are nephrotoxic if there is preexisting renal disease. Doxycycline, however, is excreted primarily by the intestine and could be safely administered to this patient.

15. The answer is C.

Rifampin is bactericidal for mycobacteria and Gram(+) pathogens. It is combined with erythromycin for *R. equi* infections. Spectinomycin is an aminocylitol used for enteric and respiratory diseases. Vancomycin is a reserve antibiotic for methicillin-resistant staphylococcal infections. Tylosin is a macrolide similar to erythromycin.

16. The answer is E.

Chloramphenicol used in food-producing animals is illegal because of the potential danger of residue-induced aplastic anemia in humans.

17. The answer is B.

Bacitracin, neomycin, and polymixin B are used topically or as nonabsorbable oral antibiotics. They are too nephrotoxic for systemic use. Bacitracin is bactericidal against Gram(+) organisms and neomycin and polymixin B are bactericidal against Gram(–) bacteria.

18. The answer is A.

Amphotericin B is nephrotoxic and renal function must be monitored weekly during long-term therapy for systemic mycoses.

19. The answer is C.

Griseofulvin's action is fungistatic and its action is slow as it inhibits fungal growth in keratin precursor cells. Infected cells are slowly shed and replaced with uninfected cells. Oral absorption is increased by fat. It inhibits mitosis by binding to microtubules to prevent spindle formation.

20. The answer is A.

Flucytosine is an antifungal that penetrates the CNS and CSF well. It is used with amphotericin B in the treatment of meningeal cryptococcosis. Ketoconazole does not penetrate the CNS well. Ketoconazole inhibits ergosterol synthesis in fungi and, at high doses, steroid synthesis in mammals. Long-term therapy is required for mycotic infections.

Chapter 16

Antiparasitic Agents

Walter H. Hsu and Richard J. Martin

I. **INTRODUCTION.** Antiparasitics are drugs that reduce parasite burdens to a tolerable level by killing parasites or inhibiting their growth. The ideal antiparasitic has a wide therapeutic index (i.e., the toxic dose is at least three times the therapeutic dose), is effective after one dose, is easy to administer, is inexpensive, and does not leave residues (an important consideration for use in food-producing animals).

A. **Mechanisms of action**

1. **Paralysis of parasites by mimicking the action of putative neurotransmitters** (Table 16-1)
2. **Alteration of metabolic processes**
   a. Inhibition of microtubule synthesis
   b. Inhibition of folic acid synthesis or metabolism
   c. Inhibition of thiamine utilization
   d. Uncoupling of oxidative phosphorylation
   e. Inhibition of chitin formation in arthropods
   f. Simulation of insect juvenile hormones
3. **Alteration of parasite reproduction**
   a. Inhibition of replication in protozoans
   b. Inhibition of egg production in nematodes

B. **Disadvantages of antiparasitics**

1. Expense
2. Development of resistant strains
3. Inhibition of host immunity

C. **Characteristics of ideal antiparasitics**

1. Effective in removing parasites from body
2. Wide therapeutic index: Toxic dose > 3× therapeutic dose
3. Economically justifiable
4. Easy to administer, for example, in feed, injections, and pour-on
5. One-dose treatment
6. No residue problems, especially in food-producing animals
7. Effective against immature form of parasites

D. **Current trends** include the use of broad-spectrum drugs and combination therapy to increase efficacy.

II. **ANTINEMATODAL DRUGS (NEMATOCIDES)** may be broad-spectrum or narrow-spectrum.

A. **Classification of antinematodal drugs**

1. Benzimidazoles
2. Nicotinic agonists: levamisole, pyrantel, morantel
3. Macrocyclic lactones: ivermectin, doramectin, eprinomectin, selamectin (avermectins), milbemycin, moxidectin (milbemycins)
4. Miscellaneous nematocides: dichlorvos, piperazine, emodepside, melarsomine

TABLE 16-1. Putative Classical Neurotransmitters of Various Parasites.*

Parasite	Excitatory	Inhibitory
Nematode	ACh, Glu	Glu, GABA
Cestode	5-HT	ACh
Trematode	5-HT	ACh, DA, NE
Arthropod	ACh, Glu	Glu, OA, GABA

Ach, acetylcholine; DA, dopamine; GABA, γ-aminobutyric acid; Glu, glutamate; NE, norepinephrine; OA, octopamine; 5-HT, serotonin.

*Note that nematodes, cestodes, trematodes, and arthropods also have a large range of excitatory and inhibitory neuropeptides. Some of the same neuropeptides are present in nematodes, trematodes, and arthropods.

B. | **Benzimidazoles (BZDs) (Figure 16-1)**

1. Thiabendazole (Figure 16-1) is the prototypical agent. It is approved for use in ruminants and horses.
   a. **Preparations.** Thiabendazole is the prototype of BZD, which is much less potent than other BZDs, and is no longer used as a nematocide. Other BZDs include **albendazole, fenbendazole, oxfendazole, oxibendazole, and febantel** (a pro-BZD that is converted to fenbendazole and oxfendazole in animals).
   b. **Chemistry.** All of BZDs, except thiabendazole, have a side chain at position 5, which prevents hydroxylation of position 5 of the BZD. Therefore, these compounds are more potent than thiabendazole as nematocides (Figure 16-2).
   c. **Mechanism of action.** BZDs inhibit microtubule synthesis in nematode cells by interfering with polymerization of β-tubulins (Figure 16-3). BZDs do not affect microtubule synthesis in animal cells, this is why these drugs are relatively safe in animals. Care should be exercised for some of the BZDs (albendazole) if the animal is in the first one-third of pregnancy.
   d. **Therapeutic uses**
      (1) **Ruminants.** Albendazole (Valbazen®), fenbendazole (Panacur®, etc.), and oxfendazole (Benzelmin®, Synanthic®) are effective against major GI worms (in both the adult and larval stages). In addition, they are effective against lungworms. However, they are ineffective against filariae.
      (2) **Horses.** Fenbendazole, oxfendazole, and oxibendazole (Anthelcide®) are effective against strongyles, but have limited activity against immature strongyles. They are not very effective against migrating larvae of *Strongylus vulgaris* and *S. edentatis*, and thus need elevated, multiple doses to treat these parasites. They are effective against *Oxyuris*, *Trichostronylus*, and *Parascaris*. They have limited activity against *Strongyloides*, *Habronema*, and *Dictyocaulus*; and thus may need elevated doses to treat these parasites. They are not effective against *Gasterophilus*.
      (3) **Swine.** Fenbendazole is effective against *Ascaris*, *Oesophagostomum*, *Hyostrongylus*, *Trichuris*, *Metastrongylus*, and *Stephanurus*. Fenbendazole usually kills both adults and larvae (L_3, L_4).

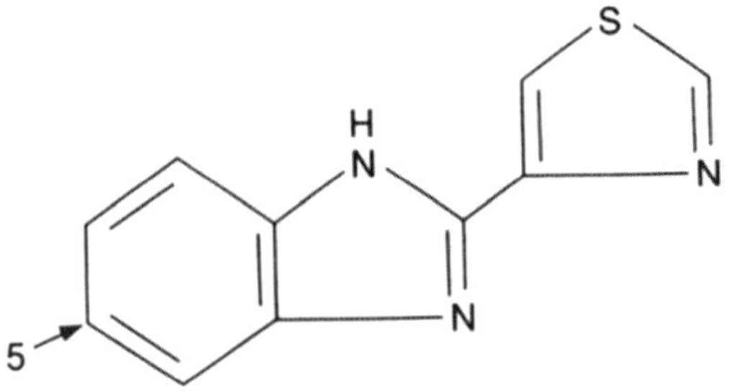

FIGURE 16-1. Chemical structure of thiabendazole, the prototypical benzimidazole. Metabolism occurs via hydroxylation at position 5. The other benzimidazoles are more potent than thiabendazole because they have a side chain, which prevents hydroxylation at position 5. (Reprint from Figure 13-1, *NVLS Pharmacology*, by Ahrens, 1996.)

Compound	Structural formula
Albendazole	
Fenbendazole	
Febantel	
Oxfendazole	
Oxibendazole	

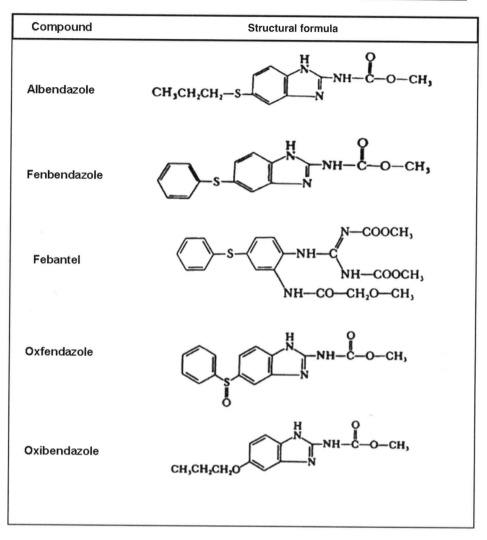

FIGURE 16-2. Chemical structures of albendazole, fenbendazole, febantel, oxfendazole, and oxibendazole. (Modified from Table 47.1, *Veterinary Pharmacology and Therapeutics*, 8th ed., by Adams, 2001).

    (4) Dogs and cats. Fenbendazole and febantel (in Drontal® Plus) are effective against ascarids, hookworms, and whipworms in both adult and larva forms.
    (5) BZDs have ovicidal activity on nematodes. In addition, production of eggs by nematodes is inhibited within 1 hour of BZD administration.
  e. Administration. BZDs are administered orally. In general, one single dose in cattle and horses, and three to five consecutive daily dosages in carnivores and omnivores.
  f. Pharmacokinetics
    (1) Absorption. GI absorption of BZDs varies, depending on the water solubility of the compound; the ones with better water solubility, for example, albendazole and oxibendazole have better GI absorption than others. Since bile can help dissolve BZDs, absorption of them will be best in animals with a full stomach. Herbivores fed fiber rather than concentrates before receiving and oral dose of BZDs have an increased area under the curve signifying better absorption. This is because the BZDs bind to the dietary fiber preventing them from passing straight through the GI tract and facilitating absorption.

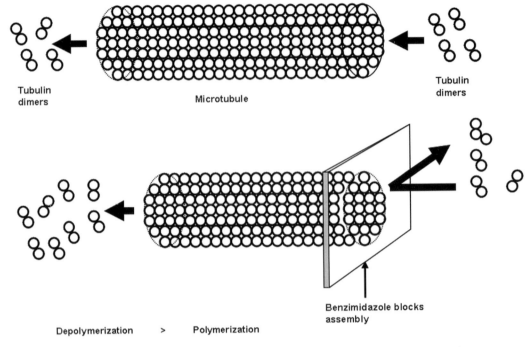

Tubulin dimers

Microtubule

Tubulin dimers

Benzimidazole blocks assembly

Depolymerization   >   Polymerization

FIGURE 16-3. Benzimidazole (BZD)-induced inhibition of microtubule synthesis in helminthes. BZD binds β-tubulin of helminthes, preventing dimerization with α-tubulin and polymerization of tubulin oligomers into microtubules. (Modified from Figure 57.2, *Human Pharmacology*, 3rd ed., by Brody, Larner, and Minneman, 1998.)

    (2) Metabolism. The degree of metabolism is related to the C5 substitution of BZD (see Figure 16-1). In general, all BZDs, except thiabendazole, are resistant to metabolism (C5-hydroxylation). Albendazole can be converted to its sulfone or sulfoxide metabolites; these metabolites are also active.

    (3) Excretion. The majority of BZDs (except thiabendazole and albendazole) are excreted unchanged in feces.

    (4) Plasma $t_{1/2}$ and drug residues and withdrawal periods

      (a) After oral administration, T_{max} for BZDs is 10–20 hours; elimination $t_{1/2}$ of albendazole in cattle is 9–14 hours; $t_{1/2}$ of fenbendazole in horses is ~10 hours, in cattle is 27–36 hours, and in sheep is 14–35 hours. $t_{1/2}$ of oxfendazole in cattle and sheep is 18 hours.

      (b) Drug residues persist for 1–3 weeks. They approach the low limit of detection in 2 days; however, residues in the liver are generally detectable in 2 weeks.

      (c) The preslaughter withdrawal period in cattle is 27 days for albendazole, 8 days for fenbendazole, and 7 days for oxfendazole. Do not use in lactating dairy cattle (exception, fenbendazole).

      (d) The preslaughter withdrawal period in swine following fenbendazole administration is 0 days.

  g. Drug resistance. Cross-resistance occurs among all BZDs.

  h. Adverse effects. These agents are generally safe, although albendazole may be teratogenic and embryotoxic. BZDs may be toxic to liver and bone marrow in dogs, particularly at high doses.

C. Nicotinic agonists

  1. Levamisole is approved for use in ruminants and pigs.

    a. Mechanism of action. Levamisole paralyzes worms by selectively activating nematode nicotinic acetylcholine (ACh) receptors, allowing entry of Na^+, Ca^{2+}, for excessive body muscle contraction, and thus induces paralysis. (Figure 16-4)

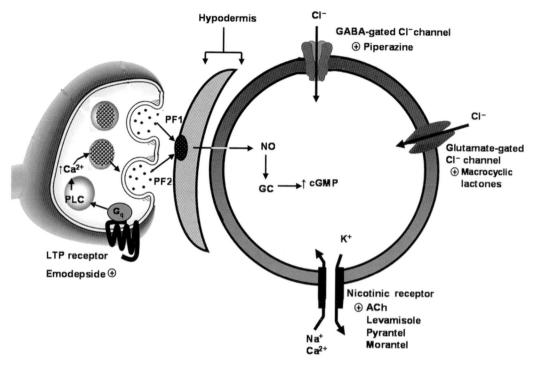

FIGURE 16-4. Mechanisms of action of antinematodal drugs that interfere with parasite nervous system. LTP = latrophilin; PLC = phospholipasec; PFI = SDPNFLRF-amide; PFZ = SADPNFLRF-amide; GC = guanylyl cyclase.

b. Therapeutic uses

    (1) Ruminants. Levamisole is effective against most mature GI worms and lungworms, but it has marginal activity against *Strongyloides* and immature GI worms.

    (2) Pigs. It is effective against ascarids, *Strongyloides*, nodular worms, lungworms, and kidney worms.

c. Pharmacokinetics

    (1) Absorption is excellent following oral, parenteral, or topical administration; it can be administered as a pour-on preparation.

    (2) In cattle, levamisole is transformed by liver into metabolites (formed by oxidation of imidazoline ring and opening of thiazolidine ring).

    (3) The plasma $t_{1/2}$ of levamisole is 4–6 hours, and the drug is eliminated from the body in 2 days after being absorbed.

    (4) More than 90% of levamisole is excreted as metabolites into urine (90%) and feces (10%) within 48 hours of administration.

    (5) The preslaughter clearance periods in cattle are 48–72 hours (PO), 7 days (SC), and 11 days (topical), respectively. The preslaughter clearance period after oral administration in pigs is 72 hours.

d. Adverse effects. Levamisole is one of the most toxic anthelmintics. It has a low safety margin, especially when given by injection. Do not administer to dairy cattle of breeding age, since milk withdrawal periods in these animals have not been determined.

    (1) Signs of levamisole poisoning include parasympathetic stimulation, convulsions, CNS depression, and asphyxia, which is primarily the result of respiratory muscle paralysis.

    (2) Atropine cannot counteract levamisole-induced depolarizing blockade of skeletal muscle; therefore, it is not an antidote for levamisole overdose.

    (3) Coadministration of levamisole and pyrantel, another nicotine-like nematocide, increases toxicity.

2. Pyrantel and morantel
a. Chemistry
(1) Pyrantel, which is inactivated in aqueous solution upon exposure to light, should be stored in tight, light-resistant containers. The drug should be used soon after the preparation of a drench solution or suspension.

(2) Morantel, the methyl ester of pyrantel, is stable in solution.

b. Preparations
(1) **Pyrantel tartrate** is approved for horses (Strongid-C®) and pigs (Banminth®).

(2) **Pyrantel pamoate** is approved for horses (Strongid-T®, Strongid-P®) and dogs (Nemex®, and in Drontal®, Heartgard®, etc.), and is used in cats as well.

(3) **Morantel** tartrate (Rumatel®) is approved for cattle.

c. Mechanism of action.
Like levamisole, pyrantel, and morantel paralyze worms by causing depolarizing neuromuscular blockade (Figure 16-4).

d. Therapeutic uses
(1) **Horses.** Pyrantel is effective against strongyles, ascarids, and pinworms, but not against bots. Pyrantel tartrate is used to prevent nematodes infestation and pyrantel pamoate is used to treat nematodes infestation.

(2) **Pigs.** Pyrantel is effective against ascarids, nodular worms, and stomach worms.

(3) **Dogs and cats.** Pyrantel is effective against all GI nematodes, but it has limited efficacy against whipworms.

(4) **Ruminants.** Morantel is used as a feed additive, which is effective against stomach worms, nodular worms, and other principal intestinal worms.

e. Pharmacokinetics
(1) **Absorption**
   (a) **Pyrantel tartrate is water soluble**; therefore, GI absorption is excellent following oral administration. Peak plasma concentrations occur 2–3 hours after dosing. Elimination $t_{1/2}$ in pigs and horses are ~6 and ~14 hours, respectively.

   (b) **Pyrantel pamoate is poorly soluble in water**, limiting GI absorption. Therefore, pyrantel pamoate is good for the treatment of bowel worms (e.g., pinworms).

   (c) **Morantel tartrate** is absorbed rapidly from the abomasum and small intestine. Peak plasma concentrations occur 4–6 hours after dosing. Plasma $t_{1/2}$ of morantel in cattle is not known.

(2) **Metabolism and excretion.** The absorbed pyrantel and morantel are rapidly metabolized (hydroxylation and conjugation) and excreted, mostly via feces, but also via urine. Preslaughter withdrawal requirements are 1 day for pyrantel tartrate in swine and 14 days for morantel in cattle.

f. Adverse effects.
At recommended doses, adverse effects are not common. However, when adverse reactions occur, they are similar to levamisole toxicity.

g. Contraindications.
Because morantel and pyrantel have the same mechanism of action as levamisole, these agents should not be used concurrently.

h. Resistance.
There is a cross-resistance among pyrantel, morantel, and levamisole.

D. Macrocyclic lactones (macrolide endectocides).
These compounds are antibiotics derived from *Streptomyces*, with activity against nematodes and arthropods. In addition to having broad-spectrum activity, they are effective at low dosages (µg/kg range).

1. General aspects of macrocyclic lactones
a. Chemistry.
There are two major groups, **the avermectins and milbemycins (Figures 16-5 and 16-6). Ivermectin, doramectin, eprinomectin, and selamectin belong to the avermectin group and have a disaccharide side chain; milbemycin and moxidectin belong to the milbemycin group and do not have the disaccharide side chain** and are more lipophilic (Figures 16-5 and 16-6).

b. Mechanism of action.
They activate the glutamate-gated chloride channels, thus inhibiting neurotransmission in nematodes (and arthropods) to induce flaccid paralysis.

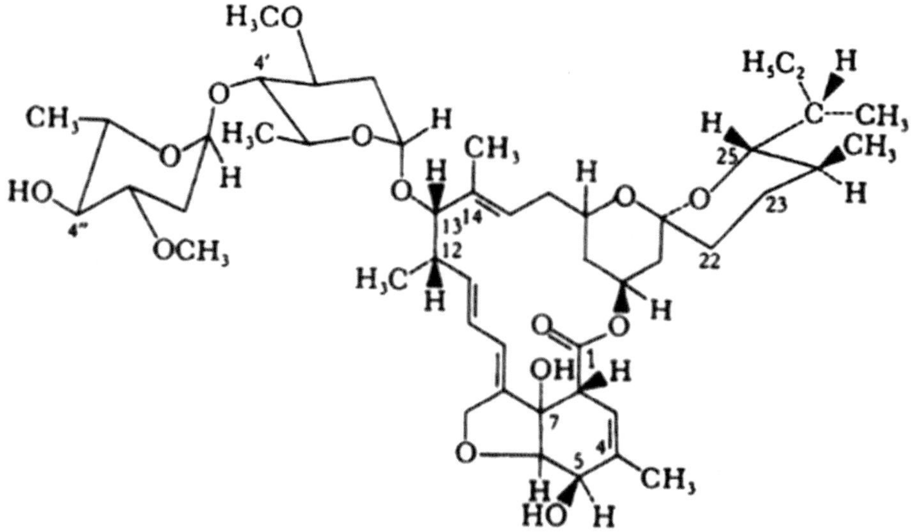

FIGURE 16-5. Structure of 22,23-dihydroavermectin B_{1a}, the major component of ivermectin. Ivermectin also contains $\leq 20\%$ 22,23-dihydroavermectin B_{1b}, which is identical except that the substituent in the 25 position is isopropyl instead of butyl. (Reprint from Fig. 47.3, *Veterinary Pharmacology and Therapeutics*, 8th ed., by Adams, 2001.)

(1) As part of the result of inhibition of neurotransmission, pharyngeal muscle of nematodes is paralyzed, this interferes with feeding; body movement is also inhibited as is egg laying.

(2) The exact site of action of the macrocyclic lactones depends on the species of the parasite and on the specific macrocyclic lactone; it is likely that there are different subtypes of receptor on the different parasite cells/tissues and selectivity for the receptor subtypes varies with the macrocyclic lactone (Figure 16-4).

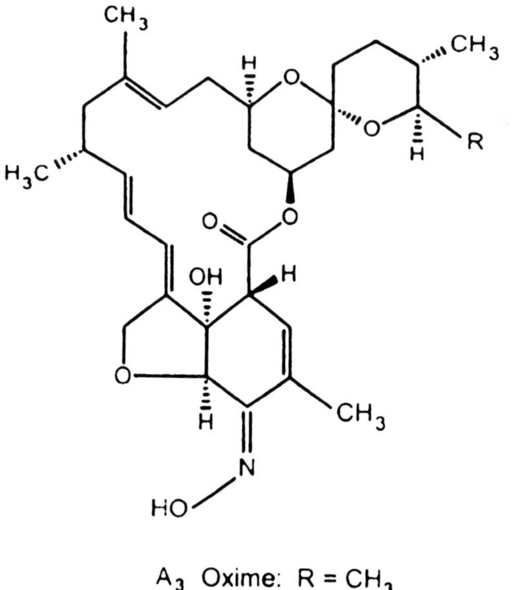

FIGURE 16-6. Structure of milbemycin oxime. (Reprint from Fig. 47.7, *Veterinary Pharmacology and Therapeutics*, 8th ed., by Adams, 2001.)

A_3 Oxime: R = CH_3
A_4 Oxime: R = C_2H_5

    c. Adverse effects. Macrocyclic lactones have a high safety margin in ruminants, horses, and swine, and are safe for use in pregnant animals and breeders. Some of the Collie dogs and Murray cattle show high sensitivity to ivermectin.

        (1) Local irritation may occur following SC administration.

        (2) CNS depression. At high doses, ivermectin may evoke CNS depression as evidenced by listlessness, mydriasis, ataxia, recumbency, and coma. Although macrocyclic lactones activate γ-aminobutyric acid (GABA)-gated Cl^- channels in animals, the GABA-receptor antagonist picrotoxin does not work well as an antidote.

    d. Resistance. Resistances to macrocyclic lactones have occurred in nematodes and arthropods. Cross-resistance among macrocyclic lactones can occur.

  2. Ivermectin. It is extracted from *Streptomyces avermitilis*. The ivermectin injectable (Ivomec®) is dissolved in propylene glycol–glycerol formal mixture.

    a. Chemistry. Ivermectin is a mixture of ~80% 22,23-dihydroavermectin B_{1a} and ~20% 22,23-dihydroavermectin B_{1b}.

    b. Therapeutic uses and administration

        (1) Ruminants. Ivermectin (Ivomec®) is effective against all major GI worms and lungworms. It is administered at 0.2 mg/kg orally or SC, and 0.5 mg/kg topically. The pour-on ivermectin is effective as a nematocide in cattle, but not in goats or sheep because of poor absorption from the skin.

        (2) Horses. It is effective against bots, stomach worms, strongyles, pinworms, and ascarids. It is administered at 0.2 mg/kg orally or SC.

        (3) Pigs. Ivermectin is effective against major GI worms, lungworms, and kidney worms. It is not effective against *Trichinella* during the muscular stage. The standard dose is 0.3 mg/kg administered SC.

        (4) Dogs

            (a) Ivermectin is effective against ascarids, hookworms, and whipworms at 0.2 mg/kg orally. However, this dose may not be safe in some breeds (e.g., Collies) and some individuals, and is therefore not approved for dogs. In the dogs, being highly susceptible to ivermectin, they have a mutation of P-glycoprotein particularly in the endothelial cells of the blood–brain barrier. P-glycoprotein, an ATP-binding cassette transporter (or multidrug transporter) found in the apical membrane of endothelial cells, is responsible for drug exit from the brain. The mutation of P-glycoprotein causes retention of drugs, particularly macrocyclic lactones, in the brain of these dogs.

            (b) Both ivermectin and selamectin are potent substrates and inhibitors of the P-glycoprotein in dogs, but moxidectin is a weak one.

            (c) Ivermectin (Heartgard®) and other macrocyclic lactones, that is, selamectin (Revolution®), milbemycin (Interceptor®, Sentinel®), and moxidectin (Proheart®) are used as heartworm preventives and are administered to dogs once a month. For this purpose, ivermectin is administered at 6–12 μg/kg. Macrocyclic lactones eliminate L_4 stage of infective larvae of *Dirofilaria immitis*.

            (d) It is effective as a microfilaricide (50 μg/kg orally). The use of ivermectin as a microfilaricide is extra-label. Ivermectin can be diluted with propylene glycol, if needed.

        (5) All species. Ivermectin is effective against all ectoparasites. It is used especially to control mites.

    c. Pharmacokinetics

        (1) After oral administration, $\leq 95\%$ of ivermectin is absorbed in monogastric animals and ~30% is absorbed in ruminants.

        (2) In swine, after oral and SC administrations of ivermectin, the peak plasma level of the drug is reached in 12 and 48 hours, respectively.

        (3) Following IV injection, the plasma $t_{1/2}$ of ivermectin is 1.6–1.8 days in dogs, and 2.7–2.8 days in ruminants.

        (4) Following SC injection, the plasma $t_{1/2}$ of ivermectin in cattle is 8 days. The long plasma $t_{1/2}$ after SC administration is probably due to the solvent system (propylene glycol–glycerol formal), which slows down the absorption from injection site.

(5) Following administration, highest concentrations of ivermectin are found in liver and bile, and lowest concentration is found in the brain.

(6) Ivermectin is metabolized in liver and fat to polar and nonpolar fatty acid esters, respectively.

(7) Fecal excretion accounts for 98% of elimination of ivermectin.

(8) Ivermectin remains in tissues with long persistency; one dose is usually effective for 2–4 weeks. Preslaughter clearance periods: swine: 5 days (PO), 18 days (SC); sheep: 11 days (PO); cattle: 35 days (SC), 49 days (topical). Ivermectin should not be administered to dairy cows that are >20 months old.

3. **Doramectin (Dectomax®)**
   a. **Chemistry.** Doramectin is an analog of ivermectin (having a cyclohexyl group at C-25). The solvent for doramectin is 90% sesame oil—10% ethyl oleate, which slows down absorption from the injection site.
   b. **Therapeutic uses.** Doramectin is used only in cattle at 0.2 mg/kg SC.
   c. **Pharmacokinetics.** Pharmacokinetics of doramectin in cattle are very similar to that of ivermectin. Preslaughter withdrawal periods are 35 days (SC) and 45 days (topical). It should not be administered to dairy cows that are >20 months old.

4. **Eprinomectin. (Eprinex®)**
   a. **Chemistry.** Eprinomectin is an analog of ivermectin (**having an epi-acetylamino group at the 4″-position**).
   b. **Therapeutic uses.** Eprinomectin is used topically in cattle (0.5 mg/kg) to control most GI nematodes, lungworms, and ectoparasites the same way as ivermectin.
   c. **Pharmacokinetics**
      (1) Eprinomectin is absorbed after topical administration and reaches peak plasma level within 2–5 days of application and declines to undetectable level in 4 weeks. The majority of the topical dose is absorbed in 7–10 days. More than 85% of eprinomectin is excreted into feces as parent compound.
      (2) No preslaughter or milk withdrawal period is required after eprinomectin treatment, since drug residue levels are below legally acceptable limits in meat and milk after topical administration.

5. **Selamectin (Revolution®)**
   a. **Chemistry.** The chemical structure of selamectin is closer to doramectin than ivermectin. There is one lactone ring short in selamectin structure when compared with those of doramectin and ivermectin.
   b. **Therapeutic uses.** It is applied topically in dogs and cats (≥6 weeks old), 6 mg/kg, once a month
      (1) **In cats**, selamectin prevents heartworms and kills ascarids, hookworms, fleas, and ear mites.
      (2) **In dogs**, selamectin prevents heartworms and kills fleas (adults, larvae, and eggs), sarcoptic mites, ear mites, and ticks. Failures have been reported for selamectin as an ectoparasiticide.
   c. **Pharmacokinetics**
      (1) After topical application, **there is 4% bioavailability in dogs and 74% bioavailability in cats.** The high bioavailability in cats is attributed to their grooming activity and slow metabolism; as a result, selamectin serves as a nematocide in cats, but not in dogs.
      (2) After topical application, plasma selamectin concentrations reach maximal in 72 hours in dogs and 15 hours in cats. Plasma $t_{1/2}$ of selamectin in dogs and cats are 14 hours and 69 hours, respectively.
      (3) After a single topical administration, clinically effective concentrations of selamectin as a heartworm preventive persist for >30 days.
      (4) After topical application, substantial amount of topical selamectin is stored in sebaceous glands to provide persistent activity against ectoparasites.

(5) Selamectin is metabolized in the liver into desmethyl selamectin, and its oxidation product. Selamectin is excreted mostly in the feces as unchanged compound along with a small amount of metabolites.

d. Adverse effects. Selamectin is safer than ivermectin in dogs; selamectin is safe in pregnant animals and ivermectin-sensitive Collies. Selamectin-treated cats may show hypersalivation, which is due to the ingestion of isopropyl alcohol, a solvent in the preparation.

6. Milbemycin (Interceptor® and in Sentinel®) is extracted from *Streptomyces hygroscopicus aureolacrimosus*.

a. Chemistry. Commercial milbemycin consists of ~80% A_4 milbemycin and ~20% A_3 milbemycin (Figure 16-6).

b. Therapeutic uses. Milbemycin is approved for use in dogs only and is effective against the infective larvae of *D. immitis*, hookworms, whipworms, and ascarids. Milbemycin at the recommended dose of 0.5 mg/kg, orally, once a month, can be used in all dog breeds, including Collies, and is safe in pregnant dogs and breeders (because it is a weak substrate of P-glycoprotein). This dose of milbemycin is effective as a microfilaricide as well.

c. Pharmacokinetics. Following oral administration, ~90% of the dose passes through the GI tract unchanged. The remaining ~10% is absorbed. It reaches peak plasma concentration within 2–5 hours after oral administration. It is subsequently excreted into the bile; close to 90% of the dose is eliminated in the feces. The plasma $t_{1/2}$ of milbemycin is 1–3 days.

d. Adverse effects. Milbemycin has a high safety margin in dogs. However, milbemycin-killed microfilaria can cause hypersensitivity manifested by lethargy, pyrexia, salivation, emesis, coughing, tachypnea, and/or shock. These adverse effects are also seen when ivermectin is used as a microfilaricide.

7. Moxidectin. It is manufactured from *Streptomyces cyanogriseus moncyanogenus* culture.

a. Chemistry. Unlike other macrocyclic lactones, moxidectin is a single compound, but not a mixture of two closely related compounds.

b. Therapeutic uses. Moxidectin is used to treat equine and bovine nematodes and ectoparasites, and as a canine heartworm preventive for once a month use. The equine preparation (Quest®) is a 2% oral gel (0.4 mg/kg), the bovine preparation (Cydectin®) is a topical solution (0.5 mg/kg), and the canine preparation (Proheart®) is in tablets (3 µg/kg, PO). There is a new moxidectin product that is in combination with a fleacide imidacloprid (Advantage Multi®) topical solutionthat is a canine and feline heartworm preventive for once a month use. The dosage is 2.5 mg/kg in dogs and 1 mg/kg in cats. This product is also effective against ascarids, hookworms, and whipworms as well as ear mites.

c. Pharmacokinetics

(1) Moxidectin is more lipophilic than ivermectin; as a result, tissue levels persist longer than ivermectin.

(2) Moxidectin is excreted mainly in feces as parent compound. Only 15% of moxidectin is present in feces as hydroxylated metabolites.

(3) Plasma $t_{1/2}$ are ~80 hours in horses and 20 days in dogs when given orally. When applied topically in dogs and cats, T_{max} are 9.3 and 1.4 days, and $t_{1/2}$ are 35 and 15 days, respectively. Information is not available for cattle after topical administration.

(4) When administered topically in cattle, no preslaughter or milk withdrawal period is required, since drug residue levels are below legally acceptable limits in meat and milk after topical administration.

d. Adverse effects. Adverse effects of moxidectin are similar to those of ivermectin. The topical product for dogs and cats should not be administered orally; the adverse effects can be very severe when administered orally.

E. **Miscellaneous antinematodal drugs**

1. Dichlorvos (Atgard®), an organophosphate, is marketed for use in pigs only.

a. **Mechanism of action.** Dichlorvos inhibits ACh breakdown by irreversibly inhibiting ACh esterase (AChE). (See Figure 2-6 for illustration.)

b. **Therapeutic uses.** Dichlorvos is effective against major GI worms, for example, whipworms, nodular worms, *Strongyloides*, hookworms, and ascarids in pigs. It has little or no activity against migrating larvae of ascarids and hookworms.

c. **Pharmacokinetics.** Dichlorvos is a lipophilic liquid that is incorporated into polyvinyl chloride resin pellets. As these pellets traverse the GI tract, dichlorvos diffuses into the intestinal fluid, allowing the drug to come into contact with nematodes. The pellets release ~50% of the drug in 48 hours. When passed into the feces, the pellets still contain ~50% of the original dose of dichlorvos, enough to kill fecal fly larvae. Information regarding elimination and $t_{1/2}$ of dichlorvos is not available.

d. **Adverse effects.** Accumulation of ACh by dichlorvos can stimulate cholinergic receptors to induce the SLUDD (salivation, lacrimation, urination, diarrhea, dyspnea) syndrome. Acute death may result from respiratory paralysis and cardiovascular arrest.

e. **Contraindications.** Dichlorvos is not to be given to weak animals, those exposed to other anti-cholinesterase (anti-ChE) agents, or those with GI disorders.

2. **Piperazine**

a. **Chemistry.** Piperazine is available in adipate, citrate, hydrochloride, tartrate, and phosphate forms. Piperazine is inactivated by moisture, CO_2, and light; therefore, containers should be tightly closed and protected from light.

b. **Mechanism of action.** Piperazine is a GABA-receptor agonist that hyperpolarizes nematode muscle, causing flaccid paralysis of worms (Figure 16-4).

c. **Therapeutic uses.** Piperazine has a limited spectrum of action but is effective against ascarids and nodular worms in all species; however, its use is limited in ruminants, because ascarids are not a significant problem in this species.

d. **Pharmacokinetics**

(1) **Absorption.** Piperazine salts are well absorbed from the GI tract.

(2) **Metabolism and excretion.** Some piperazine is metabolized in the liver and the remainder (30–40%) is excreted in the urine. Urinary excretion of piperazine starts as early as 30 minutes after dosing, and is complete within 24 hours. The plasma $t_{1/2}$ is ~2 hours.

e. **Adverse effects.** Piperazine is a safe drug, but large doses may produce vomiting, diarrhea, and ataxia. The ataxia is due to a GABA-mimetic effect of piperazine on CNS neurons and is particularly seen in young animals given high doses.

3. **Emodepside**

a. **Chemistry.** Emodepside is a semisynthetic cyclic depsipeptide.

b. **Mechanism of action.** Is a selective agonist of the presynaptic latrophilin receptor, a G_q-coupled receptor, of nematodes, which increases the release of inhibitory neuropeptides PF1 and PF2, and opens C_a^{2+}-activated K^+ channels, thereby causing flaccid paralysis of the locomotive and pharyngeal muscles in nematodes (Figure 16-4).

c. **Therapeutic uses.** It is used topically (as a spot-on product) with an anticestodal drug praziquantel (Profender®) for the treatment of nematodes in cats. Emodepside is effective against ascarids and hookworms (mature and immature adults as well as L_4 larvae). Cost of production has prevented the marketing of emodepside for large animals.

d. **Pharmacokinetics.** The drug is absorbed through the skin and enters the circulation. It appears that from the blood the drug gets deposited into adipose tissue and from these sites leaches back into the blood. The drug is eliminated via the bile and leaves in the feces mainly as unmodified emodepside. T_{max} is 40 hours and $t_{1/2}$ is 8.3 days.

e. **Adverse effects.** Alopecia may be seen at the application site. Salivation and vomiting may occur, which is due to licking the application site. Tremors may show up when cats are overdosed with emodepside. Do not use in kittens under 8 weeks of age. It is safe to be used in pregnant and lactating cats.

III. DRUGS FOR HEARTWORM PREVENTION AND THERAPY

A. **Introduction.** Treatment and prevention of heartworm involve three aspects as follows:

1. **Removal of adult heartworms** requires an adulticide.
2. Interruption of the life cycle requires a microfilaricide. Treatment to eliminate microfilaria should be initiated 3–4 weeks after the adulticide treatment. Some clinicians choose not to treat microfilaria.
   a. **Microfilaricidal treatment** reduces the incidence of glomerulonephritis, which may be induced when microfilaria are present in a large number.
   b. Microfilaricidal treatment eliminates the source of heartworm infestation (minor reason for eliminating microfilaria).
3. **Prevention of infection** requires a larvicide.

B. **Adulticides eliminate both immature (L$_5$) and adult heartworms. The heartworm adulticide melarsomine is used solely in canine species. Cats should not receive this adulticide treatment because of potential severe reactions occur when heartworms are killed in this species.**

1. **Melarsomine (Immiticide®)**
   a. **Chemistry.** Melarsomine is a trivalent arsenic compound.
   b. **Administration.** Melarsomine is administered into lumbar muscle.
      (1) The regular dose regimen is 2.5 mg/kg once a day for 2 days.
         (a) Since melarsomine is highly irritable, the first injection should be into the right lumbar muscle, and the second into the left lumbar muscle.
         (b) The two-dose regimen eliminates all adult heartworms in 60–80% of treated dogs. The regimen can be repeated in 4 months, which would increase the efficacy to 98%.
      (2) For dogs with severe infestation, a single dose (2.5 mg/kg) is followed by the full two-dose treatment 1 month later. The initial single dose would kill 88% of male and 17% of female worms, hence providing some relief of clinical signs, while reducing the risk of complication from pulmonary embolism. This regimen would remove all heartworms in 85% of treated dogs.
   c. **Mechanism of action.** Melarsomine denatures proteins/enzymes by binding to the sulfhydryl groups of cysteine residues.
   d. **Pharmacokinetics**
      (1) **Absorption.** Following IM injection, melarsomine is completely absorbed in 15 minutes and the blood concentration peaks at 8 minutes. The elimination $t_{1/2}$ is ~3 hours.
      (2) **Distribution.** Melarsomine is found in both plasma and red blood cells. The drug is widely distributed in the body, but is concentrated in the liver and kidneys.
      (3) **Metabolism and excretion.** Melarsomine is metabolized in the liver and excreted into bile. Both melarsomine and its metabolites can be found in feces and urine after administration.
   e. **Adverse effects**
      (1) Mild localized edema may occur following IM injection.
      (2) Overdose may result in distress, restlessness, pawing, salivation, vomiting, tachycardia, tachypnea, dyspnea, abdominal pain, hindlimb weakness, and recumbency. Severe cases terminate in circulatory collapse, orthopnea, coma, and death.
      (3) **Liver toxicity.** These **animals may show** anorexia, persistent vomiting, depression, melena, and jaundice. Serum alanine aminotransferase (ALT), alkaline phosphatase (AP), and bilirubin concentrations may increase.
      (4) **Nephrotoxicity.** These animals may show albuminuria, renal case and azotemia with blood urea nitrogen concentration of >100 mg/dL.
      (5) **Toxicity can be alleviated** by IM administration of 3 mg/kg **dimercaprol** (BAL) within 3 hours of the onset of symptoms. However, dimercaprol may reduce the efficacy of melarsomine.

(6) **Thromboembolic pneumonia** may be seen, which is due to dead worms accumulation within 3 weeks of treatment. Signs of pneumonia include coughing, dyspnea, hemoptysis, fever, and lethargy. The affected dogs need absolute rest for 2 weeks, and can be treated with anti-inflammatory drugs, particularly glucocorticoids and antibiotics. **Glucocorticoids can be used to prevent the adulticide-induced thromboembolic pneumonia.**

C. **Microfilaricides.** Some practitioners choose not to use microfilaricide, particularly if dogs do not harbor large number of microfilaria.

1. **Preparations.** Macrocyclic lactones, for example, ivermectin and milbemycin, are used as microfilaricides and this use is extra-label; however, these are the only drugs that may be safely and effectively used for this purpose.
2. **Administration**
   a. **Ivermectin.** Therapy entails one dose (50 μg/kg) administered orally or SC. This drug should not be used in Collies as a microfilaricide.
   b. **Milbemycin.** One dose (0.5 mg/kg) is administered orally; the treatment may be repeated in 2 weeks. This drug can be safely used in Collies.
3. **Adverse effects.** Transient weakness, pale membranes, intestinal hyperperistalsis, and tachypnea may be seen following administration of a microfilaricide, suggesting a mild cardiovascular shock resulting from reactions to dead microfilaria. The higher the microfilaria count, the greater the chance of encountering noticeable adverse effects. These adverse effects can be treated or prevented with glucocorticoids.

D. **Larvicides for heartworm prevention.** Macrocyclic lactones (e.g., ivermectin, moxidectin, milbemycin, and selamectin)

1. **Administration.** Macrocyclic lactones kill L_4 larvae. Ivermectin, moxidectin, and milbemycin are administered orally at dosages of 6–12 μg/kg, 3 μg/kg, and 500 μg/kg, respectively, once a month. The first dose is given within 1 month of the first exposure to mosquitoes. The last dose is given within 1 month following the last exposure to mosquitoes. Because it takes 2.5 months for L_4 larvae to develop into L_5 larvae, the elimination of larvae in the L_4 stage once a month is sufficient to prevent heartworm infestation.
2. **See II D 2, 5–7 for other information on mechanism of action, pharmacokinetics, and adverse effects of macrocyclic lactones.**

IV. ANTICETODAL DRUGS

A. Introduction

1. **These agents kill tapeworms and are called taeniacides**, as opposed to arecoline, an obsolete taeniafuge that only paralyzes them.
2. Worms killed by these drugs may be digested by the host animal; therefore, the killed worms may not be evident in the feces.
3. **Control of intermediate hosts** (e.g., fleas for *Dipylidium*, rodents for *Taenia* and *Echinococcus*, and mites for *Anoplocephala* and *Moniezia*.)

B. Dichlorophene

1. **Therapeutics uses.** Dichlorophene is used to treat *Taenia* and *Dipylidium* infestations in dogs and cats. Its efficacy against *Echinococcus* is variable.
2. **Administration.** Dichlorophene is best given orally after an overnight fast.
3. **Mechanism of action.** Dichlorophene causes uncoupling of oxidative phosphorylation to deplete ATP from tapeworms and disrupts the pH difference across the external tegumental membranes
4. **Pharmacokinetics.** No information is available.

5. **Adverse effects.** Vomiting and diarrhea may be seen after dichlorophene administration.

C. **Benzimidazoles. Fenbendazole, oxfendazole, and albendazole** are effective against mature *Taenia* and *Echinococcus* in dogs and cats, and *Moniezia* in ruminants. They may kill intermediate hydatid cysts of *Taenia* in infected cattle and sheep. These agents are not effective against *Dipylidium*. (See II A for basic information regarding benzimidazoles.)

D. **Praziquantel (Droncit®, Drontal®, Drontal® Plus, Zimecterin®, Equimax®, Quest® Plus)**

1. **Therapeutic uses.** Praziquantel is effective against all species of tapeworms and kills both adult and juvenile stages of the worms. However, its activity against hydatid cysts is erratic. It is also available in combination with pyrantel pamoate, ivermectin, and moxidectin to kill nematodes.

2. **Mechanism of action.** Praziquantel causes paralysis and digestion of tapeworms as well as irreversible focal vacuolization and disintegration of integument. The mechanism of action involves the selective binding of praziquantel to the β-subunit of the voltage-dependent Ca^{2+} channel of the susceptible parasites. The increased opening of the Ca^{2+} channels in the parasite mediates an excessive increase in intracellular Ca^{2+} concentrations and cell autolysis.

3. **Administration**
   a. Praziquantel is approved for dogs, cats, and horses, and has been used in other animals.
   b. Praziquantel is administered orally or SC. Fasting before oral administration is not necessary.

4. **Pharmacokinetics**
   a. **Absorption.** Praziquantel is completely absorbed within 2 hours of oral administration. The information is not available for absorption from the injection site.
   b. **Distribution.** It is distributed throughout the body, including the CNS.
   c. **Metabolism and excretion.** Praziquantel is metabolized to unknown compounds in the liver via cytochrome P450 and is excreted primarily in the urine. The elimination $t_{1/2}$ is ~3 hours in dogs. No information is available for other species.

5. **Adverse effects.** Praziquantel is the safest anticestodal drug available.
   a. Overdose induces anorexia, vomiting, salivation, diarrhea, and lethargy in <5% of animals.
   b. It exerts no teratogenic or embryotoxic effects.

E. **Epsiprantel (Cestex®)**, a praziquantel analog, is approved for use in dogs and cats. Epsiprantel is administered orally. Unlike praziquantel, epsiprantel is absorbed poorly after oral administration and most of the drug is eliminated in the feces (<0.1% of the drug is recovered in the urine after dosing).

F. **Pyrantel pamoate.** It is effective against equine tapeworms *Anoplocephala perfoliata* and is administered at 13.2 mg/kg orally (nematocide dose: 6.6 mg/kg). It is not as effective as praziquantel as an anticestodal drug, but was used frequently when praziquantel was expensive to procure. **See II C 2 for basic information regarding pyrantel pamoate.**

V. ANTITREMATODAL DRUGS

A. **General aspect.** Infestation with liver flukes (*Fasciola hepatica*) is the most common and most economically important trematode disease of domestic animals worldwide. Brief information is presented for drugs against lung flukes (*Paragonimus*) in dogs and cats.

1. **Liver fluke disease.** This disease is typically chronic and subclinical in nature.
2. **Both immature and mature liver flukes cause damages.** After metacercaria are ingested by grazing ruminants, the immature flukes emerge from the cysts, penetrate the small intestine wall, traverse the peritoneal cavity, and penetrate into liver within 4 days of infestation. These immature flukes will tunnel through liver tissues, growing rapidly. The extensive damages can cause acute clinical signs of fasciolosis, which occur within 6–8 weeks of inoculation. This stage can be fatal. Scar tissues are present after liver is damaged.
3. During the eighth week of infestation, flukes begin to penetrate the bile duct, where they become mature by 10–12 weeks after infestation. These mature flukes cause biliary inflammation and progressive occlusion.
4. Antitrematodal drugs are highly lipophilic and most of them are only effective against mature flukes, but not immature flukes, that reside in the liver.

B. **Clorsulon** (Curatrem®, Ivomec Plus®). It is a sulfonamide that is effective against both mature and immature *F. hepatica* in cattle.

1. **Therapeutic uses.** Clorsulon is the most effective drug against *F. hepatica*, killing both mature and immature flukes in cattle. However, its activity against *F. magna* is fair to poor; it is not effective against rumen flukes or lung flukes. Clorsulon is administered at 7 mg/kg orally, or 2 mg/kg SC (Ivomec Plus®). Treatment is done in late fall and early spring (in snail seasons).
2. **Mechanism of action.** Clorsulon inhibits 3-phosphoglycerate kinase and phosphoglyceromutase in the glycolytic pathway, depriving the flukes of a metabolic energy source.
3. **Pharmacokinetics.** Clorsulon is lipid soluble. After oral dosing, it is absorbed rapidly. Peak blood levels occur within 4 hours after oral administration. Biotransformation of clorsulon plays only a minor role in the elimination of this compound. Thus, clorsulon is eliminated from the body mostly in the unchanged form in both feces and urine. The preslaughter withdrawal period is 8 days. When used in combination with ivermectin (Ivomec Plus®), the preslaughter withdrawal period is 49 days, which reflects the long persistence of ivermectin. Clorsulon should not be used in lactating dairy cattle.
4. **Adverse effects.** When used as directed, adverse effects are rare. Clorsulon is safe in pregnant and breeding animals.

C. **Albendazole** (see II B) is approved for use against mature liver flukes (e.g., *F. hepatica*) in cattle. Albendazole requires a 27-day preslaughter withdrawal period. Because albendazole is a teratogen, it cannot be used in pregnant cattle during the first 45 days of gestation or in female dairy cattle of breeding age.

D. **Praziquantel** (see IV D) is effective against lung flukes in dogs. It is also effective against liver flukes; however, it is too expensive for use in ruminants.

VI. ANTHELMINTIC RESISTANCE IN LARGE ANIMALS

A. **Definition.** When a greater frequency of individuals in a parasite population no longer responds to the normal clinical dose for treatment.

1. Anthelmintic resistance ***affects agricultural incomes*** and the increase in disease also poses a ***threat to animal welfare***. The absence of alternative methods of worm control means that we should understand how resistance works and thus predict successful methods for limiting the development of resistance as much as possible.

B. **Mechanisms of resistance**

1. A change in the molecular target so that the drug no longer recognizes the target and is therefore ineffective.

2. A change in metabolism that removes the drug, for example, up-regulation of the P-glycoprotein exporter in the worm.

3. A change in the distribution of the drug in the target organism that prevents the drug from getting to its site of action.

4. Amplification of target genes to overcome the drug action.

C. **Resistance is inherited**

1. For each chemical class of anthelmintic, resistance to one member usually confers resistance to others of the same chemical class. It is possible to have *multiple resistances*, where parasites develop resistance to several anthelmintic classes.

2. When a new anthelmintic chemical class is introduced, the frequency of resistance alleles is low, and it is assumed that in the absence of treatment, resistance alleles confer a neutral or negative reproductive fitness. Resistance is a consequence of drug use, and selection for resistance will depend on the relative reproductive fitness of the susceptible and resistant alleles at the level of drug used. Thus, the development of resistance is a Darwinian process and the selection pressure is the anthelmintic.

D. **Detecting resistance**

1. Most detection of anthelmintic resistance involves the treatment of infected hosts with a recommended dose of drug followed by a *fecal egg count reduction test* that compares pretreatment egg counts with those of untreated controls. Reductions of <*95%* (based on group arithmetic means) score as clinical resistance.

2. In small ruminants, anthelmintic-resistant nematodes are now a serious problem. Resistance has arisen to all of the major families of broad-spectrum anthelmintics, the BZD, levamisole, in addition to the avermectins and milbemycins (AM) (including ivermectin, doramectin, and moxidectin).

3. In cattle, the situation is currently less severe, but there are cattle nematodes resistant to multiple anthelmintic classes in New Zealand, South America, and now in the United States.

4. In horses, BZD resistance is widespread among the cyathostomes. The AM are still effective for cyathostomes, but not for parascaris in foals. This could change as AM are used more frequently and selection pressure increases.

E. **Factors affecting the selection of resistance.** There are a number of factors that affect the selection pressure for resistance that are not under management control.

1. Parasite genetics

a. Resistance alleles might be dominant, as suggested for resistance to the avermectins and/or milbemycins. If *heterozygotes are resistant, then clinical resistance* will be apparent at much lower allele frequencies than if resistance is recessive.

b. The *fewer the genes* the faster resistance will develop.

c. The *high genetic diversity of parasitic helminthes*, coupled with their large populations, increases the likelihood that resistance alleles will already be present in a population, possibly at relatively high frequency.

d. *If resistant worms have enhanced fitness* compared to susceptible individuals, then resistance will spread faster in the population.

2. Parasite biology

a. *Parasites that have a short generation time and high fecundity* increase the speed of resistance development. Production of many individuals of several generations in a short time increases the spread of resistance alleles through the population.

b. *Direct life cycles* mean that the fitness associated with resistance alleles is not dissipated by passage through an intermediate host.

c. Parasite populations that are mobile, especially if the *hosts are moved,* increase the spread of resistance.

pool of animals releasing resistant L₃

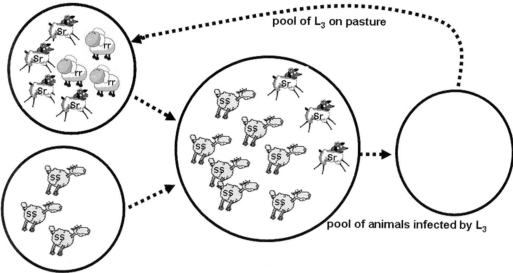

pool of animals releasing sensitive L₃

FIGURE 16-7. Diagram of the different "pools" of nematode larvae being released onto pasture. S represents dominant susceptible genes; r represents the recessive resistant genes. Infected animals release eggs that develop to infective L₃ larvae. These larvae infect preferentially young animals that have not developed immunity to the parasites. Adult parasites are then produced in these infected animals that release eggs with genes determined the infecting parasites. The aim of management procedures should be to recognize how different management procedures may produce a buildup of rr (resistant recessive) in the pool of L₃ on the pasture that lead to build up of resistant parasites.

    d. There might be low levels of resistance in untreated parasites in ***refugia.*** This slows resistance. ***What are refugia?*** They are subpopulations of parasites that are not selected by drug treatment. They are important because the higher the proportion of the population in refugia, the slower the selection for resistance. Examples of refugia are organisms in the environment (e.g., larvae on pasture) or inhibited larvae (especially encysted equine cyathostomes) that are not susceptible to the effects of some drugs (Figure 16-7).

F. **Management factors that affect the development of resistance.** Drugs should be used in ways that *maintain refugia.*

    1. It is important to ***avoid under-dosing*** and insure that treatments are fully efficacious.

    2. Treatments should be planned, through timing and management, to ***reduce the survival of free-living resistant stages in the environment***. Where practical, the access of free-living stages to the next host should be reduced by measures such as ***removal of feces and alternate grazing of different hosts.***

    3. The ***pharmacokinetics of the drug***—it is preferable to use short-acting drugs to prevent worms being exposed to the subtherapeutic concentrations that result from an extended $t_{1/2}$ of a drug, for example, a macrocyclic lactone.

    4. Use of other ***control methods to complement anthelmintics, or use alternative anthelmintics with a different mechanism of action***.

    5. The inherent ***nature of the chemical*** and its ability to select for resistance. It should be recognized that some anthelmintics allow resistance to emerge faster than others (fenbendazole is likely to be faster than ivermectin).

G. **Options available when dealing with anthelmintic resistance**

1. There is no evidence for reversion to anthelmintic susceptibility, even where the drug has been withdrawn. In the short- to medium-term, there are no realistic alternatives to the continued use of current chemicals for parasite control.
2. Pasture management can reduce the number of anthelmintic treatments required, but cannot replace them.
3. Effective vaccines, new cost-effective compounds, and nonchemical means of control are all some distance in the future—so it is vital that we maintain the efficacy of current treatments for as long as possible.
4. Reduce practices that encourage the emergence and spread of resistance. Selection pressure for resistance is largely affected by the degree of *refugia*. Experimental and field studies have suggested that **treating selected animals on the basis of infection** do not need to have negative effects on production yields and such strategies could reduce the selection pressure for resistance by increasing refugia.

H. **Management in endemic regions**

1. **Sustainability** of any approach is difficult to determine. Where **pathogenic species** such as *H. contortus* are dominant, parasite control is required and there is less choice for using nonchemical control.
2. Assuming drug use is required, there are several ways to use them to reduce the selection for resistance. Wherever possible, **treatment should be confined to animals suffering from parasitism**, and animals that can tolerate existing infections should be left untreated, thereby leaving unselected refugia. Such approaches mean that the host suffers some parasitism, and producers could experience some loss of productivity. Ideally, treatment on an individual basis requires the identification of those animals to be treated.

I. **Nonchemical methods**

1. When additional pastures or other stock (such as older sheep, cattle, or horses) are available, worms can be controlled by alternate grazing.
2. Energy and protein supplements are useful in stimulating immunity.
3. In hot moist climates, where rapid development occurs all year, rotation of pastures systems is useful.
4. For horse parasites, breaking the life cycle of the worm is a possibility. Removal of feces from pastures removes most sources of reinfection including resistant worms.
5. Host selection, through testing for worm immunity or genetic correlates, one can improve herd immunity to parasites.

J. **Quarantine**

1. Quarantine treatments, using mixtures of anthelmintic classes, are expected to exclude parasites.
2. They could theoretically select for high levels of resistance, but the alleles will be present anyway (in worms in untreated hosts).

VII. **ANTIPROTOZOAL DRUGS.** This discussion focuses on anticoccidial drugs, drugs for the treatment of equine protozoal myeloencephalitis (EPM), toxoplasmosis, giardiasis, babesiosis, and cryptosporidiosis.

A. **Aniticoccidial drugs**

1. **Introduction**
   a. **Financial implications of coccidiosis.** Coccidiosis, a prevalent disease in calves, piglets, and poultry, costs the US poultry industry >50 million dollars annually, despite the expenditures of >85 million for anticoccidial drugs. These losses are

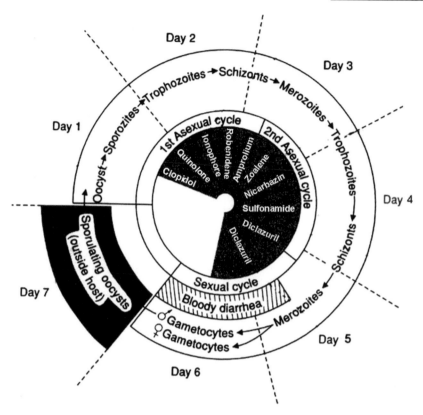

FIGURE 16-8. Life cycle of avian coccidia and the effects of anticoccidial drugs on the life cycle. All drugs are effective during the asexual cycle only, except that diclazuril is also effective during the sexual cycle. Second generation schizonts seem to play an important role in gut damages; drugs affecting this stage can be used to treat outbreak. (Modified from W. M. Reid, *Am. J. Vet. Res.*, 36:593, 1975.)

caused primarily by impaired feed conversion, slow growth, and the poor quality of carcasses at processing.

  b. Therapeutic approaches
    (1) Poultry. Most of the anticoccidial drugs discussed in this section are used in chickens.
      (a) Broilers are not vaccinated against coccidia because latent infection may retard growth.
      (b) Layers are vaccinated against coccidia. Outbreaks are usually treated with a sulfonamide or diclazuril on an as-needed basis.
    (2) Sulfonamides and ormetoprim, diclazuril can be used to treat infected animals, while clopidol, decoquinate, zoalene, amprolium, robenidine, nicarbazin, and Na^+ ionophores can be used to prevent coccidiosis.
  c. Resistance to anticoccidial drugs is minimized by using two or more drugs sequentially. Overemphasized switching may decrease immunity.
  d. Life cycle of avian coccidia (Figure 16-8)
2. Anticoccidial agents
  a. Decoquinate
    (1) Chemistry. Decoquinate is a quinolone and is lipophilic.
    (2) Therapeutic uses
      (a) Decoquinate is approved for use in cattle, sheep, goats, and broilers for the prevention of coccidiosis. It is not effective to treat clinical coccidiosis. It is usually used as a feed additive.

(b) It is effective against all species of coccidia on the sporozoites stage. Use is limited because of its tendency to induce drug resistance (due to its action on such an early stage of the asexual cycle).

(3) Mechanism of action. It halts the development of the sporozoites or trophozoites of coccidia by inhibiting the electron transport system within parasite mitochondria. This action is coccidiostatic. In addition, it may block DNA synthesis by inhibiting DNA gyrase.

(4) Pharmacokinetics. No information is located. No preslaughter withdrawal period is required. Do not feed to cows, sheep, and goats producing milk for food. Do not use in laying chickens.

(5) Adverse effects. No adverse effects are seen when the drug is used as directed.

b. Clopidol (Coyden® 25)

(1) Chemistry. Clopidol is a pyridinol derivative and is lipophilic.

(2) Therapeutic uses

(a) It is used as a feed additive to prevent coccidiosis in broilers and replacement chickens.

(b) It is effective against all species of coccidia on the sporozoites stage. Use is limited because of its tendency to induce drug resistance (due to its action on such an early stage of the asexual cycle).

(3) Mechanism of action. Clopidol may work similarly to quinolones.

(4) Pharmacokinetics. No information is located. No preslaughter withdrawal period is required.

(5) Adverse effects. No adverse effects are seen when the drug is used as directed.

c. Zoalene (dinitolmide, Zoamix®)

(1) Chemistry. It is a nitrobenzamide.

(2) Therapeutic uses

(a) Zoalene is to be fed continuously as an aid for the prevention and control of cecal and intestinal coccidiosis in chickens and intestinal coccidiosis in turkeys. It is not for use in laying birds.

(b) It is effective against all species of coccidia in chickens on the first schizont stage and can inhibit sporulation of oocysts. Zoalene is often used in combination with other coccidiostats.

(3) Mechanism of action. Unknown. It might act like nitroimidazoles; it destroys DNA of parasites.

(4) Pharmacokinetics. No information is located. No preslaughter withdrawal period is required.

(5) Adverse effects. No adverse effects are seen when the drug is used as directed.

d. Na⁺ ionophores

(1) Preparations include monensin, lasalocid, narasin, salinomycin, and semduramicin. These antibiotics are used exclusively as anticoccidial drugs.

(2) Therapeutic uses

(a) Na⁺ ionophores are effective against all coccidia species in chickens, cattle, and goats.

   i. Monensin is for use in cattle, goats, and broilers.

   ii. Lasalocid is for use in cattle and chickens for prevention of coccidiosis.

   iii. Narasin, salinomycin, and semduramicin are for use in poultry only.

   iv. Na⁺ ionophores attack the first generation of trophozoites and schizonts.

   v. The preslaughter withdrawal is not required. Do not use in veal calves. Monensin and lasalocid can be used in lactating cows; the milk from these animals can be safely consumed by humans.

   vi. Monensin and lasalocid are also used as growth promoters.

(3) Mechanism of action. Na⁺ ionophores facilitate the transport of Na⁺ and H⁺ into cells in the rumen, elevating intracellular Na⁺ and H⁺

concentrations. As a result, certain mitochondrial functions (e.g., substrate oxidations) and ATP hydrolysis are inhibited. Excess intracellular Na^+ concentrations accompanied by water can damage organelles as well.

(4) **Pharmacokinetics**

(a) **Monensin in chickens.** Following oral dosing, plasma T_{max} is ~0.5 hours and plasma $t_{1/2}$ is ~2 hours. No monensin is detectable in all tissues within 48 hours of dosing, except for liver, which becomes undetectable within 72 hours of administration.

(b) **Lasalocid in chickens.** Following oral administration, $t_{1/2}$ of serum, liver, and muscle are 11, 36, and 41 hours, respectively.

(c) **Salinomycin in chickens.** Following oral administration, residues are present only at very low concentrations in liver and muscle that fall below the limit of decision of the assay within 2 days.

(d) No information is available for narasin and semduramicin.

(e) No elimination information is available for mammals regarding Na^+ ionophores.

(f) In all species, Na^+ ionophores are metabolized in the liver by cytochrome P450 enzymes, and are excreted mostly into bile and feces as parent compound and metabolites.

(5) **Adverse effects.** These drugs may cause severe cardiovascular and skeletal muscular side effects.

(a) Increased intracellular Na^+ concentrations will damage mitochondria and Golgi body.

(b) In animal cells, intracellular Na^+ further exchanges for extracellular Ca^{2+}, thereby increasing intracellular Ca^{2+} concentrations ($[Ca^{2+}]_i$). Lasalocid may directly facilitate Ca^{2+} transport into the cells. High $[Ca^{2+}]_i$ in cardiac and skeletal muscle cells are responsible for the main toxic effects of these drugs in animals.

(c) High $[Ca^{2+}]_i$ in chromaffin cells increase catecholamine secretion can further jeopardize the cardiac arrhythmia. High $[Ca^{2+}]_i$ in endocrine cells increase various hormone secretions.

(6) **Contraindications.** Horses and turkeys are very sensitive to Na^+ ionophores. Accidental consumption by these animals can be fatal.

e. **Amprolium**

(1) **Chemistry.** Amprolium is an analog of thiamine, and is a quaternary compound.

(2) **Therapeutic uses.** Amprolium is the only anticoccidial agent that can be used in laying birds and cattle for both the prevention and treatment of outbreaks.

(a) It is effective against the first generation of trophozoites and schizonts.

(b) Amprolium is rarely used alone, because *E. maxima*, *E. mivati*, and other species are resistant to it; combination with antifolate drugs increases the efficacy of amprolium against these organisms in chickens.

(3) **Mechanism of action.** Amprolium prevents coccidia from utilizing thiamine by blocking thiamine receptors.

(4) **Pharmacokinetics**

(a) Amprolium is poorly absorbed after oral administration.

(b) No preslaughter withdrawal period is necessary.

(5) **Adverse effects.** Amprolium is a safe drug when used as directed. Neurological signs and lesions of thiamine deficiency may occur in the host following extremely high overdoses.

f. **Nicarbazin**

(1) **Chemistry.** Nicarbazin is a mixture of 4,4'-dinitrocarbanilide (DNC) and 2-hydroxy-4,6-dimethylpyrimidine (HOP).

(2) **Therapeutic uses.** Nicarbazin is approved for use in chickens to prevent coccidiosis outbreaks.

(a) It is effective against all *Eimeria* species.

(b) Its peak activity is on second-generation trophozoites.

(3) Mechanism of action. Nicarbazin's mechanism of action is unknown; however, it is thought to be via inhibition of succinate-linked NAD reduction and the energy-dependent transhydrogenase, and the accumulation of Ca^{2+} in the presence of ATP.

(4) Pharmacokinetics

   (a) Absorption. DNC and HOP are absorbed separately from the digestive tract. DNC is absorbed more rapidly but disappears more slowly from the tissues than HOP.

   (b) A 4-day withdrawal period is required before broilers are marketed.

(5) Adverse effects

   (a) Nicarbazin may bleach brown-shelled eggs, cause mottled egg yolks and poor hatchability, and impair egg production.

   (b) Medicated broilers may be more susceptible to heat stress.

g. Robenidine

   (1) Therapeutic uses. Robenidine is approved for use in chickens to prevent outbreaks of coccidiosis. It is effective against all *Eimeria* species.

   (2) Mechanism of action. The mechanism of action is undetermined. Its peak activity is on the first generation schizonts.

   (3) Pharmacokinetics. The pharmacokinetics of robenidine are not well understood.

   (4) Adverse effects. Robenidine imparts an unpleasant taste to the flesh of broilers, if therapy is not terminated 5 days before slaughter. The taste is imparted to eggs when birds are fed at dosages equal to or greater than 66 ppm. The ability of humans to taste robenidine is apparently genetically linked.

h. Sulfonamides have the longest history of use as anticoccidial drugs. These agents are discussed in detail in Chapter 15.

   (1) Preparations. Sulfonamides used most frequently as anticoccidial agents include **sulfadimethoxine, sulfamethazine, and sulfaquinoxaline** (long-acting sulfonamides).

   (2) Mechanism of action. See Chapter 15 for information.

   (3) Therapeutic uses. These drugs are used for both the prevention and treatment of coccidiosis outbreaks in all species.

   (a) They are more effective against the intestinal than cecal species of coccidia.

   (b) Their peak activity is against the second-generation schizonts.

   (c) Use of these drugs does not impair immunity development.

i. Dihydrofolate reductase inhibitors

   (1) Preparations include ormetoprim and pyrimethamine. Pyrimethamine is not approved for food animal use.

   (2) Mechanism of action. See Chapter 15 for information.

   (3) Therapeutic uses. The anticoccidial effects of ormetoprim and pyrimethamine are synergistic with sulfonamides. They are used to treat coccidiosis outbreaks. The preslaughter withdrawal period for sulfadimethoxine-ormetoprim in poultry is 5 days.

   (4) Pharmacokinetics. After oral administration, therapeutic levels of ormetoprim are maintained for ≥ 24 hours. Other information is not available for animals.

j. Diclazuril (Clinacox®)

   (1) Chemistry. It is one of benzeneacetonitriles that have potent anticoccidial activity. Diclazuril is a slightly yellowish to beige powder, and it is almost insoluble in water.

   (2) Mechanism of action. Diclazuril is effective against schizonts and gametes by inhibiting nuclear division.

   (3) Therapeutic uses. It is used as a feed additive to prevent coccidiosis in broilers. Since it is effective against later stages of coccidia, it has potential to be used for treating outbreaks of coccidiosis. It could be used in an extra-label manner to treat mammalian coccidiosis, EPM, and toxoplasmosis.

(4) Pharmacokinetics

   (a) Following oral administration to chickens, plasma concentrations of di-clazuril peak at 6 hours. The plasma and tissue $t_{1/2}$ are ~50 hours. There is a rapid equilibrium between plasma and tissue concentrations of the drug.

   (b) The tissue concentrations are 2–10 times lower than the corresponding plasma concentrations. The liver and the kidneys have the highest concentrations of the drug.

   (c) Diclazuril is excreted in the urine mostly as the parent compound. About 50% of the dose is excreted within 24 hours, and >95% after 10 days.

   (d) There is no preslaughter withdrawal time in broilers, since the tissue levels of diclazuril are below minimal limit after oral administration. Diclazuril is not for use in laying hens.

(5) Adverse effects. Diclazuril is a safe drug when use as directed.

k. Toltrazuril and ponazuril (extra-label use). Ponazuril is toltrazuril sulfone, an active metabolite of toltrazuril.

   (1) Mechanism of action. Toltrazuril and ponazuril are effective against schizonts and gametes by inhibiting nuclear division.

   (2) Therapeutic uses. These are very effective drugs against coccidia, but not yet approved by FDA for such a use. Ponazuril is approved for use to control EPM.

   (3) Pharmacokinetics of toltrazuril. After oral administration to piglets and calves, toltrazuril is absorbed slowly by the gut, which is followed by long-lasting distribution among the different compartments of the body. The plasma $t_{1/2}$ is 51 hours in piglets. Excretion is mostly into feces. There is no significant enterohepatic circulation of toltrazuril. Two metabolites of toltrazuril, both oxidation products, toltrazuril sulfoxide and toltrazuril sulfone (ponazuril), are found in the tissues and organs of piglets.

   (4) Adverse effects. They include GI disturbances (e.g., vomiting, diarrhea, and inappetence) and hypersensitivity.

l. Drugs for the control of mammalian coccidiosis. Decoquinate, amprolium, monensin, lasalocid, sulfonamides with a dihydrofolate reductase inhibitor, diclazuril, toltrazuril, and ponazuril can be used to prevent coccidiosis. Sulfonamides with a dihydrofolate reductase inhibitor, diclazuril, toltrazuril, and ponazuril can be used to treat outbreaks of coccidiosis.

B. **Drugs for the treatment of EPM**

1. Introduction. EPM is the most important equine protozoal disease in the United States, which is caused by *Sarcocystis neurona*. Opossum is the definitive host and small mammals including cats, skunks, and raccoons are intermediate hosts. Horse is considered an aberrant, dead-end host for *S. neurona*. Horses are infected by ingestion of sporocysts in contaminated feed or water. The schizonts of the asexual cycle are found in CNS, which cause cerebral damages. The signs of the infection are manifested by head tilt, ataxia, muscle weakness and atrophy, urinary incontinence, and constipation.

2. Treatment of EPM

   a. Trimethoprim-sulfadiazine and pyrimethamine, PO, daily for ≥30 days (see Chapter 15, for information on these two drugs).

   b. Ponazuril (Marquis®), PO, 5 mg/kg/day, 28–56 days.

   c. Diclazuril (Protazil®), PO, 1 mg/kg/day, 28 days.

   d. Nitazoxanide (Navigator®), PO, days 1–5: 25 mg/kg; days 6–28: 50 mg/kg.

   e. Anti-inflammatory agents. Flunixin, phenylbutazone, and glucocorticoid can be used to control inflammation.

   f. Folic acid/folinic acid for protecting bone marrow.

   g. Physical therapy following chemotherapy.

3. Anti-EPM agents

   a. Ponazuril (Marquis®)

    (1) **Chemistry.** An active metabolite of toltrazuril (sulfone). Toltrazuril is a very potent anticoccidial drug, but is not approved for use in the United States. Ponazuril is highly lipophilic.

    (2) **Therapeutic uses.** Ponazuril is for the treatment of EPM, coccidiosis, and toxoplasmosis. For the treatment of EPM, administer the drug orally, 5 mg/kg/day, for ≥4 weeks. Relapse occurs in 5–30% cases.

    (3) **Mechanism of action.** Ponazuril is against schizonts by inhibiting nuclear division.

    (4) **Pharmacokinetics.** After daily (5 mg/kg) oral administration to horses, ponazuril reaches its peak plasma levels in ~18 days and peak CSF levels in ~15 days. Peak CSF levels are 5% of those found in the plasma. Since it is a lipophilic drug, it is better absorbed on a full stomach. The drug should be given immediately after a grain meal. The elimination $t_{1/2}$ of ponazuril is 4.5 days.

    (5) **Adverse effects.** They include blisters on the nose and mouth, skin rash, hives, diarrhea, colic, and seizures. Do not use in sick or debilitated animals due to other disorders.

  b. Diclazuril (Protazil®). The therapeutic uses, mechanism of action, and adverse effects of diclazuril are the same as those of ponzuril in horses.

    (1) **Pharmacokinetics.** Diclazuril is rapidly absorbed after oral administration, with peak plasma concentrations occurring at 8–24 hours and a plasma $t_{1/2}$ of ~43 hours. When 1 mg/kg of diclazuril is administered PO daily for 21 days, mean steady-state levels of 20–70 ng/mL in the CSF is reached. The proliferation of *S. neurona* is 95% inhibited by diclazuril ≥1 ng/mL.

  c. Nitazoxanide (Navigator®)

    (1) **Chemistry.** It is a nitrothiazolyl-salicylamide derivative, which is a light yellow powder and is lipophilic.

    (2) **Mechanism of action.** Nitazoxanide is metabolized into a toxic-free radical from the "nitro" group, which blocks cellular respiration of protozoans.

    (3) **Therapeutic uses.** 32% nitazoxanide paste is used orally for the treatment of EPM. During days 1–5, 25 mg/kg; and days 6–28, 50 mg/kg. Nitazoxanide is also used in humans to treat cryptosporidiosis and giardiasis.

    (4) **Pharmacokinetics.** Following oral administration in horses, nitazoxanide is absorbed. Time to peak plasma level is 2 hours. Since it is a lipophilic drug, it is better absorbed on a full stomach. The drug should be given immediately after a grain meal. It is bound by albumin vividly. The free form of nitazoxanide is metabolized into acetyl-nitazoxanide and acetyl-nitazoxanide glucuronide and eliminated in 24 hours in the urine, bile, and feces.

    (5) **Adverse effects.** They include GI disturbances (anorexia, diarrhea, colic, etc.), enterocolitis, fever, and anaphylaxis (laminitis, edema, etc.). These signs constitute the "treatment crisis"; one may need to suspend therapy in horses with treatment crisis.

    (6) **Contraindications.** It should not be administered to horses that are <1 year old; sick or debilitated for other reasons including hepatic and renal disorders.

C. | **Metronidazole (Flagyl®)**

  1. Chemistry. A nitroimidazole antiprotozoal and antibacterial agent, metronidazole is lipophilic.

  2. Mechanism of action. A ferrodoxin-linked metabolite of metronidazole disrupts DNA synthesis in protozoans and bacteria. See Chapter 15 for more information.

  3. Therapeutic uses. Metronidazole is a broad-spectrum antiprotozoal drug that is effective against *giardia, histomonas, babesia, trichomonas,* and *ameba.* It is approved as a human drug, and has been used largely in small animals.

  4. Pharmacokinetics

    a. Absorption. The oral bioavailability of metronidazole in animals varies 50–100%. If given in food, absorption is enhanced, attributable to increased bile secretion that helps dissolve metronidazole. Peak blood levels occur within 1 hour of administration.

b. **Distribution.** Metronidazole is rapidly and widely distributed after oral absorption, because it is highly lipophilic.

c. **Metabolism and excretion.** Metronidazole undergoes hydroxylation and conjugation in the liver. Both metabolites and parent drug are eliminated in the urine and feces in 24 hours. The elimination $t_{1/2}$ is 4–5 hours in dogs.

5. **Adverse effects.** High doses of metronidazole or prolonged administration may induce lethargy, weakness, ataxia, rigidity, anorexia, vomiting, diarrhea, reversible leukopenia, and hepatotoxicity. Because metronidazole affects DNA synthesis, it may have teratogenic and carcinogenic effects.

D. **Other drugs for treatment of giardiasis—Albendazole and fenbendazole** administered orally at 25 mg/kg every 12 hours for 2 days. Albendazole may be toxic to liver and bone marrow and is a teratogen.

E. **Drugs for treatment of toxoplasmosis**

1. **Trimethoprim-sulfadiazine**, 15 mg/kg, PO, twice a day for 4 weeks.
2. **Pyrimethamine** (0.25–0.5 mg/kg) plus **sulfadiazine** (30 mg/kg), PO, twice a day for 4 weeks.
3. **Clindamycin**, 10–20 mg/kg, PO or IM, twice a day for 3–6 weeks.

F. **Drugs for the treatment of cryptosporidiosis**

1. **Paromomycin (Humatin®).** Paromomycin is an aminoglycoside for extra-label use; it can be very expensive.
   a. **Administration.** It can prevent and treat cryptosporidiosis at 50 mg/kg, PO, twice a day for 10 days.
   b. **Pharmacokinetics.** No information is available for animals. However, GI absorption after oral administration is minimal, since it is an aminoglycoside.
   c. **Adverse effects.** Paromomycin induces vomiting, diarrhea, colic, renal toxicity, and deafness.
2. **Azithromycin** (Zithromax®, 15 mg/kg, PO, twice a day for ≥7 days). It is a macrolide and inhibits protein synthesis.
3. **Nitazoxanide** in used in humans for the treatment of cryptosporidiosis.

G. **Drug for treatment of babesiosis in dogs—Imidocarb (Imizol®)**

1. **Chemistry.** Imidocarb is a diamidine derivative.
2. **Mechanism of action.** Imidocarb binds to DNA and interfere with parasite replication.
3. **Therapeutic uses.** Imidocarb is effective against *Babesia canis* when given at a single dose of 6.6 mg/kg IM or SC. Repeat the dose in 2 weeks. Imidocarb eliminates equine babesia (*B. caballi*) when given 1–2 mg/kg, twice during a 24-hour period. Although effective against bovine babesiosis, imidocarb should not be given to this species because the withdrawal times have not been determined. Feline babesiosis is refractory to imidocarb treatment.
4. **Pharmacokinetics.** Imidocarb is readily absorbed from the injection site. The elimination $t_{1/2}$ is ~3.5 hours. It is excreted mainly into urine and feces as the unchanged compound.
5. **Adverse effects**
   a. **Adverse effects** commonly seen are pain during injection and signs of parasympathetic stimulation such as salivation, nasal drip, or brief episodes of vomiting. Other effects seen less frequently are panting, restlessness, diarrhea, and injection site inflammation lasting one to several days. Atropine sulfate can be used to control the signs of parasympathetic stimulation.
   b. **Imidocarb is a teratogen and carcinogen**, since it affects DNA synthesis. Do not use in pregnant animals.

VIII. EXTERNAL ANTIPARASITICS (ECTOPARASITICIDES)

A. Introduction

1. **Clinical uses.** Insecticides are used (1) on animals to control mites, fleas, ticks, and flies, (2) on the premise to control flies and other insects, and (3) on feedstuffs.
2. **Adverse effects.** Individual animals vary in response to insecticides.
   a. **Age.** Young animals are most susceptible.
   b. **Health.** Healthy animals are least likely to experience adverse effects.
   c. **Stress** (e.g., extremely hot or humid weather) can increase susceptibility to insecticide toxicity.
   d. **Species.** Some species are especially sensitive to insecticides.
      (1) Horses tend to develop urticaria and hyperemia following application of insecticides.
      (2) Cats are very susceptible to cholinergic stimulants.
      (3) Ruminants have less blood ChE than other species; should avoid using anti-ChE agents in ruminants.
      (4) Should avoid applications in extremely hot and humid weather, due to stress-induced enhancement of insecticide toxicity.
3. **Formulations influence the degree of toxicity**, the duration of action, and the convenience of application.
   a. Sprays, dips, and shampoos are suitable when conditions are above freezing.
   b. Pour-ons and dusts can be used when temperature is below freezing.
   c. Oil sprays should be applied to the hair coat but not to the skin, in order to avoid systemic absorption.
   d. Feed additives that are absorbed are effective against bloodsucking parasites. Whether they are absorbed or not, they are effective against both the larval and pupal stages of ectoparasites in the feces.
   e. Collars and ear tags are available.

B. Organophosphates (OPs). Many OPs are still available as insecticides. The withdrawal of chlorinated hydrocarbons from the market increased the importance of OPs, since they cause nil residue problems. However, they could cause serious acute toxicity. The trend to use other safer insecticides is decreasing the use of these agents.

1. **Preparations**
   a. **Thio compounds** include coumaphos, fenthion, diazinon, ethion, famphur, phosmet, and pirimiphos.
   b. **Oxy compounds** include dichlorvos and tetrachlorvinphos.
2. **Mechanism of action.** The OP insecticides inhibit ACh breakdown by inhibiting ChE irreversibly (see Chapter 2). The thio compounds are weak ChE inhibitors and must be metabolized to oxy compounds in order to inhibit ChE effectively.
3. **Pharmacokinetics**
   a. **Absorption.** OPs are lipophilic; thus, they are well absorbed through the skin and GI tract.
   b. **Metabolism.** Metabolism of OPs occurs mainly in the liver.
      (1) Metabolism of OPs may be important for detoxification. Some of the OPs have alkyl moiety and some of them do not. The most important detoxication mechanism of OPs is the removal of the nonalkyl ester moiety by phosphatases or by oxidative reactions. The O-dealkylation of OPs is catalyzed by phosphatases, microsomal oxidases, and alkyl transferase. The hydroxylated OPs can form conjugates with glucuronide or sulfate.
      (2) Metabolism of OPs with thio- moiety into the ones with oxy- moiety will activate the compound to inhibit ChE effectively.
   b. **Excretion.** The organophosphates pose no residue problems since the metabolites are usually excreted into urine.
4. **Administration.** OPs are applied to animals topically or administered orally.

5. **Adverse effects**
   a. **Toxicity** (see Chapter 2 also)
      (1) Clinical signs include SLUDD (salivation, lacrimation, urination, defecation, and dyspnea), fasciculation, ataxia, and convulsions.
      (2) Chronic toxicity or delayed toxicity seen with some OPs is associated with a delayed onset paralysis due to a progressive demylination of motor neurons.
      (3) Treatment involves decontamination and administration of atropine sulfate. Pralidoxime methiodide (2-PAM, an ChE reactivator) may be administered along with atropine **(see Chapter 2, Figure 2-6)**. 2-PAM should not be used alone to treat organophosphate overdose, because it cannot relieve the effects of OPs on the CNS, which contribute to respiratory depression. The chronic toxicity, which is manifested by paralysis, cannot be treated.
   b. **Drug interactions** may occur with drugs that activate cholinergic receptors, skeletal muscle relaxants, and chlorinated hydrocarbons.

C. **Carbamates**

1. **Preparations.** Frequently used carbamates include carbaryl and propoxur. The carbamates are used in the treatment of ectoparasites in small animals as powder, shampoo, and collar formulations.
2. **Mechanism of action.** Carbamates inhibit ChE via carbamylation. Their effects are more reversible than those of OPs, since the binding between carbamate and ChE is noncovalent.
3. **Pharmacokinetics.** The pharmacokinetics of the carbamate insecticides are not well understood.
4. **Adverse effects** include toxicity. Carbamate poisoning is similar to acute OP poisoning. Atropine sulfate is an effective antidote. 2-PAM should not be used to treat carbamate poisoning for two reasons given below:
   a. **Carbamate binding to ChE is reversible.**
   b. **2-PAM itself inhibits ChE in a reversible manner.**

D. **Chlorinated hydrocarbons**

1. **Chlorinated ethane derivatives** (e.g., DDT, methoxychlor) are very effective synthetic insecticides. However, because of the environmental hazard posed by DDT residues, DDT has been banned by the Environmental Protection Agency (EPA) since 1972.
   a. **Mechanism of action.** These insecticides increase intracellular $[Na^+]_i$ and $[Ca^{2+}]_i$ of excitable cells via two mechanisms. High $[Na^+]_i$ causes depolarization and $[Ca^{2+}]_i$ will overstimulate neurotransmission, which paralyze the insects **(Figure 16-9)**.
      (1) They prevent the closure of Na^+ channels, leading to an increase in intracellular Na^+ concentrations.
      (2) They increase $[Ca^{2+}]_i$ by inhibiting the uptake of Ca^{2+} into the endoplasmic reticulum.
   b. **Therapeutic uses.** Methoxychlor, in powders and sprays, is to kill fleas, ticks, flies, mosquitoes, and gnats.
   c. **Pharmacokinetics**
      (1) **Absorption.** Both DDT and methoxychlor are highly lipophilic. Fat in feed promotes absorption (and, therefore, increases toxicity); however, obese animals are more resistant to insecticide toxicity, because fat adsorbs lipophilic chemicals.
      (2) **Metabolism and elimination**
         (a) **DDT is metabolized into DDD and DDE (Figure 16-10).**
            i. DDD is further metabolized into DDA, which is water soluble and is excreted in the urine.
            ii. DDE is lipid soluble and cannot be further metabolized. DDE is permanently stored in the adipose tissue of animals, causing residue problems.

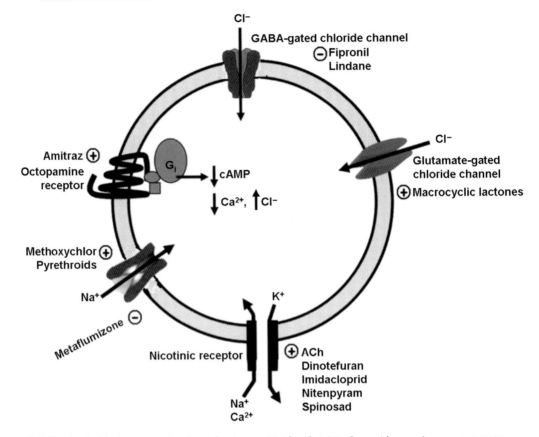

FIGURE 16-9. Mechanisms of action of ectoparasiticides that interfere with parasite nervous system.

(b) **Methoxychlor** is a biodegradable derivative of DDT that does not cause the severe residue problems associated with DDT.
  d. **Adverse effects**
    (1) **Toxicity.** Acute toxicity in animals is rare; however, overdoses can cause CNS excitation, which may lead to convulsions. Cardiac arrhythmia may be induced as well.
      (a) **Detoxification.** Activated charcoal should be administered to remove the toxicant from the gastrointestinal tract.
      (b) **Symptomatic therapy**
        i. **Anticonvulsants** can be administered for seizures. Phenobarbital, in addition to controlling seizures, induces microsomal enzymes, increasing the metabolism of chlorinated hydrocarbons.
        ii. **Artificial respiration** may be needed in cases of asphyxia.
    (2) **Drug resistance** in arthropods may be a significant problem.
    (3) **Environmental concerns.** DDT and methoxychlor pose little risk of acute toxicity in animals; however, DDT poses a hazard to the environment by persisting in the food chain, since it disrupts the actions of sex steroids.
      (a) **Eggshell thinning** results from the ability of DDT to block estrogen receptors that mediate the deposition of Ca^{2+} into the eggshell.
      (b) **Toxicity to aquatic life.**
  2. **Lindane (γ-BHC, a hexachlorocyclohexane)**
    a. Lindane is used primarily to control screwworm and ear tick infestations in cattle, horses, swine, sheep, and goats.
    b. **Mechanism of action.** Lindane increases excitability of excitable cells by blocking GABA-gated chloride channels to induce depolarization (Figure 16-9).
    c. **Pharmacokinetics.** The pharmacokinetics of the hexachlorocyclohexanes are not clear.

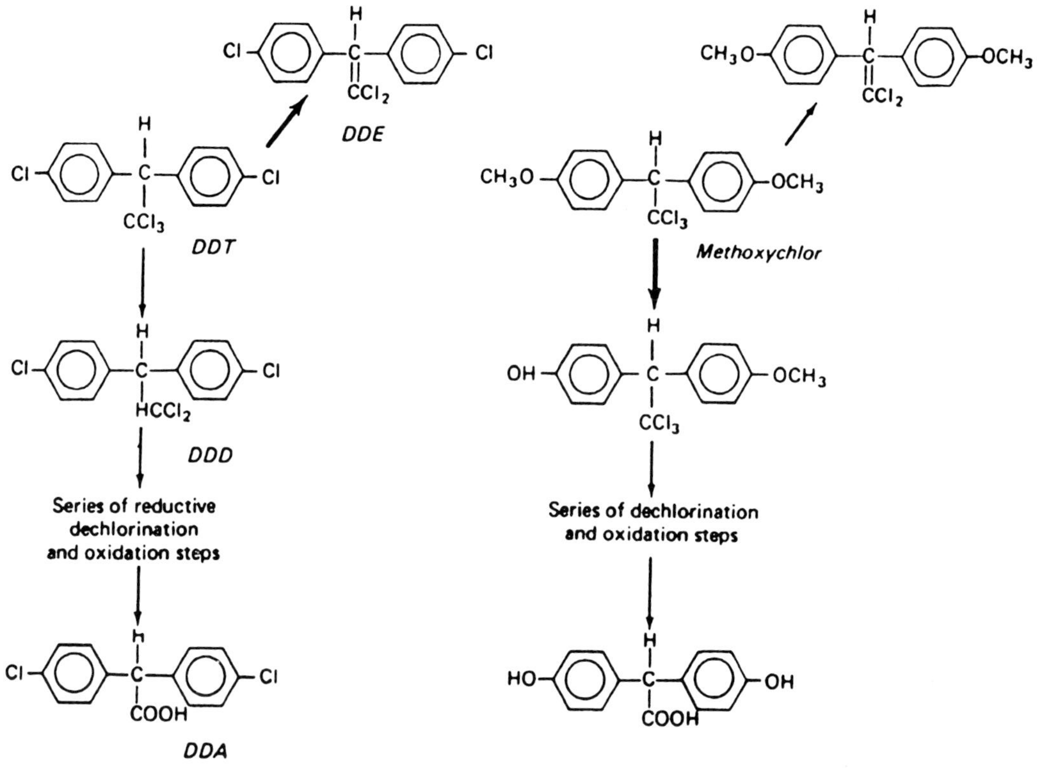

FIGURE 16-10. Major metabolic pathways of DDT and methoxychlor. (Reprint from Figure 17-5, *Toxicology: The Basic Science of Poisons*, by Casarett and Doull, 1975.)

    d. Adverse effects. Lindane is more toxic than DDT. Young animals, especially calves, and toy breed dogs are extremely sensitive to lindane poisoning.
        (1) Signs of toxicity are similar to those produced by DDT (e.g., tremors, ataxia, convulsions, prostration, and tachypnea).
        (2) Treatment of poisoning is nonspecific.

E. **Insect development inhibitors (IDIs)**
    1. Preparations. Diflubenzuron (Dimilin®, Equitrol® II) and lufenuron (Program®). Both of them are highly lipophilic compounds.
    2. Mechanism of action. IDIs inhibit chitin synthesis in larvae and eggs of insects; they have no effects on adult insects. Chitin is an important constituent of exoskeleton and eggshell.
    3. Therapeutic uses
        a. Diflubenzuron is used as a feed additive in horses (0.15 mg/kg/day) to inhibit developmental stages of flies. It is administered from early spring to fall.
        b. Lufenuron is administered orally in dogs (10 mg/kg) and cats (30 mg/kg) once a month to inhibit developmental stages of fleas. Lufenuron should be administered orally after feeding to increase the bile secretion and thus drug absorption. Lufenuron is also administered SC (10 mg/kg) once every 6 months in cats to control fleas as well. Both insecticides have no effects on adult insects.
    4. Pharmacokinetics. The GI absorption of both IDIs is increased by bile, since bile can help dissolve the insecticides. Lufenuron is accumulated readily in adipose tissues, and the release of it from fat allows maintenance of effective blood levels of drug for weeks. Following oral dosing, lufenuron reaches therapeutic concentrations in 6–12 hours and therapeutic blood levels are maintained for over a month. No other information is available.

5. **Adverse effects.** Both preparations are safe. Lufenuron is safe in young animals (>6 weeks old), in reproducing and lactating dogs and cats and their offspring. Anorexia, vomiting, and lethargy have been seen after lufenuron administration.

F. **Insect growth regulators (IGRs, juvenile hormone analogs)**

1. **Preparations** include cyromazine (Larvadex®), methoprene (in many insecticides, including Frontline® Plus), and pyriproxyfen (in many insecticide preparations).
2. **Mechanism of action.** Insect growth regulators mimic the actions of the juvenile hormones of insects. These preparations maintain persistently the larvae in an immature stage and interfere with reproductive organ differentiation.
3. **Therapeutic uses and administration**
   a. **Fecal maggot control in poultry.** Cyromazine is administered orally for 4–6 weeks to control fecal maggots in poultry. Cyromazine is also used as a spray onto surface of manure.
   b. **Flea control**
      (1) Methoprene and pyriproxyfen are sprayed in households and applied on animals to prevent eggs, pupae, and larvae from developing into adult fleas. These insecticides are effective for at least 3 months. Both of them are also available as a flea collar for dogs.
      (2) Methoprene and pyriproxyfen are mixed with pyrethroids to kill adult fleas.
4. **Pharmacokinetics.** The pharmacokinetics of these agents are not well understood.
5. **Adverse effects.** These products are safe when used as directed.

G. **Botanicals**

1. **Rotenone (Durakyl®, Ear Miticide®, etc.)**
   a. **Chemistry.** Rotenone is an alkaloid derived from the root of the *derris* plant.
   b. **Mechanism of action.** Rotenone inhibits cellular respiratory metabolism by blocking the electron generation from reduced nicotinamide adenine dinucleotide (NADH). As a result, oxidation of lactate, glutamate, and other substances is reduced and nerve conduction is inhibited.
   c. **Therapeutic uses**
      (1) Rotenone is used to kill fleas, lice, ticks, and mites. It has fast "knockdown" action on all arthropods, with little persistence.
      (2) Rotenone is also used to kill unwanted fish in ponds and lakes.
   d. **Pharmacokinetics** are not well understood. Rotenone undergoes hydroxylation by hepatic microsomal enzymes, which is followed by conjugation. The rotenone conjugates are excreted into urine.
   e. **Adverse effects** include local irritation and CNS disturbances (e.g., excitation, convulsions, depression). Do not use in reptiles.
2. **Pyrethroids**
   a. **Preparations** include pyrethrins, allethrin, cyfluthrin, cypermethrin, fenvalerate, lambdacyhalothrin, permethrin, and resmethrin.
   b. **Chemistry**
      (1) Pyrethrins are alkaloids of pyrethrum, which are among the oldest insecticides ever known.
      (2) The other pyrethroids, being synthetic, are more resistant to metabolism than pyrethrins.
   c. **Mechanism of action.** Pyrethroids increase excitability of ectoparasite neurons by prolonging the opening of Na^+ channels, thereby causing arthropod paralysis.
   d. **Therapeutic uses.** Pyrethroids are most commonly used ectoparasiticides due to their rapid "knockdown" effect with little residual activity and safety. The "knockdown" effect may or may not be fatal; therefore, these agents are usually combined with other insecticides or a synergist [e.g., piperonyl butoxide or MK264 (*N*-octyl bicycloheptene dicarboximide)] to increase insecticidal activity. Synergists inhibit induction of microsomal enzymes that degrade pyrethroids.

    e. Pharmacokinetics. The pharmacokinetics of the pyrethroids is not well understood. In humans, 1–2% of permethrin is absorbed percutaneously. Pyrethroids are metabolized through hydroxylation and almost entirely excreted in the urine in free or glucuronide-conjugated forms. In humans, permethrin is eliminated from the body within 96 hours of topical administration. No information on elimination is available for animals.

    f. Adverse effects. Pyrethroids are generally safe, but may cause local irritation, allergy, hypersalivation, nausea and vomiting, diarrhea, cardiac arrhythmia, and CNS disturbances manifested by muscle rigidity, tremors, ataxia, and convulsions. Cats are particularly susceptible to pyrethroid-induced CNS disturbances; thus, **pyrethroids should not be used in cats.** This phenomenon might be due to grooming to swallow the insecticide and poor metabolism. Anticonvulsants and central muscle relaxants such as methocarbamol can be used as antidotes.

    g. Resistance. The ectoparasites that are resistant to methoxychlor treatment may be resistant to pyrethroids.

H. **Macrocyclic lactones** (See II D for general information.)

  1. Macrocyclic lactones are effective against most ectoparasitesthat include grubs, mites, lice, ticks, and flies. However, most of them do not kill fleas at clinical doses, except selamectin, which is administered topically to dogs and cats.

  2. Macrocyclic lactones do not kill arthropods promptly, taking hours before ectoparasiticidal activity becomes apparent.

  3. Macrocyclic lactones not only kill adults and larvae of ectoparasites but also interrupt feeding, molting, and hatching of eggs.

  4. For demodicosis, ivermectin may be used in an extra-label manner at 0.4–0.6 mg/kg/day, orally, for 2–3 months to treat this disease. However, such regimen using large and frequent doses of ivermectin may be risky in some dogs. Watch for adverse effects of the treatment!

  5. For Sarcoptic mange, ivermectin may be used in an extra-label manner at 0.2 mg/kg; 2 doses, 2 weeks apart to have an effective control over this infestation.

I. **Other ectoparasiticides**

  1. **Amitraz (Mitaban®, Taktic®, ProMeris Duo®, etc.)** is a formamidine insecticide for use on dogs, pigs, and cattle.

    a. Mechanism of action. Amitraz activates octopamine receptors in arthropods, which inhibits neurotransmission, resulting in flaccid paralysis (Figure 16-9).

    b. Therapeutic uses

      (1) Amitraz is used to eliminate mites, lice, and ticks in dogs, swine, and cattle. In dog, amitraz is used as an emulsion for topical application (Mitaban®), tick collar (Preventic® Collar), and spot-on product (ProMeris®). Amitraz is used as an emulsion spray (in swine and cattle). No preslaughter withdrawal period is necessary in cattle, and it can be used on lactating dairy cattle without incurring a withdrawal period for milk following application.

      (2) Three to six biweekly treatments may be used to control demodectic mange in dogs.

    c. Pharmacokinetics. The pharmacokinetics of amitraz are not well understood.

    d. Adverse effects. In animals, amitraz activates α_2-adrenergic receptors. Therefore, the adverse effects of amitraz are similar to the pharmacological effects of xylazine (e.g., sedation, bradycardia, hyperglycemia, GI stasis). α_2-Adrenergic antagonists such as yohimbine can be used as an antidote.

    e. Contraindications

      (1) Amitraz should not be applied to swine within 3 days of slaughter.

      (2) Amitraz may cause fatal colon impaction in horses.

  2. **Insect nicotinic receptor agonists**

    a. Preparations. Imidacloprid (Advantage®), dinotefuran (Vectra 3D®), nitenpyram (Capstar®), and spinosad (Comfortis®). All of them, except spinosad, are also called neonicotinoids. Spinosad is derived from the bacterium *Saccharopolyspora spinosa.*

   b. Mechanism of action. They activate nicotinic receptors of fleas, leading to overstimulation of neurons and muscle to cause overstimulation, which is followed by paralysis (Figure 16-9). **These insecticides have very little activity on nicotinic receptors of mites, ticks, and animals.** However, spinosad has different binding sites on insect nicotinic receptors than neonicotinoids. Clinical implication for this difference is not known.

   c. Therapeutic uses. All four insecticides are used to kill adult fleas. They cause rapid detachment of fleas.

      (1) Imidacloprid is used topically (5–10 mg/kg) once a month as a spot-on product in dogs and cats that are ≥4 week old. Nearly 100% of mature fleas are killed within 12 hours of application, the fleacidal effect is persistent for 30 days, since it is stored in the sebaceous glands of the animals. It is not washed out by shampooing. Imidacloprid is also available as a mixture with permethrin (K9 Advantix®) to kill more ectoparasites, for example, ticks, in dogs and with moxidectin (Advantage® Multi) to prevent heartworms, and to kill GI nematodes, and mites in dogs and cats.

      (2) Dinotefuran is a third-generation neonicotinoid with slightly faster knockdown than imidacloprid (killing 96% fleas in 6 hours), while retaining residual activity against fleas for at least 30 days. It is available as a mixture with permethrin (to kill ticks) and pyriproxifen (to kill developing stages of fleas) for use on dogs and combined with pyriproxifen for use on cats.

      (3) Nitenpyram is used orally (1 mg/kg) for short-term control of fleas in dogs and cats. One dose can protect animals for 1–2 days. It is normally used in combination with an insect growth regulator or lufenuron to provide continuous flea control.

      (4) Spinosad is used orally at 30 mg/kg, once a month.

   d. Pharmacokinetics is not well understood for imidacloprid and dinotefuran.

      (1) Following oral administration, nitenpyram is absorbed from the GI tract rapidly. Nitenpyram undergoes hydroxylation, followed by conjugation. Nitenpyram conjugates are excreted in the urine; it is not accumulated in body tissues. The plasma $t_{1/2}$ of nitenpyram in dogs and cats are 3 and 8 hours, respectively. The longer plasma $t_{1/2}$ of nitenpyram in cats reflects the slow drug metabolism in this species.

      (2) Spinosad is readily absorbed from the GI tract after oral administration. It is rapidly metabolized and eliminated. Within 48 hours of dosing, 60–80% of spinosad or its metabolites is eliminated via the urine and feces. Depletion of spinosad residues from tissues occurs rapidly following cessation of exposure. The plasma $t_{1/2}$ in dogs is not known.

   e. Adverse effects. All four insecticides are safe, since they specifically activate insects' nicotinic receptors, but not animals'. Topical application of imidacloprid and dinotefuran may cause irritation of the skin. Spinosad may induce vomiting in dogs.

3. Fipronil (Frontline®, Frontline® Plus)

   a. Mechanism of action. Fipronil blocks GABA gated Cl⁻ channels of arthropods to cause depolarization of the neurons, thereby increasing excitability, followed by detachment (Figure 16-9).

   b. Therapeutic uses. Fipronil is a safe pesticide against fleas and ticks for topical use in dogs (≥8 weeks old) and cats (≥12 weeks old); 6.5–13 mg/kg topically. It is available as a spray and a spot-on product and is applied once every 4 weeks. Fipronil is persistent even in animals subjected to shampooing. The mixture with methoprene (Frontline® Plus) is to kill the developing stages of fleas.

   c. Pharmacokinetics. When used topically, it is stored in sebaceous glands and follicles of the animal, and is slowly released to kill ectoparasites. No other information is available for animals.

    d. Adverse effects. Fipronil is safe when use as directed; only local irritation and hypersalivation have been reported.

    e. Drug Resistance. Fipronil may cause cross-resistance with lindane.

4. Metaflumizone (ProMeris®, ProMeris® Duo)

    a. Mechanism of action. Metaflumizone attacks the nervous system of the flea by blocking neuronal Na^+ channels to cause hyperpolarization of the neuronal membrane, which results in reduced feeding, flaccid paralysis, and death of the flea.

    b. Therapeutic uses. Metaflumizone is a fleacide for topical spot-on use in dogs and cats that are ≥8 weeks old. It should be applied at the 4–6 week intervals. In combination with amitraz, ProMeris® Duo can kill both fleas and ticks in dogs.

    c. Pharmacokinetics. Metaflumizone is rapidly distributed throughout the surface of the skin. Maximum concentrations in the hair generally reach 1–2 days posttreatment and gradually decline through 56 days posttreatment. Only very small amounts of metaflumizone are absorbed systemically from dermal application.

    d. Adverse effects. It is safe when use as directed; only lethargy has been reported when over-dosed.

J. Resistance to ectoparasiticides

1. Introduction. Some arthropods are resistant to the lethal effects of ectoparasiticides following continuous exposure to them. This resistance is increasing prevalent; more than 500 species of arthropods are resistant to one or more ectoparasiticides. Approximately 200 of resistant species are either parasites of animals or humans.

2. Mechanisms of resistance. There are two classes of mechanisms, physiological and behavior mechanisms.

    a. Behavioral mechanisms. After exposing to a particular ectoparasiticide, the pests would develop the behavior to avoid the agent.

    b. Physiological mechanisms. These are more important than behavioral mechanisms, which affect selection and effective use of ectoparasiticides.

        (1) Decreased penetration into target organism.

        (2) Increased metabolism (detoxication) of ectoparasiticides.

        (3) Decreased sensitivity of the target site (or receptor).

3. Strategies to reduce the resistance development to ectoparasiticides. These include the following:

    a. Appropriate selection of ectoparasiticides. One should target chemistry that does not favor a higher level of resistance and/or agents that are less persistent.

    b. Reduction in the number of treatments. It is best achieved by an integrated approach to parasite management in which chemicals are combined with other means of controlling parasites.

    c. Use of ectoparasiticide rotations and mixtures. Rotation of agents across several generations of target ectoparasite may be superior to rotation over single generations. Mixing of agents usually results in redundant killing in which each agent is used alone. On the contrary, mixtures often are variable in their persistence following application, resulting in a shorter period of redundant efficacy.

    d. Limited interactions with agronomical pesticides. Increased frequency of exposure of target ectoparasites to agronomical pesticides may accelerate the development of resistance. It is prudent to consider integrating procedures for managing agronomical and animal pests to avoid promoting resistance against currently effective agents.

    e. Resistance monitoring. It can be useful in determining continuing efficacy of agents or the effectiveness of resistance management program.

SUGGESTED READING

Craig TM. 2003. Treatment of external and internal parasites of cattle. *Vet Clin North Am Food Anim Pract* 19:661–678.

Hsu WH, Kakuk TJ. 1984. Effect of amitraz and chlordimeform on heart rate and pupil diameter: Mediated by α_2-adrenoreceptors. *Toxicol Appl Pharmacol* 73:411–415.

Hsu WH, Lu ZX, Hembrough FB. 1986. Effect of amitraz on heart rate and aortic blood pressure in conscious dogs: Influence of atropine, prazosin, tolazoline, and yohimbine. *Toxicol Appl Pharmacol* 84:418–422.

Hsu WH, McNeel SV. 1985. Amitrazinduced prolongation of gastrointestinal transit and bradycardia in dogs and their antagonism by yohimbine: Preliminary study. *Drug Chem Toxicol* 8:239–253.

Lindsay DS, Blagburn BR. 2001. "Antiprotozoan drugs." In *Veterinary Pharmacology and Therapeutics.* Edited by Adams HR. 8th ed., pp. 992–1016. Ames, IA: Iowa State University Press.

Martin RJ. 1997. Modes of action of anthelmintic drugs. *Br Vet J* 154:11–34.

Martin RJ, Purcell J, Day T, Robertson AP. 2003. "Neurotransmitters." In *Molecular Medical Parasitology.* Edited by Marr JJ, Nielsen T, Komuniecki R. pp. 349–394. New York: Academic Press.

Plumb DC. 2005. *Veterinary Drug Handbook.* 5th ed. Ames, IA: Blackwell Publishing.

Pritchard R, Tait A. 2001. The role of molecular biology in veterinary parasitology. *Vet Parasitol* 98:169–194.

Reid WM. 1976. Progress in the control of coccidiosis with anticoccidials and planned immunization. *Am J Vet Res* 31:593–596.

Reinermeyer CR, Courtney CH. 2001. "Antinematodal drugs." In *Veterinary Pharmacology and Therapeutics.* Edited by Adams HR. 8th ed., pp. 947–979. Ames, IA: Iowa State University Press.

Robertson AP, Bjorn H, Martin RJ. 1999. Levamisole resistance resolved at the single-channel level. *FASEB J* 13:749–760.

Schaffer DD, Hsu WH, Hopper DL. 1990. The effects of yohimbine and four other antagonists on amitrazinduced depression of shuttle avoidance responses in dogs. *Toxicol Appl Pharmacol* 104:543–547.

Wolstenholme AJ, Fairweather I, Pritchard R, von Samson-Himmelstjerna G, Sangster NC. 2004. Drug resistance in veterinary helminthes. *Trends Parasitol* 20:469–476.

STUDY QUESTIONS

DIRECTIONS: Each of the numbered items or incomplete statements in this section is followed by answers or by completion of the statement. Select the **one** lettered answer or completion that is **best** in each case.

1. Of the following drugs used in heartworm therapy or prevention, which one has the greatest potential for causing icterus and bilirubinuria?

(A) Selamectin
(B) Ivermectin
(C) Milbemycin
(D) Melarsomine

2. Which one of the following antinematodal drugs is effective against equine bots (*Gasterophilus*)?

(A) Fenbendazole
(B) Ivermedtin
(C) Piperazine
(D) Pyrantel

3. Which one of the following ectoparasiticides may cause xylazine-like effects in animals?

(A) Amitraz
(B) Lindane
(C) Methoxychlor
(D) Permethrin
(E) Rotenone

4. Which one of the following anthelmintics requires the longest preslaughter withdrawal period when used in beef cattle?

(A) Albendazole
(B) Clorsulon
(C) Ivermectin
(D) Levamisole
(E) Morantel

5. A 5-year-old Arabian mare is diagnosed with a *Strongylus vulgaris* infection. Repeated dosings with oxibendazole have failed to improve the mare's condition that suggests that the worms are resistant to the treatment. The veterinarian decides to use another nematocide to treat the mare for this condition. Under the circumstances, which one of the following drugs should be avoided?

(A) Fenbendazole
(B) Ivermectin
(C) Moxidectin
(D) Pyrantel

6. Clinical signs of a coccidiosis outbreak are detected in a flock of layers. Which one of the following anticoccidial drugs would be most appropriate?

(A) Sulfadimethoxine
(B) Lasalocid
(C) Decoquinate
(D) Amprolium

7. Which of the following antinematodal drugs is also used in the treatment of giardiasis dogs?

(A) Fenbendazole
(B) Ivermectin
(C) Levamisole
(D) Piperazine
(E) Pyrantel

8. Which of the following antinematodal drugs used in cats works by increasing the release of inhibitory neuropeptides?

(A) Piperazine
(B) Febantel
(C) Pyrantel pamoate
(D) Selamectin
(E) Emodepside

9. Which one of the following antitrematodal drugs is most effective against immature (i.e., less than 14 weeks old) *Fasciola hepatica* in cattle?

(A) Albendazole
(B) Clorsulon
(C) Praziquantel

10. Which one of the following antinematodal drugs does *not* have significant activity against hookworms in dogs?

(A) Febantel
(B) Fenbendazole
(C) Milbemycin
(D) Piperazine
(E) Pyrantel

11. All of the following anticoccidial drugs have shown good results in the control of mammalian coccidiosis except:

(A) amprolium.
(B) decoquinate.
(C) monensin.
(D) robenidine.
(E) sulfaquinoxaline.

12. All of the following are toxic effects of metronidazole except:

(A) convulsions.
(B) carcinogenicity.
(C) cardiac arrhythmia.
(D) diarrhea.
(E) reversible leukopenia.

13. Which of the following anticestodal drugs has consistent efficacy against *Taenia*, *Dipylidium*, and *Echinococcus* in dogs?

(A) Dichlorophene
(B) Fenbendazole
(C) Praziquantel
(D) Pyrantel

14. Piperonyl butoxide is a "synergist" that is usually found in which of the following ectoparasiticide preparations?

(A) Rotenone
(B) Pyrethrins
(C) Fipronil
(D) Lufenuron
(E) Methoprene

15. Pralidoxime (2-PAM) is an acetylcholinestrase regeneratorthat has been used as an

antidote in the treatment of overdose of cholinesterase inhibitors as ectoparasiticides. However, 2-PAM is not effective in overdose.

(A) dichlorvos
(B) carbaryl
(C) coumaphos
(D) fenthion
(E) phosmet

16. Which of the following anticoccidial drugs can be legally used in laying chickens?

(A) Amprolium
(B) Clopidol
(C) Nicarbazin
(D) Diclazuril
(E) Sulfadimethoxine and ormetoprim

17. Which of the following fleacides act by blocking neuronal Na^+ channels that leads to flaccid paralysis of the parasites?

(A) Fipronil
(B) Imidacloprid
(C) Metaflumizone
(D) Nitenpyram
(E) Permethrin

18. Which of the following drugs for the treatment of equine protozoal myeloencephalitis (EPM) acts by forming a toxic-free radical in order to block cellular respiration of the protozoans?

(A) Trimethoprim-sulfadiazine
(B) Ponazuril
(C) Nitazoxanide

19. Which of the following ectoparasiticides is not effective in killing ticks?

(A) Fipronil
(B) Rotenone
(C) Amitraz
(D) Imidacloprid
(E) Permethrin

ANSWERS AND EXPLANATIONS

1. The answer is D.
Melarsomine is hepatotoxic. Signs of toxicity include persistent vomiting, bilirubinuria, hyperbilirubinemia, icterus, melena, stupor, and coma. Affected animals may show increased serum concentrations of alkaline phosphatase and alanine transaminase. Selamectin, ivermectin, and milbemycin are not hepatotoxic.

2. The answer is B.
Macrocyclic lactones, such as ivermectin, are effective against bots. Benzimidazoles, piperazine, and pyrantel are not.

3. The answer is A.
Like xylazine, amitraz is an α_2-adrenergic agonist. Therefore, it can cause sedation, bradycardia, and hyperglycemia in animals. Other ectoparasiticides do not have this activity.

4. The answer is C.
In cattle, the preslaughter withdrawal period for ivermectin (35 days following SC administration and 49 days following topical administration) is longer than that for albendazole (27 days), clorsulon (8 days), levamisole (2 days, oral; 7 days, SC; 11 days, topical), and morantel (14 days).

5. The answer is A.
Cross-resistance occurs among all benzimidazoles. Thus, if a nematode species becomes resistant to oxibendazole, one should avoid using another benzimidazole as an alternative nematocide. Ivermectin, moxidectin, and pyrantel are not benzimidazoles; thus, cross-resistance with oxibendazole is not a problem.

6. The answer is A.
Aulfa drug with or without ormetoprim is recommended for the treatment of coccidial outbreaks in poultry. Diclazuril, not mentioned in the question, can also be used to treat coccidiosis outbreak. Lasalocid, amprolium, and decoquinate are used for prevention only.

7. The answer is A.
Benzimidazoles, for example, fenbendazole, are used for the control of giardiasis. Other antinematodal drugs are not effective against *Giardia*.

8. The answer is E.
Emodepside activates the presynaptic latrophilin receptor, which increases the release of inhibitory neuropeptides PF1 and PF2, thereby causing flaccid paralysis of muscles in nematodes. Piperazine activates GABA receptors of nematodes to cause flaccid paralysis. Selamectin activates glutamate-gated chloride channels, which also causes flaccid paralysis. Febantel is a pro-benzimidazole, which is metabolized into fenbendazole and oxfendazole. Benzimidazoles inhibit microtubule synthesis. Pyrantel pamoate is a nicotine-like nematocide, which activates nicotinic receptors to increase muscle contraction, which is followed by paralysis.

9. The answer is B.
Clorsulon has excellent activity against both mature and immature *F. hepatica*. Albendazole is used to kill mature *F. hepatica* only. Praziquantel has not been tested for activity against liver flukes in cattle for economic reasons.

10. The answer is D.
Piperazine is effective against ascarids and nodular worms in all species, but it has no activity against hookworms. Febantel, fenbendazole, milbemycin, and pyrantel are effective against hookworms.

11. The answer is D.
Sulfonamides and ormetoprim, amprolium, decoquinate, and sodium ionophores, for example, monensin are used as anticoccidial drugs in mammals. Robenidine is approved for use in birds only.

12. The answer is C.
Cardiac arrhythmia is not an adverse effect of metronidazole. However, metronidazole may induce lethargy, weakness, ataxia, rigidity, anorexia, vomiting, diarrhea, and, rarely, reversible leukopenia. Metronidazole may be hepatotoxic, teratogenic, and carcinogenic.

13. The answer is C.
Praziquantel is effective against all three species of tapeworms in the dog. Dichlorophene is effective against *Taenia* and *Dipylidium*, but not *Echinococcus*. Fenbendazole is effective against *Taenia* and *Echinococcus*, but not *Dipylidium*. Pyrantel at high doses is effective against horse tapeworm *Anoplocephala perfoliata*, but there is no evidence that it kills canine tapeworms.

14. The answer is B.
Piperonyl butoxide inhibits cytochrome P450 enzymes in ectoparasites, which will help protect pyrethrins and thus increase the efficacy of this botanical ectoparasiticide. Piperonyl butoxide is usually found in the pyrethroid preparations, but not in other ectoparasiticides.

15. The answer is B.
2-PAM is effective in regenerating cholinesterase that is bound covalently by organophosphates. Since carbamates such as carbaryl do not form covalent bond with cholinesterase, it is not effective in regenerating the enzyme.

16. The answer is A.
Amprolium is a quaternary compound that is minimally absorbed from the gut of animals. As a result, it is legally used in laying chickens. All other anticoccidial drugs are absorbed significantly in the gut, and thus cannot be used in laying chickens.

17. The answer is C.
Metaflumizone is a newly developed fleacide, which causes flaccid paralysis of the fleas by blocking neuronal Na^+ channels. Permethrin prolongs the opening of neuronal Na^+ channels, which causes depolarizing neuromuscular blockade of the ectoparasites. Imidacloprid and nitenpyram overstimulate nicotinic receptors of fleas. Fipronil blocks GABA-gated Cl^- channels to cause depolarization of the neurons that paralyzes the fleas.

18. The answer is C.
Nitazoxanide forms a toxic-free radical from the "nitro" group, which blocks cellular respiration of protozoans. Trimethoprim-sulfadiazine inhibits folate synthesis and metabolism. Ponazuril is effective against schizonts and gametes by inhibiting nuclear division.

19. The answer is D.
Imidacloprid is effective against fleas but not ticks. All other ectoparasiticides mentioned in the question are effective in killing both fleas and ticks.

Chapter 17

Antineoplastic Drugs

Leslie E. Fox

I. **GENERAL PRINCIPLES OF CANCER CHEMOTHERAPY**

A. The goal of treatment with chemotherapy in veterinary medicine is to increase the length and quality of life of patients based on an accurate histologic diagnosis of the tumor and the clinical stage or extent of the neoplastic process.

B. Chemotherapy is best used as treatment for systemic disease, palliation for metastatic, or nonresectable disease, large tumor size reduction, making them more amenable to surgery and/or radiation therapy called neoadjuvant chemotherapy, adjuvant therapy after surgery and/or radiation therapy to slow metastasis or kill residual tumor cells, and to increase tumor cell sensitivity to the lethal effects of radiation therapy.

C. The kinetics of chemotherapy drug-induced cell kill is *first-order*—a constant percentage (not a constant number) of cells is killed with each dose. Antineoplastic drugs are most effective when the tumor is small (microscopic) and is rapidly growing (high growth fraction).

D. Because tumor cells undergo a high spontaneous mutation rate, up to 1 in every 10,000 tumor cells may have acquired mutations that can confer resistance at the time of diagnosis, even in the absence of previous exposure to chemotherapeutic agents. Thus, multimodality and multiagent therapy administered as early in the course of disease as is possible, is likely to be the most helpful.

E. Drug resistance develops in neoplastic cells with mechanisms similar to those observed in antibiotic resistant bacteria. These include the following:

  1. Decreased cell permeability or uptake, or increased efflux of drugs
  2. Increased production of enzymes which degrade the drug
  3. Increased capacity to repair or bypass the effects of the drug
  4. Decreased binding of drug to receptors or target enzymes

F. In general, multidrug protocols are more efficacious than single drug protocols. They are designed using drugs with different mechanisms of action to augment cell kill and slow the development of resistance. Additionally, the nonoverlapping adverse effects of each drug decrease overall toxicity to the patient. The drugs are given at the maximum dose and schedule with acceptable or no adverse effects for optimal tumor cell kill.

G. Most drugs are dosed on the basis of body surface area (BSA) in square meters (an estimate of metabolic rate), because of the narrow therapeutic index of antineoplastic drugs. The BSA method of dosage calculation overestimates the metabolic rate of smaller dogs and cats therefore increased toxicity (and perhaps, efficacy) is seen in smaller animals with some drugs. Doxorubicin is an example of a drug that is more toxic to smaller patients (<10–15 kg body weight) when dosed using BSA than when calculated on using milligrams per kilogram body weight. Some overweight pets may need dosage calculation based on their lean body weight.

$$\text{BSA} = M^2 = \frac{k \times \text{weight (in grams)}^{2/3}}{10^4}$$

$$k = 10.0 \text{ for dogs and } 10.1 \text{ for cats}$$

FIGURE 17-1. The cell cycle. Mitosis (M) is followed by the first growth phase (G$_1$), or by a resting phase (G$_0$). During the S phase, DNA synthesis takes place. The S phase is followed by a second growth phase (G$_2$). (From Figure 12-1, *NVMS Pharmacology*.)

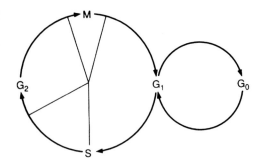

H. Rapidly multiplying and growing cells are most susceptible to drug effects. These include the normal cells of the hair follicles, gastrointestinal tract, and bone marrow. Thus, hair loss, vomiting and diarrhea, and leucopenia and thrombocytopenia are common side effects of therapy.

I. Minimum baseline assessment consists of a physical examination, complete blood count, serum biochemical panel, and urinalysis. A complete blood count should be performed before each subsequent dose. Treatment should be temporarily suspended if the neutrophil count falls below 3,000/mm^3 or platelet count below 100,000/mm^3 for dogs depending on the normal range for each laboratory.

J. Collie-type breeds and others (long-haired whippet) have a higher risk of toxicity reactions from antineoplastic drugs that are actively transported by the p-glycoprotein membrane pump. Natural products (doxorubicin, vinca alkaloids, actinomycin-D, and the taxanes) cause increased toxicity when given to dogs with a mutation of the multidrug resistance 1 (MDR 1) allele coding for p-glycoprotein, because the mutation diminishes the excretion of drugs dependent on p-glycoprotein.

K. Chemotherapeutic drugs have the potential to be mutagenic, embryotoxic, teratogenic, carcinogenic, and cytotoxic. They are skin irritants and can enter the body by absorption through mucous membranes (oral especially), the eyes (including soft contact lenses), and the skin, or by inhalation. To prevent accidental exposure, appropriate handling techniques for hazardous drugs are necessary based on the Occupational and Safety Health Administration guidelines (found on the United States Department of Labor website).

II. THE CELL CYCLE

Knowledge of the cell cycle is essential to the understanding of the action of antineoplastic drugs. Many drugs are cell cycle specific in that they kill tumor cells in specific phase of the cell cycle (Figure 17-1).

A. **G$_1$ phase**. In the G$_1$ phase there is synthesis of proteins (enzymes) and RNA required for DNA replication in the S phase. The duration of the G$_1$ phase varies from hours to days depending on the cell type.

B. **S phase**. DNA synthesis occurs in the S phase. Its duration usually is 2–4 hours. Many drugs act at this phase of the cycle.

C. **G$_2$ phase**. The G$_2$ phase is characterized by the synthesis of proteins and RNA required for mitosis and cell division. Its duration usually is 3–8 hours.

D. **M phase**. Mitosis: its duration is 1 hour.

E. **G_0 phase.** The G_0 phase is the resting phase. The nonproliferating cells in G_0 are resistant to the cytotoxic action of drugs. The duration is variable, hours to weeks depending on the cell type. Most normal cells are found in this phase.

III. ALKYLATING AGENTS

A. **Chemistry.** Alkylating agents contain one or more alkyl groups ($R\text{-}CH_2\text{-}CH_2\text{-}X$) which are converted to reactive intermediates to form covalent bonds with compounds containing hydroxyl, amino, phosphate, sulfhydryl, or other nucleophilic groups. The alkyl radical ($R\text{-}CH_2\text{-}CH_2^+$) replaces a hydrogen atom on these groups.

B. **Mechanism of action**

1. Alkylating agents cross-link DNA and inhibit replication.
2. Alkylation labelizes DNA and increases breakdown of the molecule.
3. Alkylation of proteins and RNA may also occur. These drugs are considered non-cell cycle specific.

C. **Nitrogen mustards**

1. **Cyclophosphamide (Cytoxan®)**
   a. **Therapeutic uses.** Cyclophosphamide is the most commonly used alkylating agent in veterinary medicine. It is used for immunosuppression and alone or in combination protocols for lymphoreticular neoplasms, mammary gland and other carcinomas, soft tissue sarcomas, multiple myelomas, and mast cell tumors.
   b. **Pharmacokinetics**
      (1) Cyclophosphamide is inactive until being hydroxylated in the liver by microsomes as the first step in conversion to phosphoramide mustard and acrolein, the active metabolites. Thus, it should not be injected directly into tumors.
      (2) Cyclophosphamide is well absorbed orally, widely distributed except to the CNS, and the parent compound and metabolites are slowly excreted by the kidneys over 48–72 hours.
      (3) After IV injection, the $t_{1/2}$ of cyclophosphamide is ~4–12 hours.
   c. **Administration.** Cyclophosphamide may be administered orally or IV at intervals which vary with the type of cancer and the protocol employed. A common regimen is once a day (in the AM, see below) for 4 consecutive days/weeks or once a week IV. The oral form is coated with a protective layer and should not be broken or crushed. A CBC is required before administration and periodic urinalyses.
   d. **Adverse effects.** Myelosuppression (white blood cell nadir of 7 days) is most common. Mild alopecia in susceptible breeds, and sterile hemorrhagic cystitis are less common side effects. GI signs (nausea, vomiting, diarrhea) are infrequent. A rare complication is transitional cell carcinoma of the bladder. Cystitis is most common in dogs and is due to the irritant effects of acrolein and other metabolites. Concurrent administration of furosemide (IV most effective) with cyclophosphamide decreases the risk (to <1%) and/or delays the onset of cyclophosphamide-induced hemorrhagic cystitis. Administration of cyclophosphamide in the morning, stimulation of water intake and frequent voiding will reduce the frequency of cystitis. Initial treatment includes discontinuation of diuresis (no furosemide or corticosteroids) and cyclophosphamide.
2. **Chlorambucil (Leukeran®)**
   a. **Therapeutic uses and administration.** Chlorambucil is most commonly used as an immunosuppressive agent and for treatment of lymphocytic leukemia, gastrointestinal lymphoma (cats), multicentric lymphoma (dogs and cats), multiple myeloma, and polycythemia vera. Chlorambucil is administered orally every 2 days. Initially, a CBC is required every 1–2 weeks.

b. Pharmacokinetics.
   (1) Chlorambucil is a slow-acting nitrogen mustard, which is well tolerated following oral administration. The peak plasma concentration reaches maximum within 1 hour of oral administration.
   (2) A total of 99% of circulating chlorambucil is bound by albumin. It is metabolized by the liver to form active metabolite, phenylacetic acid mustard.
   (3) The $t_{1/2}$ is 1.5 hours (chlorambucil) and 2.4 hours (phenylacetic acid mustard). A total of 15–60% is excreted in urine after 24 hours.
c. Adverse effects. Chlorambucil is very well tolerated. Cumulative myelosuppression with chronic administration is the most common adverse effect in cats and dogs. Chlorambucil may be used as a substitute for cyclophosphamide when hemorrhagic cystitis has developed.

3. Melphalan (Alkeran®)
   a. Therapeutic uses and administration. Melphalan has been used predominantly in the treatment of multiple myeloma and other lymphoreticular neoplasms, as well as, anal sac adenocarcinoma. Melphalan is administered orally. Initially, a CBC is required every 7–14 days.
   b. Pharmacokinetics. Melphalan does not require hepatic metabolism for activation like cyclophosphamide. Its oral absorption is variable. It is eliminated mainly by hydrolysis in the plasma. In humans, terminal $t_{1/2}$ is ~90 minutes. In humans, 10% is excreted in the urine.
   c. Adverse effects. Myelosuppression is the most common adverse effect. It may be cumulative when used with other myelosuppressive drugs.

4. Mechlorethamine HCl (Mustargen®)
   a. Therapeutic uses and administration. This drug is most commonly used for treatment of relapsed lymphoreticular neoplasms or given intracavitary for pleural and peritoneal effusions. Although available in an ointment, it is highly immunosuppressive and topical administration is not recommended. It is most commonly given IV. Immediate administration is required as mechlorethamine is highly unstable. Deactivation of the remaining drug is required after dosing as it is highly toxic.
   b. Pharmacokinetics. It is widely distributed in tissues despite rapid (minutes) deactivation in tissues.
   c. Adverse effects. Bone marrow depression and GI toxicity (nausea and vomiting) are most common in dogs and cats. Hair loss and hepatotoxicity are possible. Tissue necrosis occurs with extravasation. A CBC is required before each treatment and periodic serum biochemical panel assessment.

5. Nitrosoureas. Nitrosureas are lipid soluble and cross the blood–brain barrier.
   a. Lomustine (CCNU, CeeNU®)
      (1) Therapeutic uses and administration. Lomustine is useful in the management of CNS neoplasms, relapsed lymphoma, histiocytic sarcoma, mycosis fungoides, and mast cell tumors in cats and dogs. Lomustine is well tolerated when administered orally. A CBC is needed prior to and 7–10 days after administration. Assessment of serum liver enzymes should be done before each treatment or before alternate treatments (see toxicity).
      (2) Pharmacokinetics. Lomustine is readily absorbed following oral administration and metabolized by the liver into active metabolites. In humans, the elimination $t_{1/2}$ of lomustine is ~20 minutes, whereas the plasma $t_{1/2}$ of the metabolites is ~16 hours to 2 days. A total of 60–70% of the total dose is excreted in the urine in 96 hours. It has high lipid solubility.
      (3) Adverse effects. In dogs, lomustine may cause delayed, cumulative dose-related, chronic, irreversible hepatotoxicity and should not be used in patients with preexisting hepatic disease. Reversible hepatic enzyme increase is far more frequent (4 times elevation in ALT is indication for drug discontinuation). Hepatotoxicity may be delayed, prevented, or treated with S-adenosyl methionine (anecdotal) or other antioxidants. Hepatic toxicity is infrequent in cats.

Potentially, severe neutropenia may be found in dogs and cats treated with lomustine. Neutrophil nadirs are variable for dogs (1–4 weeks after administration, typically 1 week) and cats (1–5 weeks after administration). Thrombocytopenia lasting 4–6 weeks is possible with cumulative dosing. Dose escalation based on a nadir neutrophil count of $>2{,}000$ cells/μL (dogs) helps avoid severe neutropenia. Starting dose for dogs (50 mg/m^2 increasing to 90 mg/m^2 every 3 weeks) and cats (40 mg/m^2 increasing to 60 mg/m^2 every 4 weeks). GI complications are rare. Alopecia is seen in susceptible breeds.

  b. Carmustine (BiCNU®)

    (1) Therapeutic uses and administration. Like lomustine, carmustine is also useful for treatment of lymphoma and CNS malignancies (anecdotal in cats). Carmustine is given IV every 6 weeks for brain tumors or orally for lymphoma. Carmustine crosses the blood–brain barrier.

    (2) Pharmacokinetics. Carmustine is rapidly degraded in plasma into active metabolites. In humans 60–80% of the total dose is excreted in urine. It is lipophilic and crosses the blood–brain barrier.

    (3) Adverse effects. Potentially severe neutropenia (7-day nadir) is the predominant potential toxicity in dogs.

6. Streptozocin (Zanosar®)

  a. Mechanism of action. Streptozocin activity is not well understood, but it is thought to alkylate and thus, inhibit DNA formation.

  b. Therapeutic uses. As streptozocin selectively, typically, and irreversibly destroys the pancreatic β-cells in dogs resulting in diabetes mellitus (species-specific characteristic). It is used investigationally for treatment of insulinomas when complete surgical excision is not possible.

  c. Pharmacokinetics. After IV administration, it is distributed to most tissues; concentrations in the pancreas are higher than those found in the plasma. Streptozocin is metabolized, probably in the liver. Both unchanged and metabolized drug are excreted in the urine. After rapid IV injection, unchanged drug is rapidly cleared from the plasma with $t_{1/2}$ of 35 minutes in humans.

  d. Administration. IV administration with extensive saline diuresis both before and after streptozocin administration to decrease the potential for severe renal toxicity. Antiemetic therapy is necessary both before and for 72 hours after streptozocin infusion as severe, prolonged vomiting is possible.

  e. Adverse effects—See **d.** Nausea and vomiting and renal toxicity may be frequent and severe. Like doxorubicin, extravasation causes intense tissue necrosis. Less common and less serious are myelosuppression and increases in liver enzymes. Hypoglycemia-induced weakness may occur after infusion. Before each treatment, a complete blood count, biochemical panel, and urinalysis is needed. Risk for renal insufficiency is greater if the patient is dehydrated or concurrently receiving other potentially nephrotoxic drugs.

7. Procarbazine (Matulane®)

  a. Therapeutic uses and administration. Procarbazine is used in combination with other drugs for treatment of relapsed and CNS lymphoma as well as granulomatous meningoencephalitis. It is well absorbed orally and is given daily often in combination with other antineoplastic drugs. Adverse effects in cats and dogs may necessitate every other day dosing (see toxicity below).

  b. Pharmacokinetics. Procarbazine is an alkylator that crosses the blood–brain barrier. It is also a monoamine oxidase inhibitor. No information is available for animals. In humans, procarbazine is well absorbed after oral administration and rapidly equilibrates between the CSF and plasma. Peak levels in plasma reach in 60 minutes; in the CSF, about 30–90 minutes after administration. It is metabolized in the liver and kidney. Metabolic products are cytotoxic and excreted in the urine (mostly as N-isopropylterephthalamic acid, less than 5% as unchanged). Plasma $t_{1/2}$ is ~10 minutes after IV administration.

  c. Adverse effects. Myelosuppression (thrombocytopenia, leukopenia) and gastrointestinal effects (nausea, vomiting, and hemorrhagic gastroenteritis in dogs, anorexia most common in cats) are the most common adverse effects. These signs may be enhanced when procarbazine used in combination with other anticancer agents. CNS toxicity may be noted in some dogs. Monitor weekly CBC and monthly renal and hepatic function.

8. **Ifosfamide (Ifex®)**
   a. **Therapeutic uses and administration.** Ifosfamide use is investigational, but it has activity against lymphoma and soft tissue sarcoma in dogs and cats. It is administered IV every 3 weeks.
   b. **Pharmacokinetics.** Ifosfamide is inactive until metabolized by the liver into active metabolites via hydroxylation. In humans, $t_{1/2}$ is 7–15 hours. A total of 70–90% of metabolites and unchanged drug are excreted in the urine.
   c. **Adverse effects.**
      (1) Neutropenia (7 days and with repeated dosing, 14–21 days), hypersalivation (nausea) during infusion, and anorexia after treatment and potential nephrotoxicity were most common in cats.
      (2) Dogs exhibited neutropenia (nadir 7 days) which was dose-limiting and mild GI adverse effects.
      (3) When given IV to dogs and cats, extensive saline diuresis before and after drug administration minimizes nephrotoxicosis, while concurrent Mesna (2-mercaptoethanesulfonate, a free radical scavenger) prevents hemorrhagic cystitis (caused by irritant metabolites acrolein and 4 hydroxy-ifosfamide) in dogs and cats.

9. **Dacarbazine (DTIC-Dome®)**
   a. **Mechanism of action.** Exact mechanism is undetermined, but acts like an alkylating agent and requires hepatic activation for activity.
   b. **Therapeutic uses and administration.** Dacarbazine has activity in relapsed lymphoma, epitheliotrophic lymphoma in dogs. **It is not given to cats, because they may not have adequate hepatic metabolism.** Dacarbazine may be given IV (over 4–6 hours) every 2–4 weeks with premedication with antiemetics (single dose dolasetron or ondansetron is ... effective).
   c. **Pharmacokinetics.** It is metabolized into 5-amino-imidazole-4 carboxamide. In humans, the distribution $t_{1/2}$ is ~20 minutes and elimination $t_{1/2}$ is 5 hours; 40% is excreted unchanged in urine in 6 hours.
   d. **Adverse effects.** Acute GI toxicity is expected consisting of vomiting during and immediately after administration. Other GI toxicity includes anorexia and diarrhea. Extravasation causes painful tissue. Neutropenia and thrombocytopenia (nadir in several weeks after administration) is usually asymptomatic.

D. **Infrequently used alkylating agents**

1. **Busulfan** is an alkylsulfonate, which is well absorbed orally used for polycythemia and chronic myelogenous leukemia. Parent drug (25–50%) is eliminated as metabolites in the urine of humans in 48 hours.
2. **Hydroxyurea (Hydrea®)**
   a. **Therapeutic uses and administration.** Hydroxyurea is used for treatment of polycythemia vera, chronic myelogenous leukemia, meningioma, feline hypereosinophilic syndrome and mast cell tumor. Daily or alternate day oral administration is useful.
   b. **Pharmacokinetics.** Hydroxyurea is well absorbed after oral administration and crosses the blood–brain barrier. In humans, up to 50% of oral dose is metabolized. In addition, hydroxyurea is degraded by urease by intestinal bacteria. A total of 40–80% is excreted in urine within 12 hours. Elimination $t_{1/2}$ is 3–4.5 hours.
   c. **Adverse effects.** Toenail sloughing (dogs) and myelosuppression are most frequent. Myelosuppression is more problematic for cats. Renal insufficiency, stomatitis, GI signs, and exacerbation of urate urolithiasis secondary to increased serum urea are infrequent. Monitor with a CBC every 1–2 weeks initially, then every 3 months. More frequent monitoring for cats. Renal function is assessed initially and then every month or two.

IV. PLATINATING AGENTS

A. **General considerations.** Like alkylating agents, cisplatin and carboplatin act similarly since they cross-link DNA and prevent replication of DNA. They are cell cycle non-specific.

B. **Cisplatin (cis-diaminodichloroplatinum, CDDP, Platinol-AQ®)**

1. **Mechanism of action.** Cisplatin acts like a bifunctional alkylating agent producing inter- and intrastrand crosslinks in DNA through binding to guanine residues.
2. **Therapeutic uses.** In dogs, cisplatin is administered IV alone or in combination protocols for carcinomas and sarcomas.
3. **Pharmacokinetics.** Cisplatin is not absorbed orally. Following parenteral administration, it accumulates in kidneys, liver and the GI tract. Renal excretion occurs as free platinum (80% of dose in urine in 48 hours). It has a biphasic elimination profile with a distribution plasma $t_{1/2}$ of 20 minutes and a long terminal phase of 120 hours in dogs.
4. **Administration.** No aluminum needles should be used for administration.
   a. **Dogs.** IV saline must be given for 4 hours before and 2 hours after IV cisplatin. It is given once every three weeks. Slow IV infusion is also required to decrease nephrotoxicity. It may be given intracavitary along with saline diuresis.
   b. **Horses.** Intratumoral injection of cisplatin in sesame oil once every 2 weeks is the usual protocol for sarcoids, squamous cell carcinoma/papillomas, and melanomas.
5. **Adverse effects.** Nausea and vomiting is the most common acute toxicity requiring pre- and posttreatment antiemetic therapy. Renal toxicity (due to platinum accumulation but reduced by saline infusions), and myelosuppression (thrombocytopenia and/or neutropenia) are more common side effects. Rarely, ototoxicity or neurotoxicity may occur. Pretreatment CBC, BUN, serum creatinine concentrations, and urine specific gravity are minimum monitoring parameters.
   Note: Cisplatin causes fatal pulmonary toxicity in cats and should not be used.
6. **Special formulation.** Cisplatin may be delivered locally as a slow release formulation in a biodegradable, impregnated open-cell-polylactic acid polymer (OPLA-PT sponge). It has improved survival of dogs with osteosarcoma and nasal adenocarcinoma. Cisplatin is released for 21 days with no systemic side effects.

C. **Carboplatin (Paraplatin®)**

1. **Mechanism of action.** Acts like a bifunctional alkylating agent causing inter- and intrastrand crosslinks.
2. **Therapeutic uses.** Similar to cisplatin (carcinomas, sarcomas), except carboplatin can be safely administered to cats. When compared with cisplatin, carboplatin may be less effective against transitional cell carcinoma and more effective against malignant melanoma.
3. **Pharmacokinetics.** After IV administration, carboplatin is well distributed throughout the body; highest concentrations are found in the liver, kidney, skin and tumor tissue. Less protein bound than cisplatin, its elimination $t_{1/2}$ is shorter. The parent drug is degraded into platinum and platinum-complex compounds that are primarily eliminated into the urine. In dogs, 50% of the dose is excreted in the urine within 24 hours.
4. **Administration**
   a. **Intravenous.** Carboplatin is given by slow IV infusion without saline diuresis every 21 days for dogs and every 28 days for cats.
   b. **Intratumor.** Carboplatin may be mixed with sterilized sesame oil and given intratumorally every 4 weeks to cats with nasal cutaneous squamous cell carcinoma.
5. **Adverse effects.** When compared with cisplatin, carboplatin is much less emetogenic and nephrotoxic. The most common adverse effects still include GI abnormalities and myelosuppression. Neutrophil nadir is 14 days in dogs and 14–21 days in cats. Like cisplatin, a CBC with BUN and serum creatinine concentrations and

urine specific gravity are the minimum monitoring parameters obtained prior to each treatment.

V. ANTIMETABOLITES

A. **General considerations.** Antimetabolites are structural analogs of normal cellular molecules such as folic acid, purines, or pyrimidines; they impair DNA synthesis and are primarily S phase specific.

B. **Methotrexate (Rheumatrex Dose Pack®)**

1. **Mechanism of action.** Methotrexate inhibits dihydrofolate reductase and prevents conversion of dihydrofolic acid (DHFA) to tetrahydrofolic acid (THFA). THFA is essential for purine and pyrimidine synthesis.
2. **Therapeutic uses and administration.** Previously, methotrexate has been used in protocols for lymphomas, carcinomas, and sarcomas. It is more commonly given for immunosuppressive effects. In dogs and cats, methotrexate is typically given IV or orally, alone or in combination with other drugs.
3. **Pharmacokinetics.** Methotrexate exhibits dose-dependent oral absorption with variability in peak concentration and bioavailability. It is widely distributed except to the CNS. Plasma $t_{1/2}$ is <10 hours; generally 2–4 hours. Almost all is eliminated via renal tubular secretion and glomerular filtration (no hepatic metabolism).
4. **Adverse effects.** Adverse effects include nausea, vomiting, and diarrhea most commonly and less frequently, myelosuppression. A pretreatment CBC along with regular assessment of renal function and hepatic enzymes is recommended. Important potential adverse drug-methotrexate interactions should be evaluated before treating a patient with methotrexate.

C. **5-Fluorouracil (5-FU, Adrucil®)**

1. **Mechanism of action.** 5-FU is a pyrimidine analog. It is phosphorylated in cells to F-dUMP which block thymidylate synthase reactions and thus inhibits DNA synthesis. Also, 5-FU is incorporated into RNA and DNA.
2. **Therapeutic uses.** 5-FU is used in chemotherapy of carcinoma of the GI tract, mammary gland, liver and lungs. Sarcoids (horses) and cutaneous squamous cell carcinoma (dogs, cats, horses) respond to intralesional 5-FU.
3. **Pharmacokinetics.** 5-FU is administered parenterally since oral absorption is unpredictable. Distribution is wide and the drug readily enters CSF. Metabolism by reduction of the pyrimidine ring occurs primarily in the liver. Plasma $t_{1/2}$ after IV administration in humans is ~20 min. Information in animals is not available.
4. **Administration.**
   a. **Intravenous.** In dogs and cats, 5-FU is administered IV once a week.
   b. **Intratumoral.** 5-FU can be injected directly into tumor tissue every 2 weeks for 7 treatments.
5. **Adverse effects.** 5-FU cannot be used in cats because it produces severe, potentially irreversible and fatal neurotoxicity. In dogs, diarrhea, other GI tract mucosal toxicity, and myelosuppression are common side effects. CNS toxicity may occur in dogs and is characterized by excitement, ataxia, tremors, and convulsions.

D. **Cytosine arabinoside (Cytarabine, CytosarU®)**

1. **Mechanism of action.** Cytosine arabinoside is a pyrimidine analog which is phosphorylated in cells to Ara CMP and incorporated into DNA, resulting in labile linkages.
2. **Therapeutic uses.** Cytarabine is used in dogs and cats for lymphoreticular neoplasms, myeloproliferative disease, granulomatous meningoencephalitis and CNS lymphoma (crosses the blood–brain barrier).

3. **Pharmacokinetics.** Cytosine arabinoside is activated and metabolized by deaminase mainly the liver, but is also converted in the kidneys, intestinal mucosa, and granulocytes into uracil arabinoside (ara-U). Its metabolism is quite rapid (minutes), requiring continuous infusion over hours. ~80% of a dose is excreted in the urine within 24 hours (90% as ara-U and 10% as unchanged cytarabine).
4. **Administration.** Cytarabine is administered IV (by continuous infusion) or SC once a day to dogs and cats.
5. **Adverse effects.** Myelosuppression is the most common toxicity (neutropenia nadir at 5–7 days) and anemia and thrombocytopenia may also occur.

E. Gemcitabine (Gemzar®)

1. **Mechanism of action.** Gemcitabine is metabolized intracellularly to diflurodeoxycytidine monophosphate (dFdCMP) that is then converted into diphosphate (dFdCDP) and triphosphate (dFdCTP). The diphosphate inhibits ribonucleotide reductase. The triphosphate competitively inhibits incorporation of with deoxycytidine triphosphate (dTCP) for incorporation into DNA strands.
2. **Therapeutic uses.** Gemcitabine efficacy is questionable in veterinary medicine and considered investigational use. It may have activity in hepatocellular carcinoma and pancreatic adenocarcinoma in dogs and cats.
3. **Pharmacokinetics.** Plasma $t_{1/2}$ of 1.5 hours is in the dog after IV bolus injection. The drug is excreted into urine (>90% as metabolites).
4. **Administration.** Gemcitabine is given in a biweekly IV bolus. Slower IV infusion may improve antitumor activity by prolonging duration of action.
5. **Adverse effects.** Gemcitabine may cause myelosuppression particularly neutropenia and thrombocytopenia. Monitoring consists of a CBC before each treatment along with periodic assessment of liver and kidney function.

F. Azathioprine (Imuran®)

1. **Mechanism of action.** Azathioprine is converted to the active metabolite 6-mercaptopurine (6-MP) in the liver. It interferes with the *de novo* synthesis of purine nucleotides.
2. **Therapeutic uses and administration.** Azathioprine is used primarily as an immunosuppressive agent in the treatment of immune-mediated diseases and perianal fistulas in dogs. Clinical response is typically 3–5 weeks. Azathioprine is given orally once a day in dogs.
3. **Pharmacokinetics.** Azathioprine is absorbed from the GI tract. Conversion of 6-MP metabolites by thiopurine methyltransferase is essential for azathioprine detoxification; however, cats and 10% of dogs have low enzyme activity. In these patients, low activity should be identified early so that doses are decreased and bone marrow toxicity avoided. Azathioprine is rapidly eliminated from blood. In humans, no azathioprine is detectable in urine after 8 hours of administration.
4. **Adverse effects.** Neutropenia, thrombocytopenia, and anemia can result from azathioprine. In dogs, GI toxicity (self-limiting nausea and diarrhea) and hepatotoxicity are seen. Pancreatitis, possibly exacerbated by concurrent steroid administration, has been reported. Monitor CBC every one to 2 weeks initially and renal and liver function monthly.

G. 6-Mercaptopurine (6-MP, Purinethol®)

1. **Mechanism of action.** 6-MP is a purine analog which is phosphorylated in cells. It inhibits multiple steps of DNA and RNA synthesis.
2. **Therapeutic uses and administration.** 6-MP is used in dogs and cats for acute lymphocytic leukemia, granulocytic leukemia, and lymphosarcoma. 6-MP is administered orally once a day.
3. **Pharmacokinetics**
   GI absorption after oral dosing is variable and incomplete. Absorbed 6-MP and its metabolites are widely distributed in the body. The drug crosses the blood–brain barrier, but not in concentrations high enough to treat CNS neoplasms.

6-MP, via the enzyme xanthine oxidase, is rapidly metabolized in the liver to 6-thiouric acid, which along with the parent compound and other metabolites are principally excreted in the urine. In humans, ~50% of 6-MP is excreted in urine within 24 hours as parent drug and metabolites. Plasma $t_{1/2}$ is ~45 minutes in adults.

4. **Adverse effects**. Leukopenia and thrombocytopenia are the most common side effects.

H. **6-Thioguanine (6-TG, Thioguanine Tabloid®)**

1. **Mechanism of action**. 6-TG is a purine analog with actions similar to 6-MP.
2. **Therapeutic uses**. 6-TG is used in dogs and cats for acute leukemia. 6-TG is administered orally once a day.
3. **Pharmacokinetics.**
   a. 6-TG is administered orally, but GI absorption is variable. In humans, only ~30% of a dose is absorbed.
   b. 6-TG is distributed into the DNA and RNA of bone marrow, but several doses may be necessary for this to occur. It does not apparently enter the CNS.
   c. 6-TG is rapidly metabolized primarily in the liver to methylate derivative that is less active than the parent compound. This and other metabolites are then eliminated in the urine.
   d. The short $t_{1/2}$ of 6-TG of ~2 hours in humans support the notion that it is rapidly metabolized.
4. **Adverse effects**. Leukopenia and thrombocytopenia are the most common side effects.

VI. MITOTIC SPINDLE INHIBITORS

A. **General Considerations.** Vincristine and vinblastine are extracts of the common periwinkle plant (vinorelbine is semisynthetic). The taxanes are from the Japanese yew tree.

B. **Vincristine/Vinblastine**

1. **Mechanism of action.** The vinca alkaloids, vincristine and vinblastine bind to tubulin in the mitotic spindle to prevent cell division during metaphase. They are active in the G2 and M phases of the cell cycle.
2. **Therapeutic uses**
   a. **Vincristine (Vincasar PFS®).** Vincristine is the most commonly used mitotic inhibitor in veterinary medicine. It is employed in the treatment of lymphoreticular neoplasms, carcinomas, and sarcomas in dogs and cats and transmissible venereal tumors (TVT) in dogs.
   b. **Vinblastine (Velban®).** Vinblastine has been used to treat lymphomas and mast cell tumors in dogs and cats.
   c. **Vinorelbine (Navelbine®).** Vinorelbine has been used to manage pulmonary carcinomas in dogs and cats.
3. **Pharmacokinetics.** The vinca alkaloids are not absorbed orally. After IV administration, they are rapidly distributed except to the CNS. ~75% is bound to tissue proteins. They are metabolized by the liver and mainly excreted in the bile/feces. Maximum tissue concentration attained in one hour. In dogs, elimination $t_{1/2}$ is 75 minutes for vincristine and ~4 hours for vinblastine.
4. **Administration.** The vinca alkaloids are administered IV every 7–14 days, usually in combination protocols except for TVT. Note: The vinca alkaloids are severe vesicants if injected perivascularly.
5. **Adverse effects**
   a. The vinca alkaloids, especially vincristine, may produce a peripheral neurotoxicity, (neural tissue has a high concentration of tubulin protein), neuromuscular weakness, and constipation secondary to autonomic neuropathy.

b. Myelosuppression may occur, but is less severe than that produced by other antineoplastic drugs. In order of decreasing myelosuppression in dogs are vinorelbine, vinblastine, and vincristine.

c. Biliary excretion may be inhibited by cholestasis requiring a dose reduction if serum bilirubin is >2.0 mg/dl.

d. Extravasation results in severe tissue necrosis.

C. Taxanes

1. **Paclitaxel (Taxol®)**

   a. **Mechanism of action.** Microtubule dissolution (depolymerization) is inhibited. This stability inhibits the normal dynamic reorganization of the microtubule network that is essential for vital interphase and mitotic cellular functions.

   b. **Therapeutic uses.** Investigational use suggests activity against mammary carcinoma, osteogenic osteosarcoma, and histiocytosis in dogs. Its use is not recommended because of severe adverse effects.

   c. **Pharmacokinetics.** There is no information in animals.

   (1) In humans, 89–98% of paclitaxel is bound by plasma proteins following IV administration. It is also extensively bound by tissues during extravascular distribution.

   (2) Paclitaxel is metabolized primarily to 6α-hydroxypaclitaxel 3-p-hydroxypactlitaxel and 6α,-p-dihyroxypaclitaxel by cytochrome P450 enzymes in the liver.

   (3) The metabolites and unchanged drug are excreted mainly in feces (71%) and lesser in urine (14%). Following 3- and 24-hour infusions, the $t_{1/2}$ of paclitaxel is 13–53 hours.

   d. **Administration.** Paclitaxel is given via IV administration every 3 weeks. Premedication with corticosteroids and antihistamines (H1 and H2 blockers) is imperative one hour prior to administration. The calculated dose of paclitaxel is diluted in 0.9% NaCl at a concentration of 0.6–0.7 mg taxol/mL and administered IV over 2 hours. Slow infusion if adverse reactions occur.

   e. **Adverse effects.** Myelosuppression can be severe with a nadir at day 3 with gastrointestinal adverse effects (vomiting, anorexia especially). Anaphylactoid reactions (sometimes severe) caused by diluent (Cremphor EL) and somnolence by (alcohol) are most problematic acutely and may be severe. Some adverse reactions may be fatal. Severe alopecia is seen in susceptible canine breeds. Paclitaxel has been given to few cats. The same (often fatal) reaction to Cremaphor EL vehicle occurs in cats.

VII. TOPOISOMERASE INHIBITORS OR ANTITUMOR ANTIBIOTICS

A. Doxorubicin (Adriamycin®)

1. **Mechanism of action.** Doxorubicin is an anthracycline antibiotic that inhibits topoisomerase II, an enzyme is involved in the cleavage, unwinding, and rejoining of segments of DNA. It also intercalates DNA (forms a stable complex), inhibits DNA helicase, and generates oxygen free radicals, leading to oxidative damage to cell membranes and DNA. It is non-cell cycle specific (inhibits DNA and RNA synthesis) but is most active in the S phase.

2. **Therapeutic uses.** Doxorubicin is used in the treatment of carcinomas and sarcomas in dogs and cats, especially lymphoma, thyroid and mammary gland carcinoma and osteosarcoma.

3. **Pharmacokinetics.**

   a. Doxorubicin is not absorbed orally. It causes severe tissue necrosis if given SC or IM. Following IV administration, it is rapidly and widely distributed throughout the body except to the CNS. It is highly bound to plasma and tissue proteins.

   b. It is metabolized by the liver and other tissues via aldo-keto-reductase primarily to an active metabolite, doxorubicinol, and other inactive metabolites. Doxorubucin and its metabolites are primarily excreted in bile and feces.

   c. Doxorubucin is eliminated in a triphasic manner: During the first phase ($t_{1/2}$ 0.6 hours) doxorubicin is rapidly metabolized, via the "first-pass" effect followed by a second phase ($t_{1/2}$ 3.3 hours). The third phase has a much slower elimination $t_{1/2}$ of ~15 hours for doxorubicin and ~30 hours for metabolites), probably due to the slow release of the drug from tissue proteins. Less than 5% is excreted in the urine of dogs. Plasma $t_{1/2}$ in dogs is ~1 hour.

4. **Administration.** Doxorubicin is administered IV every 21 days as part of a multidrug protocol. Limit total dose to 180–240 mg/m^2 or simultaneously treat with desroxazone) to avoid cardiomyopathy. Dose reductions of 50% required for serum bilirubin concentrations >2.0 mg/dl in dogs. Do not give to hyperbilirubinemic cats.

5. **Adverse effects.** Extravasation produces severe tissue necrosis. Complete blood count and ECG are minimal pretreatment requirements.

   a. Dogs. In addition to leucopenia and thrombocytopenia (nadir at 7–10 days), anaphylactoid reaction, and gastroenteritis (diarrhea, anorexia, hemorrhagic enterocolitis 2–5 days after administration), doxorubicin may produce chronic, irreversible, dose-dependent cardiomyopathy via free radical myocardial damage.

   b. Cats. Nephropathy and renal insufficiency with cumulative doses, leukopenia, thrombocytopenia, prolonged anorexia, and vomiting are not uncommon side effects.

6. **Other Formulations. Liposome-encapsulated doxorubicin (Doxil®).** When compared with doxorubicin, liposome-encapsulated (PEG) doxorubicin given IV every 3–4 weeks has increased half-life, less cardiotoxicity, similar leukopenia and thrombocytopenia, similar anaphylactoid reactivity, less GI toxicity, more renal toxicity and alopecia. A unique toxicity, palmar-plantar erythrodysesthesia syndrome (hand-foot syndrome) occurs, but its onset and severity in dogs may be reduced by administering pyridoxine (vitamin B6) concurrently. It has a similar activity spectrum to native doxorubicin.

B. Mitoxantrone (Novantrone®)

1. **Mechanism of action.** By intercalation between base pairs and nonintercalative electrostatic interactions, mitoxantrone inhibits both DNA and RNA synthesis. It may also function as an inhibitor of topoisomerase II. Mitoxantrone is not considered cell-cycle phase specific, but appears to be most active during the S phase.

2. **Therapeutic uses and administration.** Mitoxantrone indications include lymphoma (naïve and relapsed), squamous cell carcinoma, soft tissue sarcomas, mammary gland carcinoma, transitional cell carcinoma, other carcinomas/sarcomas. It is given IV every 3 or 4 weeks in dogs and cats.

3. **Pharmacokinetics.** In humans, it is rapidly taken up by tissues when given intravenously and slowly released from tissues over days. Highest concentrations of mitoxantrone are found in the liver, heart, thyroid and red blood cells. In humans, ~80% of the drug is bound to plasma proteins. It is metabolized in the liver, but the majority of the drug is excreted unchanged in the urine. The $t_{1/2}$ of the drug in humans is ~5 days as a result of the drug being bound by, and then slowly released from tissues.

4. **Adverse effects.** Cardiotoxicity has not been reported in dogs and cats. The most frequently noted toxicities are myelosuppression (neutrophil nadir about 10 days) and GI disturbances (vomiting, anorexia, and diarrhea). When compared with doxorubicin, extravasation is less damaging to tissue and anaphylactoid reaction is not reported. A CBC should be performed prior to each treatment. Additional liver and renal function assays may be needed in nonhealthy patients.

C. Actinomycin D (Dactinomycin, Cosmegen®)

1. **Mechanism of action.** Actinomycin D intercalates with the DNA helix and blocks transcription by RNA polymerase. It is not cell cycle specific.

2. **Therapeutic uses and administration.** In dogs and cats, lymphoma (naïve and relapsed), soft tissue and bone sarcomas, and some carcinomas may be treated with actinomycin D. Actinomycin D is administered IV once a week in dogs and every 3–4 weeks in cats.

3. **Pharmacokinetics.**
   a. Actinomycin D is poorly absorbed when given orally; it must be administered IV. It is rapidly distributed, but the distribution does not extend to the CNS.
   b. It is excreted mostly unchanged in the urine and bile. In humans, only ~30% of the drug is excreted within 7 days of administration. The $t_{1/2}$ of the drug is ~36 hours. No information is available in animals.

4. **Adverse effects.** Nausea, vomiting, diarrhea, and leucopenia (particularly thrombocytopenia) are common side effects. Extravasation causes tissue necrosis. A CBC and liver enzyme tests are recommended before each treatment.

D. **Etoposide (Topscar®)**

1. **Mechanism of action.** Etoposide is a semisynthetic analog of the natural product podophyllotoxins, found in mandrake plants. Although it binds to tubulin and inhibits polymerization like mitotic inhibitors, etoposide is a DNA topoisomerase II inhibitor that stops the action of topoisomerase II after it creates a nick in one strand of the DNA. The nicked DNA is unable to unwind and eventually breaks.

2. **Therapeutic uses and administration.** Intravenous etoposide administration is too toxic to be given to dogs; however, etoposide for injection can be safely given orally to dogs.

3. **Pharmacokinetics.** In humans, etoposide is eliminated by hepatic glucuronidation and approximately 40 percent of the drug is excreted unchanged in the urine. Oral absorption occurs, but is variable.

4. **Adverse effects.** When given orally, adverse hematologic and gastrointestinal effects were mild.

VIII. **HORMONES**

A. **Glucocorticoids**

1. **General considerations.** Glucocorticoids cause apoptosis of lymphocytes and thus are lympholytic. They are cell cycle nonspecific. In dogs and cats, lymphoreticular neoplasms including lymphomas of CNS and mast cell tumors respond to glucocorticoids. They are frequently employed in cancer therapy with other drugs for their symptomatic improvement of appetite and well-being. See Chapter 12 for more information.

IX. **ENZYMES**

A. **L-Asparaginase (Elspar®)**

1. **Mechanism of action.** L-asparaginase is an enzyme which hydrolyses L-asparagine to deplete circulating levels and thus, inhibit protein synthesis. Normal cells synthesize sufficient L-asparagine for protein synthesis, but certain neoplastic cells require an exogenous source of this amino acid, and its depletion results in cell death. It is G1 phase specific.

2. **Therapeutic uses.** Acute lymphoblastic leukemia and multicentric lymphoma in dogs and cats respond to L-asparaginase. It is used in multidrug protocols.

3. **Pharmacokinetics.**
    a. In humans, after IM administration, the time to reach peak plasma concentrations is 14–24 hours. Plasma $t_{1/2}$ after IM and IV administrations are 39–49 hours and 8–30 hours, respectively. Half-life in dogs is 12–40 hours, but asparagine plasma concentrations remain depressed for 1–3 weeks after administration. It is not absorbed orally.
    b. The metabolic fate of asparaginase is not known. It is probably metabolized by proteases in the liver and kidneys. Only trace amounts are found in bile and urine of dogs.
4. **Administration.** To decrease the incidence and severity of anaphylactic reaction to a "foreign" protein, L-asparaginase is administered IM or SC once a week.
5. **Adverse effects.** Anti-L-asparaginase antibodies are present in some dogs prior to any l-asparaginase administration, anaphylactic reaction is possible to the first dose of l-asparaginase. Pancreatitis may develop in susceptible dogs and should not be given to patients with a history of pancreatitis. Myelosuppression occurs if given with vincristine.

X. MISCELLANEOUS

A. Piroxicam (Feldene®)

1. **Mechanism of Action.** Although not fully determined, the mechanism of action of piroxicam (a NSAID that inhibits both COX-1 and COX-2) is thought to relate to inhibition of COX-2 activity expressed on transitional cell carcinoma cells and to inhibition of tumor angiogenesis.
2. **Therapeutic uses.** Piroxicam can be used as a single agent or as an adjunctive therapy against transitional cell carcinoma (dogs and cats) and oral squamous cell carcinoma (dogs), canine mammary gland carcinoma, and canine nasal carcinomas. It is administered PO.
3. **Pharmacokinetics.**
    a. After oral administration, piroxicam is well absorbed from the gut. The presence of food will decrease the rate of absorption.
    b. Peak levels occur in ~3 hours. Elimination $t_{1/2}$ is ~12 hours.
    c. Piroxicam is highly bound to plasma proteins. In humans, piroxicam has a very long plasma (~50 hours). The drug is mainly excreted as metabolites in the urine after hepatic biotransformation.
4. **Adverse effects.** Adverse effect include GI irritation and nephrotoxicity. These difficulties may be more severe in cats than dogs. Regular evaluation of PCV, BUN, creatinine, and urine specific gravity are advised in order to monitor for renal toxicity and GI bleeding.

B. Mitotane (O,P'-DDD, Lysodren®)

1. **Mechanism of action.** Mitotane is a chlorinated hydrocarbon which is selectively cytotoxic to the cells of the adrenal cortex. See Chapter 12 III B4, page 269 for further information.

C. Bleomycin (Blenoxane®)

1. **Mechanism of action.** Bleomycin is a mixture of glycopeptide antibiotics which bind to DNA and cause chain scission and fragmentation via generation of free radicals. Cells accumulate in the G_2 phase and the antibiotic is G_2 specific.
2. **Therapeutic uses and administration.** Bleomycin is rarely used in veterinary medicine; however, responses have been seen for squamous cell carcinoma and relapsed lymphoma in dogs and cats. A common protocol is IV or SC administration of bleomycin daily for 3–4 days, then once a week.

3. **Pharmacokinetics.** Bleomycin is not absorbed orally. Distribution is wide with high concentrations in skin and lungs, but it does not cross the blood–brain barrier and is found in low concentrations in bone marrow. It is degraded by tissue hydrolase. Bleomycin is excreted by the kidneys. In patients with normal renal function, elimination $t_{1/2}$ is ~2 hours. In humans, 60–70% of a dose is excreted as intact drug in the urine.

4. **Adverse effects**. Myelosuppression is minimal. However, nausea and a delayed pulmonary fibrosis and/or skin ulcers may develop.

SUGGESTED READING

Frimberger AE. 2005. "Principles of chemotherapy." In *Textbook of Veterinary Internal Medicine.* Edited by Ettinger SJ, Feldman EC. 6th ed., pp. 708–712. Philadelphia, PA: Saunders. http://www.drugs.com

Lucroy MD. 2001. Chemotherapy safety in veterinary practices: Hazardous drug preparation. *Compend Contin Educ Pract Vet* 23:860–870.

Lucroy MD. 2002. Chemotherapy safety in veterinary practices: Hazardous drug administration. *Compend Contin Educ Pract Vet* 24:140–147.

Moore AS. 2005. "Practical chemotherapy." In *Textbook of Veterinary Internal Medicine.* Edited by Ettinger SJ, Feldman EC. 6th ed., pp. 713–720. Philadelphia, PA: Saunders.

Plumb DC. 2005. *Veterinary Drug Handbook.* 5th ed. Ames, IA: Blackwell Publishing.

■ STUDY QUESTIONS

DIRECTIONS: Each of the numbered items or incomplete statements in this section is followed by answers or by completions of the statement. Select the **one** lettered answer or completion that is **best** in each case.

1. Which one of the following statements about antineoplastic drugs is true?

(A) They kill a constant number of cancer cells with each dose.
(B) They are most effective against cells in the G_0 phase of the cell cycle.
(C) They kill malignant cells quickly and thus resistance seldom develops.
(D) The dosage is based on body surface area.
(E) They are not carcinogenic, teratogenic, and genotoxic.

2. Which one of the following is an alkylating agent used in the treatment of lymphoma in cats and dogs?

(A) 5-Fluorouracil
(B) Methotrexate
(C) Vincristine
(D) Doxorubicin
(E) Cyclophosphamide

3. Which one of the following is true about cytosine arabinoside?

(A) Stops neoplastic cell division in metaphase
(B) Blocks purine synthesis by inhibiting dihydrofolate reductase
(C) Is used primarily for adrenal tumors
(D) Is cell cycle nonspecific
(E) Is a pyrimidine analog which is phosphorylated in cells to Ara CMP

4. The high concentration of tubulin protein in neural tissue may be the basis for neuromuscular weakness and constipation observed in cancer chemotherapy with:

(A) Vincristine
(B) Doxorubicin
(C) Chlorambucil
(D) Methotrexate
(E) 5-Fluorouracil

5. Which one of the following statements is true about cyclophosphamide?

(A) Tends to produce less myelosuppression than other classes of antineoplastics
(B) Is usually injected directly into body cavities or tumor masses
(C) Readily crosses the blood–brain barrier
(D) Cross-links DNA
(E) Is excreted by the liver

6. Which one of the following drugs is given because it inhibits COX-2 and is considered a nonsteroidal anti-inflammatory drug?

(A) L-asparaginase
(B) Cyclophosphamide
(C) Lomustine
(D) Cyclophosphamide
(E) Piroxicam

7. Which one of the following drugs is a mitotic inhibitor which would arrest lymphoma cells in metaphase?

(A) Vincristine
(B) 6-Mercaptopurine
(C) Chlorambucil
(D) Doxorubicin
(E) Cisplatin

8. Furosemide may slow the onset and severity of hemorrhagic cystitis resulting from which one of the following drugs?

(A) Cyclophosphamide
(B) L-asparaginase
(C) Melphalan
(D) Doxorubicin
(E) Methotrexate

9. Two antineoplastic drugs *should not* be used in cats because of severe pulmonary toxicity and neurotoxicity respectively. Which pair below cannot be given to cats?

(A) Chlorambucil and methotrexate
(B) Cisplatin and 5-fluorouracil
(C) Vincristine and bleomycin
(D) Mitotane and 6-thioguanine

10. Cardiomyopathy may accompany myelo-suppression and gastroenteritis in dogs treated with one of the following drugs?

(A) 6-Mercaptopurine
(B) Vincristine
(C) Doxorubicin
(D) Actinomycin D
(E) Ifosfamide

11. IV saline infusions prior to and following drug administration are necessary to reduce renal toxicity of which one of the following drugs?

(A) Melphalan
(B) Vinblastine
(C) Methotrexate
(D) Cisplatin
(E) Chlorambucil

12. Phosphorylation in cells to a derivative which blocks thymidylate synthetase characterizes the action of which one of the following drugs?

(A) 5-Fluorouracil
(B) Actinomycin-D
(C) Carmustine
(D) Bleomycin
(E) Cyclophosphamide

13. An alkylating agent which must be activated in the liver to cytotoxic metabolites before it can kill tumor cells is which one of the following drugs?

(A) L-asparaginase
(B) Vincristine
(C) Lomustine
(D) Cyclophosphamide
(E) Cisplatin

14. Which one of the following statements about chlorambucil is true?

(A) It is a rapid-acting nitrogen mustard.
(B) Its toxicity such as myelosuppression is potentially milder when compared with cyclophosphamide.
(C) It is more effective than cyclophosphamide in rapidly growing tumors.
(D) It is not absorbed orally.
(E) It may be used instead of cyclophosphamide in patients who have cyclophosphamide-induced hemorrhagic cystitis.

15. When given as a single agent, which one of the following drugs is least myelotoxic?

(A) Azathioprine
(B) L-asparaginase
(C) Actinomycin-D
(D) Paclitaxel
(E) Mitoxantrone

16. Which one of the following drugs is cell-cycle phase specific?

(A) Vincristine
(B) Lomustine
(C) Chlorambucil
(D) Doxorubicin
(E) Cisplatin

17. Which one of the following drugs does not readily cross the blood–brain barrier?

(A) Doxorubicin
(B) Cytosine arabinoside
(C) Corticosteroids
(D) Lomustine
(E) Procarbazine

ANSWERS AND EXPLANATIONS

1. The answer is D.
Antineoplastic drugs are dosed based on body surface area in most instances. Doxorubicin is an exception where smaller dogs and also cats, are dosed on a milligram/kilogram basis. Chemotherapeutic drugs have the potential to be mutagenic, embryotoxic, teratogenic, carcinogenic, and cytotoxic. Most drugs are not effective during the G_0 phase of the cell cycle because the cells are resting (normal cells are found in this phase). Drug resistance develops in neoplastic cells with mechanisms similar to those observed in antibiotic resistant bacteria. Drugs kill a constant percentage of cancer cells with each dose.

2. The answer is E.
The only alkylating agent in the group listed is cyclophosphamide. It is also used in the treatment of immune-mediated disorders such as, immune-mediated hemolytic anemia.

3. The answer is E.
Cytosine arabinoside is a pyrimidine analog which is phosphorylated to Ara CMP in cells. It is an antimetabolite which works primarily in the S phase of the cell cycle. It is used in dogs and cats for lymphoreticular neoplasms, myeloproliferative disease, granulomatous meningoencephalitis and CNS lymphoma (crosses the blood–brain barrier).

4. The answer is A.
The vinca alkaloids, especially vincristine, may produce a peripheral neurotoxicity (neural tissue has a high concentration of tubulin protein), neuromuscular weakness, and constipation secondary to autonomic neuropathy.

5. The answer is D.
Cyclophosphamide is inactive until being hydroxylated in the liver by microsomes as the first step in conversion to phosphoramide mustard and acrolein, the active metabolites. Thus, it should not be injected directly into tumors. It cross-links DNA and thus inhibits replication. It is myelosuppressive and does not cross the blood–brain barrier readily.

6. The answer is E.
Piroxicam is a NSAID that inhibits both COX-1 and COX-2 receptors. Its antitumor mechanism is thought to relate to inhibition of COX-2 activity expressed on transitional cell carcinoma cells and to inhibition of tumor angiogenesis.

7. The answer is A.
Vincristine is a mitotic inhibitor which arrests cells in metaphase.

8. The answer is A.
Cystitis is most common in dogs and is due to the irritant effects of acrolein and other metabolites. Concurrent administration of furosemide (IV most effective) with cyclophosphamide decreases the risk (to <1%) and/or delays the onset of cyclophosphamide-induced hemorrhagic cystitis. Administration of cyclophosphamide in the morning, stimulation of water intake and frequent voiding will reduce the frequency of cystitis. Initial treatment includes discontinuation of diuresis (no furosemide or corticosteroids) and cyclophosphamide.

9. The answer is B.
Cisplatin causes fatal pulmonary edema and 5-flourouracil causes intractable seizures. Neither drug should be used systemically in cats.

10. The answer is C.
In dogs, leucopenia and thrombocytopenia (nadir at 7–10 days), anaphylactoid reactions, gastroenteritis (diarrhea, anorexia, hemorrhagic enterocolitis 2–5 days after administration of doxorubicin), and chronic, irreversible, dose-dependent cardiomyopathy via free radical myocardial damage.

11. The answer is D.
IV saline must be given for 4 hours before and 2 hours after IV cisplatin once every three weeks. Slow IV infusion is also required to decrease nephrotoxicity. It may be given intracavitary if saline diuresis is administered concurrently.

12. The answer is A.
5-FU is a pyrimidine analog that is phosphorylated in cells to F-dUMP which block thymidylate synthase reactions and thus inhibits DNA synthesis.

13. The answer is D.
Cyclophosphamide must be converted to phosphoramide mustard and acrolein by hepatocytes.

14. The answer is B.
Chlorambucil is a slow-acting alkylating agent that is well absorbed orally. It is less effective than cyclophosphamide, but is less myelosuppressive and does not cause hemorrhagic cystitis.

15. The answer is B.
L-asparaginase has no myelosuppressive effect unless given with myelosuppressive drugs such as, vincristine. Normal cells synthesize sufficient L-asparagine for protein synthesis, but certain neoplastic cells require an exogenous source of this amino acid, and its depletion results in cell death.

16. The answer is A.
Cell-cycle phase specific drugs include those which kill cells predominantly in one phase of the cell cycle. The taxanes and vinca alkaloids kill in the cell phase when the mitotic spindle is formed.

17. The answer is A.
Doxorubicin does not cross the blood–brain barrier appreciably. Whereas, lomustine and procarbazine cross readily thus are useful for treating brain tumors. Corticosteroids and cytosine arabinoside penetrate the brain and are used to treat lymphoma and granulomatous meningoencephalitis.

Chapter 18

Fluid and Blood Therapy

Walter H. Hsu

I. BIOCHEMICAL BASIS OF FLUID THERAPY

A. Body water

1. **Water content** is 55–60% of body weight in mature animals, 70–75% in immature animals, and 50% in obese animals.
2. **Intracellular fluid (ICF)** represents 40% of the body weight.
3. **Extracellular fluid (ECF)** consists of:
   a. **Plasma water:** 5% of the body weight.
   b. **Interstitial fluid:** 14% of the body weight.
   c. **Transcellular fluid:** 1–6% of the body weight.
4. **Body water turnover**
   a. It is regulated by thirst and drinking control centers and vasopressin (antidiuretic hormone [ADH]), responding to osmolarity and blood volume changes: the higher the osmolarity and the lower the blood volume, the more stimulation of the drinking control centers and vasopressin secretion. As a result, large volume of water is being drunk.
   b. **Body water turnover** is 50–130 mL/kg/day, 65 mL/kg/day in mature animals.
   c. **The role of skin and body surface.** Skin is the largest organ of the body. The smaller the size of an animal, the larger the body surface is; thus, the higher the body water turnover rate. This is why dehydration has a much greater impact on young animals than mature animals.

B. Concept of milliequivalents (mEq)

1. Most of the electrolyte concentrations are expressed as mEq/L; mEq is calculated as mg of chemical divided by its equivalent weight. For example, the equivalent weight of NaCl is 58.5; 1 mEq of NaCl = 58.5 mg.
2. Total concentration of cations in the plasma is equal to that of anions.
3. Calcium and phosphorus in the plasma are measured as mg%, ~50% of plasma calcium is in the free ionized form and ~50% is bound by plasma proteins. Plasma phosphorus is present as $H_2PO_4^-$, HPO_4^{2-}, and PO_4^{3-}.

C. Osmosis and osmolarity

1. **Role of semipermeable membranes in osmosis.** Fluid compartments are separated by semipermeable membranes, which allow free passage of water but restrict particles. Water moves to the compartment with the highest number of particles (osmotic pressure).
2. **Osmolarity** is to describe properties related to the number of particles in solution and is expressed as mOsm/L of body fluid.
3. **Calculation of mOsm/L from mM**
   a. **For electrolyte solutions.** Since NaCl dissociates into two particles, Na^+ and Cl^-, 1 mmol/L (1 mmolar or 1 mM) of NaCl solution yields 2 mOsm/L. A total of 1 mmol of NaCl contains 58.5 mg since its molecular weight is 58.5.
   b. **For nonelectrolyte solutions.** Since glucose does not dissociate, 1 mM of glucose solution yields 1 mOsm/L.
4. **Osmolarity of an isotonic solution is ~300 mOsm/L.** One should be able to determine if a solution in mM is isotonic depending on whether the chemical can dissociate in the solvent. For example, 150 mM NaCl and 300 mM glucose solutions are isotonic.

D. **Role of the kidney in water and electrolyte regulation**

1. A total of 80–90% of water, Na^+, Cl^-, and so forth, is reabsorbed from the proximal tubule.
2. Information on renal physiology is presented in Chapter 9, I B (Review of nephron ion and water transport).

E. **Acid–base regulation**

1. **Definition of acid, base, and pH** Acid is a proton (H^+) donor and base is a H^+ acceptor. Thus, HCl is an acid, and HCO_3^- is a base, so is NH_3; chloride (Cl^-) is not an acid and Na^+ is not a base. pH is $-\log [H^+]$. If $[H^+] = 10^{-7}$ M, pH = 7.
2. **Use of Henderson–Hasselbalch equation** to calculate the ratio between base and acid

$$pH = \frac{pKa + \log[A^-]}{[HA]}$$

Since $pKa = 6.1$ for the $[HCO_3^-] - [H_2CO_3]$ pair, and if pH is 7.4:

$$7.4 = 6.1 + \log [HCO_3^-]/[H_2CO_3], \text{ the } \log [HCO_3^-]/[H_2CO_3]$$

$$= 1.3; \text{ the antilog of } 1.3 \text{ is } 20$$

$$\text{Thus, } \frac{[HCO_3^-]}{[H_2CO_3]} = \frac{20}{1} \text{ at pH } 7.4.$$

When this ratio is disturbed, the result is either acidosis or alkalosis.

3. **Buffer systems in the body**
   a. **Intrinsic buffering system.** Bicarbonate, hemoglobin, phosphate, and proteins (amino acids) constitute 53, 35, 5, and 7% of the intrinsic buffering system, respectively.
   b. **The cellular component of the buffering system** takes place during the first stage of the abnormality.
      (1) **Na^+–H^+–K^+ exchanges** (Figure 18-1). Normally, H^+ generated during cellular metabolism is removed via Na^+–H^+ antiport, which exports H^+ and imports Na^+. The increased $[Na^+]_i$ will then exchange for $[K^+]_o$ via Na^+, K^+-ATPase. Thus, **the net result of the reaction is one molecule of H^+_{in} exchanges for one molecule of K^+_{out}.** During acidosis (acidemia), this exchange process is inhibited by low pH, and thus more H^+ stays in the cells and more K^+ stays in the ECF. During alkalosis (alkalemia), this exchange is accelerated, and thus more H^+ is lost to the ECF and more K^+ enters the cells.
      (2) **Cl^-–HCO_3^- exchange.** The plasma membranes of animal cells contain an anion exchange protein, which exports HCO_3^- and imports Cl^-. The activity

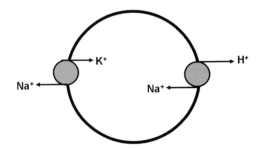

FIGURE 18-1. The compensatory mechanisms for acid–base disturbances involving intra- and extracellular H^+, Na^+, and K^+ exchanges. As a result of these exchanges, acidosis and alkalosis can lead to hyperkalemia, and hypokalemia, respectively. By the same token, hyperkalemia and hypokalemia can lead to acidosis and alkalosis, respectively.

Hyperkalemia $(\uparrow[K^+]_o) \to \uparrow[K^+]_i \ [Na^+]_o \to \uparrow[H^+]_o$

Hypokalemia $(\downarrow[K^+]_o) \to \downarrow[K^+]_i \ [Na^+]_o \to \downarrow[H^+]_o$

Acidemia $(\uparrow[H^+]_o) \to \downarrow[Na^+]_i \to \downarrow[K^+]_i, \uparrow[K^+]_o$

Alkalemia $(\downarrow[H^+]_o) \to \uparrow[Na^+]_i \to \uparrow[K^+]_i, \downarrow[K^+]_o$

$$\text{Normal pH:} \quad \frac{[HCO_3^-]}{[H_2CO_3]} = \frac{20}{1}$$

Metabolic compensation
↓

$$\text{Hypoventilation} \atop \text{(Resp. acidosis)} \quad : \quad \frac{20}{1+1} = \frac{20}{2} \rightarrow \frac{20+20}{2} = \frac{40}{2} = \frac{20}{1}$$

Respiratory compensation
↓

$$\text{Metabolic acidosis:} \quad \frac{20-10}{1} = \frac{10}{1} \rightarrow \frac{10}{1-0.5} = \frac{10}{0.5} = \frac{20}{1}$$

Metabolic compensation
↓

$$\text{Hyperventilation} \atop \text{(Resp. alkalosis)} \quad : \quad \frac{20}{1-0.5} = \frac{20}{0.5} \rightarrow \frac{20-10}{0.5} = \frac{10}{0.5} = \frac{20}{1}$$

Respiratory compensation
↓

$$\text{Metabolic alkalosis:} \quad \frac{20+20}{1} = \frac{40}{1} \rightarrow \frac{40}{1+1} = \frac{40}{2} = \frac{20}{1}$$

FIGURE 18-2. The compensatory mechanisms for simple acid–base disturbances as explained by the changes in the Henderson–Hasselbalch equation.

of this protein is stimulated to lower intracellular pH once it rises above 7.0 (normal intracellular pH is <7.0). With alkalosis, this exchange process is active and thus more HCO_3^- is expelled to keep the cells less alkaline. With acidosis, this exchange process is inhibited and thus less HCO_3^- is expelled, resulting in the cells being less acidic.

(3) **Renal regulation of H^+ and K^+.** Renal regulation of H^+ and K^+ occurs at the distal renal tubule level, where **one molecular of Na^+ is reabsorbed into the tubular cell at the expense of one molecule of H^+ or K^+. With acidosis, more H^+ than K^+ is expelled (secreted) into the lumen, resulting in hyperkalemia as part of the compensatory process.** By the same token, alkalosis would lead to hypokalemia through this same process.

c. **Respiratory and metabolic components**

Since H_2CO_3–HCO_3^- is the major buffering system in the body, **respiratory and renal control of the blood CO_2 and HCO_3^- concentrations intends to keep body pH normal. Under normal physiological condition, the ratio of blood [HCO_3^-] and [H_2CO_3] is 20:1, where HCO_3^- is the metabolic component and H_2CO_3 (or dissolved CO_2) is the respiratory component.** This ratio will change by addition or loss of CO_2 and HCO_3^- to the system. Figure 18-2 depicts changes in the ratio of [HCO_3^-] and [H_2CO_3] that might occur during simple acid–base disturbances.

During hypoventilation (respiratory acidosis), retention of CO_2 will lower the ratio. In order to return the ratio to 20:1, the body must retain more HCO_3^- through metabolic compensation.

During metabolic acidosis, loss of HCO_3^- will decrease the ratio. In order to return the ratio to 20:1, body must expel more CO_2 to lower the ratio through respiratory compensation.

These changes in [HCO_3^-]/[H_2CO_3] also account for the compensatory processes during respiratory alkalosis (hyperventilation) and metabolic alkalosis (Figure 18-2).

4. **Acid–base parameters and terminology**

  a. At pH 7.4, the ratio of $\dfrac{[HCO_3^-]}{[H_2CO_3]} = 20:1$

b. **Base deficit/excess** is defined as the titratable acid or base, respectively, needed to titrate the blood to a pH of 7.4 under standard conditions of PCO_2 (40 mm Hg), temperature (38°C), and complete hemoglobin oxygenation.

c. **Acidemia and alkalemia.** Acidemia is defined as arterial pH of <7.35 and alkalemia is defined as arterial pH of >7.45.

d. **Anion gap.** The difference between the ECF concentration of Na^+ (140 mEq/L) and the sum of the concentrations of HCO_3^- (25 mEq/L) and Cl^- (105 mEq/L). The normal anion gap varies with the species, but is 13–25 in dogs and cats. Metabolic acids contribute to the anion gap. Untreated cases of metabolic acidosis may have high anion gaps.

II. GENERAL CONCEPTS OF FLUID AND ELECTROLYTE THERAPY

A. **Institution of fluid therapy.** Fluid therapy should be instituted for the following conditions: dehydration, acid–base disturbances and/or electrolyte imbalances, nutritional problems, and loss of body fluids.

1. **Basis for institution of fluid therapy**
   a. **Accurate diagnosis** based on clinical examination and laboratory data is important for fluid therapy.

   The clinical signs for detection of dehydration include: loss of skin elasticity, dry buccal mucosa and tongue, and sunken eyeballs should be taken into account.

   b. Signs of vomiting, diarrhea, abnormal respiratory pattern, and CNS depression or excitation may help with the diagnosis of acid–base disturbances.
   c. Blood gas and urine analyses are useful for the precise diagnosis of acid–base and electrolyte disturbances.

2. **Dehydration**
   a. **General considerations. Dehydration may be considered in three general categories:**
      (1) **Hypertonic dehydration,** which is attributable to loss of pure water or hypotonic fluid.
      (2) **Isotonic dehydration,** which is attributable to loss of isotonic body fluids. However, isotonic dehydration is only seen in acute cases, since with some degree of water replacement, isotonic dehydration will become hypotonic dehydration.
      (3) **Hypotonic dehydration.** The loss of a hypertonic fluid or loss of isotonic fluid with water replacement results in hypotonic dehydration.
   b. **Causes**
      (1) Decreases in water intake usually lead to hypertonic dehydration.
         (a) Lack of water source.
         (b) Disorders and pain of the buccal cavity and pharynx.
         (c) CNS disturbances.
      (2) Increases in body fluid excretion usually lead to hypotonic dehydration.
         (a) **Polyuria.** Diabetes, nephrosis, hypoaldosteronism, and diuretics. Diabetes insipidus will cause hypertonic dehydration.
         (b) Respiratory loss of water during high temperature may lead to hypertonic dehydration.
         (c) Profuse sweating in horses.
         (d) Vomiting/diarrhea.
         (e) **Third space loss.** Body fluid lost to the body cavities and hollow organs.
   c. **Role of electrolytes on hydration states and acid–base balance:**
      (1) ↑ $[Na^+]$ in ECF → water retention
      (2) Changes in $[K^+]$ in ECF result in changes in acid–base balance:
         (a) ↑ $[K^+]$ in plasma→↑$[K^+]$,↓$[H^+]$ in urine → Acidemia
         (b) ↓ $[K^+]$ in plasma→↓$[K^+]$,↑$[H^+]$ in urine → Alkalemia.

Average weights for breeds are shown

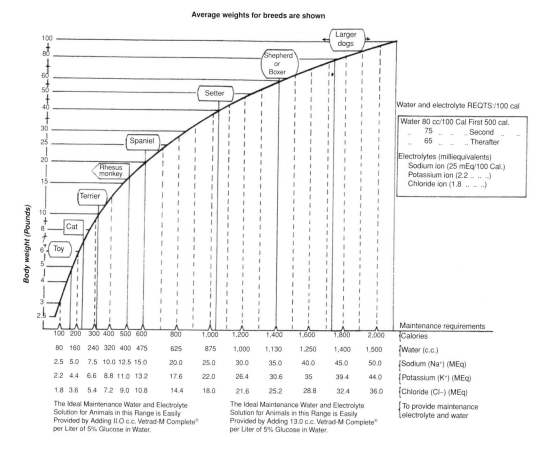

FIGURE 18-3. Daily water, calorie, and electrolyte requirements for dogs and cats. (Reprinted with permission from *Fluid, Electrolyte, and Acid–Base Disorders,* 3rd ed. Edited by DiBartola S. P. Saunders/Elsevier, 2006, Figure 14-1. This figure was modified from Harrison J. B., Sussman H. H., and Pickering D. E. Fluid and electrolyte therapy in small animals. *JAVMA* 137:637–645, 1960, Figure 1.)

    d. Role of carbohydrate metabolism on hydration states and acid–base balance:
        (1) ↓ Carbohydrate utilization → Hyperglycemia → Glucosuria→ Polyuria → Dehydration
        (2) ↓ Carbohydrate utilization →↑ Gluconeogenesis → Ketoacidosis
        (3) ↑ Carbohydrate intake (grain overload) in herbivores →↑ Lactic acid production → Acidosis.
    e. Treatment (amount of fluid to be used) must be based on the body water maintenance plus replacement of the deficit and ongoing loss
        (1) Amount of body water maintenance
            (a) On the basis of body water turnover
            (b) A total of 50–75 mL/kg/day (average 65 mL/kg/day)
            (c) For more precise estimation of water maintenance doses in dogs and cats, see Figure 18-3.
        (2) Determination of water deficit (dehydration)
            (a) Dehydration of 4, 6, 8, and 12% (of body weight), only **loss >4%** needs a replacement
            (b) A total of 4% dehydration (mild)
                i. Animals with 4% dehydration have a history of fluid loss, but without significant signs of dehydration.
                ii. No replacement is needed.

  (c) **A total of 6% dehydration (moderate)**
      i. Animals with 6% dehydration have decreased skin turgor. In dogs and cats, **when the skin over the lateral thorax is picked into a tented fold, it will return to normal slowly**; in species having tight skin, pinch the dorsal eyelid to do the test.
      ii. A decrease in skin elasticity is also seen in cachexia; thus, one cannot conduct this test in cachectic animals.
      iii. Animals with 6% dehydration have dull haircoat and **dry mucous membranes.**
  (d) **About 8–10% dehydration (severe).** The animals with 8–10% dehydration have the following signs:
      i. The skin lacks pliability. In dogs and cats, when the skin is pinched into a tented fold, it will tent and stay after the pinch is released.
      ii. Dry mucous membranes and tongue.
      iii. Soft eyeballs that are sunken into the orbit.
      iv. Cold extremities.
      v. Capillary refill time >3 seconds (normal <2 seconds).
  (e) **About 12% dehydration (extremely severe).** The animals with 12% dehydration have following signs:
      i. All the signs seen with 8–10% dehydration.
      ii. Circulatory collapse (shock).
(3) **Estimation of water deficit.** The replacement volume for the initial deficit is estimated according to the following equations:

$$\text{Replacement volume}\,(L) = \%\,\text{dehydration} \times \text{body weight}\,(kg)$$

(4) **The composition of replacement fluid** should be similar to the volume of fluid lost. For example, if the deficit is due to loss of the electrolyte-rich GI fluid, then a balanced salt solution containing Na^+, K^+, Ca^{2+}, Cl^-, and HCO_3^- (or indirect alkalinizing agents) should be used. See Table 18-1 for the compositions of commonly used replacement fluids of crystalloid in nature. In contrast, if the deficit is due to loss of pure water, volume can be replaced with 5% dextrose (glucose in water) over 24–72 hours. An isotonic solution of 2.5% dextrose and 0.45% NaCl can also be used.
(5) The ongoing loss must be taken into account when estimating the fluid therapy volume. The ongoing loss of fluid via vomiting, diarrhea, and polyuria must be estimated and replaced.
(6) **Additional factors need to be considered**
    (a) Dehydration affects young animals much faster than adult animals.
    (b) Old animals with chronic diseases require more water than younger adult animals.
    (c) Physical and weather conditions may affect the requirement, particularly when it is hot and humid.
    (d) Drugs will alter requirements, particularly diuretics and mineralocorticoids can affect water and electrolyte balances.
(7) The volume to be used for treatment of dehydration is considered an estimate, since it is based on clinical signs to estimate the body water deficit. **Despite the importance of good data collection and application of principles of fluid therapy, the adjustment of volume based on the "reassess" process is needed for each individual case.**
3. **Therapy in acid–base disturbances**
   a. **Metabolic acidosis**
      (1) **Causes**
          (a) **Gain of acid.** Severe tissue breakdown, grain overload, ketosis, poor tissue perfusion, hyperkalemia, lactic acid overproduction, and drug overdose, for example, acidic NSAIDs, chemical poisonings, for example, ethylene glycol (which is metabolized into oxalic acid in the body).
          (b) **Loss of base.** Severe diarrhea, severe salivation, renal insufficiency, and so forth.
      (2) **General signs.** Hyperpnea, CNS depression.

TABLE 18-1. Composition of Selected Fluid Therapy Solutions

Type	Solution	Characteristics		Ion Composition (mEq/L)					Glucose (g/L)	Alkalinizing Equivalents (mEq/L)
		pH	Osmolarity (mOsm/L)	Na$^+$	K$^-$	Cl$^-$	Ca^{++}	Mg^{++}		
Replacement										
Acidifying BES	Ringer's	5.4	309	147	4	155	4	0	0	0
Acidifying BES	Normal saline (0.9%)	5.0	308	154	0	154	0	0	0	0
Alkalinizing BES	Lactated Ringer's	6.6	273	130	4	109	3	0	0	28 (lactate)
Alkalinizing BES	Normosol-R	6.6	294	140	5	98	0	3	0	27 (acetate) 23(gluconate)
Alkalinizing BES	Plasma-Lyte A	7.4	294	140	5	98	0	3	0	27 (acetate) 23 (gluconate)
Maintenance										
Acidifying	2.5% dextrose/water in 0.45% saline plus potassium addition (16 mEq/L)	4.5	280	77	16	77	0	0	25	0
	Equal volumes 5% dextrose/water and lactated Ringer's plus potassium addition (16 mEq/L)	5.0	309	65.5	18	55	1.5	0	25	14 (lactate)
	Normosol-M with 5% dextrose	5.0	363	40	13	40	0	3	50	16 (acetate)
	Plasma-Lyte M with 5% dextrose	5.5	377	40	16	40	5	3	50	12 (lactate) 12 (acetate)
Other solutions	5% dextrose/water	4.0	252	0	0	0	0	0	5	0
	50% dextrose/water	4.2	2,780	0	0	0	0	0	50	0
	7.5% saline	—	2,566	1,283	0	1,283	0	0	0	0
	8.4% NaHCO$_3$	—	2000	1,000	0	0	0	0	0	1,000
	14.9% KCl	—	4,000	0	2,000	2,000	0	0	0	0

BES, balanced electrolyte solution.

443

(3) **Laboratory data and pathogenesis.** ↑ Blood $[H^+]$, ↓$[HCO_3^-]$ (**Base deficit >4 mEq/L**).

(4) **Therapy. Treatment of the underlying disease and the use of alkalinizing agents.**

(a) **Direct alkalinizing agents:** $NaHCO_3$ and THAM (Tris). $NaHCO_3$ is used commonly in animals, but THAM is not frequently used.

   i. Advantage of $NaHCO_3$: It directly works to neutralize excess of H^+.

   ii. Disadvantages of $NaHCO_3$:
- It has a short shelf life of 2 years in solution. Discard the solution when it is cloudy.
- It cannot be autoclaved, since heat will cause:
$$2NaHCO_3 \rightarrow Na_2CO_3 + H_2O + CO_2$$
- Oral dosing of $NaHCO_3$ decreases gastric acidity, which will interfere with milk clot formation, resulting in poor milk digestion.

(b) **Indirect alkalinizing agents.** Na lactate, lactated Ringer's, Na gluconate, Na acetate, acetated polyionic solution, and Na citrate. **The most frequently used indirect alkalinizing agents are Na acetate and Na lactate. The onset of alkalinizing action for an indirect agent is ~30 minutes.**

   i. How do they alkalinize? See Figure 18-4.

   ii. Most of commercial lactate solutions are the mixture of D- and L-forms (racemic form). D-lactate is minimally metabolized, thus is eliminated mostly via renal excretion.

   iii. Other indirect agents do not have the problem with D-form of the chemical as with Na lactate.

   iv. Lactate is metabolized in the liver (Krebs cycle), whereas Na acetate is used throughout the body, especially by the muscle. Thus, acetate is metabolized to form HCO_3^- more efficiently than lactate.

   v. Acetate can induce vasodilation, which may be detrimental when it is administered IV to patients in shock.

   vi. Do not use Na lactate in patients with lactic acidosis, who already have had a problem metabolizing lactate.

   vii. Do not use Na acetate in patients with ketoacidosis, since acetate can form ketone bodies.

   viii. Since the acidotic animals usually have K^+ deficit, supplement of alkalinizing agents with K^+-containing solutions.

   ix. Dose of $NaHCO_3$ to be administered, if base deficit (BD) is known: mEq of $NaHCO_3$ administered = BW (kg) × 0.3 × BD

   x. The $NaHCO_3$ should be administered via IV infusion for over a few hours, and the blood gas reevaluated before making a decision on further therapy.

   xi. Dose of $NaHCO_3$, if base deficit is not known: 1–2 mEq/kg in a balanced electrolyte solution can be administered.

   xii. It is rather difficult to over-alkalinize the body using an indirect agent in a patient with normal renal function. Excess $NaHCO_3$ produced can easily be excreted in the urine.

$$D,L\text{-}NaC_3H_5O_3 \text{ (Na Lactate)} \rightarrow \rightarrow \rightarrow NaHCO_3$$

$$C_3H_5O_3^- + H^+ \rightleftharpoons HC_3H_5O_3$$

$$HC_3H_5O_3 + 3O_2 \xrightarrow{\text{Krebs Cycle}} 3H_2O + 3CO_2$$

$$3H_2O + 3CO_2 \xrightarrow{\text{C. A.}} 3H_2CO_3 \rightarrow 3HCO_3^- + 3H^+$$

FIGURE 18-4. The metabolism of lactate into bicarbonate by the Krebs cycle.

b. Metabolic alkalosis
    (1) Causes. Gain of base, excessive gastric vomiting, GI stasis or obstruction, hypokalemia, excess of aldosterone or diuretics, urea poisoning in cattle, and so forth.
        (a) How does GI stasis lead to metabolic alkalosis? $NaHCO_3$ and HCl are produced in the parietal cell of the stomach. Once being made, $NaHCO_3$ is diffused into ECF, and HCl is released into the gastric lumen.

$$H_2CO_3 + NaCl \rightarrow NaHCO_3 + HCl$$

        HCl will then be absorbed from the small intestine. GI stasis will prevent/delay the absorption of HCl into the circulation, thereby resulting in metabolic alkalosis.
        (b) How does urea poisoning lead to metabolic alkalosis?

$$CO(NH_2)_2 + H_2O \overset{Urea}{\underset{Cycle}{\rightarrow}} 2\,NH_3 + CO_2$$
$$NH_3 + HCl\,(strong\ acid) \rightarrow NH_4Cl\,(weak\ acid)$$

        Alkalosis becomes apparent when a large amount of HCl is converted into NH_4Cl.
    (2) General signs. Hypopnea, excitation including tetany, tremors, convulsions, and muscle rigidity may or may not be seen.
    (3) Laboratory data. $\downarrow$ blood $[H^+]$, $\uparrow[HCO_3^-]$ (Base excess >4 mEq/L), alkaluria or paradoxical aciduria (particularly in the presence of hyponatremia).
    (4) Therapy
        (a) Treat etiology
        (b) Chloride-responsive alkalosis. NaCl, KCl + NaCl, Ringer's solution, NH_4Cl + NaCl. It is best to use solutions containing NaCl and KCl, since affected animals usually have K^+ deficit.
        (c) Chloride-resistant alkalosis. This is usually due to hyperaldosteronism, and thus the mineralocorticoid receptor antagonist spironolactone can be used to treat Cl^--resistant alkalosis. However, this condition is rarely seen in animals.
        (d) H_2-antihistamines or omeprazole, an H^+ blocker, to stop the loss of H^+ into the GI tract. See Chapters 3 and 11 for more information about these drugs.
        (e) Oral KCl in patients with heart failure receiving furosemide, who may have hypokalemia.
    (5) How does NH_4Cl acidify the body?
        Through urea cycle:

$$2NH_4Cl + CO_2 \Leftrightarrow \underset{(urea)}{CO(NH_2)_2} + H_2O + 2HCl$$

    (6) How does NaCl acidify the body?
        (a) Normal renal function. Reabsorption in distal tubule: $Cl^- > HCO_3^-$.
        (b) Supplying a large volume of normal saline $\rightarrow$ More Cl^- than HCO_3^- is reabsorbed from the distal tubule $\rightarrow \uparrow$ plasma $[Cl^-]$, $\downarrow$ plasma $[HCO_3^-]$.
c. Respiratory acidosis
    (1) Causes. Respiratory distress/pulmonary diseases, CNS depression resulting in inhibition of the respiratory center (disease or drug overdose), and so forth.
    (2) General signs. Respiratory distress, cyanosis, CNS depression, and tachycardia.
    (3) Laboratory data. $\uparrow$ Blood $[H^+]$, P_aCO_2 (>45 mm Hg).
    (4) Therapy. Proper ventilation, alkalinizing agent is optional and can be used when ventilation alone will not correct the condition (e.g., pulmonary obstructions).

d. Respiratory alkalosis

(1) **Causes.** Overheat, fever, hyperventilation (particularly if there is overactive positive pressure ventilation during anesthesia), central neurologic disease, CNS stimulant overdose, and salicylate poisoning/overdose.

(2) **General signs.** Hyperpnea with and without panting, CNS stimulation with and without tremors/spasms/convulsions.

(3) **Laboratory data.** ↓ Blood [H^+], ↓P_aCO_2 (<35 mm Hg).

(4) **Therapy.** Correction of hyperventilation; underlying etiologic factors must be eliminated; administration of sedatives may help in cases of CNS excitation; administration of an acidifying agent is optional.

e. Mixed acid–base disturbances occur much more frequently because of the development of compensation processes. Treatment may convert one type of acid–base disturbance into another; close monitoring is necessary. **At arterial blood pH of <7.2 or >7.6, then steps must be taken to correct the pH imbalance.**

f. In cases of combined metabolic and respiratory acidosis (which is a very severe form of acidosis), one must try to restore ventilation as the top priority; subsequently, an alkalinizing agent preferably $NaHCO_3$ can be administered to help raise blood pH. In the presence of high P_aCO_2, $NaHCO_3$ cannot work effectively as an alkalinizing agent.

g. In the field situation, if acid–base status is unclear, Ringer's solution should be administered. Lactated Ringer's solution or an acetated polyionic solution is the second choice.

h. Hypokalemia

(1) **Causes.** Reduced intake, loss via the GI tract, kidney, loss of interstitial fluid, excess of aldosterone or diuretics, and so forth.

(2) **General signs.** CNS depression and weak muscle contraction are attributable to hyperpolarization of the excitable membranes, cardiac arrhythmia.

(3) **Laboratory data.** ↓ Blood [K^+], [H^+], ↑[HCO_3^-], ↑Urine[H^+], ↓[HCO_3^-].

(4) **Electrocardiogram (ECG) findings in hypokalemia-induced cardiac arrhythmia:**

(a) ↑ Amplitude of QRS complex and P wave.

(b) Prolongation of QT interval.

(c) Flattened or inverted T waves.

(5) **Mechanisms underlying hypokalemia-induced cardiac arrhythmia.** Hypokalemia evokes an increase in myocardial [Na^+] via Na^+, K^+-ATPase mechanism. High myocardial [Na^+] increases Ca^{2+} influx via the Na^+–Ca^{2+} exchange mechanism (see Chapter 8, Figure 8-2). **Most of the ECG findings are attributable to the increase in myocardial [Ca^{2+}].**

(6) **Therapy for hypokalemia**

(a) Only for severe acute hypokalemia (**<2.5 mEq/L**) or chronic hypokalemia.

(b) KCl or K gluconate, PO, SC, or IV (**≤0.5 mEq/kg/h**). **Parenteral fluids containing KCl (≤35 mEq/L) can be used safely by the SC route.**

(c) **Watch out for KCl-induced hyperkalemia by** monitoring signs of hyperkalemia.

(7) **Drug interaction. Severe cardiac arrhythmias may occur in patients with hypokalemia when given digoxin.**

i. Hyperkalemia

(1) **Causes.** Reduced urinary excretion, acidosis, hypoadrenocorticism, diabetes mellitus (early phase), excessive cell/tissue damage, increased intake, and so forth.

(2) **General signs**

(a) Increased neuromuscular excitability.

(b) Skeletal muscle twitching, irritability, and muscle weakness.

(c) **Cardiac disturbances due to decreased resting membrane potential and a decreased myocardial [Ca^{2+}].**

(3) **Laboratory data.** Similar to metabolic acidosis.

(4) Therapy for hyperkalemia
- **(a)** Ca gluconate administration to replenish myocardial [Ca^{2+}]
- **(b)** Cation-exchange resin
- **(c)** Peritoneal dialysis
- **(d)** Diuretic administration
- **(e)** $NaHCO_3$ (1–2 mEq/kg) or dextrose to effect; insulin for diabetes mellitus.

B. **Route and rate of administration**

1. Oral route
  a. Advantages
    (1) Rapid administration is possible.
    (2) Adverse reactions are minimal.
    (3) Economical.
    (4) Caloric needs may be easily met.
  b. Disadvantages
    (1) May be contraindicated if GI disease is present.
    (2) Utilization is slower than by some other routes.

2. Intravenous route
  a. Advantages
    (1) Rapid dispersion of fluid occurs.
    (2) Precise dosage is possible.
    (3) Hypertonic or hypotonic solution may be administered.
  b. Disadvantages
    (1) The procedure may be time-consuming.
    (2) A limited number of sites are available.
    (3) A greater chance of adverse reactions.
  c. Rates of intravenous infusion
    (1) If the heart, lungs, and kidneys are normal, the maximal rate of administration is **90 mL/kg/h** for an isotonic solution.
    (2) Rate of infusion should be high if the fluid loss was rapid and should be low if the fluid loss was gradual/slow. **Infusion rate of 15 mL/kg/h is appropriate for most cases.**
    (3) Rapid administration of glucose (>4 mg/kg/min) will result in hyperglycemia.
    (4) Rate of infusion should be slowed down after the first hour of administration especially if anuria is present (a catheter should be placed in urinary bladder in critically ill patients). Every attempt must be made to establish renal function. After ≥4 hours of infusion without urine flow, the rate of infusion must be decreased to 2 mL/kg/h.
    (5) **Watch for adverse reactions due to pulmonary edema and vagal stimulation. Central venous pressure (CVP) monitoring may aid in avoiding a volume overload (normal CVP is 0–3 cm of water). The infusion rate should be adjusted for each patient.**

3. Subcutaneous route
  a. Advantages
    (1) It is convenient.
    (2) Solution with high K^+ concentrations, for example, 35 mEq/L may be given using this route.
    (3) Large quantities of a warm solution can be given to dogs and cats, particularly to very young or small size animals (hypodermoclysis).
  b. Disadvantages
    (1) Limited to isotonic solutions.
    (2) Irritating solutions cannot be given.
    (3) Absorption may be poor in patients with edema or shock.
    (4) Five percent glucose, SC, is not a good idea, especially in animals in shock.

4. Intraperitoneal route
  a. Advantage. Relatively rapid absorption.

      b. Disadvantages
         (1) May induce peritonitis or injury to viscera.
         (2) Limited to isotonic solutions.
  5. Rectal route
      a. Advantage. It is convenient, especially in very young or small size animals, for example, birds. It is a viable alternative for fluid resuscitation in hypovolemic shock. This easy and noninvasive method of fluid replacement may be useful when standard IV access is impossible. Warm the solution to facilitate the absorption.
      b. Disadvantages
         (1) Erratic absorption.
         (2) Contraindicated if diarrhea is present.
  6. Intramedullary route. This is a rarely used route of fluid administration.
      a. Advantages
         (1) Rapid absorption.
         (2) May be easier than IV route in neonates and birds.
      b. Disadvantages
         (1) May cause osteomyelitis.
         (2) The procedure may be painful.

C. **Products for fluid therapy**

  1. Crystalloids (Table 18-1)
      a. Replacement solutions. Ringer's, normal saline, lactated Ringer's, acetated polyionic solutions (Normosol-R®; Plasma-Lyte A®).
      b. The composition of the replacement fluids should reflect the composition of the fluid lost. For example, if the loss is due to diarrhea, then a solution containing Na^+, K^+, Cl^-, and HCO_3^- with concentrations similar to those of the body fluid should be administered.
      c. Maintenance fluids are needed when a patient does not voluntarily ingest adequate amount of food and water to keep up with the daily maintenance dose requirements.
      d. For the practical purpose, the maintenance fluid can be infused at the dose of 50–75 mL/kg/24 h for mature animals and 75–130 mL/kg/24 h for immature/young animals; the high dose of 130 mL/kg/24 h is reserved for very young animals.
      e. Maintenance solutions (diluted electrolyte solutions using dextrose/water). These solutions usually contain high K^+ (13–18 mEq/L) and low Na^+ (40–80 mEq/L). Other factors affecting body water maintenance should be taken into consideration (see II A2 e (6)].
      f. Other solutions: 5% dextrose, 50% dextrose, 7.5% saline, 8.4% (1 M) $NaHCO_3$, 14.9% (1 M) KCl, 5 M Na lactate, 2 M Na acetate, and so forth.
  2. Colloids (plasma expanders)
      a. General consideration
         (1) The critical distribution of body water between plasma and interstitial fluid is maintained in part by the colloid osmotic pressure (COP) of plasma proteins, primarily albumin. This force pulls and holds body water into capillaries and balances the hydrostatic pressure driving water out. This forms the basis for IV colloid therapy.
         (2) The crystalloids do not exert COP, and they are minimally retained in the vascular space, since they are small molecules. As a result, crystalloids cause much smaller volume of expansion than colloids.
      b. Therapeutic uses
         (1) Colloids are usually included in fluid regimens for small-volume resuscitation during shock (see below), management of hemorrhage, and improvement of microcirculatory flow and capillary integrity during systemic inflammatory response syndrome.

TABLE 18-2. Activity of Colloids on Plasma Expansion

Fluid (1 liter)	Plasma Volume Expansion (liter)	Expansion Duration (hours)
Plasma	1.000	
L. Ringer's	0.194	2
6% Hetastarch	0.710	24–36
6% Dextran 70	0.800	24
10% Dextran 40	1.000	4–6

L. Ringer's, Lactated Ringer's solution.

(2) Colloids must be used in combination with a crystalloid solution to replenish the interstitial and ICF deficits. In fact, the appropriate use of colloids can reduce the required amount of crystalloid solution by 40–60%.

(3) **Care must be taken to adjust the amount and rate of all fluids to prevent overload and edema.** COP can be monitored by using a colloid osmometer (normal being 20–25 mm Hg).

a. **Preparations.** Plasma, dextran 40, dextran 70, hetastarch, and polygelatins (Table 18-2).

  (1) **Dextrans**

    (a) These are polysaccharides produced by *Leuconostoc* bacteria. Dextrans 40 and 70 have sizes of 40 and 70 kDa, respectively.

    (b) Dextrans 40 and 70 have plasma $t_{1/2}$ of 1–3 and 2–6 hours, respectively.

    (c) Elimination. In normal dogs, 70% of the dextran 40 dose and 40% of the dextran 70 dose are excreted unchanged within 24 hours. The remaining dextrans are metabolized slowly to glucose by hepatic dextranase. Some of the molecules can remain in the body for weeks after administration.

  (2) **Hetastarch**

    (a) It is a synthetic glucose polymer. It is very slowly metabolized by α-amylase if size is >59 kDa, whereas smaller molecules (<59 kDa) are excreted by the kidneys or taken up by macrophages and slowly metabolized by lysozymes.

    (b) In dogs, 24 hours after administration, ~40% of hetastarch remains in the plasma and ~30% is excreted in the urine.

  (3) **Polygelatins**

    (a) Gelatins are prepared by degradation of bovine collagen and are available in several forms, oxypolygelatin, succinated gelatin, and urea-linked gelatin. 5% oxypolygelatin is the only polygelatin available in the United States for fluid therapy.

    (b) The plasma $t_{1/2}$ of oxypolygelatin is ~24 hours.

    (c) Gelatins are metabolized by proteolytic enzymes in the liver with ~70 and ~15% of the end products being excreted in the urine and feces, respectively.

b. **Rate of colloid infusion**

  (1) In acute situations, for example, shock or hemorrhage, 10–40 mL/kg IV bolus to effect, followed by a constant-rate infusion (CRI) to maintain a mean arterial pressure (MAP) of 80 mm Hg.

  (2) In chronic situations, use CRI to maintain MAP of 80 mm Hg.

  (3) Since cats are more likely to show signs of allergic reactions, especially when synthetic colloids are infused rapidly, only small volumes are infused at slower rates (5 mL/kg increments given over 5–10 minutes, repeated to effect at ≤20 mL/kg).

c. **Adverse effects**

  (1) Volume expansion may dilute blood constituents.

  (2) Rapid volume expansion may be detrimental to patients with acute renal failure or congestive heart failure.

(3) Dextran 40 may cause acute renal failure.

(4) Colloids may cause antigen–antibody reactions (<0.1% in humans).

(5) Dextrans and hetastarch may interfere with **fibrin clot formation by diluting and reducing clotting factors and interfering with platelet function. Thus, they should not be used before or during major surgery. However, some hetastarch preparations have Ca^{2+} in the medium, which may reduce clotting abnormalities. Gelatins have less anticoagulatory effects than other colloids.**

3. **Hypertonic solutions** (e.g., 7.5% NaCl)

   a. **Therapeutic uses.** These solutions are used for the resuscitation of animals suffering from shock (plasma volume expansion), and treatment of head injury and burns.

   b. **Hypertonic solutions are used in combination with colloids**; for example, 7% NaCl–6% dextran 70 (4–8 mL/kg).

   c. **Other actions.** Hypertonic solutions decrease afterload (due to vasodilatation), increase catecholamine release, and increase oxygen delivery to the heart. Hypertonic solutions could have positive inotropic effects and immunomodulatory effects.

   d. **Adverse effects.** Volume overload and edema.

   e. **Contraindications.** Patients with hypernatremia or coagulation problems should not receive hypertonic solutions.

D. **Parenteral nutritional therapy.** It is used in animals who cannot voluntarily consume food because of a GI, pancreatic, or hepatic disease. This technique is to prevent malnutrition and to treat animals that are malnourished.

1. **Total parenteral nutrition (TPN).** The IV infusion of glucose, lipid, amino acids, trace elements, and vitamins (usually only B-complex) in adequate amounts to meet the nutritional needs.

2. **Partial parenteral nutrition.** In some cases, enteral nutrition is provided in combination with parenteral nutrition. These animals are more likely to survive compared with animals not receiving any enteral nutrition.

3. **Most companion animals receive parenteral nutrition for short time, average 3–4 days**. Occasionally, parenteral nutrition is administered for prolonged periods, but the risk/benefit ratio must be considered for these cases.

4. **Two premises for performing TPN because of the administration of hypertonic solutions (700–1,000 mOsm/L):**

   a. **Infusion into a large bore vein, that is, the jugular vein.**

   b. **Continuous (24 hours) infusion of the solution.**

5. **Formulation of parenteral nutrition requirements**

   a. **Calorie requirements.** The determination of daily calorie requirement in each dog or cat can be performed by using the information in Figure 18-3 or by calculating the resting energy requirement (RER) in Figure 18-5.

      (1) One should avoid using the linear regression in Figure 18-5 for animals >25 kg, since it will overestimate their energy requirement; the exponential regression can estimate more precisely their calorie needs than the linear regression.

      (2) Sources for calories: Glucose (dextrose) and lipid are major sources for calories. Glucose and lipid generate 4 and 9 kcal/g, respectively.

      (3) The maintenance doses of calories in dogs and cats are presented in Figure 18-3. For example, a 10-kg dog would require 700 kcal for daily maintenance, which can be generated by 175 g of glucose or 78 g of lipid. Glucose is usually used for the supply of calories. However, lipid solution can provide essential fatty acids.

      (4) For the calorie requirements, 50% dextrose instead of 5% should be used; the latter is too diluted to meet the daily maintenance requirement.

      (5) **The glucose infusion rate should be ≤4 mg/kg/min to avoid hyperglycemia.** In diabetic patients, the insulin dose will require adjustment in order to maintain normoglycemia.

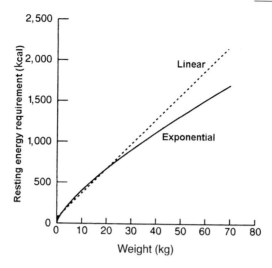

FIGURE 18-5. Comparison of resting energy requirements (RERs), as calculated using a linear equation [(30 × body weight) + 70] versus an exponential equation [70 (body weight)$^{0.75}$]. Note that the equations yield similar results for animals weighing between 3 and 25 kg. For animals that weight >25 kg, the linear equation overestimates the animal's RER. (Reprint with permission from *Fluid, Electrolyte, and Acid-Base Disorders*, 3rd ed. Edited by DiBartola S. P. Saunders/Elsevier, 2006, Figure 25-5.)

6. **Amino acid requirements.** Animals need a nitrogen source to induce positive nitrogen balance and essential amino acids; these requirements can be met by using an amino acid solution that is available 3.5–15% (Aminosyn®, Travasol®, Noramine®, FreAmine®, and ProcalAmine®) containing all essential amino acids, except taurine. Most amino acid solutions are available in two formulations: one with electrolytes and one without.
   a. **Dosages: 40–50 mg amino acids/kcal/day for dogs and 60 mg/kcal/day for cats (Note: dosage is based on kcal requirement, but not body weight).**
   b. Animals with large draining wound or hypoproteinemia should use higher quantity of amino acids than heretofore recommended.
   c. The amino acid dosages should be reduced in patients with protein intolerance, for example, those with hepatic encephalopathy or renal failure.
   d. **Calories must be provided at the same time** to prevent the gluconeogenesis from amino acids.
7. **Lipid requirements.** Lipid emulsions are occasionally used in TPN as an energy source and to provide essential fatty acids.
   a. **Lipid generates 9 kcal/g.** The lipid preparations used include soybean oil/safflower oil, egg yolk phospholipids, glycerin, and water.
   b. Since high doses of lipid can cause immunosuppression via granulocyte and reticuloendothelial cell dysfunction, and inflammation due to increased formation of eicosanoids, the **doses should be limited to 2 g/kg/day.** Patients with high blood levels of triglyceride should not receive a lipid emulsion.
   c. Animals have a need for essential fatty acids; **dogs need linoleic acid and cats need arachidonic acid.** The fatty acids can be provided by a lipid emulsion. In parenteral nutrition, fatty acids are usually not required, unless the animals remain on prolonged nutritional treatment.
8. **Other nutritional requirements.** Electrolytes, vitamin B-complex, and trace elements may be added to the parenteral nutrition. Because most animals are on short duration of parenteral nutrition, fat-soluble vitamins are usually not included in the formulation. Adjustments to the nutritional plan may include Na^+ restriction for cardiac patients, protein restriction for encephalopathic patients, and end-stage renal failure patients.
9. **Problems associate with parenteral nutrition** include infection (sepsis), hyperglycemia, and mechanical complications.

III. BLOOD THERAPY

A. Blood transfusions

1. **Major indications for whole blood therapy**
   a. **Hemorrhage or shock:** Keep in mind that **normal blood volume is ~75 mL/kg** and **normal plasma volume is ~50 mL/kg**
   b. **Anemia**
   c. **Coagulation abnormalities**
   d. **Provision of antibodies**
2. **Donor selection. To find a healthy donor with compatible erythrocytes.**
   a. **Three strong hemagglutinin antigens in dogs:** dog erythrocyte antigen (DEA) **1.1, DEA1.2, and DEA7; DEA7 is an isoantibody** and is active only below 37°C. **The ideal dog blood donor has to be healthy, and should be free of these strong hemagglutinin antigens.**
   b. **Two hemagglutinin antigens in cats**
      (1) **A and B: These are isoantibodies.**
      (2) **Type A (anti-B):** Weak; Siamese and 99% of domestic cats in the United States.
      (3) **Type B (anti-A):** Cats with type B blood have strong anti-A antibody; 20% of pure bred cats are type B. One milliliter of type A blood given to a type B cat can be fatal, even without prior sensitization. Type A kittens born to and allowed to nurse from type B queens suffer from neonatal isoerythrolysis.
      (4) **Type AB (no antibody):** 0.1% of cats in the United States belong to type AB.
   c. **For horses, male ponies with no previous history of blood transfusion can serve as donors**, if cross-matching technique is not practical in the field.
   d. **Other species also have isoantibodies; one can do cross-matching to determine agglutination** (see below).
   e. **Cross-matching technique**
      (1) **Major technique:** Potential donor's RBCs are mixed with recipient's serum to determine agglutination.
      (2) **Minor technique:** Potential donor's serum is mixed with recipient's RBCs to determine agglutination.
3. **Blood collection and storage**
   a. **Collection:** 20% of blood from a donor at 2–4 weeks intervals.
   b. Collection in plastic bags with an anticoagulant solution: **CPD (citrate–phosphate–dextrose) or CPDA-1 (citrate–phosphate–dextrose–adenine).** CPDA-1 is the most commonly used anticoagulant in human medicine for the collection and storage of whole blood. The commercially available canine and feline whole blood products (from Animal Blood Bank, Inc.) are also preserved in CDPA-1.
   c. **CPD or CDPA-1: 14 mL is needed to collect 100 mL of blood.**
   d. **The blood using CPD and CPDA-1 as the anticoagulant can be preserved for 3 and 7 weeks, respectively, at 4°C.**
   e. **Sterile (autoclaved) 3.5% Na citrate** solution can be used as an inexpensive anticoagulant, particularly in large animals (1 part of 3.5% Na citrate to 9 parts of blood). The blood collected using Na citrate should be utilized as soon as possible, since it does not have any additives (dextrose, phosphate, or adenosine) to preserve the blood cells.
   f. **Sodium citrate may induce vomiting** in nonherbivores.
   g. **Plasma** can be separated from blood cells before the bag of blood is expired.
   h. **Heparin** should not be used as an anticoagulant to collect blood for transfusion. Heparin has following problems.
      (1) Heparinized blood cannot be stored, since heparin is inactivated in 24–48 hours in the blood.
      (2) Heparin activates platelets, rendering them nonfunctional.

4. **Administration and dosages**
   a. **Administer when PCV <20%.**
   b. The blood should be filtered to remove possible blood clots and warmed to 37°C before being transfused into a recipient.
   c. One should conduct cross-matching whenever possible before administration.
   d. Administer IV, IP, or intramedullary.
   e. Dosages: **10–20 mL/kg** or using the formula: **mL of blood infused = 1 mL/lb × % PCV change desired.**
   f. **Rate of administration** depends on clinical signs and the dose: **60 mL/min (large animals), 5–10 mL/min (small animals), and 40–50 mL/30 min (cats).**
5. **Plasma**
   a. **Therapeutic uses.** Plasma is used to expand plasma volume, or to increase plasma proteins, for example, albumin and globulin in patients with hepatic dysfunction, and to provide clotting factors and platelets.
   b. **Preparations.** Plasma is available either as a fresh or frozen preparation.
      (1) Fresh plasma **contains platelets** and clotting factors, and must be used within 4 hours of preparation because of the risk of bacterial contamination at room temperature.
      (2) Fresh frozen plasma contains clotting factors (freeze at <–40°C, good for 1 year; at −20°C, good for 3 months), which are destroyed if the unit has been thawed for >8 hours, **but contains no platelets.**
   c. **Administration**
      (1) **Administer when serum albumin concentration is <1.5 g/dL.**
      (2) **Dosages: 5–10 mL/kg, IV infusion.**
6. **Adverse effects.** Hemoglobinemia, hemoglobinuria, jaundice, thrombocytopenia, leucopenia, fever, emesis, incontinence, urticaria and/or weakness, hypocalcemic tetany, and circulatory overload. Neonatal animals may develop hemolysis after nursing due to the development of antibodies to erythrocyte antigen in the colostrum.
7. **Interspecies transfusion** is prohibited because of incompatibility.
8. **Polymerized bovine hemoglobin (Oxyglobin®)**
   a. **Preparation**: 13 g/dL in lactated Ringer's solution.
   b. **Therapeutic uses.** For the treatment of anemia in dogs: 30 mL/kg, IV, at a rate of ≤10 mL/kg/h. **It is particularly useful in dogs with autoimmune hemolytic anemia shortly before an immunosuppressant is given.**
   c. **Elimination $t_{1/2}$: 30–40 hours** (90% being eliminated in 5–7 days).
   d. **Adverse effects.** Discoloration/GI and CV disturbances, pulmonary edema, anaphylaxis, and death.
   e. **Contraindications.** Do not use this product in patients with a cardiac or renal disease.
   f. **Warnings**
      (1) Do not use this product repeatedly in the same dog, since the repeated use of this product can cause anaphylaxis.
      (2) Must finish the product within 4 days once it is opened; otherwise, it may form methemoglobin.

IV. SPECIAL TOPICS IN FLUID THERAPY

A. Horses

1. Cases of severe diarrhea, shock, intestinal obstruction, or esophageal obstruction may predispose to severe metabolic acidosis.
2. The respiratory acidosis may be associated with inhalation anesthesia.
3. A severe hyponatremia may be associated with dehydration.
4. A severe hyperkalemia (plasma K^+ concentrations of ≥7 mEq/L) may be associated with acidosis in foals.

B. Cattle

1. The metabolic alkalosis may be associated with an abomasal disease.
2. A severe metabolic acidosis and dehydration and sometimes severe hyperkalemia may be associated with grain overload and calf diarrhea.
3. A severe K^+ deficit may be present in anorectic animals.
4. The oral fluid therapy should be administered to treat neonatal diarrhea whenever possible.

C. Problems seen in all species

1. **Effects of anesthesia and surgery**
   a. Anesthetic and surgical effects
      (1) General anesthetics depress the cardiovascular system and the glomerular filtration rate.
      (2) Inhalation anesthetics cause vasodilatation.
      (3) Fluid loss may increase during general anesthesia and surgery.
      (4) Third spacing may occur during surgery.
      (5) IV fluids cause reduction in plasma protein concentrations and blood cell counts.
      (6) Patients may have volume overload and hypertension during postsurgical period.
2. **Heat exhaustion and prostration.** Excessive heat will cause the loss of a large amount of NaCl from the ECF. As a result, K^+ is released from the cells to compensate for the loss of Na^+. Renal excretion of NaCl diminishes, but water excretion continues. The body has a severe deficit of Na^+, K^+, Cl^-, and dehydration. Hyperventilation in response to heat may lead to respiratory alkalosis. All measures are needed to lower the high body temperature. In addition, an electrolyte solution (e.g., Ringer's, lactated Ringer's, or acetated polyionic solution) should be administered. If hypertonic dehydration, maintenance crystalloid solutions with low Na^+ and high K^+ should be administered.
3. **Burns.** With burns, more electrolyte than water is lost, which leads to hypotonic dehydration. Hypertonic solution can be used to treat patients with burns.

D. Oral fluid therapy in neonatal calf and piglet diarrhea

1. **Generation considerations.** Oral fluids are indicated for the correction of diarrhea-associated dehydration in neonatal animals that still retain the suck reflex.
   a. In general, neonatal animals that can stand and have a suck reflex are good candidates for oral fluid therapy. Calves that are weak and have poor suck reflex often benefit from oral fluids, but they may have to be administered via the stomach tube.
   b. Recumbent neonatal calves that do not have suck reflex and/or show rapidly progressing signs of severe dehydration should not be treated with oral fluid; instead, they should be treated with IV fluids. As a rule of thumb, neonatal animals not clinically improved within 1–2 hours of oral fluid administration are likely candidates for IV fluid administration.
   c. The effectiveness of oral fluids depends on their composition, the severity of the condition under treatment, and the aggressiveness of the treatment regimen. Oral crystalloid solutions containing electrolytes, glucose, glycine, and alkalinizing agents are highly efficacious in treating calves and piglets with severe diarrhea. Table 18-3 shows the composition of four commercially available preparations.
      (1) **Utilization of the action of cotransporters** (glucose–Na^+, amino acid–Na^+) into the gut mucosa. Rehydration depends on Na^+ absorption. Numerous glucose–Na^+ and amino acid–Na^+ cotransporters are found in the gut mucosa. These cotransporters are stimulated by glucose and neutral amino acids, respectively, to facilitate the transport of glucose, amino acids, and Na^+. Glycine is the neutral amino acid most frequently used in oral crystalloid solutions.

TABLE 18-3. Composition of Four Oral Electrolyte Solutions Designed to Be Fed to Diarrheic Calves

Product	Glucose (mmol/L)	Glycine (mmol/L)	Na+ (mEq/L)	K+ (mEq/L)	Cl− (mEq/L)	Alkalinizing Ability (mEq/L)	HCO₃⁻ (mEq/L)	Citrate (mEq/L)	Acetate (mEq/L)
Electrolyte Powder®	110	0	139	10	101	48	48*	0	0
Electrolyte with Thickener®	220	25	184	38	46	110	110*	0	0
Hydra-Lyte®	405	16	118	30	45	103	0	4	99
Resorb®	120	44	78	17	78	0	0	1	0

*Interferes with milk clotting.

(2) Inclusion of alkalinizing agents. $NaHCO_3$ and the indirect alkalinizing agents Na acetate, Na gluconate, and Na citrate are used in oral fluids. The addition of alkalinizing agents to the oral fluids has decreased the mortality in neonatal calves and piglets. Alkalinizing agents are usually added to the oral fluids at the rate of 40–100 mEq/L.

    (a) $NaHCO_3$ can directly neutralize acid, but it also decreases gastric/abomasal) acidity, which may predispose to bacterial overgrowth in the small intestine, and may interfere with milk digestion by preventing its clot formation.

    (b) The advantage of indirect alkalinizing agents is that they will not affect gut pH. The disadvantage of indirect alkalinizing agents is decreased utilization in diarrheic animals with severe dehydration.

(3) Inclusion of KCl. In diarrheic neonatal animals, there is a severe K^+ deficit. The addition of KCl to the oral fluids may save the life of neonatal animals. KCl is usually found in the oral fluids at the rate of 10–40 mEq/L.

(4) Inclusion of gelling agents. These agents are found in some of the commercial preparations (e.g., Electrolyte with Thickener®). They are indigestible mucopolysaccharides. Despite claims that they can slow down the flow and elimination of oral fluids, which reduce the severity of diarrhea, no scientific evidence supports these claims.

(5) Milk consumption. Milk is the most easily digestible food source for neonatal animals and should be reintroduced early in the treatment of diarrhea. It provides the most nutrition of all types; it provides calories, protein, vitamins, minerals, and water. Milk contains 500–600 kcal/L. Studies have shown that enterocyte repair is increased in diarrheic calves after they drank milk. Frequent milk feedings (1 liter, 2–4 times a day), in addition to oral fluid therapy, usually facilitates the recovery from calf diarrhea rather well.

(6) Dosages of oral fluids. The diarrheic neonatal calves should be fed with oral fluids 2–4 times a day with total intake of 4 liters.

SUGGESTED READING

Constable P. 2003. Fluid and electrolyte therapy in ruminants. *Vet Clin North Am Food Anim Pract* 19:577–597.

DiBartola SP. 2006. *Fluid, Electrolyte, and Acid–Base Disorders in Small Animal Practice.* 3rd ed. St. Louis, MD: Saunders.

Kochevar DT. 2001. "Drugs affecting renal function and fluid-electrolyte balance." In *Veterinary Pharmacology and Therapeutics.* Edited by Adams HR. 8th ed., pp. 501–533. Ames, IA: Iowa State University Press.

Naylor JM. 1990. Oral fluid therapy. *Vet Clin North Am Food Anim Pract* 6:51–67.

Tromp AM. 1990. A practitioner's view on fluid therapy in calves. *Vet Clin North Am Food Anim Pract* 6:103–110.

STUDY QUESTIONS

DIRECTIONS: Each of the numbered items or incomplete statements in this section is followed by answers or by completions of the statement. Select the **one** lettered answer or completion that is **best** in each case.

1. Which of the following blood transfusion practices in cats may pose the most serious hemagglutination problem?

(A) The type A donor donates blood to the type B recipient.
(B) The type B donor donates blood to the type A recipient.
(C) The type A donor donates blood to the type AB recipient.
(D) The type AB donor donates blood to the type A recipient.

2. Which of the following statements regarding sodium bicarbonate as an alkalinizing agent is correct?

(A) It is an indirect alkalinizing agent.
(B) It can be autoclaved for sterilization without losing its alkalinizing ability.
(C) It does not alkalinize well in combined metabolic and respiratory acidosis.
(D) It does not interfere with milk digestion in calves when administered orally.

3. Which of the following statements regarding route of administration for fluid therapy is correct?

(A) The oral route causes more adverse effects than most of other routes.
(B) The rectal route may be useful when standard IV access is impossible.
(C) KCl in the concentration of 30 mEq/L is best given IV if parenteral administration is necessary.
(D) The SC route is versatile in dogs and cats because it can be used to administer a large amount of isotonic, hypertonic, or hypotonic solution.

4. If you decide to perform a blood transfusion in a dog with severe blood loss, the appropriate dosage should be

(A) 4–5 mL/kg.
(B) 10–20 mL/kg.
(C) 40–50 mL/kg.

(D) 60–70 mL/kg.
(E) 90–100 mL/kg.

5. Which of the following statements regarding hypokalemia is correct?

(A) It is usually accompanied by acidemia.
(B) One of the causes is hypoaldosteronism.
(C) In an acute case, an animal with plasma K^+ concentration of 3.5 mEq/L or less requires KCl treatment.
(D) There is usually an increase in the amplitude of QRS and P waves in ECG.

6. How much of a 50% glucose solution would be needed to meet the daily maintenance requirement of a 10-kg adult dog who is off feed and recumbent?

(A) 25 mL
(B) 45 mL
(C) 90 mL
(D) 185 mL
(E) 370 mL

7. Consider the patient in Question 6. How much of an 8.5% of amino acids solution should be given to this dog on daily basis, if one decides to perform TPN?

(A) 22 mL
(B) 55 mL
(C) 110 mL
(D) 220 mL
(E) 550 mL

8. Which of the following statements regarding sodium acetate as an alkalinizing agent is **false**?

(A) Acetate can cause vasodilatation, which is detrimental to patients in shock.
(B) Acetate can be metabolized into bicarbonate throughout the body.
(C) Acetate is contraindicated in the treatment of lactic acidosis.
(D) Acetate is more efficient than lactate in forming sodium bicarbonate.

9. Which of the following sodium acetate solutions is **isotonic**? The molecular weight of this chemical is 82.

(A) 0.31%
(B) 0.62%
(C) 1.23%
(D) 2.46%
(E) 4.92%

10. Which of the following is a **false** statement with regard to special problems in fluid therapy?

(A) Severe K^+ deficit is usually seen in anorectic cattle.
(B) Hypertonic dehydration is usually seen in a patient with burns.
(C) Metabolic acidosis is usually associated with grain overload in cattle.
(D) Patients may have volume overload and hypertension during postsurgical period.

11. Which of the following is a **correct** statement regarding blood collection and storage?

(A) Heparin is a potent anticoagulant, and thus is good for blood storage.
(B) Forty percent of blood volume can be safely collected from a healthy donor every 2–4 weeks.
(C) The blood that is collected using CPDA-1 can be stored longer than the one that is collected using CPD.
(D) The blood that is collected using 3.5% sodium citrate can be stored at 4°C for 3 weeks.

12. Which of the following colloid solutions has the shortest duration of action?

(A) 6% hetastarch
(B) 6% dextran 70
(C) 10% dextran 40
(D) 5% oxypolygelatin

ANSWERS AND EXPLANATIONS

1. The answer is B.
Cats with type B blood have strong anti-A antibody. One milliliter of type A blood given to a type B cat can be fatal, even without prior sensitization. Type A kittens born to and allowed to nurse from type B queens suffer from neonatal isoerythrolysis. Cats with type A blood have weak anti-B antibody, which does not cause a serious hemagglutination problem. Cats with type AB blood have no isoantibody against either A or B antigen, and thus they do not cause any hemagglutination problems when serving as a donor.

2. The answer is C.
Sodium bicarbonate is a direct alkalinizing agent that neutralizes H^+. However, in combined metabolic and respiratory acidosis, excess of CO_2 and carbonic acid interferes with the reaction between HCO_3^- and H^+. Therefore, for treatment of this situation, one must treat respiratory acidosis immediately. Sodium bicarbonate cannot be autoclaved for sterilization, since heat will convert this chemical to sodium carbonate and lose its alkalinizing ability. Sodium bicarbonate will decrease gastric acidity; the acidity is important for milk clot formation, which is needed for milk digestion.

3. The answer is B.
The rectal route may be an alternative when IV access is unobtainable, for example, during shock. In fact, the rectal route has been considered as a viable route for treating hypovolemic shock. However, one must recognize the fact that the rectal route may cause erratic absorption, and it cannot be used in the presence of diarrhea. The oral route causes fewer adverse effects than most of other routes. KCl at high concentrations is not safe when given IV. The SC route is not versatile and only isotonic solution should be administered SC.

4. The answer is B.
The recommended dosage for blood transfusion is 10–20 mL/kg.

5. The answer is D.
In hypokalemia, because of higher resting potential and myocardial Ca^{2+} concentrations,

there is an increase in the amplitude of QRS and P waves. Hypokalemia is usually accompanied by metabolic alkalosis (not acidosis). One of the causes of hypokalemia is hyperaldosteronism, which increases the excretion of K^+ and H^+ in the urine. In acute hypokalemia, an animal with plasma K^+ concentration of ≤ 2.5 mEq/L (not 3.5 mEq/L) needs to be treated with a K^+ solution.

6. The answer is D.
According to Figure 18-5, the maintenance calorie requirement for a 10-kg dog is $10 \times 30 + 70 = 370$ kcal. Since each gram of glucose can generate 4 kcal, 92.5 g of glucose can generate 370 kcal. A total of 50% glucose has 50 g glucose in 100 mL. Thus, 185 mL of 50% glucose has 92.5 g glucose in the solution.

7. The answer is D.
The amino acid's requirement in the dog that needs parenteral nutrition is 40–50 mg/kcal/day. Since this is a small size dog, the dog should receive 50 mg/kcal/day. The calorie requirement for this dog is 370 kcal, and thus $50 \, mg \times 370 = 18,500 \, mg$ or 18.5 g of amino acids should be administered. The 8.5% amino acid's solution contains 8.5 g/100 mL. Thus, 218 mL ($\sim$220 mL) of the 8.5% solution will provide 18.5 g of amino acids.

8. The answer is C.
Sodium acetate is contraindicated in the treatment of ketoacidosis, but not lactic acidosis. Acetate can be used to form ketone bodies.

9. The answer is C.
Since sodium acetate dissociates into two particles (Na^+ and acetate) in water, 150 mM of sodium acetate solution is isotonic. A total of 150 mM of sodium acetate = 150 mmol/L = 150×82 mg/L = 12,300 mg/L = 12.3 g/L = 1.23 g/100 mL = 1.23%.

10. The answer is B.
Patients with burns would have had a great deal of loss of hypertonic or isotonic body fluid by the time they receive treatment. As a result of the body fluid loss, they

would have hypotonic, but not hypertonic, dehydration.

11. The answer is C.
The blood that is collected using CPDA-1 can be stored for 7 weeks, while the one collected using CPD can be stored for 3 weeks. Heparin is not a good anticoagulant for blood collected for storage; it is inactivated in the blood within 48 hours, and it activates platelets, rendering them nonfunctional. A total of 20% of blood volume can be safely collected from a healthy donor every 2–4 weeks. The blood that is collected using 3.5% sodium citrate should be used for transfusion soon after being collected, because this anticoagulant solution does not contain phosphate buffer, glucose, or adenine.

12. The answer is C.
Dextran 40 solution has a shorter duration of action as a plasma expander than dextran 70, hetastarch, and oxypolygelatin solutions. Dextran 40 solution contains dextran molecules at 40 kDa, which can leave the vascular space more effectively than other colloids by penetrating through the capillaries.

Chapter 19

Drug Interactions and Adverse Drug Reactions

Walter H. Hsu and Franklin A. Ahrens

A. Introduction

1. Drug interactions are defined as an altered pharmacological response to one drug caused by the presence of second drug. The expected response may be increased or decreased as a result of the interaction.
   a. **Pharmacokinetic interactions** are those in which plasma and/or tissue levels of a drug are altered by another drug.
   b. **Pharmacodynamic interactions** are those in which the action or effect of one drug is altered by a second drug.
   c. **Pharmaceutic interactions** or drug incompatibilities result from chemical or physical reactions of drugs mixed in vitro.

B. Pharmacokinetic interactions

1. **Interactions affecting absorption**
   a. **Gastric emptying.** Drugs that increase gastric motility hasten delivery to the small intestine and increase the rate of intestinal absorption. Conversely, drugs that delay gastric emptying decrease the rate of intestinal absorption.
      For example, metoclopramide and cisapride promote gastric emptying by increasing acetylcholine release from the vagus nerve. Atropine slows down gastric emptying by blocking muscarinic receptors.
   b. **Gastric pH.** Some drugs reduce gastric acidity and slow the absorption of certain other drugs. Antacid, H_2-antihistamines, and omeprazole reduce gastric acidity and thus decrease the absorption of weak acids, for example, tetracycline, salicylates, and ketoconazole.
   c. **Complex formation.** Some drugs form insoluble complexes with divalent cations, which are poorly absorbed from the GI tract. For example, tetracycline forms a complex with Ca^{2+}.
2. **Interactions affecting distribution (plasma protein binding of drugs).** Many drugs are highly bound to plasma albumin. Displacement of bound drugs may occur when a second drug with greater binding affinity is added. The resulting increase in free drug concentration may produce an exaggerated response. For example, the anticoagulant effect of coumarins is potentiated by the presence of a NSAID. The barbiturate-induced anesthesia is prolonged by the presence of a sulfonamide, NSAID, or doxycycline.
3. **Interactions affecting drug metabolism**
   a. **Inhibition of metabolism**
      (1) Drugs that inhibit hepatic microsomal (cytochrome P450) enzymes may prolong the action of drugs, which normally are inactivated by microsomal oxidation (phase I) reactions. **Examples:** chloramphenicol, enrofloxacin, ketoconazole, cimetidine, ranitidine, prednisolone, and quinidine are enzyme inhibitors.
      (2) Drugs that inhibit other enzymes than hepatic microsomal enzymes may prolong the action of drugs, which normally are inactivated by the specific enzymes. For example, imipenem is metabolized by renal dihydropeptidase-1 (DHP-1) in the proximal tubule. Plasma $t_{1/2}$ of imipenem is prolonged by cilastatin, which is a DHP-1 inhibitor.
      (3) Drugs that inhibit enzymes of organisms may prolong the action of anti-infective action of the drugs. For example, clavulanate, a β-lactam, prolongs

the antibacterial action of amoxicillin by inhibiting β-lactamase. Piperonyl butoxide prolongs the action of a pyrethroid ectoparasiticide by inhibiting cytochrome P450 enzymes of the ectoparasites.

b. Increased rate of metabolism

Drugs that induce hepatic microsomal enzymes diminish the efficacy and duration of action of drugs metabolized by the cytochrome P450 enzyme system. **Examples include** phenobarbital, phenytoin, griseofulvin, phenylbutazone, rifampin, and chlorinated hydrocarbons (lindane and methoxychlor), which can induce cytochrome P450 enzymes.

4. Interactions affecting renal excretion

a. Decreased active secretion. Acidic and basic drugs are actively secreted into urine by the renal tubular transport system. Competition for active transport between drugs may slow the rate of excretion.

(1) Acidic drugs. Examples: penicillins, cephalosporins, chlorothiazide, ethacrynic acid, furosemide, probenecid, and the following NSAIDS: aspirin, phenylbutazone, meclofenamic acid, flunixin, ketoprofen, carprofen, and etodolac.

(2) Basic drugs. Examples: histamine, serotonin, procainamide, neostigmine, trimethoprim, and atropine.

b. Increased passive excretion. Altering urinary pH increases the excretion of ionizable drugs by ion-trapping and preventing their reabsorption from tubular urine filtrate. Urinary alkalinizers (e.g., sodium bicarbonate) increase the excretion of acidic drugs and urinary acidifiers (e.g., ammonium chloride) increase the excretion of basic drugs.

c. Diuretics increase urine flow and hasten the excretion of many drugs by decreasing their reabsorption from the nephron.

C. Pharmacodynamic interactions

1. Antagonistic effects. Specific receptor antagonists are available to be used therapeutically to block or reverse agonist activity. The antagonistic effects could be pharmacological or physiological. Examples include concurrent use of the following:

a. A miotic drug and an H₁-antihistamine. Most H$_1$-antihistamines have the side effect of blocking muscarinic receptors to evoke mydriasis, which will antagonize the effect of a miotic drug (physiological antagonism).

b. An α-adrenergic agonist, for example, epinephrine, phenylephrine or phenylpropanolamine and a phenothiazine tranquilizer, for example, acepromazine or chlorpromazine. A phenothiazine can block α-adrenergic receptors to antagonize the effects of an α-adrenergic agonist (pharmacological antagonism). Blockade of the α-adrenergic action of epinephrine may produce hypotension by unmasking the β-adrenergic action of epinephrine. This effect is known as **epinephrine reversal.**

c. Tetracycline and a β-lactam antibiotic. A β-lactam antibiotic works most effectively in rapidly growing bacteria. Tetracycline inhibits bacterial growth, thereby reducing the antibacterial effect of a β-lactam (physiological antagonism).

2. Additive effects. Drugs that have a similar mechanism of action may exhibit additive effects in combination. The end point of the pharmacological effect is the algebraic sum of each drug's action. Additive interactions are observed with many classes of drugs.

3. Synergistic effects. Drug combinations that produce a therapeutic or toxic effect, which is greater than the sum of each drug's action, are termed synergistic. **Examples (concurrent use of):**

a. A sulfonamide and an inhibitor of dihydrofolate reductase (trimethoprim, ormetroprim) potentiate the antibacterial effect of the sulfonamide.

b. A furosemide and an aminoglycoside antibiotic may potentiate the nephrotoxic effect of the aminoglycoside.

c. A furosemide and a digitalis may potentiate the inotropic effect of the digitalis. Furosemide can induce hypokalemia.

d. An inhalant anesthetic and an aminoglycoside may potentiate the skeletal muscle-relaxing effect of the inhalant anesthetic. Aminoglycosides can inhibit acetylcholine release from the somatic nerve.

D. **Pharmaceutic interactions (drug incompatibilities)**

1. **General.** Physical and/or chemical incompatibility between drugs is common and may result in inactivation or increased toxicity. Drugs should never be mixed in a syringe or added to parenteral solutions unless the components are known to be compatible. Visual indicators of incompatibilities such as cloudiness or precipitation may or may not be evident.

2. **Physical incompatibilities** are usually manifested as insolubility. **Examples:**
   a. A macrocyclic lactone diluted in water or aqueous solution will form precipitate (propylene glycol should be used as a diluent).
   b. Amphotericin B is insoluble in water, but can be dissolved in sodium desoxy-cholate.

3. **Chemical incompatibilities**
   a. **pH.** The stability of many drugs in solution is pH dependent. Alkaline solutions (sulfonamides, aminophylline, or barbiturates) are incompatible with acidic solutions (penicillin G, cephalosporins, xylazine HCl, ketamine HCl, gentamicin sulfate, etc.) or alkaloid salts such as atropine sulfate.
   b. **Oxidation–reduction.** Redox reactions may result in loss of drug potency. Tetracyclines are oxidized by riboflavin; phenothiazine tranquilizers are oxidized by ferric salts.
   c. **Complex formation.** Multivalent cations may form insoluble complexes with anionic drugs. **Examples:** Ca^{2+} reacts with $NaHCO_3$, tetracyclines, cephalosporins, barbiturates, fluoroquinolones, penicillins, furosemide, and the following NSAIDS: aspirin, phenylbutazone, meclofenamic acid, flunixin, ketoprofen, carprofen, and etodolac.

II. **ADVERSE DRUG REACTIONS (ADRs)**

A. **General. Three types of adverse drug reactions:**

1. **Drug toxicity** (Type A; reported adverse effects of the drug)
2. **Drug allergy** (Type B)
   a. Immune mediated—previous sensitizing exposure.
   b. Reaction occurs in only a fraction of animal population.
   c. Minute drug dose may cause reactions.
   d. Manifestations differ from pharmacological effects of the drug.
   e. Small molecules, such as most drugs, are not immunogenic. Therefore, they or their metabolites must covalently bind to macromolecules (proteins) and act as haptens or the drug may alter the structure of a macromolecule.
   f. **Allergic or hypersensitivity reactions are classified as:**
      (1) **Type 1 or immediate hypersensitivity reactions result from interaction of the allergen (drug) with IgE antibody on the surface of mast cells and basophils.** The target organs for Type 1 reactions include skin, airway, GI tract, and vasculature. The resulting release of chemical mediators (autacoids) such as histamine, kinins, and prostaglandins increases contraction of smooth muscle and capillary permeability to induce edema. Clinical signs may range from skin wheals and urticaria, rhinitis, bronchoconstriction, and diarrhea to life-threatening anaphylactic shock. Penicillin allergy is the most common Type 1 reaction observed clinically.
      (2) **Type 2 hypersensitivity reactions are complement fixing reactions involving antibody (IgM, IgG) binding to antigen (drug–macromolecular complex) followed by deposition on cell surfaces of circulating blood cells resulting in lysis.** Clinical effects include hemolytic anemia, agranulocytosis,

and thrombocytopenic purpura. Type 2 reactions have been observed with NSAIDs, phenothaizine tranquilizers, and sulfonamides.

(3) **Type 3 hypersensitivity reactions result from the deposition of antigen–antibody complex on target tissue cells (e.g., skin, joints, kidneys), activation of complement, release of lysosomal enzymes and tissue damage.** Clinical signs include fever, arthralgia, skin eruptions, and glomerulonephritis. Type 3 reactions have been observed with cephalosporins, penicillins, sulfonamides, and erythromycin.

(4) **Type 4 hypersensitivity reactions are cell-mediated and are delayed allergic reactions. They result from the direct interaction of an allergen (drug) with sensitized lymphocytes (T cells). This produces a release of cytokines and cellular damage.** Clinical signs include eczema and contact dermatitis, and, in severe cases, granocytopenia, hepatitis, and nephritis. Type 4 reactions have been observed with phenytoin, phenobarbital, sulfonamides, NSAIDS, and many topically applied drugs.

3. **Drug idiosyncrasy** (Type C). The manifestations of the ADR differ from pharmacological effects of the drug for unknown reasons.

B. **Prominent examples of ADRs in small animals based on the summary of FDA–Center for Veterinary Medicine (CVM) accumulated reports (1987–2005, unless otherwise indicated) are listed in Table 19-1. In the FDA reporting system, one report can describe the involvement of many animals.**

Most of the ADR signs reported to FDA–CVM belong to the known adverse effects of the drug; less frequently, drug allergy and idiosyncrasy have also been reported.

C. **Drug toxicity in cats.** Compared to other species, cats are particularly vulnerable to drug toxicity. This is mainly due to the fact that cats have a deficiency in metabolizing drugs/chemicals.

1. **Deficient metabolism in cats as a cause of adverse drug reactions**
   a. **Phase I metabolism**—hepatic microsomal—cytochrome P450 enzymes oxidize, reduce, or hydrolyze drugs. Cats, in general, have lower activity of phase I metabolizing enzymes than other species.
   b. **Phase II metabolism**—conjugation of drug with glucuronide, sulfate, glutathione, or acetyl groups. Cats have a deficiency in glucuronyl transferase. Drugs containing a –OH, –COOH, $-NH_2$, –NH, or –SH group are usually glucuronated, for example, opioids, NSAIDs, phenols, chloramphenicol, and aromatic acids such as benzoic acid.
      Cats tend to have better conjugation activity with acetyl groups than other species.

2. **Other reasons for increased toxicity of certain drugs in cats**
   a. Active metabolites formation, for example, acetyl-procainamide.
   b. Susceptibility of hemoglobin to oxidation (methemoglobinemia).
   c. Anaphylactic reactions to IV administration of ionic drugs, for example, iodide contrast materials in radiology and amphotericin B.
   d. Respiratory distress in drug-induced anaphylaxis.

3. **Drugs not to be used in cats**
   a. **Acetaminophen.** Cats are deficient in glucuronyl transferase; as a result, acetaminophen cannot form a conjugate with glucuronide. Acetaminophen undergoes phase I metabolism to form toxic metabolites that are conjugated by glutathione and that overwhelms the glutathione scavenger system. Methemoglobinemia is the most common indication of toxicity.
   b. **Methylene blue.** Methylene blue is used for treatment of methemoglobinemia. However, feline hemoglobin is more susceptible to oxidative denaturation than other species. Methylene blue is only marginally effective to treat feline methemoglobinemia. Ascorbic acid as a reducing agent can be used in cats.
   c. **Phosphate enemas.** Phosphate enemas can induce severe hyperphosphatemia and hypocalcemia in cats.

TABLE 19-1. Prominent Examples of Adverse Drug Reactions in Small Animals Reported to the FDA–Center for Veterinary Medicine (1987–2005)

Drug	Species	Route	Reports	Treated	Reacted	Died
Antiparasitics						
Ivermectin	Cats	Oral	62	88	83	16
	Cats	Parenteral	42	55	52	17
	Dogs	Oral	869	1,084	981	149
	Dogs	Parenteral	63	84	75	28
Milbemycin	Dogs	Oral	1,675	2,384	2,299	129
Milbemycin-Lufenuron	Dogs	Oral	914	1,039	971	48
Moxidectin	Dogs	Oral	253	394	356	62
	Dogs	Parenteral	5,269	6,042	5,473	599
Selamectin	Cats	Topical	3,168	4,578	3,991	292
	Dogs	Topical	9,661	9,737	9,545	223
Pyrantel	Cats	Oral	52	79	75	16
	Dogs	Oral	217	795	613	214
Melarsomine	Dogs	Parenteral	1,362	1,429	1,409	293
Amitraz	Dogs	Topical	149	161	160	57
Antibacterials						
Amoxicillin	Cats	Oral	199	804	344	33
	Dogs	Oral	291	365	319	62
Enrofloxacin	Cats	Oral	270	310	294	19
	Cats	Parenteral	141	154	151	15
	Dogs	Oral	189	235	225	43
	Dogs	Parenteral	44	47	47	13
CNS depressants and antagonists						
Medetomidine	Cats	Parenteral	99	181	145	41
	Dogs	Parenteral	774	910	882	165
Atipamezole	Cats	Parenteral	50	58	58	18
	Dogs	Parenteral	272	310	290	75
Ketamine	Cats	Parenteral	889	9,966	4,746	426
	Dogs	Parenteral	159	1,159	653	62
Tiletamine-Zolazepam	Cats	Parenteral	567	5,089	1,476	269
	Dogs	Parenteral	372	2,219	983	143
Isoflurane	Cats	Inhalation	92	373	311	50
	Dogs	Inhalation	401	636	401	23
NSAIDS						
Carprofen	Cats	Oral	404	459	400	11
	Dogs	Oral	12,901	13,607	13,202	2,655
Deracoxib	Cats	Oral	53	53	53	26
	Dogs	Oral	3,177	3,278	3,198	740
Etodolac	Dogs	Oral	1,566	1,907	1,760	190
Meloxicam	Cats	Oral	222	228	227	44
	Dogs	Oral	686	695	694	75

  d. Benzyl-containing products. Benzyl alcohol, benzocaine, benzoic acid (in pet food preservative) can induce CNS toxicosis in cats, with the following signs: ataxia, hyperesthesia, fasciculation, coma, convulsions, respiratory failure, and death. These compounds are poorly metabolized by cats.

  e. Cisplatin. Cisplatin is a platinum complex used as an antineoplastic drug. Cisplatin causes severe pulmonary toxicity in cats, which is manifested by vasculitis in alveolar capillaries. Carboplatin does not cause this adverse effect in cats.

  f. 5-Fluorouracil. 5-Fluorouracil is an antineoplastic drug, and is particularly neurotoxic to cats.

TABLE 19-2. Prominent Examples of Adverse Drug Reactions in Large Animals Reported to the FDA–Center for Veterinary Medicine (1987–2005)

Drug	Species	Route	Reports	Treated	Reacted	Died
Antiparasitics						
Albendazole	Cattle	Oral	47	13,491	1,937	171
	Sheep	Oral	26	2,567	673	101
Fenbendazole	Cattle	Oral	22	2,863	1,356	87
	Pigs	Oral	8	2,061	No report	101
Dichlorovos	Pigs	Oral	9	1,820	222	120
Famphur	Cattle	Topical	80	12,268	3,277	217
Doramectin	Cattle	Parenteral	54	15,884	6,612	74
	Cattle	Topical	402	131,054	49,658	44
	Pigs	Parenteral	68	94,362	21,334	395
	Pigs	Topical	6	8,880	2,130	70
Ivermectin	Cattle	Parenteral	55	2,965	798	58
	Cattle	Oral	9	2,022	21	18
	Cattle	Topical	83	23,359	4,793	60
	Horses	Oral	117	478	279	53
	Pigs	Oral	27	4,821	916	53
Moxidectin	Cattle	Topical	212	75,002	51,302	94
	Goats	Oral	5	150	32	22
	Horses	Oral	965	3,029	1,249	111
Lasalocid	Cattle	Oral	4	2,049	2,029	150
Monensin	Cattle	Oral	213	99,405	25,712	3,876
	Goats	Oral	6	756	411	103
	Horses	Oral	50	1,328	251	134
	Sheep	Oral	29	4,660	1,396	615
	Pigs	Oral	6	4,756	3,378	1,174
Levamisole	Cattle	Topical	95	14,207	2,531	86
	Cattle	Parenteral	34	3,384	1,084	82
	Goats	Oral	6	735	43	32
	Pigs	Oral	3	64	27	3
	Sheep	Oral	19	5,726	194	103
Antibacterials						
Ceftiofur	Cattle	Parenteral	75	7,578	1,591	297
	Horses	Parenteral	19	60	24	13
Enrofloxacin	Cattle	Parenteral	12	336	125	29
	Cattle	Unknown	9	650	232	105
Oxytetracycline	Cattle	Parenteral	219	6,352	1,800	251
	Cattle	Unknown	28	1,307	299	44
	Pigs	Parenteral	6	255	243	27
Procaine Penicillin G	Cattle	Parenteral	80	5,155	361	122
	Horses	Parenteral	88	237	135	52
	Pigs	Parenteral	34	4,693	3,407	533
Spectinomycin	Cattle	Parenteral	8	409	124	120
Spectinomycin-Lincomycin	Cattle	Parenteral	166	9,033	1,725	1,224
Tiamulin	Pigs	Oral	18	14,505	822	224
Tilmicosin	Cattle	Parenteral	249	15,962	4,017	627
Tylosin	Cattle	Oral	11	62,019	18,311	758
	Cattle	Parenteral	16	519	67	38
	Pigs	Oral	27	226,286	9,207	484
	Pigs	Parenteral	15	748	510	420
Drugs affecting nutrition/metabolism						
Ractopamine	Cattle	Oral	30	98,715	5,209	124
	Pigs	Oral	209	No report	143,867	5,015
Iron Dextran	Pigs	Parenteral	57	7,912	1,685	618
	Cattle	Parenteral	4	624	100	37
Selenium-Vitamin E	Cattle	Parenteral	111	9,356	1,233	140
	Horses	Parenteral	88	347	209	50
	Pigs	Parenteral	3	130	42	22
	Sheep	Parenteral	19	807	534	198
Edetate	Cattle	Parenteral	7	2,087	107	104
Sometribove	Cattle	Parenteral	1,759	179,785	54,196	379
Isoflupredone	Cattle	Parenteral	22	463	180	162

g. **Primidone.** Primidone must be metabolized to phenobarbital for its action as an anticonvulsant. Cats have very limited ability to convert primidone to phenobarbital.

h. **Synthetic pyrethroids**, especially as spot-on products. Cats are very sensitive to the CNS effects of pyrethroids. Although the exact mechanisms are not known, this may be due to their deficiency in drug metabolism.

4. **Drugs requiring low dosage/increased interval in cats compared to dogs** since cats are more sensitive to these drugs than dogs:
   a. **Morphine and other opioids**
   b. **Salicylates**
   c. **Chloramphenicol**
   d. **Organophosphates**
   e. **Lidocaine**

D. Prominent examples of ADRs in large animals based on the summary of FDA–CVM accumulated reports (1987–2005) are listed in Table 19-2. In the FDA reporting system, one report can describe the involvement of many animals. Most of the ADR signs reported to FDA–CVM belong to the known adverse effects of the drug; less frequently seen are drug allergy and idiosyncrasy. In general, the number of cases reported for a specific drug in food animals is lower than in other species, but the number of animals reported in each case is higher than other species.

SUGGESTED READING

Boothe DM. 1990. Drug therapy in cats: Mechanisms and avoidance of adverse drug reactions. *J Am Vet Med Assoc* 196:1297–1305.

Boothe DM. 1990. Drug therapy in cats: A therapeutic category approach. *J Am Vet Med Assoc* 196:1659–1669.

Boothe DM. 1990. Drug therapy in cats: Recommended dosing regimens. *J Am Vet Med Assoc* 196:1845–1850.

http://www.fda.gov/cvm/index/ade.html

Maddison JE, Page SW. 2008. "Adverse drug reactions." In *Small Animal Clinical Pharmacology*. Edited by Maddison JE, Page S, Church D. 2nd ed., pp. 41–51. St. Louis, MD: Saunders.

Naranjo CA, Shear NH, Busto U. 1998. "Special topics in pharmacology." In *Principles of Medical Pharmacology*. Edited by Kalant H, Roschlau WHE. 6th ed., pp. 792–793. New York: Oxford University Press.

Taniguchi CM, Armstrong SR, Green LC, Golan DE, Tashjian AH, Jr. 2008. "Drug toxicity." In *Principles of Pharmacology: The Pathophysiologic Basis of Drug Therapy*. Edited by Golan DE, Tashjian AH, Jr, Armstrong EJ, Armstrong AW. 2nd ed., pp. 63–69. Baltimore, MD: Lippincott Williams & Wilkins.

Vomand KC, Sumano H. 1990. Adverse drug reactions in cattle. *J Am Vet Med Assoc* 197:899–905.

■ STUDY QUESTIONS

DIRECTIONS: Each of the numbered items or incomplete statements in this section is followed by answers or by completions of the statement. Select the **one** lettered answer or completion that is **best** in each case.

1. A dog that is maintained on phenobarbital for the control of epilepsy may not respond to antifungal therapy with griseofulvin because phenobarbital

(A) forms an insoluble complex with griseofulvin.
(B) blocks uptake of griseofulvin by keratin precursor cells.
(C) increases renal blood flow, hastening the excretion of griseofulvin.
(D) induces hepatic microsomal enzymes, increasing griseofulvin metabolism.

2. The efficacy of pilocarpine, a miotic, may be reduced in the presence of

(A) phenytoin.
(B) H_1-antihistamines.
(C) glucocorticoids
(D) nonsteroid anti-inflammatory drugs.

3. A pharmacodynamic interaction resulting in drug antagonism may be caused by the concurrent administration of penicillin G and

(A) cephalexin.
(B) gentamicin.
(C) doxycycline.
(D) enrofloxacin.

4. Drugs that inhibit hepatic microsomal metabolism (Type I metabolism) include all of the following, except:

(A) phenylbutazone.
(B) ketoconazole.
(C) chloramphenicol.
(D) enrofloxacin.
(E) cimetidine.

5. All of the following are examples of combinations that would result in pharmaceutic interaction incompatibility, except:

(A) amphotericin B—sodium desoxycholate.
(B) tetracycline—riboflavin.
(C) ketamine HCl—thiopental sodium.
(D) penicillin G—sulfadimethoxine.

6. Adverse reactions to penicillin in animals are manifested as clinical signs ranging from skin wheals, urticaria, rhinitis, bronchoconstriction, diarrhea to life-threatening anaphylactic shock. These adverse reactions suggest which type of immune-mediated drug allergy?

(A) Type I
(B) Type II
(C) Type III
(D) Type IV

7. Which of the following drug pairs inhibit hepatic microsomal enzymes and thus, may prolong the action of other drugs?

(A) Phenylbutazone and phenobarbital
(B) Chloramphenicol and griseofluvin
(C) Ketoconazole and prednisolone
(D) Cimetidine and lindane
(E) Enrofloxacin and phenytoin

8. All of the following drugs should not be used in cats, except:

(A) acetaminophen.
(B) benzocaine.
(C) cisplatin.
(D) meloxicam.
(E) permethrin.

9. All of the following drugs should be used in lower dosages/interval than dogs, except:

(A) chloramphenicol.
(B) lidocaine.
(C) morphine
(D) aspirin.
(E) gentamicin.

10. According to FDA ADE reports (1987–2005), which of the following drug groups cause more adverse drug reactions than other groups?

(A) Sedatives/analgesics
(B) Cardiovascular drugs
(C) Antiparasitic drugs
(D) Antimicrobial drugs
(E) Anti-inflammatory drugs

ANSWERS AND EXPLANATIONS

1. The answer is D.
Phenobarbital is a potent inducer of hepatic microsomal enzymes involved in the oxidative metabolism of many drugs, including griseofulvin. The resulting rapid metabolism may reduce or eliminate drug effects on target tissues or organisms. Phenobarbital does not alter the uptake, excretion, or solubility of griseofluvin.

2. The answer is B.
H_1-anthhistamines have weak antimuscarinic activity that may antagonize the miotic action of parasympathomimetic drugs used in the treatment of glaucoma (e.g., pilocarpine). This is an example of a pharmacodynamic drug interaction.

3. The answer is C.
Concurrent administration of a penicillin and a tetracycline can reduce the efficacy of the penicillin. The bactericidal action of penicillins is greatest in rapidly dividing microorganisms. Tetracyclines, which are bacteriostatic antibiotics, inhibit protein synthesis, slowing bacterial growth. Cephaloxin, gentamicin, and enrofloxacin are bacteriocidal.

4. The answer is A.
Phenylbutazone induces enzymes of the cytochrome P450 system (microsomal enzymes), thus increasing the rate of metabolism of drugs inactivated by this pathway. Cimetidine, chloramphenicol, ketoconazole, and enrofloxacin inhibit microsomal enzymes and may prolong the action of drugs that are metabolized by these enzymes.

5. The answer is A.
Amphotericin B is not incompatible with sodium desoxycholate. In fact, sodium desoxycholate is the recommended diluent for amphotericin B to form a stable colloidal suspension. Tetracyclines are oxidized by riboflavin. Ketamine HCl and penicillin G, acidic solutions, form precipitates when exposed to alkaline solutions such as thiopental and sulfadimethoxine.

6. The answer is A.
The clinical signs of adverse drug reactions to penicillin, including skin wheals, urticaria, rhinitis, asthma, diarrhea, and anaphylactic shock suggest Type I drug allergy.

7. The answer is C.
Chloramphenicol, enrofloxacin, ketoconazole, cimetidine, ranitidine, prednisolone, and quinidine are inhibitors of cytochrome P450 enzymes, whereas phenylbutazone, Phenobarbital, griseofulvin, lindane, and phenytoin are inducers of these enzymes.

8. The answer is D.
Meloxicam, an NSAID, is approved for use in cats. Acetaminophen forms toxic metabolites in cats, which lead to oxidative damages, for example, methemoglobinemia. Bezocaine is poorly metabolized in cats, and can cause serious CNS disturbances. Cisplatin causes severe pulmonary toxicity in cats, which is manifested by vasculitis in alveolar capillaries. Cats are very sensitive to pyrethroid ectoparasiticides by showing tremors, muscle rigidity, and seizures (see Chapter 16 for further information).

9. The answer is E.
Cats have problems metabolizing chloramphenicol, lidocaine, morphine, aspirin, and many other drugs, and thus these drugs should be used in lower dosages/interval than dogs. The dosage of gentamicin in cats (3 mg/kg, IV, IM, or SC, q8h) is similar to that in dogs, since the elimination of aminoglycosides does not require drug metabolism.

10. The answer is C.
According to FDA CVM ADE reports, antiparasitic drugs cause more adverse reactions than other groups of drugs. This is attributable to the frequent use of antiparasitic drugs. In addition, many of the anthelmintics and ectoparasiticides affect neuromuscular function of parasites and animals.

Chapter 20

Legal Aspects of Medication Usage in Veterinary Medicine

Stephen D. Martin

I. **INTRODUCTION.** It is important for the practitioner to be aware of the rules, regulations, and standards that impact how they dispense, prescribe, or administer medications. While the objective of this chapter is to present an overview of these topics, it is beyond the scope of this chapter to include every regulation; therefore, the appropriate agency should be consulted for further explanation and completeness if necessary.

II. **REGULATORY AGENCIES.** There are both state and federal agencies, which govern how drugs are used in veterinary medicine.

A. **Federal agencies**

1. **Food and Drug Administration (FDA).** An agency of the United States Department of Health and Human Services. The 1938 Federal Foods, Drugs and Cosmetics Act (and subsequent amendments) gives the FDA the authority and responsibility for regulating a wide range of products to insure the safety and efficacy of foods, drugs, and cosmetics in the United States.
2. **Center for Veterinary Medicine (CVM).** A subdivision of the FDA which is responsible for regulating the drugs, devices, and food additives administered to animals.
3. **Drug Enforcement Agency (DEA).** A division of the United States Department of Justice which is responsible for the enforcement of the Controlled Substance Act (CSA) of 1970.

B. **State agencies**

1. **Board of Veterinary Medicine (BVM).** It protects the health and safety of the public and animals through the regulation of the practice of veterinary medicine as expressed in the state's veterinary practice act. A state's BVM contact information can be found at www.aavsb.org under "Boards and Agencies."
2. **Board of Pharmacy (BOP).** It regulates the wholesale and the pharmacy distribution of pharmaceutical products (including veterinary drugs). The BOP also regulates licensed veterinarians engaged in the prescribing and distribution of controlled substances used in veterinary practice. A state's BOP contact information can be found at www.nabp.net under "Boards of Pharmacy."

III. **PRESCRIPTION WRITING.** Definitions are as follows:

A. **Prescription.** An order for a medication (or device) issued by a licensed medical practitioner. The prescription is a legal document.

B. **Prescription blanks.** Printed forms on which the prescription is written. Prescription blanks are often preprinted with the name, address, and telephone number of the clinician or clinic. Some states require specialized prescription blanks for controlled substances.

C. **Prescription drug.** A drug or device that is required by state or federal law to be dispensed on prescription only, or is restricted to use by a practitioner only. Such products are identified by one of the following statements or legends appearing on the manufacturer's label.

1. "Rx Only."
2. "Caution: Federal law prohibits dispensing without a prescription."
3. "Caution: Federal law restricts this drug to use by or on the order of a licensed veterinarian."

D. **Prescription drugs** are sometimes called legend drugs because of these statements. A prescription, however, can also be written for nonprescription drugs (over-the-counter or OTC drugs) by the clinician.

E. **Required information on a prescription**

1. Date
2. Owner's name, address, and animal species or identification
3. Name, strength, and quantity of drug/device prescribed
4. Directions for use
5. Name, address, and signature of the prescriber
6. DEA number if a controlled drug is ordered
7. Refill information (how many times the prescription can be refilled) is optional, however, if not indicated the prescription cannot be refilled

F. **Medication error prevention.** A medication error, defined by the American Society of Health System Pharmacists, is "any preventable event that may cause or lead to inappropriate medication use or patient harm, while the medication is in the control of the healthcare professional, patient, or consumer. These events can be related to professional practice, health care products, procedures and systems, including prescribing, order communication, product labeling, packaging, nomenclature, compounding, dispensing, distribution, education, monitoring, and use." Prescribing and dispensing are two of the most common sources of a medication error.

G. **Prescribing errors** can be categorized as errors of omission or errors of commission.

1. **Errors of omission** are caused by missing or incomplete information, examples include:
   a. Failure to specify the quantity to dispense or the duration of therapy.
   b. Failure to specify the dose or dosage regimen.
   c. Failure to write legibly.
   d. Failure to provide all legally required information (example: DEA number for controlled substance).
   e. Incomplete specification of dosage form or strength or the specification of an unavailable dosage form or strength.
2. **Errors of commission** are caused by incorrect information, examples include:
   a. Incorrect dose or regimen.
   b. Incorrect drug or indication for use.
   c. Incorrect dosage form.
   d. Incorrect quantity or duration of therapy.
   e. Therapeutic duplication.
   f. Incorrect patient name on the prescription.
   g. Use of outdated references.
   h. Drug interactions or contraindications.

H. **Dispensing errors** include the errors of commission listed above as well as errors of omission.

1. Failure to counsel the owner about the medication prescribed.

I. **Medication error prevention in prescription writing**

1. When specifying a strength or dose, use a zero before the decimal point for an amount less than a whole unit (i.e., 0.1 mg, not a .1 mg); do not use trailing

zeros after the decimal point for whole numbers (i.e., 1 mg, not 1.0 mg). The use of a "naked decimal" (.1 mg and 1.0 mg) could cause misinterpretation of the intended amount by a factor of ten (1 mg and 10 mg).

2. Many drug names (brand and generic names) look alike or sound alike; care should be taken to insure the correct drug is selected (i.e., hydralazine vs. hydroxyzine, Celebrex® vs. Celexa®).

3. The prescription information must be legible; poor or illegible handwriting can be misinterpreted and be a source of a medication error.

4. The metric system should be used to express strengths and quantities (i.e., Phenobarbital 30 mg); the use of outdated weight and measures should not be used (i.e., Phenobarbital ½ grain).

5. Vague directions for use (i.e., "take as directed") should be avoided; the directions should be concise and include what the medication is used for infection, cough, and so forth, and for nonmaintenance drugs, the length of the treatment 1 week, 10 days, and so forth.

6. The use of abbreviations should be minimized or eliminated in prescription writing. Abbreviations can be misinterpreted, especially if penmanship is poor, leading to a medication error. Some abbreviations have been banned from use in human hospitals because they have frequently been the source of medication errors. (For a complete list of hazardous abbreviations and explanations refer to the Error-Prone Abbreviation List at the Institute for Safe Medication Practices' website www.ismp.org.)

   a. For example, both abbreviations "QOD" (every other day) and "QD" (daily) have been mistaken for the abbreviation "QID" (four times daily).

   b. Veterinarians should avoid using nonstandardized abbreviations when writing a prescription to be taken to a human pharmacy. The abbreviation "SID" (once daily) is only used in veterinary medicine veterinarians—it is not used by any other healthcare profession. As a result, it has been mistaken for "QID" (four times daily) and "BID" (twice daily) by community pharmacists.

J. **Issuance of the prescription.** The information on a prescription can generally be communicated to a pharmacy by any of the three methods: written, oral, or electronic format.

1. **Written format.** The prescription information is written on a prescription blank and then is given to the animal's owner to present to a pharmacy.

   a. The prescription should always be written in ink or printed via computer; never written with a pencil.

   b. Alterations and changes should be avoided; rewrite on new prescription blank if necessary.

2. **Oral format.** The prescription is telephoned to the pharmacy by the veterinarian or their agent and the information is recorded on a prescription blank by a pharmacist. Prescriptions for C-II drugs (next section) cannot be given over the phone.

3. **Electronic format.** Requirements and restrictions for this format may vary from state to state; the veterinarian should check with their state's BOP before using this format.

   a. Facsimile transmission: written information is faxed to the pharmacy and the information is processed the same as a written or oral prescription.

   b. Computer to computer and handheld devices: prescription information is communicated electronically to the pharmacy's computer system.

IV. **CONTROLLED SUBSTANCES.** Controlled substances are drugs (legal and illegal) and chemicals under the jurisdiction of the federal Controlled Substance Act (CSA) which regulates the manufacture, distribution, and dispensing of controlled substances. The Drug Enforcement Administration (125) enforces the CSA through the regulations found in Title 21, Code of Federal Regulations (CFR), Parts 1300-end. A Practitioner's Manual is available on the DEA website (www.deadiversion.usdoj.gov) under "publications" to

Drug Enforcement Administration
Practitioner's Manual

DEPICTION of PAGE 1 of DEA FORM-222
U.S. OFFICIAL ORDER FORM - SCHEDULES I & II

See Reverse of PURCHASER'S Copy of Instructions	No order form may be issued for Schedule I and II substances unless a completed application form has been received, (21 CFR 1305.04).	OMB APPROVAL No. 1117-0010

TO: *(Name of Supplier)*   STREET ADDRESS

CITY and STATE	DATE	TO BE FILLED IN BY SUPPLIER
		SUPPLIERS DEA REGISTRATION No.

L I N E No.	No. of Packages	Size of Package	Name of Item	National Drug Code	Packages Shipped	Date Shipped
1						
2						
3						
4						
5						
6						
7						
8						
9						
10						

TO BE FILLED IN BY PURCHASER

◀ **LAST LINE COMPLETED** *(MUST BE 10 OR LESS)*   SIGNATURE OR PURCHASER OR ATTORNEY OR AGENT

Date Issued	DEA Registration No.	Name and Address of Registrant
Schedules		
Registered as a	No. of this Order Form	

DEA Form-222 (Oct. 1992)

U.S. OFFICIAL ORDER FORMS - SCHEDULES I & II
DRUG ENFORCEMENT ADMINISTRATION
SUPPLIER'S Copy 1

Note: The graphic illustrated above is not intended to be used as an actual order form.

2006 Edition

FIGURE 20-1. Depiction of page 1 of DEA Form-222. U.S. official order form—Schedules I and II.

assist the practitioner in their understanding of the CSA and CFR; the manual summarizes the requirements for prescribing, administering, and prescribing controlled substances.

A. **Registration requirements for controlled substances**

1. Registration with both the DEA and the state BOP is a requirement for any practitioner that will dispense, administer, or prescribe any controlled drug.
   a. DEA (federal) registration needs renewal every 3 years; refer to the Practitioner's Manual for the registration process.

    b. State registration forms are available from the state's BOP. The renewal period may vary from state to state.

  2. Registration certificates must be maintained at the registered location in a readily retrievable manner.

  3. Separate registration is required for each principal business or practice where controlled substances are dispensed, administered or stored; separate registration is not required for locations where controlled substances are prescribed but not dispensed, administered, or stored.

  4. The practitioner must notify both the DEA and the state's BOP if there is a change in their practice or business address.

B. **Schedules of controlled substances.** The drugs and chemicals that are considered controlled substances are divided into five schedules based on abuse potential, safety, and accepted medical use in the United States.

  1. Schedule I. These substances have no current accepted medical use in the United States, have a lack of accepted safety when used, and have a high abuse potential. Examples: heroin, methamphetamine, LDS, and marijuana.

  2. Schedule II. These substances have a high abuse potential and an accepted medical use in the United States. This schedule includes narcotics, depressants, and stimulants.
    a. Examples used in veterinary medicine: morphine, dihydomorphine, fentanyl, and pentobarbital.

  3. Schedule III. These substances have an accepted medical use in the United States and less abuse potential than Schedule I and II.
    a. Examples used in veterinary medicine: ketamine, boldenone, buprenorphine, and hydrocodone with homatropine.

  4. Schedule IV. These substances have a lower potential for abuse relative to the Schedule III substances.
    a. Examples used in veterinary medicine: butorphanol, diazepam, and phenobarbital.

  5. Schedule V. These substances have the lowest abuse potential of the controlled substances.
    a. Examples used in veterinary medicine: phenylpropanolamine.

  6. The amount of the controlled substance in a product also may influence into which schedule it fit; also, the combination of a controlled substance with a noncontrolled substance may affect the scheduling.
    a. Example: codeine 30 mg tablets are Schedule II, codeine 30 mg/acetaminophen 325 g tablets are Schedule III, products with codeine 200 mg or less per 100 mL or 100 g are Schedule V.

  7. The term "class" which is symbolized by the letter "C" is used interchangeably with "Schedule"; for example, a Schedule II drug and a C-II drug represent the same classification. Manufacturers use the "C" symbol on their label to identify the product as a controlled substance.

C. **Controlled substance recordkeeping.** The CSA created a closed distribution system in which all legitimate handlers of controlled substances: researchers, manufacturers, distributors, practitioners, pharmacies, with the exception of the ultimate user, must be registered. Under this distribution system, strict recordkeeping for accountability of all controlled substance transactions must be maintained.

  1. Recordkeeping
    a. All controlled substance records must be maintained in a readily retrievable manner separate from other business records.
    b. All controlled substance records must be kept available for inspection for a minimum of 2 years. This includes invoices, credit memos, dispensing transactions, and administration records.
    c. All Schedule II records must be kept separate from Schedule III to V records.
    d. A practitioner that dispenses or administers controlled substances must take a beginning controlled substance inventory on the date they initially start to

dispense or administer and take a new inventory every 2 years from when the beginning inventory was taken (a biennial inventory).

 e. A perpetual inventory system is recommended for the practitioner to use when recording a controlled substance that is purchased, dispensed or administered.

 f. The practitioner should contact their regional DEA office or their state's BOP for disposal of controlled substances which are unusable (i.e., damaged, out-of-date, and unwanted) if they cannot be returned to the manufacturer or distributor. Copies of all records documenting the return or disposal of controlled substances should be maintained for at least 2 years.

D. Ordering controlled substances for inventory

1. A practitioner can order Schedule III through Schedule V drugs for their clinic by either phoning the manufacturer or distributor or by faxing or mailing them an order.
2. All orders for Schedule II drugs must be ordered on a special DEA order form (DEA-222). See example DEA 222 form (Figure 20-1).
3. DEA 222 forms may be ordered online at www.deadiversion.usdoj.gov or by contacting a regional DEA office for assistance.
4. The forms come in packets of seven sequentially numbered forms and should be used in sequence.
5. The DEA-222 form must be filled out in ink and cannot have any alterations or erasures.
6. The form can only be signed by the registrant whose name appears on the form unless power of attorney has been granted to an authorized individual.
7. The form is in triplicate with copies 1 and 2 going to the supplier; copy 3 is kept by the purchaser and when the order is received the date and the quantities received must be recorded on this copy. Copy 3 is filed in sequential order with a invoice copy attached.
8. Ordering Schedule II drugs electronically using the DEA's CSOS system may also be an option if the supplier accepts this format and the practitioner has a CSOS certificate. More information on CSOS is available at www.deadiversion.usdoj.gov.

E. Prescribing controlled drugs

1. The practitioner's DEA number and practice address is required information for a prescription for a controlled substance in addition to the information listed under Required Information on a Prescription section.
2. A written prescription is required for Schedule II drugs. Schedule III, IV, and V prescriptions may be written or phoned. Electronic transmission requirements of Schedule III–V may vary from state to state.
3. Refills are not allowed on Schedule II prescriptions—a new prescription is required each time. Schedule III–V prescriptions may be refilled, if authorized on the prescription, up to five times within 6 months for the date the prescription was written.

F. Security measures

1. Practitioners must store controlled substances in a securely locked cabinet or safe.
2. Keep controlled substance inventory to a minimum level; restrict inventory access to a minimal number of employees.
3. Any theft or loss of a controlled substance must be reported to the DEA and the state's BOP.
4. Keep prescription blanks in a secure place away from public access.
5. Use tamper-resistant prescription blanks. (Some states require special prescription blanks for controlled drugs-check with the BOP.)
6. Do not make alterations on the prescription; write out the amount prescribed in addition to the number quantity, that is, #12 (twelve).

  A state's controlled substance regulations are often the same as the federal controlled substance regulations; however, there can be some differences. If the practitioner complies with the most stringent set of regulations (federal or state) they will be assured of being in compliance with both sets of regulations (federal and state).

V. **EXTRA-LABEL USE OF MEDICATIONS.** Extra-label use (also called "off-label use") of a medication is defined in 21 CFR, Part 530, as the actual or intended use of a medication in an animal in a manner that is not in accordance with the approved labeling.

A. **Background on extra-label use.** As a result of legislation passed by Congress in 1958 (The Food Additives Amendment to the Federal Food, Drug, and Cosmetic Act of 1938), animal drugs were also considered food additives because they could become a component of meat, milk, or eggs. Since the amendment required FDA approval of a food additive prior to its inclusion in food, the extra-label use (ELU) of drugs in animals became illegal. Therefore, unlike the physician, the veterinarian could not prescribe or treat their patients (food animal and nonfood animal) with medications in a manner other than stated on the manufacturer's label without violating federal law and placing themselves at risk of regulatory action. In the 1980s, the FDA issued Compliance Policy Guides (CPG) to their personnel as guidance for regulatory action and enforcement priorities regarding ELU, especially in food animals, in an effort to balance the needs of the patient while protecting the public's health. However, the CPG were for FDA internal guidance only and did not confer or grant any rights or privileges for ELU to the veterinarian, leaving them still in violation. In 1994, the CPG were codified in law when Congress passed the Animal Medicinal Drug Use Clarification Act.

B. **Animal Medicinal Drug Use Clarification Act (AMDUCA) of 1994**

1. Implemented in 1996 by the regulations in 21 CFR, Part 530—Extralabel Drug Use in Animals.
2. AMDUCA and 21 CFR, Part 530 can be accessed at www.fda.gov/cvm/ amduca-toc.htm; highlights are discussed below.
3. AMDUCA allows veterinarians to treat their patients with approved animal drugs and approved human drugs in an extra-label manner.
4. ELU is allowed only if a valid veterinarian–client–patient relationship (VCPR) exists. A valid VCPR exists when:
   a. A veterinarian has assumed the responsibility for making decisions for the health and treatment of the animal for which the owner has agreed to follow.
   b. The veterinarian is familiar enough with the animal, having recently seen and examined the animal and is acquainted with its keeping and care, to make a general diagnosis of the animal's condition.
   c. The veterinarian is readily available if an adverse reaction or treatment failure occurs.
5. ELU is only permitted on the order of a licensed veterinarian within the context of a valid VCPR; a lay person outside of a valid VCPR is not permitted to use drugs in an extra-label manner.
6. ELU is limited to the treatment of an animal when suffering or death may result if not treated or when the animal's health is threatened.
7. ELU of drugs is not permitted in or on animal feed; when a residue may be a risk to the public health; or when ELU results in residues exceeding established safe levels or concentrations.
8. Although the emphasis of AMDUCA is ELU in food-producing animals, AMDUCA also permits ELU in nonfood producing animals if:
   a. There is not an approved drug, concentration, or dosage form available.
   b. In the veterinarian's judgment, the approved drug is not clinically effective.
   c. When the public health is not threatened.
9. ELU is permitted in food-producing animals:
   a. If there is not an approved animal drug available or if the approved drug is not, in the veterinarian's judgment, an effective treatment.

    b. A careful diagnosis is made before prescribing or dispensing a drug to be used in an ELU manner.

    c. A withdrawal interval has been established prior to marketing the edible product.

    d. The identity of the animal is maintained.

    e. Measures have been taken to assure compliance with the established withdrawal time and there is no illegal drug residue from ELU in the treated animal.

    f. Additionally, if the drug is an approved human drug or an animal drug not approved for use in food animals, the following requirements must be met:

        (1) The ELU must be in accordance with appropriate medical rationale.

        (2) In the absence of scientific information on human food safety from the ELU use of a drug, the veterinarian must take appropriate measures to keep the animal and its food products out of the human food supply.

        (3) ELU of an approved human drug is not permitted if a drug approved for food animals can be used an extra-labeled manner.

  10. ELU record requirements

    a. The veterinarian is required to keep records of ELU for at least 2 years unless Federal or State law requires longer.

    b. The FDA may request access to ELU records to determine if the ELU presents a risk to public health.

    c. The ELU records should be maintained in an orderly and timely manner, and are readily retrievable if requested for review or inspection.

    d. The ELU record must contain documentation of:

        (1) The animal's identification either as an individual or for food animals by group (herd, flock, or by client).

        (2) The established name of the drug and its active ingredient.

        (3) The condition being treated.

        (4) The species of the animal being treated.

        (5) The number of animals being treated.

        (6) The dose administered.

        (7) Duration of treatment.

        (8) The specified withdrawal, withholding, or discard time for meat, milk, eggs or any food derived from any food animal treated.

  11. ELU labeling requirements

    a. Human or animal drugs intended for ELU must be labeled properly or accompanied by the labeling information to assure safe and proper use.

    b. ELU labeling is required of the veterinarian dispensing the product or the pharmacist dispensing the product pursuant to an order from a veterinarian.

    c. The required labeling information must include:

        (1) The name and address of the prescribing/dispensing veterinarian.

        (2) If the drug is dispensed by a pharmacy on the order of a veterinarian, the pharmacy label must include the pharmacy name and address and the prescribing veterinarian's name (the veterinarian's address is optional).

        (3) The established name of the drug or established names of each active ingredient if formulated with more than one.

        (4) Any directions specified by the veterinarian including the class/species or animal identification or group (herd, flock, pen, and so forth) being treated.

        (5) The dosage, frequency, and duration of treatment.

        (6) Any cautionary statements.

        (7) The veterinarian's specified withdrawal, withholding or discard time for any food items (meat, milk, eggs, and so forth).

  12. Compounded drug preparations are considered ELU drugs

    a. Permitted if there is no approved new animal drug or no approved new human drug in an available dosage form or concentration that can be used.

    b. Human drugs cannot be compounded for food animal use if an approved animal drug can be used for the compounding.

    c. Compounding from bulk drugs is not permitted.

  13. Prohibition of ELU Drugs

a. **The FDA can prohibit ELU in nonfood animals if there is a risk to public health.**
b. **The FDA can prohibit ELU in food animals if:**
   (1) ELU is risk to the public health or
   (2) If acceptable analytical methods have not been established or cannot be established to quantify safe levels and residue levels.
   (3) ELU can be prohibited for a specific drug or a class of drugs or the prohibition can be limited to a species, indication, dosage form or route of administration or any combination of these conditions in food animals.
   (4) Drugs prohibited for ELU in food animals
       (a) Adamantane derivatives (amantadine and rimantadine) and neuraminidase inhibitors (oseltamivir and zanamivir) in chickens, turkeys, and ducks
       (b) Chloramphenicol
       (c) Clenbuterol
       (d) Diethylstilbesterol (DES)
       (e) Dimetridazole
       (f) Ipronidazole
       (g) Other nitroimidazoles
       (h) Furazolidone, nitrofurazone, other nitrofurans
       (i) Fluoroquinolones
       (j) Glycopeptides (example: vancomycin)
       (k) Phenylbutazone in female dairy cattle 20 months of age or older
       (l) Sulfonamide drugs in lactating cattle—except approved use of sulfadimethoxine, sulfabromomethazine, and sulfaethoxypridazine
       (m) Estradiol cypionate
   (5) Changes to the prohibited list are posted at http://www.fda.gov/cvm website.

VI. DRUG RESIDUE.

VI. DRUG RESIDUE. An additional consideration for the veterinarian when treating a food–animal patient with medications is the potential for the medication to be present in the edible tissue (meat, milk, eggs) of the animal.

Drug residue is a subset of the chemical contamination threat to the human food supply chain—a significant food safety issue. In addition to drugs, pesticides, herbicides, industrial and agricultural chemicals, and other environmental contaminants also present risks to the food supply. Human exposure to these chemicals and/or their metabolites as residues in the food supply is a public health concern because of their potential risk of being carcinogens, mutagens, teratogens, allergens, or contributing to the development of bacterial resistance to antibiotics.

A. **Safe concentrations** (or tolerance levels) of a drug in edible tissue are determined by the FDA through toxicology testing and estimating an acceptable daily intake of the edible tissue or milk. When the drug residue concentration is at or below the determined safe concentration, the food product containing the drug residue is not considered a public health risk. The Environmental Protection Agency (EPA) establishes safe concentrations for pesticides and other chemicals in the edible tissue of food animals.

B. **Withdrawal times** are calculated by the FDA from residue studies and pharmacokinetic data submitted by the drug sponsor (manufacturer) following FDA guidelines. Withdrawal time is the period after treatment that is needed to insure that drug concentrations in target tissues (tissues with the slowest depletion rate of the residue) reach a safe concentration; at this point the edible tissues are considered safe for human consumption. Statistically, withdrawal time is expressed as the point that can be predicted with a 95% confidence interval that the residue concentration in the target tissue of 99% of the animals have decreased to concentrations below the established safe concentration. Withdrawal times for drugs approved by the FDA for use in food animals are specific to species, route of administration, dose, duration of treatment, and product formulation submitted by the drug sponsor. The withdrawal time information is found on the approved food animal product's label or packaging (also see Appendix I).

After a food animal drug is approved by the FDA and is marketed, the United States Department of Agriculture (USDA) and its division, the Food Safety Inspection Service (FSIS) become the regulatory agencies for insuring the compliance of animal-derived foods with the established safe concentrations for drug residues (as well as for pesticides and other chemical residues). The primary cause for noncompliance with the established safe concentrations is the failure to observe approved withdrawal times. However, if a drug is used in an extra-label manner, the withdrawal times stated by the manufacturer no longer apply. Extra-label use is allowed under AMDUCA (see section IV) if the veterinarian can establish an appropriate withdrawal interval to insure that the edible tissues are safe for human consumption.

 C. **FARAD** (Food Animal Residue Avoidance Databank) is a database the veterinarian can use to establish withdrawal intervals to minimize drug residues. (www.farad.org).

The FARAD program was developed by pharmacologists and toxicologists at the University of California at Davis, North Carolina State University, the University of Florida, and the University of Illinois as a repository of residue avoidance information.

The veterinarian should also take into consideration general condition of the animal since the withdrawal time or withdrawal interval is a pharmacokinetic value (elimination half-life) which can be influenced by renal function, hydration status, and so forth, and therefore may require a more conservative withdrawal time or interval. Once the withdrawal time or interval has been determined the veterinarian should test the tissue for drug residue levels; if the levels are above the safe concentration, the withdrawal time or interval should be extended until they are at the safe concentration.

 VII. **DRUG IMPORTATION OF FDA-UNAPPROVED VETERINARY DRUGS.** Veterinary drugs (but not human drugs) which are available in other countries and are unapproved by the FDA for use in the United States can be imported into the United States for companion animal use if permission is obtained from the FDA-CVM.

A. **Permission request.** The first step of importation requires the veterinarian to submit a letter to the FDA-CVM requesting permission to import the drug. The letter must contain the following information:

1. Veterinarian's name, address, and phone number
2. Clinic name and address
3. Client's name and address
4. Patient name and nonfood species
5. Name of drug
6. Drug family or class
7. Name and address of drug supplier
8. Legal status of the drug in the foreign country
9. Amount of drug to be imported (full bottles; small quantities allowed-maximum of a 90-day supply)
10. Disease condition to be treated
11. Reason why an approved human or animal drug will not treat this disease condition
12. A statement that:
    a. The DVM will notify the animal owner that the drug is not approved;
    b. The drug will not be used in any food animal;
    c. The DVM agrees to notify the FDA if there are any adverse reactions.
13. How the DVM learned of the existence of this drug. The letter should be submitted to: Division of Compliance HFV-230, Center for Veterinary Medicine, Food and Drug Administration, Metro Park North, 7500 Standish Place, Rockville, MD

20855. Attn: Mr. Michael Zimmerman or faxed to: 240.276.9241. Additional contact information: ph 240.276.9209; Michael.Zimmerman@fda.hhs.gov.

B. **FDA guidelines.** The FDA has developed policy guidelines for the personal importation of unapproved drugs which FDA personnel use in determining whether to allow a drug to be imported; the guidelines include:

1. The drug is intended for use for a serious condition for which effective treatment is not available in the United States;
2. There is no known commercialization or promotion of the drug to persons residing in the United States by those distributing the drug;
3. The drug is not considered to present an unreasonable risk;
4. The individual seeking to import the drug affirms in writing that the drug is for a specific patient's use (usually not more than a 90-day supply).

C. **FDA permission to import.** The approval process takes 2–4 weeks; if the request to import is approved, the FDA will send a permission to import letter to the DVM. A copy of this letter must be forwarded to the supplier along with the product order. Without the permission to import letter the drug may be seized by the U.S. Customs Service or refused entry into the country. If the animal is to continue beyond the 90 days supply, a new letter requesting permission to import must be sent to the FDA-CVM and the new FDA-CVM permission letter must accompany the reorder.

SUGGESTED READING

"Animal Medicinal Drug Use Clarification Act of 1994." January 2007. http://www.fda.gov/cvm/ amducatoc.htm.

Botsoglou N, Fletouris D. 2001. *Drug Residues in Foods: Phamracology, Food Safety, and Analysis.* New York: Marcel Dekker.

Brown SA. 2001. "Dosage forms, drug prescription orders, and veterinary feed directives." In *Veterinary Pharmacology and Therapeutics.* Edited by Adams HR. 8th ed., pp. 1157–1165. Ames, IA: Iowa State University Press.

Committee on Drug Use in Food Animals, Comp. 1999. *The Use of Drugs in Food Animals Benefits and Risks.* Washington, DC: National Academy Press.

"Error Prone Abbreviation List." Institute for Safe Medication Practices. March 2007. http://www.ismp.org.

"FARAD." May 2007. http://www.farad.org/gen.html.

"Practitioner's Manual." DEA Office of Diversion Control. Department of Justice. April 2007. hppt://www.deadiversion.usdoj.gov/pubs/manuals/pract/index.html.

■ STUDY QUESTIONS

DIRECTIONS: Each of the numbered items or incomplete statements in this section is followed by answers or by completions of the statement. Select the **one** lettered answer or completion that is **best** in each case.

1. The Drug Enforcement Administration is the division of the FDA, which is responsible for the safety and efficacy of prescription drugs.

(A) True
(B) False

2. According to both state and federal laws, over-the-counter medications cannot be ordered on a prescription blank.

(A) True
(B) False

3. Which of the following is **not** required information on a veterinary prescription?

(A) Owners' name
(B) Number of authorized refills
(C) Directions for using the medication
(D) All of the above information is required.

4. Which of the following is **not** considered an error of omission in prescription writing?

(A) The quantity to be dispensed is not specified
(B) Illegible handwriting
(C) Wrong patient/owner information
(D) None of the above are errors of omission
(E) All of the above are errors of omission

5. Which of the following measures can prevent medication errors?

(A) Use a "naked decimal" to express a strength or dose in order to avoid clutter on the prescription.
(B) Make sure handwriting is legible or print the information on the prescription.
(C) Make certain the abbreviations "QOD" (every other day), "QD" (daily), and "SID" (once a day) are neatly written on the prescription.
(D) All of the above

6. Which of the following statements about controlled substances is **true**?

(A) A practitioner is required to have both state and federal registrations in order to write a prescription for a controlled substance.
(B) Schedule V substances have the highest abuse potential.
(C) All controlled substances to be dispensed or administered to patients in a clinic need to be ordered from the supplier on a special DEA order form.

7. According to AMDUCA which of the following is **false**?

(A) Extra-label drug use is permitted only if a valid client–patient relationship exists.
(B) The extra-label use of drugs is permitted in both food animal and nonfood animal patients.
(C) Using an approved drug for beef cattle at a higher dose than the dose on the manufacturer's label would not be considered extra-label use as long as beef cattle are still being treated.

8. According to AMDUCA, the FDA can no longer prohibit the veterinarian from using drugs in an extra-label manner.

(A) True
(B) False

9. To establish a withdrawal interval for a drug used in an extra-label manner, which of the following would be the **best** resource for the veterinarian?

(A) FSIS
(B) FDA
(C) EPA
(D) FARAD

10. Drugs not approved by the FDA for use in the United States may be legally imported if:

(A) The drug will not be used in any food animal.

(B) The DVM requests permission from the CVM to import the medication.

(C) The animal's owner is informed that the drug is not approved in the United States.

(D) All of the above.

ANSWERS AND EXPLANATIONS

1. The answer is B.
The Drug Enforcement Administration is a division of the Department of Justice and is responsible for the enforcement of the CSA. The FDA is responsible for the safety and efficacy of prescription drugs.

2. The answer is B.
A clinician may write a prescription for over-the-counter medications. This is often done when special patient instructions are required or unusual quantities are needed.

3. The answer is B.
Refill information is optional information. Owner information and the medication directions is required information.

4. The answer is C.
Wrong patient/owner information is an error of commission; incorrect information was provided. Missing the quantity to dispense and illegible handwriting are considered errors of omission.

5. The answer is B.
Handwriting should be legible or the information neatly printed; the information on the prescription should be clearly understood. Using a "naked decimal" (.1 in place of 0.1 or 1.0 in place of 1) is a source of a medication error which could result in the patient receiving an inappropriate dose; the abbreviations "QOD" and "QD" are considered dangerous and have been banned from use in human hospitals because they can be mistaken for "QID" especially if poorly written. The abbreviation "SID" is not used outside of veterinary medicine and should not be used in prescription writing; it has been mistaken for "BID" and "QID."

6. The answer is A.
Both state- and federal-controlled substance registration are required in order for a clinician to write a prescription for a controlled substance. Schedule II substances have the highest abuse potential in descending order down to Schedule V, the lowest abuse

potential. Only Schedule II drugs for clinic use are required to be ordered on the special DEA form 222.

7. The answer is C.
Using a dose different than what is on the manufacturer's label would be considered extra-label use. Using a drug in a manner inconsistent with the manufacturer's packaging or label is extra-label use.

8. The answer is B.
Under AMDUCA the FDA can prohibit extra-label use in both non-food animals and food animals if there is a risk to public health.

9. The answer is D.
FARAD (Food Animal Residue Avoidance Databank) is a comprehensive database of residue avoidance information; it would be the most useful to establish a withdrawal interval for extra-label use. FSIS (Food Safety and Inspection Service),is the part of the USDA responsible for making sure the commercial supply of meat, poultry, and eggs is safe and correctly packaged, but would not be a resource for withdrawal intervals. Although the FDA's responsibilities include establishing safe concentrations and withdrawal times, it would not be a resource for extra-label use. The EPA (Environmental Protection Agency) is responsible for protecting human health and the environment by enforcing environmental laws; it would not be a source of information on extra-label drug use.

10. The answer is D.
All of them are correct. The importation process of an unapproved drug into the Unites States begins with a permission to import letter sent to the FDA-CVM. In the letter, the veterinarian must include the statements: (1) The drug will not be used in any food animal. (2) The DVM will notify the animal's owner that the drug is not approved. (3) The DVM agrees to notify the FDA if there are any adverse reactions.

Appendix I

Withdrawal Time Charts

The following pages contain a reference table listing generic names alphabetically. The document summarizes information on withdrawal times for food products (meat and milk) according to the species and the route of administration. The withdrawal times listed correspond to label dosages of the drug and directions. Deviations from label recommendations may lead to drug residues in food products.

DISCLAIMER: Every effort has been made to ensure the accuracy of the information published. However, it remains the responsibility of the readers to familiarize themselves with the information contained on the product label or package insert. The author (W. H. Hsu) cannot be responsible for publication errors or any consequence that could result from the use of published information.

Generic name	Species	Route of administration	Meat	Milk
Acepromazine maleate (Recommended by FARAD)	Cattle	IM, IV	7d	48h
	Sheep	IM, IV	7d	48h
	Swine	IM, IV	7d	
	Goat	IM, IV	7d	48h
Albendazole	Cattle	Oral	27d	
	Sheep	Oral	7d	
Altrenogest	Swine	Oral	21d	
Amitraz	Cattle	Topical	0d	0d
	Swine	Topical	3d	
Amoxicillin	Cattle	IM, SC	25d	96h
	Dairy cattle	IMM	12d	60h
Ampicillin	Cattle	IM	6d	48h
Amprolium	Cattle	idw, oral	24h	
Carbaryl	Poultry	Topical	7d	
Ceftiofur hydrochloride	Dairy cattle	IMM	0–3d	0–72h
Ceftiofur sodium	Cattle	IM, SC	0d	0d
	Goat	IM	0d	0d
	Sheep	IM	0d	0d
	Poultry	SC	0d	
	Swine	IM	4d	
Cephapirin benzathine	Dairy cattle	IMM	42d	72h
Cephapirin sodium	Dairy cattle	IMM	4d	96h
Chlortetracycline	Poultry	idw	1d	
	Swine	idw	5d	
	Cattle	idw	24h	
Chlortetracycline + Penicillin G + Sulfamethazine	Swine	In the feed	15d	
Chlortetracycline + Sulfamethazine	Beef cattle	In the feed	7d	
Clorsulon	Cattle	Oral	8d	

(continued)

(*Continued*)

Generic name	Species	Route of administration	Meat	Milk
Cloxacillin benzathine	Dairy cattle	IMM	28d	
Cloxacillin sodium	Dairy cattle	IMM	10d	48h
		IMM	30d	
Coumaphos	Cattle	Topical	0d	0d
	Swine	Topical	0d	
Dexamethasone	Cattle	IM, IV		
Dichlorvos	Swine	In the feed	0d	
	Cattle	Premise	1d	
Diclazuril	Chickens	in the feed	0d	
Dinoprost	Cattle	IM	0d	0d
	Swine	IM	0d	
Docusate sodium	Cattle	Oral	3d	96h
	Goat	Oral	3d	96h
	Sheep	Oral	3d	96h
Doramectin	Cattle	IM, SC	35d	
	Swine	IM	24d	
Enrofloxacin	Beef cattle	SC	28d	
Erythromycin	Cattle	IM	14d	72h
	Dairy cattle	IMM	14d	36h
	Sheep	IM	3d	
	Swine	IM	7d	
	Poultry	idw	1d	
Fenbendazole	Cattle	Oral	8d	
	Beef cattle	Oral	11d	
	Cattle	In the feed	13d	0d
	Swine	In the feed	0d	
Florfenicol	Cattle	IM	28d	
	Cattle	SC	38d	
Flunixin meglumine	Cattle	IV	4d	36h
	Swine	IM	12d	
Furosemide	Cattle	IM, IV	48h	48h
Gentamicin	Swine	Oral	14d	
	Swine	IM	40d	
	Swine	idw	10d	
	Chickens	SC	35d	
	Turkeys	SC	63d	
Hetacillin potassium	Dairy Cattle	IMM	10d	72h
Isoflupredone acetate	Cattle	IM	7d	
	Swine	IM	7d	
Ivermectin	Cattle	Topical	48d	
	Cattle	SC	35d	
	Swine	SC	18d	
Lasalocid	Cattle	In the feed	0d	
Levamisole	Swine	idw	72h	
	Cattle	SC	7d	
Lincomycin	Chickens	idw	0d	
	Swine	idw	0d	
	Swine	IM	48h	
Magnesium hydroxide	Dairy cattle	Oral		12–24h
	Goat	Oral		12–24h
	Sheep	Oral		12–24h
Magnesium oxide	Dairy cattle	Oral		24h
Melengestrol acetate	Cattle	in the feed	48h	
Morantel tartrate	Cattle	In the feed	14d	0d
Moxidectin	Cattle	SC	21d	
Narasin + Nicarbazin	Chickens	In the feed	5d	

Generic name	Species	Route of administration	Meat	Milk
Neomycin	Cattle	idw	1d	
	Goat	idw	3d	
	Sheep	idw	2d	
	Swine	idw	3d	
Nicarbazin	Chickens	In the feed	4d	
Novobiocin	Dairy cattle	IMM	30d	
Oxfendazole	Cattle	IR, SC	7d	
Oxytetracycline	Cattle	IM, IV	28d	96h
	Swine	IM	28d	
	Swine	idw	7–14d	
	Poultry	idw	7–14d	
	Sheep	IM, SC	28d	96h
	Goat	IM, SC	28d	96h
Oxytetrecycline + Neomycin	Cattle	Oral	30d	
		mr	30d	
Penicillin G	Cattle	IM	10d	48h
	Sheep	IM	9d	
	Swine	IM	7d	
Penicillin G procaine	Dairy cattle	IMM	3d	60h
Penicillin G + Novo-biocin	Dairy cattle	IMM	30d	
Penicillin G benzathin + Penicillin G procaine	Beef cattle	SC	30d	
Permethrin	Swine	Premise, topical	5d	
	Cattle	Topical	0d	0d
	Goat	Topical	0d	0d
	Sheep	Topical	0d	
Phosmet	Cattle	Topical	3d	
	Swine	Topical	1d	
Piperazine	Poultry	idw	14d	
	Swine	idw	21d	
Pirlimycin HCl	Dairy cattle	IMM	9d	36h
Propylene glycol	Dairy cattle	IR, oral		96h
Pyrantel tartrate	Swine	In the feed	24h	
Robenidine hydrochloride	Chicken	Oral	5d	
Roxarsone	Poultry	In the feed	5d	
	Swine	In the feed	5d	
	Poultry	idw	5d	
	Swine	idw	5d	
Spectinomycin	Cattle	SC	11d	
	Swine	Oral	21d	
	Chickens	idw	5d	
Streptomycin	Cattle	idw	2d	
	Chickens	idw	4d	
Sulfachlorpyridazine	Cattle	idw	7d	
	Swine	idw	4d	
Sulfadimethoxine	Cattle	Oral, idw	7d	60h
	Cattle	IV	5d	60h
	Poultry	idw	5d	

(continued)

Generic name	Species	Route of administration	Meat	Milk
Sulfamethazine	Cattle	Oral	12d	
Sulfaquinoxaline sodium	Cattle	idw	10d	
	Poultry	idw	10d	
Tetrachlorvinphos	Cattle	Topical	0d	
	Poultry	Premise, topical	0d	
	Swine	Topical	0d	
Tetracycline	Cattle	idw	5d	
	Poultry	idw	4d	
	Swine	idw	4d	
Tiamulin	Swine	idw	3–7d	
	Swine	In the feed	0–7d	
Tilmicosin	Swine	In the feed	7d	
	Cattle	SC	28d	
	Sheep	SC	28d	
Tolazoline (Recommended by FARAD)	Cattle	IV	8d	48h
Tripelennanime HCl	Cattle	IM, IV	4d	24h
Tulathromycin	Cattle	SC	18d	
	Swine	IM, IV	5d	
Tylosin	Cattle	IM	21d	
	Swine	IM	14d	
Xylazine (Recommended by FARAD)	Cattle	IM	4d	24h
Zeranol	Cattle	Ear implant	0d	
	Sheep	Ear implant	40d	
Zilpaterol	Cattle	in the feed	48h	

Abbreviations: d, day(s); h, hour(s); idw, in drinking water; IM, intramuscular; IMM, intramammary; IR, intraruminal; IV, intravenous; mr, milk replacer; SC, subcutaneous; FARAD, Food Residue Avoidance Databank.
All withdrawal times are determined by the FDA, except those for three drugs that are recommended by the FARAD.

Appendix II
Dosage Table

DISCLAIMER: Dosages listed in this table are based on best available evidence at the time of table preparation; however, the author (W. H. Hsu) cannot ensure the efficacy of drugs used according to recommendations in this table. Adverse effects may be possible from drugs listed, of which author was not aware at the time of table preparation. Veterinarians using this table are encouraged to check current literature, product label, and the manufacturer's disclosure for information regarding efficacy and any known adverse effects or contraindications.

Chapter 2: Drugs Acting on Peripheral Nervous System

Name of drugs	Species	Route	Dose	Notes
Adrenergic agonists				
Catecholamines				
Epinephrine (Epinject®, etc.)	Dog	IV, IM, SC	20 mcg/kg or 0.1–0.5 mL of 1:1,000	
		IV	10–20 mcg/kg	Anaphylaxis
	Cat	IV, IM, SC	20 mcg/kg or 0.1–0.5 mL of 1:1,000	
	Horse	IM, SC	3–5 mL of 1:1,000/450 kg	
	Foal	IV	0.1 mL/kg of 1:1,000	Resuscitation
		IV	10–20 mcg/kg	Cardiopulmonary resuscitation
	Ruminants	SC, IM	0.5–1.0 mL of 1:1,000/45 kg	Anaphylaxis
	Swine	SC, IM	0.5–1.0 mL of 1:1,000/45 kg	Anaphylaxis
Dopamine (Intropin®)	Dog, cat	IV	2–10 mcg/kg/min (prepare 40 mg in 500 mL Lactated Ringer's solution)	
	Horse	IV	1–5 mcg/kg/min (200 mg in 500 mL saline infused at 0.45 mL/kg/h)	
Isoproterenol (Isuprel®)	Dog	IV	0.04–0.08 mcg/kg/min	
		IM, SC	0.1–0.2 mg q4h	
	Cat	IV	0.4 mg in 250 mL saline drip slowly to effect	
		IV	0.2 mg in 100 mL of saline to effect q8h	Asthma
	Horse	IV	0.4 mcg/kg	Short-term bronchodilation
		IV	0.05–1 mcg/kg/min	Resuscitation

(continued)

(*Continued*)

Name of drugs	Species	Route	Dose	Notes
Norepinephrine (Levophed®)	Dog, cat	IV slowly	0.05–0.3 mcg/kg/min, CRI	
	Horse	IM	10 mcg/kg	
Non-catecholamines				
Albuterol (Proventil®, Ventolin®)	Dog	PO	20–50 mcg/kg q8h	
	Cat	Inhalation	90–110 mcg/puff aerosol albuterol inhaler	
	Horse	PO	8 mcg/kg q12h	
		Inhalation	2–3 mcg/kg using a specially designed mask	
Clenbuterol (Ventipulmin®)	Horse	PO	0.8–3.2 mcg/kg q12h	
		IV	0.8 mcg/kg q12h	
Dobutamine (Dobutrex®)	Dog	IV	2.5–20 mcg/kg/min	
	Cat	IV	2.5–5 mcg/kg/min	
	Horse	IV	1–10 mcg/kg/min	
Ephedrine (Broncholate®)	Dog	PO	1–2 mg/kg q8–12h	
	Cat	PO	2–4 mg/kg q8–12h	
	Horse	PO	0.7 mg/kg q12h	
Phenylephrine (Neo-Synephrine®)	Dog	IV	1–3 mcg/kg/min 0.9% NaCl	
	Cat	IV	1–3 mcg/kg/min 0.9% NaCl	
	Horse	IV	0.1–0.2 mcg/kg/min; total dose not over 10 mcg/kg	
Phenylpropanolamine (Propalin®, PPA®)	Dog	PO	1–2 mg/kg q12h	
	Cat	PO	1 mg/kg q12h	
Ractopamine (Optaflexx®, Paylean®)	Cattle	In feed	200 mg/head/d	
	Swine	In feed	5–20 ppm	
Terbutaline (Brethine®)	Dog			
	Small	PO, SC	0.625–1.25 mg/dog q8–12h	
	Medium	PO, SC	1.25–2.5 mg/dog q8–12h	
	Large	PO, SC	2.5–5 mg/dog q8–12h	
	Cat	PO, SC	0.312–0.625 mg/cat q12h	
	Horse	PO, IV or inhalation	0.02–0.06 mg/kg q12h	
Zilpaterol (Zilmax®)	Cattle	In feed	60 mg/head/d	
Adrenergic antagonists ***α-Adrenergic antagonists***				
Atipamezole (Antisedan®)	Dog	IV	35–100 mcg/kg	Reversal of actions of α_2-agonists, e.g., detomidine, medetomidine, xylazine, and amitraz

(*Continued*)

Name of drugs	Species	Route	Dose	Notes
	Cat	IM	50–200 mcg/kg	
		IV	50–150 mcg/kg	
		IM	150–400 mcg/kg	
	Horse	IV	50–100 mcg/kg	
Phenoxybenzamine (Dibenzyline®)	Dog	PO	0.25–0.5 mg/kg q8h	
	Cat	PO	2.5–7.5 mg/cat q12–24h	
	Horse	IV	0.71 mg/kg in 500 mL saline q6–8h	
Phentolamine (Regitine®)	Dog, cat	IV	0.02–0.1 mg/kg	
Prazosin (Minipress®)	Dog	PO	1 mg/15 kg q8–24h	
	Cat	PO	0.25–0.5 mg/cat q12–24h	
		IV	0.03 mg/kg	
Tolazoline (Tolazine®)	Horse, ruminants	IV slowly	2–4 mg/kg	Reversal of actions of α_2-agonists, e.g., detomidine, romifidine, and xylazine
Yohimbine (Yobine®, Antagonil®)	Dog, cat	IV slowly	0.1 mg/kg	Reversal of actions of α_2-agonists, e.g., detomidine, medetomidine, romifidine, xylazine, and amitraz
	Horse	SC, IM	0.25–0.5 mg/kg	
		IV slowly	0.075 mg/kg	
β-Adrenergic antagonists				
Atenolol (Tenormin®)	Dog	PO	0.25–1 mg/kg q12–24h	
	Cat	PO	0.5–3 mg/kg q12–24h	
	Ferret	PO	6.25 mg (total dose) q24h	
Esmolol (Brevibloc®, Miniblock®)	Dog	IV	50–500 mcg/kg bolus q5min	
	Cat	IV slowly	200–500 mcg/kg over 1 min; followed by 25–200 mcg/kg/min	
Propranolol (Inderal®)	Dog	IV	20–60 mcg/kg over 5–10 min q8h	
		PO	0.2–1 mg/kg q8h	
	Cat	PO	0.4–1.2 mg/kg q8–12h	
		IV slowly	20 mcg/kg q8–12h	
	Horse	PO	0.38–0.78 mg/kg q8h	
		IV	0.05–0.16 mg/kg q12h	
	Ferret	PO, SC	0.5–2 mg/kg q12–24h	

(*continued*)

(*Continued*)

Name of drugs	Species	Route	Dose	Notes
Cholinergic agonists				
Bethanechol (Myotonachol®)	Dog	PO	5–25 mg/dog q8h	
	Cat	PO	1.25–7.5 mg/cat q8h	
	Horse	SC	0.025–0.1 mg/kg q6–8h	
		PO	0.3–0.4 mg/kg q6–8h	
	Cattle	IV	0.7 mg/kg	
Pilocarpine (E-Pilo®)	Dog, cat	Topical	1 drop (2%) into eye q8–12h	Glaucoma
Anticholinesterase agents				
Demecarium (Humorsol®)	Dog, cat	Topical	1 drop (0.125 or 0.25%) into eye q12–48h	Glaucoma, miosis
Edrophonium (Tensilon®, Enlon®)	Dog	IV	0.11–0.22 mg/kg	
	Cat	IV	0.1 mg/kg	
Neostigmine (Prostigmin®)	Dog	PO	0.5–1 mg/kg q6–12h	
		IM	0.04–0.05 mg/kg q6h	
	Cat	IM	0.04 mg/kg q6h	
	Horse	SC	0.004–0.02 mg/kg	
	Cattle	SC	0.02 mg/kg	
	Swine	IM	0.03 mg/kg	
	Sheep, goat	SC	0.01–0.02 mg/kg	
Pyridostigmine (Mestinon®)	Dog	PO	0.5–3 mg/kg q8–12h	Antimyasthenic
		IV	0.02–0.04 mg/kg q2h	Antimyasthenic
	Cat	PO	1–3 mg/kg q8–12h	
Echothiophate iodide (Phospholine Iodide®)	Dog, cat	Topical	1 drop (0.03–0.06%) into eye q12–48h	Glaucoma, miosis induction
Cholinergic antagonists				
Aminopentamide (Centrine®)	Dog	IM, SC, PO	0.01–0.03 mg/kg q8–12h	
		SC, IM	0.1–0.4 mg q8–12h	Antiemetic
	Cat	IM, SC	0.02 mg/kg q8–12h	
		SC, IM	0.1–0.4 mg q8–12h	Antiemetic
Atropine (Atroject®, etc.)	Dog, cat	IM, SC	0.022–0.044 mg/kg	
	Horse	IV, IM, SC	0.01–0.1 mg/kg	
	All species	IV, SC, IM	0.2–0.5 mg/kg	Anti-ChE toxicity
	Cattle	IM	0.06–0.12 mg/kg	Preanesthetic
	Swine	IV, IM, SC	0.01–0.1 mg/kg	Preanesthetic
	Sheep, goat	IM	0.15–0.3 mg/kg	Preanesthetic
Glycopyrrolate (Robinul®-V)	Dog	IV, IM	5–10 mcg/kg q8–12h	
		SC	10–20 mcg/kg	
	Cat	IV, IM	5–10 mcg/kg	
		SC	10–20 mcg/kg	
	Horse	IV	5–10 mcg/kg	

Name of drugs	Species	Route	Dose	Notes
Propantheline (Pro-Banthine®)	Dog	PO	0.25–0.5 mg/kg q8–12h	
	Cat	PO	0.25–0.5 mg/kg q12–24h	
	Horse	IV	0.04 mg/kg	
Scopolamine (Hyoscine®)	Dog, cat	IM, SC	0.03 mg/kg q6h	Antiemetic
Tropicamide (Mydriacyl®)	Dog, cat	Topical	1 drop (0.5–1%) into each eye; repeat in 5 min	Mydriatic, ophthalmic examination

Neuromuscular blocking drugs

Name of drugs	Species	Route	Dose	Notes
Atracurium (Tracrium®, Sitrac®)	Dog	IV	0.22–0.5 mg/kg, then 0.1–0.25 mg/kg	
	Cat	IV	0.22 mg/kg	
		IV	0.11 mg/kg	Intraoperative dose
	Horse	IV	0.055 mg/kg	Intraoperative dose
Pancuronium (Pavulon®)	Dog, cat	IV	0.044–0.11 mg/kg	
	Swine	IV	0.11 mg/kg	
	Horse	IV	0.04–0.066 mg/kg	
Succinylcholine (Anectine®, etc.)	Dog	IV	0.07–0.22 mg/kg	
	Cat	IV	0.06–0.11 mg/kg	
	Horse	IV, IM	0.088–0.11 mg/kg	
Vecuronium (Norcuron®)	Dog	IV	10–20 mcg/kg	
	Cat	IV	20–40 mcg/kg	

Chapter 3: Autacoids and Their Antagonists

Name of drugs	Species	Route	Dose	Notes
H₁ antihistamines				
Cetirizine (Zyrtec®)	Dog	PO	5–10 mg	
	Cat	PO	1 mg/kg	
Dimenhydrinate (Dramamine®)	Dog	IV, IM, PO	4–8 mg/kg q8h	
	Cat	IV, IM, PO	12.5 mg/cat q8h	
Diphenhydramine (Benadryl®)	Dog	IV, IM, SC, PO	2–5 mg/kg q6–8h	
	Cat	IM, SC, PO	2–5 mg/kg q6–8h	
	Horse	IV, IM	0.25–1 mg/kg	
	Cattle	IM, IV	0.5–1 mg/kg	
Fexofenadine (Allegra®)	Dog	PO	2–5 mg/kg q24h	
Hydroxyzine (Atarax®, Vistaril®)	Dog	PO	0.5–2.2 mg/kg q6–8h	
	Cat	PO	5–10 mg (total dose)	
	Horse	PO, IM	0.5–1 mg/kg q12h	
Loratadine (Claritin®)	Dog			
	Small	PO	5 mg q12h	
	Medium	PO	10 mg q24h	
	Large	PO	10 mg q12h	

(continued)

Name of drugs	Species	Route	Dose	Notes
Meclizine (Antivert®, etc.)	Dog	PO	<10 kg: 12.5 mg q24h	
		PO	≥10 kg: 25 mg q24h	
	Cat	PO	4 mg/kg q24h	
Pyrilamine (Histall®, etc.)	Dog	PO	12.5–25 mg q6h	
		IM	25–125 mg	
	Horse	IV, IM, SC	1 mg/kg	
	Cattle	IM	0.5–1.5 g	
	Sheep	IM	0.25–0.5 g	
	Swine	IM	0.25–0.5 g	
Tripelennamine (Azaron®, Etono®)	Dog, cat	PO, IM	1 mg/kg q12h	
	Horse	IV, IM	1 mg/kg	
	Cattle	IV, IM	1 mg/kg	
	Swine	IV, IM	1 mg/kg	
H_2 antihistamines				
Cimetidine (Tagamet®)	Dog, cat	IV, IM, SC, PO	5–15 mg/kg q6–12h	
		IV, PO	2.5–5 mg/kg q12h	Renal failure patients
	Horse	IV	6.6 mg/kg q4–6h	
		PO	8–10 mg/kg q8h	
	Cattle	PO	8–16 mg/kg q8h	
	Swine	In feed	300 mg/swine q12h	
Famotidine (Pepcid®)	Dog, cat	IV, SC, PO	0.5–1.1 mg/kg q12–24h	
	Horse	PO	3.3 mg/kg q8h	
		IV	0.35 mg/kg q12h	
Nizatidine (Axid®)	Dog, cat	PO	2.5–5 mg/kg q24h	
	Horse	PO	6.6 mg/kg q8h	
Ranitidine (Zantac®)	Dog	IV, PO	2–4 mg/kg q8–12h	
	Cat	IV	2.5 mg/kg q12h	
		PO	3.5 mg/kg q12h	
	Horse	PO	6.6 mg/kg q8h	
		IV, IM	1.5–2 mg/kg q6–8h	
Histamine release inhibitors				
Cromolyn sodium (Cromolom®, etc.)	Dog, cat	Topical	1 drop (4%) q4–6h	
	Horse	Inhalation	80–300 mg	
5-HT agonists and antagonists				
Cisapride	Dog	PO	0.1–0.5 mg/kg q8–12h	
	Cat	PO	2.5–5 mg q8–12h	
	Horse	IM	0.1 mg/kg	
		PO	0.5–0.8 mg/kg for 7d	
Cyproheptadine (Periactin®)	Dog	PO	0.3–2 mg/kg q12h	
	Cat	PO	1–4 mg/cat q12–24h	
	Horse	PO	0.5 mg/kg q12h	
Metoclopramide (Reglan®, Clopra®)	Dog, cat	IM, SC, PO	0.2–0.4 mg/kg q6–8h	
		IV	1–2 mg/kg/d, CRI	
		IV	0.02 mg/kg/h, CRI	
	Horse	IV	0.1–0.25 mg/kg/h, CRI	
		PO	0.6 mg/kg q4h	

Chapter 4: Drugs Acting on the Central Nervous System

Name of drugs	Species	Route	Dose	Notes
Anticonvulsants				
Barbiturates				
Pentobarbital (Nembutal®, etc.)	Dog, cat	IV	25–30 mg/kg	General anesthesia
		IV	5–15 mg/kg to effect	Status epilepticus
		IV	1–4 mg/kg	Sedative
	Horse	IV	2–20 mg/kg	
Phenobarbital (Solfoton®, etc.)	Dog	IV slowly	10–20 mg/kg	Status epilepticus
		IV, IM, PO	2.2–5 mg/kg q12h	Seizure disorders
		PO	2–8 mg/kg q12h	Sedative
	Cat	IV slowly	10–20 mg/kg	Status epilepticus
		PO	1–2 mg/kg q12h	
	Horse	IV slowly	5–25 mg/kg in 30 mL saline	
	Cattle	PO	5 g for 3–4 wk, off 3–4 wk, then repeat for 3–4 more wk	Hydrocarbon insecticide toxicity
Primidone (Neurosyn®, etc.)	Dog	PO	8–22 mg/kg q8–12h	
	Cat	PO	11–22 mg/kg q8h	
	Horse	PO	1–2 g/foal q6–12h	
Benzodiazepines				
Clonazepam (Klonopin®, Clonax®)	Dog	PO	0.5–1.5 mg/kg q8–12h	
		IV	0.05–0.2 mg/kg	Injectable not available in United States
		PO	0.05–0.25 mg/kg q12–24h	Anxiolytic
	Cat	PO	0.5–1.5 mg/kg q8–12h	
		PO	0.05–0.2 mg/kg q12–24h	Anxiolytic
Diazepam (Valium®, Diastat®)	Dog	IV slowly	0.3–0.5 mg/kg; repeat prn	Status epilepticus
			0.6–0.8 mg/kg rectally	Status epilepticus
		PO	1–2 mg/kg q8h	Anticonvulsant
		IV slowly	0.1–0.5 mg/kg	Preanesthetic
		PO	0.25 mg/kg q12h	Urethral hyperreflexia
	Cat	IV	0.05–0.15 mg/kg (maximum 5 mg) prn	Appetite stimulant
		PO	1–2 mg q12–24h	Appetite stimulant
		PO	1.25–7.5 mg q12–24h	Urethral hyperreflexia

(continued)

(Continued)

Name of drugs	Species	Route	Dose	Notes
	Horse	IV slowly	0.03–0.5 mg/kg; repeat in 30 min prn	
	Cattle, sheep, goat	IV slowly	0.02–0.08 mg/kg	
Midazolam (Versed®, Zolamid®)	Dog, cat	IV, IM	0.1–0.25 mg/kg	Status epilepticus
		IV	0.1–0.3 mg/kg/h, CRI	
	Horse	IV, IM	0.05–0.2 mg/kg	
Miscellaneous anticonvulsants				
Gabapentin (Neurontin®)	Dog, cat	PO	10–30 mg/kg q8h	
Levetiracetam (Keppra®)	Dog	PO	7–24 mg/kg q8h	
Felbamate (Felbatol®)	Dog	PO	15–65 mg/kg q8h	
Zonisamide (Zonegran®)	Dog	PO	5–10 mg/kg q12h	
Phenytoin (Phenytek®)	Dog	PO	20–35 mg/kg q8h	
		IV	10 mg/kg	Antiarrhythmic
	Cat	PO	2–3 mg/kg q24h	
	Horse	IV	5–10 mg/kg	Convulsing foals
		IV, IM, PO	1–5 mg/kg for maintenance 4h	
		PO	10–22 mg/kg q12h	Digoxin-induced arrhythmias
Potassium bromide	Dog, cat	PO	15–30 mg/kg q12h	
Sodium bromide	Dog	PO	20–60 mg/kg q24h	
Valproic acid (Depakene®)	Dog	PO	60–200 mg/kg q8h	
	Cat	PO	60 mg/kg q8h	
Benzodiazepine antagonist				
Flumazenil (Romazicon®)	Dog, cat	IV	10–20 mcg/kg	
CNS stimulants				
Doxapram (Dopram-V®)	Dog	IV	5–10 mg/kg	
		SC, IV	1–5 mg	Neonates
	Cat	IV	5–10 mg/kg	
		SC, IV	1–5 mg	Neonates
	Horse	IV	0.5–1 mg/kg at 5 min intervals	Not over 2 mg/kg in foals
	Cattle	IV	5–10 mg/kg	
	Swine	IV	5–10 mg/kg	
Phenothiazine derivatives				
Acepromazine (Aceproject®, PromAce®)	Dog	IV	0.025–0.2 mg/kg; maximum 3–4 mg	Restraint, sedative
		IM, SC	0.1–0.25 mg/kg; maximum 3–4 mg	Restraint, sedative
		PO	0.55–2.2 mg/kg q8h	Restraint, sedative
	Cat	IV	0.05–0.10 mg/kg; maximum 1 mg	
		PO	1.1–2.2 mg/kg q8h	
	Horse	IM	0.03–0.066 mg/kg	

(*Continued*)

Name of drugs	Species	Route	Dose	Notes
		IV	0.033–0.055 mg/kg followed by 0.055–0.066 mg/kg butorphanol	
		IV	0.04 mg/kg followed by 0.6 mg/kg meperidine	
	Cattle	IV	0.01–0.02 mg/kg	
		IM	0.03–0.1 mg/kg	
	Swine	IV, IM, SC	0.1–0.2 mg/kg	
	Sheep, goat	IM	0.05–0.1 mg/kg	
Chlorpromazine (Thorazine®)	Dog	IM, SC	0.5 mg/kg q6–8h	
	Cat	IM, SC	0.5 mg/kg q6–8h	
	Cattle	IV	0.22–1.0 mg/kg	
		IM	1.0–4.4 mg/kg	
	Swine	IV	0.55–3.3 mg/kg	
		IM	2–4 mg/kg	
	Sheep, goat	IV	0.55–4.4 mg/kg	
		IM	2.2–6.6 mg/kg	
Prochlorperazine (Compazine®, etc.)	Dog	IM	0.25–0.5 mg/kg q8–12h	
		PO	1 mg/kg q12h	
	Cat	IM	0.13 mg/kg q12h	
		PO	0.5 mg/kg q12h	
Promethazine (Phenergan®)	Dog, cat	IV, IM, PO	0.2–0.4 mg/kg q6–8h (maximum 1 mg/kg)	
Trimeprazine (Panectyl®)	Dog, cat	PO	0.5–2 mg/kg q12h	
α_2-*Adrenergic agonists*				
Detomidine (Dormosedan®)	Horse	IV, IM	20–40 mcg/kg	
	Cattle	IV, IM	30–60 mcg/kg	
Medetomidine (Domitor®)	Dog	IV	7–20 mcg/kg	
		IM, SC	10–40 mcg/kg	
	Cat	IV	10–30 mcg/kg	
		IM, SC	30–80 mcg	
Romifidine (Sedivet®)	Horse	IV	40–120 mcg/kg	
Xylazine (Rompun®, etc.)	Dog	IV	1.1 mg/kg	Sedative
		IM, SC	1.1–2.2 mg/kg	Sedative
		IM	0.1–1 mg/kg	Emetic
	Cat	IM	1.1 mg/kg	Sedative
		IM, IV	0.44 mg/kg	Emetic
		IV	0.05–0.1 mg prn	Analgesic
	Horse	IV	0.2–1.1 mg/kg	
		IM	2.2 mg/kg	
	Cattle	IV	0.05–0.15 mg/kg	
		IM	0.10–0.33 mg/kg	
Opioids				
Opioid agonists				
Alfentanil (Alfenta®, Rapifen®)				
	Dog	IV	2–5 mcg/kg	Analgesic, preanesthetic

Name of drugs	Species	Route	Dose	Notes
Fentanyl (Sublimaze®)	Dog	IV, IM, SC	20–40 mcg/kg q2h	Analgesic
		IV, IM, SC	10 mcg/kg (with acepromazine or diazepam)	Preanesthetic
	Cat	IV	2–5 mcg/kg/h	Analgesic
	Horse	IV	10 mcg/kg	Analgesic
	Small ruminants	IV	5–10 mcg/kg	Analgesic
Hydromorphone (Dilaudid-HP®, etc.)	Dog	IV, IM, SC	0.1–0.2 mg/kg prn	
	Cat	IV, IM	0.02–0.1 mg/kg q6–8h	
		IV	0.01–0.03 mg/kg/h, CRI	
Methadone (Dolophine®, etc.)	Dog	IV	0.1 mg/kg prn	
		IM	0.11–0.55 mg/kg prn	
	Cat	IV, IM	0.1–0.5 mg/kg q4–5h	
Morphine	Dog	IV, IM, SC	0.05–0.1 mg/kg q2–3 min or prn	Analgesic, sedative
		IV	0.1–0.5 mg/kg/h, CRI	Analgesic, sedative
		IM, SC	0.2–0.6 mg/kg q4h	Orthopedic pain
		IM, SC	0.1–0.25 mg/kg q4–6h	Pulmonary edema
	Cat	IV, IM, SC	0.1–0.5 mg/kg q3–4h	Analgesic, sedative
		IM, SC	0.1–0.2 mg/kg q4h	Orthopedic pain
		IM, SC	0.05–0.1 mg/kg q6–8h	Pulmonary edema
	Horse	IV, IM	0.2–0.6 mg/kg	
	Swine	IM	0.2–0.9 mg/kg	
	Sheep, goat	IM	Up to 10 mg total dose	
Oxymorphone (Numorphan®)	Dog	IV, IM	0.02–0.1 mg/kg (maximum 3 mg) prn	Sedative
		IM, SC	0.025–0.05 mg/kg	Preanesthetic
		IV, IM, SC	0.1–0.2 mg/kg q2–6h (60 mg maximum dose)	Analgesic
	Cat	IV, IM, SC	0.02–0.1 mg/kg q2–6h	Analgesic
	Horse	IM	0.02–0.03 mg/kg	
Sufentanil (Sufenta®)	Dog, cat	IV	2–5 mcg/kg titrated to effect	
Tramadol (Ultram®)	Dog	PO	1–4 mg/kg q8–12h	
	Cat	PO	4 mg/kg q12h	
Opioid partial agonists				
Butorphanol (Torbutrol®, etc.)	Dog	PO	0.5–1.1 mg/kg q6–12h	Antitussive
		IV	0.1–0.2 mg/kg	Analgesic
		IM, SC	0.1–0.4 mg/kg	Analgesic
		IV, IM, SC	0.2–0.6 mg/kg	Antiemetic

Name of drugs	Species	Route	Dose	Notes
	Cat	IV	0.05–0.2 mg/kg	Analgesic
		IM, SC	0.1–0.3 mg/kg	Analgesic
	Horse	IV, IM	0.01–0.1 mg/kg	Analgesic
	Cattle	IV	20–30 mg	Preanesthetic
Opioid agonist–antagonist drugs				
Buprenorphine (Buprenex®)	Dog	IV, IM, SC	5–30 mcg/kg q4–8h	Analgesic
	Cat	IV, IM, SC	5–10 mcg/kg q4–8h	Analgesic
	Horse	IV	4–6 mcg/kg	Analgesic
Nalbuphine (Nubain®)	Dog	IV, IM, SC	0.5–2 mg/kg q1–6h prn	Analgesic
	Cat	IV, IM, SC	0.5–1.5 mg/kg	Analgesic
Opioid antagonists				
Naloxone (Narcan®)	Dog	IV, IM, SC	0.04 mg/kg prn	
	Cat	IV, IM, SC	0.05–0.1 mg/kg prn	
	Horse	IV	0.01–0.02 mg/kg	
Naltrexone (ReVia®)	Dog	PO	1–4 mg/kg q12–24h	
	Cat	PO	25–50 mg/cat q24h	

Chapter 5: Behavior Modifying Drugs

Name of drugs	Species	Route	Dose	Notes
Anxiolytics				
Alprazolam (Xanax®)	Dog	PO	0.05–0.1 mg/kg q12h or prn	
	Cat	PO	0.125–0.25 mg/kg q12h	
Chlordiazepoxide (Librium®, Mitran®)	Dog	PO	2.5–5 mg q12–24h	
	Cat	PO	0.5–1 mg/kg q12–24h	
Clorazepate (Tranxene®), Gen-Xene®)	Dog	PO	0.5–1 mg/kg q8h	Epilepsy, refractory
	Cat	PO	0.2–0.5 mg/kg q12–24h	Anxiety, compulsive behaviors
Diazepam (Valium®)	Dog	IV slowly	0.3–0.5 mg/kg; repeat prn	Status epilepticus
			0.6–0.8 mg/kg rectally	Status epilepticus
		PO	1–2 mg/kg q8h	Anticonvulsant
		IV slowly	0.1–0.5 mg/kg	Preanesthetic
		PO	0.25 mg/kg q12h	Urethral hyperreflexia
	Cat	IV	0.05–0.15 mg/kg (maximum 5 mg) prn	Appetite stimulant
		PO	1–2 mg q12–24h	Appetite stimulant
		PO	1.25–7.5 mg q12–24h	Urethral hyperreflexia
	Horse	IV slowly	0.03–0.5 mg/kg; repeat in 30 min prn	Sedative

(continued)

(*Continued*)

Name of drugs	Species	Route	Dose	Notes
	Cattle	IV slowly	0.02–0.08 mg/kg	Sedative
	Sheep, goat	IV slowly	0.02–0.08 mg/kg	Sedative
Lorazepam (Ativan®)	Dog, cat	PO	0.05–0.1 mg/kg	
Oxazepam (Serax®)	Dog	PO	0.2–1 mg/kg q12–24h	
	Cat	PO	0.2–0.5 mg/kg q12–24h	
Antidepressants				
Tricyclic antidepressants				
Amitriptyline (Elavil®)	Dog	PO	2.2–4.4 mg/kg q12–24h	
	Cat	PO	0.5–2.2 mg/kg q12–24h	
Clomipramine (Clomicalm®)	Dog	PO	1–3 mg/kg q12–24h (not over 200 mg/d)	
	Cat	PO	0.5 mg/kg q24h	
Doxepin (Sinequan®)	Dog	PO	1–5 mg/kg q12h (maximum 150 mg q12h)	
	Cat	PO	0.5–1 mg/kg q12–24h. Up to 25–50 mg/cat	
Imipramine (Tofranil®, etc.)	Dog	PO	2.2–4.4 mg/kg q12–24h	
		PO	5–20 mg q12h	Urinary incontinence
	Cat	PO	2.5–5 mg q12h	
	Horse	PO	100–600 mg q12h for 2 wk	Improves ejaculation
		IM, IV	0.55 mg/kg q8h	
		PO	1.5 mg/kg q8h	
Selective serotonin reuptake inhibitors				
Fluvoxamine (Luvox®, Fevarin®)	Dog	PO	0.5–2 mg/kg q12h	
	Cat	PO	0.25–0.5 mg/kg q24h	
Fluoxetine (Reconcile®, etc.)	Dog	PO	1 mg/kg q12–24h	
	Cat	PO	0.5–1 mg/kg q24h	
Paroxetine (Paxil®)	Dog	PO	1–2 mg/kg q12–24h	
	Cat	PO	0.5–1 mg/kg q12–24h	
Sertraline (Zoloft®, Serlain®)	Dog	PO	1–4 mg/kg q12–24h for ≥ 8 wk	
	Cat	PO	0.5–1 mg/kg q12–24h	
Monoamine oxidase inhibitors				
Selegiline (Anipryl®)	Dog	PO	0.5–1 mg/kg q24h	
Novel antidepressants				
Buspirone (BuSpar®)	Dog, cat	PO	0.5–1 mg/kg q8–12h	
Hormones (Progestins)				
Medroxyprogesterone acetate (Provera®, Amen®)	Dog	IM, SC	10 mg/kg	One dose lasts 30d
	Cat	SC	10–20 mg/kg	

Name of drugs	Species	Route	Dose	Notes
Megestrol acetate (Ovaban®)	Dog	PO	1.1–4.4 mg/kg q24h for 2 wk, then 0.5–1.1 mg/kg q24h for 2 wk	
	Cat	PO	2 mg/kg/d for 5d, then 1 mg/kg/d for 5d, then 0.5 mg/kg/d for 5d	

Chapter 6: Anesthetics

Name of drugs	Species	Route	Dose	Notes
Inhalant anesthetics				
Desflurane (Suprane®)	Dog	Inhalation	MAC 7.2%	
	Cat	Inhalation	MAC 9.79%	
Isoflurane (Aerrane®, etc.)	Dog, cat	Inhalation	5% for induction	
		Inhalation	1.5–2.5% for maintenance	
Sevoflurane (SevoFlo®, Ultane®)	Dog	Inhalation	MAC 2.36%	
	Cat	Inhalation	MAC 2.58%	
Injectable anesthetics				
Ultrashort-acting barbiturates				
Methohexital (Brevital®)	Dog, cat	IV	11 mg/kg, 1/2 the dose rapidly and then titrate to effect	
		IV	5.5–6.6 mg/kg, 10–30% is given rapidly IV and then the remainder titrated to effect	If preanesthetic was used
Thiopental (Pentothal®)	Dog	IV	10–26 mg/kg	
	Cat	IV	5–10 mg/kg	
	Horse	IV	6–12 mg/kg	
	Cattle	IV	8–15 mg/kg	
	Swine	IV	5.5–11 mg/kg	
	Sheep	IV	10–15 mg/kg	
	Goat	IV	20–22 mg/kg	
Short-acting barbiturates				
Pentobarbital (Nembutal®, etc.)	Dog, cat	IV	25–30 mg/kg (to effect)	
	Cattle	IV	30 mg/kg (to effect)	
	Swine	IV	30 mg/kg (to effect)	
	Sheep, goat	IV	20–30 mg/kg (to effect)	
Cyclohexylamines				
Ketamine (Ketaset®, Vetalar®, etc.)	Dog	IV	10 mg/kg (+ Diazepam 0.5 mg/kg)	
	Cat	IM	22–44 mg/kg	
		IV	2.2–4.4 mg/kg (with atropine)	

(continued)

(*Continued*)

Name of drugs	Species	Route	Dose	Notes
	Cattle	IV	2 mg/kg, premedicate with atropine and xylazine	
	Horse	IV	2 mg/kg, premedicate with xylazine (1 mg/kg IV or 2 mg/kg IM)	
	Swine	IM	11–22 mg/kg premedicate with atropine and acepromazine	
	Sheep	IM	22 mg/kg, premedicate with atropine (0.22 mg/kg) and acepromazine (0.55 mg/kg)	
	Goat	IM	11 mg/kg, premedicated with atropine 0.4 mg/kg, followed by xylazine 0.22 mg/kg	
Tiletamine + Zolazepam (Telazol®)	Dog, cat	IM, SC IV	3–10 mg/kg 2–5 mg/kg	
	Horse	IV	1.65–2.2 mg/kg premedicated with xylazine (1.1 mg/kg IV)	
Miscellaneous injectable anesthetics				
Propofol (Rapinovet®, PropoFlo®)	Dog, cat	IV IV	6–8 mg/kg to effect 0.51–0.81 mg/kg/min CRI for maintenance	
Etomidate (Amidate®)	Dog, cat	IV IV	0.5–3 mg/kg 0.5–1 mg/kg when given with opioids	
Central muscle relaxants				
Guaifenesin (Guailaxin®)	Dog	IV	44–88 mg/kg	
	Horse	IV	55–110 mg/kg	
	Cattle	IV	55–110 mg/kg	
	Swine	IV	44–88 mg/kg	
	Goat	IV	66–132 mg/kg	
	Dog	PO	15–20 mg/kg, q8h	Intervertebral disk disease
Methocarbamol (Robaxin®V)	Dog, cat	PO	Initially, 132 mg/kg/d, divided q8h–q12h, then 61–132 mg/kg, divided q8h–q12h. If no response in 5 d, discontinue	Moderate conditions
		IV	50–220 mg/kg	Strychnine, pyrethroid toxicosis, tetanus; repeat 1/2 dose prn

Name of drugs	Species	Route	Dose	Notes
	Horse	PO	30–75 mg/kg	
		IV slowly	15–25 mg/kg, may repeat up to 4 times/d if needed	
	Cattle	IV	110 mg/kg	CNS hyperactivity

Chapter 7: Nonsteroidal Anti-inflammatory Drugs (NSAIDs)

Name of drugs	Species	Route	Dose	Notes
Nonselective cap inhibitors				
Aspirin	Dog	PO	10–25 mg/kg q8–12h	Analgesic
		PO	20–40 mg/kg q12h	Anti-inflammatory
		PO	5–10 mg/kg q24–48h	Antiplatelet
	Cat	PO	10 mg/kg q48h	Analgesic
		PO	10–20 mg/kg q48h	Anti-inflammatory
	Horse	PO	10–100 mg/kg q12h	
	Cattle	PO	50–100 mg/kg q12h	
	Swine	PO	10 mg/kg q4–6h	
Carprofen (Rimadyl®)	Dog	PO	4.4 mg/kg q24h	Osteoarthritis
		IV, SC, PO	2.2 mg/kg q12h	
	Cat	SC	4 mg/kg q24h	Osteoarthritis
		IV, SC	1–2 mg/kg q12h	Analgesic
	Horse	IV	0.7 mg/kg q24h	
Etodolac (EtoGesic®, Lodine®)	Dog	PO	10–15 mg/kg q24h	
	Horse	PO, IV	10–15 mg/kg q24h	
Flunixin meglumine (Banamine®, etc.)	Dog	IV	0.5–1 mg/kg q12h	
		IV, IM	0.5–1 mg/kg q24h for 1–3d	Analgesic
	Cat	SC	0.25 mg/kg q24h	Analgesic
	Horse	PO, IM, IV	0.25–1.1 mg/kg q8–24h	
	Cattle	IV slowly	1.1–2.2 mg/kg	
Ketoprofen (Ketofen®, Oruvail®)	Dog	IV, IM, SC, PO	1.1–2 mg/kg q24h for 5d	
	Cat		1–2 mg/kg SC q24h for 3d	
	Horse	IV, IM	2.2 mg/kg	
Meclofenamic acid (Meclomen®)	Dog	PO	1.1–2.2 mg/kg q24h for 5–7d	
	Horse	PO	2.2 mg/kg q12h for 5–7d	
Meloxicam (Metacam®)	Dog	PO, SC, IV	0.2 mg/kg once; then 0.1 mg/kg q24h	
	Cat	PO, SC, IV	0.2 mg/kg once; then 0.1 mg/kg q24h × 3d; then 0.05 mg/kg × 10d; then 0.025 mg/kg q24–48h	

(*continued*)

Name of drugs	Species	Route	Dose	Notes
Naproxen (Naprosyn®)	Horse	PO, IV	10 mg/kg q12–24h	
Phenylbutazone	Dog	IV	10–15 mg/kg q12h; not over 4 doses	
		PO	10–22 mg/kg q8h; maximum 800 mg/d	
	Horse	PO, IV	2–4.4 mg/kg q12h	
	Cattle	PO	4–8 mg/kg	
		IV	2–5 mg/kg	
	Swine	PO	4–8 mg/kg	
		IV	2–5 mg/kg	
Cap-2 selective inhibitors				
Deracoxib (Deramaxx®)	Dog	PO	3–4 mg/kg q24h for less than 7d	
		PO	1–2 mg/kg q24h	Chronic use
Firocoxib (Previcox®)	Dog	PO	5 mg/kg q24h	
Dual inhibitors				
Tepoxalin (Zubrin®)	Dog	PO	20 mg/kg q24h for 1 time; then 10 mg/kg q24h	
Miscellaneous anti-inflammatory drugs				
Dimethyl sulfoxide (Domoso®)	Dog	PO	125–300 mg/kg (10% soln) q24h	
		SC	80 mg/kg 3 times/wk	
		IV	1 g/kg of 10% soln over 45 min q6–8h	CNS trauma
		IV slowly	1.1 g/kg q12h, diluted 1:4 in 0.9% saline	Shock therapy
	Cat	IV slowly	550 mg/kg q12h, diluted 1:4 in 0.9% saline	Shock therapy
	Horse	IV	0.1–1 g/kg (diluted in 5% dextrose); q8–12h	
Hyaluronate sodium (Legend®, Hycoat®)	Dog	IV	20 mg/kg prn	
	Horse	Topical	20–120 mg around inflamed tendon	
		Intraarticular	20–50 mg	
Glycosaminoglycan (Glyco-Flex®)	Dog, cat	IM	1.1–4.8 mg/kg q 4d	
	Horse	IM	500 mg q4d	

Chapter 8: Drugs Acting on the Cardiovascular System

Name of drugs	Species	Route	Dose	Notes
Drugs for chronic CHF management **Diuretics**				
Chlorothiazide (Diuril®)	Dog, cat	PO	20–40 mg/kg q12h	
Furosemide (Lasix®, etc.)	Dog	PO	1–3 mg/kg q8–24h; use smallest effective dose	
	Cat	PO	1–2 mg/kg q8–12h; use smallest effective dose	

(Continued)

Name of drugs	Species	Route	Dose	Notes
Hydrochlorothiazide (Oretic®, Ezide®)	Dog Cat	PO PO	2–4 mg/kg q12h 1–2 mg/kg q12h	
Spironolactone (Aldactone®)	Dog, cat	PO	0.5–1 mg/kg q12–24h	
ACE inhibitors				
Benazepril (Lotensin®)	Dog, cat	PO	0.25–0.5 mg/kg q12–24h	
Captopril (Capoten®)	Dog	PO	0.5–2.0 mg/kg q8–12h (low initial dose)	
	Cat	PO	0.5–1.25 mg/kg q12–24h	
Enalapril (Enacard®)	Dog Cat	PO PO	0.5 mg/kg q12–24h 0.25–0.5 mg/kg q12–24h	
Fosinopril (Monopril®)	Dog	PO	0.25–0.5 mg/kg q24h	
Imidapril (Tanatril®)	Dog	PO	0.25 mg/kg q24h	
Lisinopril (Prinivil®, etc.)	Dog	PO	0.25–0.5 mg/kg q12–24h	
	Cat	PO	0.25–0.5 mg/kg q24h	
Ramipril (Altace®)	Dog	PO	0.125–0.25 mg/kg q24h	
Other vasodilators				
Amlodipine (Norvasc®)	Dog	PO	0.05 (initial) to 0.3 (−0.5) mg/kg q12–24h	
	Cat	PO	0.3125–0.625 mg/cat q12–24h	
Hydralazine (Apresoline®)	Dog	PO	0.5–2 mg/kg q12h (to 1 mg/kg initial)	
	Cat	PO	2.5 (up to 10) mg/cat q12h	
Isosorbide dinitrate (Isorbid®, etc.)	Dog	PO	0.5–2 mg/kg q8–12h	
Isosorbide mononitrate (Monoket®)	Dog	PO	0.25–2 mg/kg q12h	
Nitroglycerin (2%) (Nitrol®)	Dog	Topical	0.5–4 cm cutaneously q4–6h	
	Cat	Topical	0.5–1 cm cutaneously q4–6h	
Positive inotropic agents				
Digoxin (Cardoxin®, Lanoxin®, etc.)	Dog <22 kg	PO	5–8 mcg/kg q12h; Decrease by 10% for elixir. Maximum: 0.5 mg/d or 0.375 mg/d for Doberman Pinchers	
	Dog ≥22 kg	PO	3–5 mcg/kg q12h. Decrease by 10% for elixir. Maximum: 0.5 mg/d or 0.375 mg/d for Doberman Pinchers	
	Cat	PO	7 mcg/kg q48h	

(continued)

(*Continued*)

Name of drugs	Species	Route	Dose	Notes
Pimobendan (Vetmedin®, Acardi®)	Dog	PO	0.1–0.3 mg/kg q12h, start low; give at least 1h before feeding	
	Cat	PO	1.25 mg/cat q12h	
Drugs for diastolic dysfunction				
Atenolol (Tenormin®)	Dog	PO	0.2–1 mg/kg q12–24h	
	Cat	PO	6.25–12.5 mg/cat q12–24h	
Diltiazem (Cardizem®, Tiazac®)	Dog	PO	0.5–2 mg/kg q8h	
	Cat	PO	1.5–2.5 mg/kg q8h; sustained release: diltiazem (Dilacor), 30 mg/cat q12–24h; or Cardizem, 10 mg/kg q24h	
Antiarrhythmic drugs				
Class I antiarrhythmics				
Flecainide (Tambocor®)	Dog	PO	1–5 mg/kg q8–12h	
Lidocaine	Dog	IV	Initial boluses of 2 mg/kg slowly, up to 8 mg/kg; or rapid infusion at 0.8 mg/kg/min; if effective, then 25–80 mcg/kg/min CRI	
	Cat	IV	initial bolus of 0.25–0.5 (or 1.0) mg/kg slowly; can repeat boluses of 0.15–0.25 mg/kg, up to total of 4 mg/kg; if effective, 10–40 mcg/kg/min CRI	
Mexiletine (Mexitil®)	Dog	PO	4–10 mg/kg q8h	
Phenytoin (Phenytek®)	Dog	IV slowly	10 mg/kg	
		PO	30–50 mg/kg q8h	
	Cat		Do not use	
Procainamide (Procanbid®, etc.)	Dog	IV	6–10 (up to 20) mg/kg over 5–10 min; 10–50 mcg/kg/min CRI	
		IM	6–20 (up to 30) mg/kg q4–6h	
		PO	10–25 mg/kg q6–8h	
	Cat	IV slowly	1–2 mg/kg or 10–20 mcg/kg/min CRI	
		IM, PO	7.5–20 mg/kg q6–8h	
Propafenone (Rythmol SR®)	Dog	PO	3–4 mg/kg q8h	
Quinidine	Dog	IM	6–20 mg/kg q6h (loading dose, 14–20 mg/kg)	

Name of drugs	Species	Route	Dose	Notes
		PO	6–16 mg/kg q6h; sustained action preparations: 8–20 mg/kg q8h	
	Cat	IM, PO	6–16 mg/kg q8h	
Class II antiarrhythmics				
Atenolol (Tenormin®)	Dog	PO	0.2–1.0 mg/kg q12–24h	
	Cat	PO	6.25–12.5 mg/cat q12–24h	
Carvedilol (Coreg®)	Dog	IV slowly	0.05–0.1 mg/kg q24h, up to 0.2–0.3 mg/kg q12h or as tolerated	
Esmolol (Brevibloc®)	Dog, cat	IV	0.1–0.5 mg/kg over 1 min (loading dose), followed by infusion of 0.025–0.2 mg/kg/min	
Metoprolol (Lopressor®)	Dog	PO	initial dose, 0.1–0.2 mg/kg q8–12h, up to 1 mg/kg q8–12h; or as tolerated	
Propranolol (Inderal®)	Dog	IV slowly	0.02 mg/kg (up to maximum of 0.1 mg/kg)	
		PO	0.1–0.2 mg/kg q8h, up to 1 mg/kg q8h	
	Cat	IV slowly	0.02 mg/kg (up to maximum of 0.1 mg/kg)	
		PO	2.5–10 mg/cat q8–12h	
Class III antiarrhythmics				
Amiodarone (Cordarone®, Pacerone®)	Dog	IV slowly	3–5 mg/kg slowly (over 10–20 min), can repeat but do not over 10 mg/kg/h	
		PO	10 mg/kg q12h for 7d, then 8 mg/kg q24h	
Sotalol (Betapace®)	Dog	PO	1–3.5 (–5) mg/kg q12h	
	Cat	PO	2–4 mg/kg q12h	
Class IV antiarrhythmics				
Diltiazem (Cardizem®)	Dog, cat	PO	0.5 mg/kg (up to 2+ mg/kg) q8h or loading dose: 0.5 mg/kg followed by 0.25 mg/kg q1h to a total of 1.5 (–2.0) mg/kg or conversion	

(continued)

Name of drugs	Species	Route	Dose	Notes
		IV	0.15–0.25 mg/kg over 2–3 min, can repeat every 15 min until conversion or maximum 0.75 mg/kg; CRI: 5–15 mg/kg/h	Supraventricular tachycardia
Verapamil (Calan®, Verelan®)	Dog	PO	0.5–2 mg/kg q8h	
		IV slowly	0.02–0.05 mg/kg, can repeat q5min up to a total of 0.2 mg/kg	
	Cat	PO	0.5–1 mg/kg q8h	
		IV slowly	0.025 mg/kg, can repeat q5min up to a total of 0.2 mg/kg	
Anticholinergics				
Atropine	Dog, cat	PO	0.04 mg/kg q6–8h	
		IV, IM, SC	0.02–0.04 mg/kg	
Glycopyrrolate (Robinul®)	Dog, cat	IV, IM	0.005–0.01 mg/kg	
		SC	0.01–0.02 mg/kg	
Hyoscyamine (Levsin®)	Dog	PO	3–6 mcg/kg q8h	
Propantheline (Pro-Banthine®)	Dog	PO	3.73–7.5 mg q8–12h	
β-Adrenergic agonists				
Isoproterenol (Isuprel®)	Dog, cat	IV	0.045–0.09 mcg/kg/min CRI	
Terbutaline (Brethine®)	Dog	PO	2.5–5 mg/dog q8–12h	
	Cat	PO	1.25 mg/cat q12h	
Other agents				
Adenosine (Adenocard®)	Dog	IV rapidly	up to 12 mg	
Digoxin	Dog <22 kg	PO	5–8 mcg/kg q12h; Decrease by 10% for elixir. Maximum: 0.5 mg/d or 0.375 mg/d for Doberman Pinchers	
	Dog ≥22 kg	PO	3–5 mcg/kg q12h. Decrease by 10% for elixir. Maximum: 0.5 mg/d or 0.375 mg/d for Doberman Pinchers	
	Cat	PO	7 mcg/kg q48h	
Edrophonium (Tensilon®, Enlon®)	Dog, cat	IV	0.05 to 0.1 mg/kg	
Phenylephrine (Neo-Synephrine®)	Dog, cat	IV	4–10 mcg/kg	
Drugs used to treat hypertension				
ACE inhibitors				
Benazepril (Lotensin®)	Dog, cat	PO	0.25–0.5 mg/kg q24–12h	

(Continued)

Name of drugs	Species	Route	Dose	Notes
Captopril (Capoten®)	Dog	PO	0.5–2.0 mg/kg q8–12h	
	Cat	PO	0.5–1.25 mg/kg q12–24h	
Enalapril (Enacard®)	Dog	PO	0.5 mg/kg q24–12h	
	Cat	PO	0.25–0.5 mg/kg q24h	
Ramipril (Altace®)	Dog	PO	0.125–0.25 mg/kg q24h	
Calcium channel blocker				
Amlodipine (Norvasc®)	Dog	PO	0.1–0.3 mg/kg q24–12h	
	Cat	PO	0.1–0.2 mg/kg q24–12h	
β-Adrenergic antagonists				
Atenolol (Tenormin®)	Dog	PO	0.2–1.0 mg/kg q12–24h (start low)	
	Cat	PO	6.25–12.5 mg/cat q12–24h	
Propranolol (Inderal®)	Dog	PO	0.1–1.0 mg/kg q8h (start low)	
	Cat	PO	2.5–10 mg/cat q8–12h	
α₁-Adrenergic antagonists				
Phenoxybenzamine (Dibenzyline®)	Dog	PO	0.2–1.5 mg/kg q8–12h	
	Cat	PO	0.2–0.5 mg/kg q12h	
Prazosin (Minipress®)	Dog	PO	0.05–0.2 mg/kg q8–12h	
Diuretics				
Furosemide (Lasix®, etc.)	Dog	PO	0.5–3 mg/kg q8–24h	
	Cat	PO	0.5–2 mg/kg q12–24h	
Hydrochlorothiazide (Naquasone®, etc.)	Dog	PO	1–4 mg/kg q12–24h	
	Cat	PO	1–2 mg/kg q12–24h	
Drugs for hypertensive crisis				
Acepromazine (Aceproject®, etc.)	Dog, cat	IV	0.05–0.1 mg/kg (up to 3 mg total)	
Esmolol (Brevibloc®)	Dog, cat	IV	50–75 mcg/kg/min CRI	
Hydralazine (Apresoline®)	Dog, cat	PO	0.5–2.0 mg/kg q12h (titrate up to effect)	
		IV, IM	0.2 mg/kg, repeat q2h prn	
Labetolol (Normodyne®, Trandate®)	Dog, cat	IV	0.25 mg/kg over 2 min, repeat up to total dose of 3.75 mg/kg, followed by CRI of 25 mcg/kg/min	
Nitroprusside (Nitropress®)	Dog, cat	IV	0.5–1 mcg/kg/min CRI (initial) to 5–15 mcg/kg/min	

(continued)

Name of drugs	Species	Route	Dose	Notes
Phentolamine (Regitine®)	Dog, cat	IV	0.02–0.1 mg/kg, followed by CRI to effect	
Propranolol (Inderal®)	Dog, cat	IV slowly	0.02 mg/kg (initial) to 0.1 mg/kg	
Drugs used for thromboembolic disease **Antiplatelet therapy** Aspirin	Dog Cat	PO PO	0.5 mg/kg q12h 81 mg/cat 2–3 times/wk or 5 mg/cat q72h	
Clopidogrel (Plavix®)	Dog Cat	PO PO	2–4 mg/kg q24h 18.75 mg/cat q24h	
Anticoagulant therapy Dalteparin (Fragmin®)	Dog, cat	SC	150 IU/kg q4–12h	
Enoxaparin (Lovenox®)	Dog, cat	SC	1.5 mg/kg q6–12h	
Sodium heparin	Dog, cat	IV	200–250 IU/kg, followed by 200–300 IU/kg SC q6–8h for 2–4d or prn	
Thrombolytic therapy Rt-PA (Recombinant tissue plasminogen activator)	Dog Cat	IV IV	1 mg/kg q1h for 10 doses 0.25–1 mg/kg/h (up to a total of 1–10 mg/kg)	
Streptokinase (Streptase®)	Dog, cat	IV slowly	90,000 IU over 20–30 min, then at 45,000 IU/h for 3h or more	

Chapter 9: Diuretics

Name of drugs	Species	Route	Dose	Notes
Loop (high-ceiling) diuretics Bumetanide (Bumex®)	Dog, cat	IV	0.02–0.1 mg/kg q8–24h	
Ethacrynic acid (Edecrin®)	Dog, cat	IV, IM	0.2–0.4 mg/kg q4–12h	
Furosemide (Lasix®, etc.)	Dog	IV, IM, SC, PO	2–6 mg/kg q8–12h	
	Cat	IV, IM, SC, PO	1–4 mg/kg q12h	
	Horse	IV, IM	1–3 mg/kg q12h	
	Cattle	IV	2.2–4.4 mg/kg q12h	
Thiazide diuretics (benzothiadiazides) Chlorothiazide (Diuril®, Diurigen®)	Dog, cat Cattle	PO PO	20–40 mg/kg q12h 4–8 mg/kg q12–24h	
Hydrochlorothiazide (Oretic®, Esidrix®)	Dog Cat Horse Cattle	PO PO PO IV, IM	2–4 mg/kg q12h 1–2 mg/kg q12h 250 mg/450 kg q24h 125–250 mg q12–24h	

Name of drugs	Species	Route	Dose	Notes
Trichlormethiazide	Horse	PO	200 mg/450 kg q24h	
Osmotic diuretics				
Dimethyl sulfoxide (Domoso®)	Dog	IV slowly	1 g/kg of 10% soln over 45 min q6–8h	
	Horse	IV slowly	1 g/kg (20% solution), for 30 min q24h for 3d	
Glycerol	Dog, cat	PO	1–1.5 g/kg initially, then 500 mg/kg q8h	
	Horse	IV slowly	0.5–2 g/kg for brain edema	
Mannitol	Dog, cat	IV slowly	1–3 g/kg, over 30–60 min	Glaucoma, acute
		IV slowly	0.25–0.5 g/kg over 15–60 min q4–6h	Renal failure
		IV slowly	1–3 g/kg over 30–60 min	Cerebral edema
		IV slowly	1 g/kg over 30 min; repeat q4–6h	Diuretic, osmotic
	Horse	IV	0.25–2.0 g/kg (20% solution)	
	Cattle	IV	1–3 g/kg	
	Swine	IV	1–3 g/kg	
	Sheep	IV	1–3 g/kg	
	Goat	IV	1–3 g/kg	
Carbonic anhydrase inhibitors				
Acetazolamide (Diamox®, etc.)	Dog	PO	5–10 mg/kg q8–12h	
	Cat	PO	7 mg/kg q8h	
	Horse	PO	2.2 mg/kg q12h–6h	
	Cattle	IV, IM, SC	6–8 mg/kg	
	Swine	IV, IM, SC	6–8 mg/kg	
Dichlorphenamide (Daranide®)	Dog	PO	2.2–5 mg/kg q8–12h	
	Cat	PO	1 mg/kg q8–12h	
	Horse	PO	1 mg/kg q12h	
Ethoxzolamide (Cardrase®)	Dog, cat	PO	4–5 mg/kg q8–12h	
Methazolamide (GlaucTabs®)	Dog, cat	PO	2–6 mg/kg q8–12h	
	Horse	PO	2–4 mg/kg q8–12h	
Potassium-sparing diuretics				
Spironolactone (Aldactone®)	Dog, cat	PO	1–4 mg/kg q12h	
Triamterene (Dyrenium®)	Dog, cat	PO	1–2 mg/kg q12h	
Methylxanthines				
Aminophylline (Truphylline®)	Dog	IV slowly	2–5 mg/kg over 30–60 min q12h	
		IM, PO	10–11 mg/kg q6–8h	
	Cat	IV slowly	2–5 mg/kg over 30–60 min q12h	
		PO	5–6 mg/kg q12h	
	Horse	PO	5–10 mg/kg q12h	
Theophylline (Elixophyllin®)	Dog	IV, IM, PO	5–10 mg/kg q6–8h	
	Cat	IV, IM, PO	4–4.5 mg/kg q8–12h	
	Horse	PO	1 mg/kg q6h	

(continued)

Chapter 10: Respiratory Pharmacology

Name of drugs	Species	Route	Dose	Notes
Theophylline sustained action (Slo-bid®, Theo-Dur®)	Dog Cat	PO PO	20–30 mg/kg q12h 20–25 mg/kg q12h	
Acidifying salts Ammonium chloride (Uroeze®, etc.)	Dog Cat	PO PO	100 mg/kg q12h 800 mg/cat	
Removal of hypersecretions N-acetylcysteine (Mucomyst®, Mucosil-10®)	Dog, cat	IV	50 mg/h for 30–60 min q12h by nebulization	
Expectorants Guaifenesin (Guailaxin®)	Horse	PO	3 mg/kg	
Potassium Iodide (Pima syrup®, SSKI®)	Dog Cat Horse	PO PO PO	40 mg/kg q8h 20 mg/kg q12–24h 2–20 g q24h	
Leukotriene receptor antagonists Zafirlukast (Accolate®)	Cat	PO	1–2 mg/kg q12–24h	
Serotonin receptor inhibitors Cyproheptadine (Ciplactin®, etc.)	Dog, cat	PO	0.25–1.1 mg/kg q8–12h	Antihistamine
	Cat	PO	2 mg q8–24h	Appetite stimulant
	Horse	PO PO	2 mg q8–12h 0.5 mg/kg q12h	Asthma
Immunosuppressants Cyclosporine (Atopica®)	Dog	PO	7.5–15 mg/kg q12–24h	
	Cat	PO	7.5 mg/kg q12h	
Cough suppression Codeine	Dog, cat	PO, SC PO	1–4 mg/kg q6–12h 1–2 mg/kg q6–12h	Analgesic Antitussive
Hydrocodone (Hycodan®, etc.)	Dog, cat	PO	0.22 mg/kg q6–12h	Antitussive
Dextromethorphan	Dog, cat	PO	1–2 mg/kg q6–8h	Antitussive
Bronchodilators Theophylline (Elixophyllin®)	Dog Cat	PO, IV, IM PO, IV, IM	5–10 mg/kg q6–8h 4–4.5 mg/kg q8–12h	
Drug for pulmonary hypertension control Sildenafil (Viagra®)	Dog	PO	0.5–1 mg/kg q24h	

Chapter 11: Drugs Acting on the Gastrointestinal Tract

Name of drugs	Species	Route	Dose	Notes
Control of visceral pain Buscopan	Horse	IV	0.3 mg/kg	Control of colic
Butorphanol (Torbutrol®)	Horse	IV	0.01–0.02 mg/kg alone or in combination with xylazine	

Name of drugs	Species	Route	Dose	Notes
Flunixin meglumine (Banamine®)	Horse	IV or IM	1.1 mg/kg q24h for up to 5d	Control of colic
Morphine	Dog Cat Horse	IM, SC IM, SC	0.5–2 mg/kg q6h 0.05–0.02 mg/kg q6h 0.05–0.02 mg/kg	
Xylazine (Rompun®, etc.)	Horse	IV IM	1.1 mg/kg 2.2 mg/kg	Control of colic Control of colic
Appetite stimulants Cyproheptadine (Cyheptine®, etc.)	Cat	PO	2 mg/cat q12–24h	
Diazepam (Valium®)	Cat	PO, IV, IM	0.2 mg/kg q12–24h	
Oxazepam (Serax®)	Cat	PO	2.5 mg/kg q24h	
Glucocorticoids Prednisone (Meticorten®, etc.)	Cat	PO	0.25–0.5 mg/kg	Only ~10% of prednisone is converted to prednisolone in cats for action
Prednisolone (Prelone®, etc.)	Cat	PO	0.25–0.5 mg/kg	
Anti-obesity drugs Dirlotapide (Slentrol®)	Dog	PO	0.05 mg/kg q24h	
Gastric secretory inhibitors **H₂ antikistamines** Famotidine (Pepcid®, etc.)	Dog, cat	PO	0.5–1.0 mg/kg q24h	
Ranitidine (Zantac®)	Dog, cat	PO, IV	2 mg/kg q12h	
Proton pump inhibitor Omeprazole (Prilosec®, Gastrogard®)	Dog, cat horse	PO PO	0.7 mg/kg q24h 4 mg/kg, q24h, for 4 wk followed by 2 mg/kg, q24h, for ≥4 wk	Gastric ulcer control
Mucosal cytoprotectants Misoprostol (Cytotec®)	Dog	PO	3–5 mcg/kg q8h	
Sucralfate (Carafate®)	Dog Cat	PO PO	0.5–1 g q8h 0.25–0.5 g q12h	
Prokinetic drugs Cisapride	Dog, cat	PO	0.1–0.5 mg/kg q8h	
Erythromycin (E-Mycin®, etc.)	Dog, cat	PO	0.5–1.0 mg/kg q8h	
Metoclopramide (Reglan®, Clopra®)	Dog, cat	PO	0.2–0.4 mg/kg q8h	30 min before meals
Ranitidine (Zantac®)	Cat	PO	1–2 mg/kg q12h	
Digestants Pancrelipase (Viokase-V®)	Dog Cat	In feed In feed	1–1.5 tsp (2.8–3.2 g)/meal 0.5 tsp (1.4 g)/ meal	

(continued)

Name of drugs	Species	Route	Dose	Notes
Drugs to treat hepatic encephalopathy				
Lactulose (Cephulac®, Chronulac®)	Dog	PO	5–15 mL (3.3–10 g) q8h to induce soft stools	
	Cat	PO	0.5 mL (0.33 g)/kg q12h	
Metronidazole (Flagyl®, etc.)	Dog, cat	PO	10–20 mg/kg q12h	
Emetics				
Apomorphine HCl (Apokyn®, Apokinon®)	Dog	IV, IM	0.03 mg/kg	
Xylazine (Rompun®, etc.)	Dog	IM	0.6 mg/kg	
	Cat	IM	0.44 mg/kg	
Antiemetics				
Aminopentamide (Centrine®)	Dog	IM, SC, PO	0.01–0.03 mg q8–12h	
	Cat	SC,IM	0.1–0.4 mg	
Chlorpromazine (Thorazine®)	Dog, cat	IM, IV, SC	0.5 mg/kg q8h	
Diphenhydramine (Benadryl®, etc.)	Dog, cat	PO	2–4 mg/kg q8h–12h	
Maropitant (Cerenia®)	Dog	SC	1 mg/kg/d q24h	
Metoclopramide (Reglan®, etc.)	Dog	PO, SC,IM	0.2–0.4 mg/kg q8h	
		IV slowly	1.1–2.2 mg/kg over 24h	Intractable vomiting
	Cat	PO, SC, IM	0.2–0.4 mg/kg q8h	
		IV slowly	1.1–2.2 mg/kg over 24h	Intractable vomiting
Ondansetron (Zofran®)	Dog	PO	0.1–1.0 mg/kg q24h–q12h	
	Cat	PO	0.22 mg/kg q8–12 h	
Prochlorperazine (Compazine®)	Dog, cat	IM	0.1 mg/kg q8h	
Laxative agents				
Docusate sodium	Dog	PO	25–50 mg q24h–q12h	
	Cat	PO	25 mg q24h	
Lactulose (Cephulac®, Cholac®)	Dog, cat	PO	0.5 mL (0.33 g)/kg q8–12h	
Polyethylene glycol in Electrolyte solution	Dog	Gastric intubation	20 mL (0.15 g)/kg–dosage may be repeated for colonoscopy	
Anti-diarrheal drugs				
Bismuth Subsalilate (Bismusal®)	Dog	PO	3.5 mg/kg q8h	
Diphenoxylate + Atropine (Lomotil®)	Dog	PO	0.05 mg/kg q8h	
Loperamide (Imodium®)	Dog	PO	0.1–0.2 mg/kg q8–12h	
Drugs for therapy of inflammatory bowel disease				
Metronidazole (Flagyl®, etc.)	Dog, cat	PO	20 mg/kg q12h	

(Continued)

Name of drugs	Species	Route	Dose	Notes
Olsalazine (Dipentum®)	Dog	PO	10–20 mg/kg q8h	
Sulfasalazine (Azulfidine®)	Dog	PO	20–30 mg/kg q8–12h	
Tylosin (Tylan®)	Dog	PO	10 mg/kg q8h	

Chapter 12: Endocrine Pharmacology

Name of drugs	Species	Route	Dose	Notes
Growth hormones				
Somatotropin	Dog	SC	0.1 IU (0.05 mg)/kg	
Sometribove (Posilac®)	Bovine	SC	500 mg/2 wk	
Gonadotropins **GnRH**				
Deslorelin (Ovuplant®)	Horse	SC	implant in the neck (2.1 mg)	
Gonadorelin (Factrel®)	Dog	IM	50–100 mcg/dog q24–48h	
	Cat	IM	25 mcg/cat once	
	Horse	SC	50 mcg 2.5h prebreeding	For low libido
		IM	40 mcg 6h prebreeding	Induces ovulation
	Cattle	IM, IV	100 mcg/cow	
	Sheep, goat	IM	100 mcg/sheep	
Leuprolide (Lupron®, Eligard®)	Ferret		100 mcg/month	Adrenocortical disease
	Bird		375 mcg/month	Inhibits ovulation
HCG	Dog	IM	500–1000 IU; repeat in 48h	Luteinization of follicular cysts
		IM	25–100 IU twice weekly for 4–6 wk	Induces descent of inguinal testis
		SC	500 IU twice weekly for 4 wk	Male hypogonadism
		IM	22 IU/kg q24h for 2d following FSH	Induces ovulation
	Cat	IM	100–500 IU	
		IM	250 IU, following FSH or after mating	Induces ovulation
	Horse	IV	1,000–5,000 IU	
	Cattle	IV	2,500–5,000 IU	
		IM	10,000 IU	
	Sheep, goat	IV, IM	250–1,000 IU	
	Swine	IM	200 IU	PG600®
PMSG (ECG) (PG600®)	Swine	IM	400 IU	
Sex steroids **Estrogens**				
Diethylstilbestrol (Apstil®, etc.)	Dog, cat	PO	0.1–1 mg q24h	

(continued)

(*Continued*)

Name of drugs	Species	Route	Dose	Notes
Estradiol cypionate (ECP®, Depo-Estradiol®)	Dog	IM	0.02–0.04 mg/kg (total dose not over 1 mg)	
	Cat	IM	0.25 mg/cat	
	Horse	IM	4–8 mcg/kg q2d	Urinary incontinence
	Cattle	IM	4–20 mg	
Zeranol (Ralgro®)	Cattle	SC	Ear implant (72 mg)	
	Sheep	SC	Ear implant (12 mg)	
Anti-estrogens				
Tamoxifen (Nolvadex®)	Dog	PO	10–20 mg q12	
Progestins				
Altrenogest (Regu-Mate®, Matrix®)	Horse	PO	0.044 mg/kg q24h for 15d	Estrus synchronization
		PO	0.044 mg/kg	Prevents aggression
		PO	0.044 mg/kg q24h	Pregnancy maintenance
	Swine	PO	15 mg/gilt for 14d	Estrus synchronization
Medroxyprogesterone (Provera®, Amen®)	Dog, cat	IM	1.1–2.2 mg/kg q7d	
		IM, SC	11 mg/kg 3 times yearly	Aggression
Megestrol (Oraban®)	Dog	PO	2.2 mg/kg q24h for 32d	Contraceptive
	Cat	PO	2.5–5 mg/cat for 1 wk	
Melengestrol (MGA®)	Cattle	In feed	0.25–0.5 mg/cattle/d	
Progesterone (Depo-Provera®, Provera®)	Dog, cat	IM	1.1–2.2 mg/kg q7d	
		IM, SC	11 mg/kg 3 times yearly	Aggression
	Cattle	Implant	100–200 mg	
	Horse	IM	150 mg q24h	Suppresses estrus
			300 mg q24h	Maintains pregnancy
Androgens				
Boldenone (Equipoise®)	Horse	IM	1 mg/kg repeated at 3 wk intervals	
Danazol (Danocrine®)	Dog, cat	PO	5–10 mg/kg q12h	
Stanozolol (Winstrol-V®)	Dog	PO	1–4 mg/dog q12h	
		IM	25–50 mg/dog/wk	
	Cat	PO	1 mg/cat q12h	
		IM	25 mg/cat/wk	
	Horse	IM	0.5 mg/kg, up to 4 doses q1–2 wk	
Testosterone aqueous	Horse	SC	0.1–0.2 mg/kg q48h for 2 wk	Inadequate libido
Testosterone cypionate (Andro-Cyp®)	Dog, cat	IM	1–2 mg/kg q2–4 wk	
Testosterone propionate (Malogen®, Testex®) (Synovex-H®)	Dog, cat	IM	0.5–1 mg/kg 2–3 times/wk	
	Cattle	IM	200–1,000 mg	
Trenbolone (Synovex®)	Cattle	SC	Ear implant (200 mg)	

(Continued)

Name of drugs	Species	Route	Dose	Notes
Anti-androgens				
Finasteride (Proscar®)	Dog	PO	0.5–5 mg/kg q24h	
Uterine contractants				
Cabergoline (Dostinex®)	Dog	PO	5 mcg/kg q24h for 5–10d	Estrus induction
	Dog, cat	SC	1.7 mcg/kg q24h for 6d	Abortifacient
		PO	5–15 mcg/kg q24h for 5d	Abortifacient
Bromocriptine (Parlodel®)	Dog	PO	10–100 mcg/kg	
	Horse	IM	5 mg q12h	
Ergonovine (Ergotrate®)	Dog	IM, PO	0.2 mg/kg once	
	Horse	IM	1–3 mg	
Oxytocin	Dog	IM	5–20 IU/dog q30min	
	Cat	IM	3–5 IU/cat	
	Horse	IV	2.5–5 IU/450 kg as bolus q20min	
		IV slowly	80–100 IU in 500 mL saline	
		IM, IV	10–20 IU/450 kg	
		IV	1–3 IU/450 kg	Milk let down
		IV	0.5–10 IU/kg	Induces parturition
	Cattle	IM	20–60 IU	
	Swine	IM	20–50 IU	
		IV	5–10 IU	
	Sheep, goat	IM	10–20 IU	
Prostaglandin $F_2\alpha$ and analog				
Cloprostenol (Estrumate®)	Dog	Not specified	1–5 mcg/kg q24h	
	Horse	IM	100 mcg/horse	
	Cattle	IM	500 mcg/cattle	
	Swine	IM	175 mcg	
	Sheep	IM	62.5–125 mcg	
	Goat	IM	62.5–125 mcg	
Dinoprost tromethamine (Lutalyse®)	Dog, cat	SC	0.1–0.25 mg/kg q24h	
	Horse	IM	1 mg/45 kg	
	Cattle	IM	25–30 mg	
	Swine	IM	5–25 mg	
	Sheep, goat	IM	2.5–20 mg	
Corticosteroids				
Glucocorticoids				
Betamethasone (Betasone®)	Dog, cat	PO	0.1–0.2 mg/kg q 12–24h	
	Horse	IM or PO	0.02–0.1 mg/kg	
		Intralesional	4–10 mg	
Dexamethasone	Dog, cat	IV, IM, PO	0.1–0.2 mg/kg q12–24h	Anti-inflammation
		IV	2.2–4.4 mg/kg	Shock

(continued)

(*Continued*)

Name of drugs	Species	Route	Dose	Notes
	Horse	IV, IM, PO	0.02–0.2 mg/kg q24	
		IV	0.5–2 mg/kg	Septic shock
		IV	100 mg/450 kg q24h for 5d	Induces parturition
	Cattle	IV, IM	1–2 mg/kg q4h	Insect bites
		IM	5–40 mg/cattle for 2–3d	
			20–25 mg + 25 mg PGF2α	Abortion
	Swine	IV, IM	1–10 mg	
Fludrocortisone (Florinef-Acetate®)	Dog	PO	0.2–0.8 mg/dog (0.02 mg/kg) q24h	
	Cat	PO	0.1 mg/cat q24h	
Flumethasone (Flucort®)	Dog	IV, IM, SC, PO	0.0625–0.25 mg/dog q24h	
	Cat	IV, IM, SC, PO	0.03–0.125 mg/cat q24h	
	Horse	PO	2–8 mcg/kg	
Fluoroprednisolone (Isoflupredone)	Horse	IM	5–20 mg/450 kg	
Predef® 2X	Cattle	IM	10–20 mg	
	Swine	IM	5 mg/140 kg	
Hydrocortisone (Cortef®, Hydrocortone®, etc.)	Dog, **cat**	PO	1 mg/kg q12h	Replacement therapy
		PO	2.5–5 mg/kg q12h	Anti-inflammatory
	Horse	IV drip	1–4 mg/kg	
	Cattle	IV, SC	100–600 mg in 1,000 mL of 10% dextrose saline	For Photosensitization
Methylprednisolone (Medrol®)	Dog	PO	0.22–0.44 mg/kg q12–24h	
Methylprednisolone acetate (Depo-Medrol®)	Dog	IM	1 mg/kg q1–3 wk	
	Cat	IM	10–20 mg q1–3 wk	
	Horse	IM	0.2–0.7 mg/kg	
Methylprednisolone sodium succinate (Solu-Medrol®)	Dog, cat	IV	30 mg/kg, repeat at 15 mg/kg in 2–6h	
	Horse	IV	30 mg/kg, then 5.4 mg/kg/h for 23h	CNS trauma
		Subconjunctival Intraarticular	20 mg up to 100 mg	
Prednisolone	Dog	IV, IM, PO	0.5–1 mg/kg q12–24h initially then taper to q48h	Anti-inflammatory
	Cat	IV, IM, PO	2.2 mg/kg q12–24h initially then taper to q48h	Anti-inflammatory
	Dog, cat	IV, IM, PO	initially 2.2–6.6 mg/kg then taper to 2–4 mg/kg q 48h	Immunosuppressive
	Horse	PO, IM	0.2–4.4 mg/kg q12–24h	
	Cattle	IM, IV	0.2–1 mg/kg	
		IM, IV	1–4 mg/kg	Cerebral edema

(Continued)

Name of drugs	Species	Route	Dose	Notes
Prednisolone sodium succinate	Dog, cat	IV	15–30 mg/kg then repeat in 4–6 h	Shock
		IV	15–30 mg/kg then taper to 1–2 mg/kg q12h	CNS trauma
	Horse	IV	2–5 mg/kg	Septic shock
	Swine	IM, IV	0.2–1 mg/kg	
Prednisone	Dog	IV, IM, PO	0.5–1 mg/kg q12–24h initially then taper to q48h	Anti-inflammatory
	Cat	IV, IM, PO	2.2 mg/kg q12–24h initially then taper to q48h	Anti-inflammatory, only ~10% of prednisone is converted to prednisolone in cats for action
	Dog, cat	IV, IM, PO	2.2–6.6 mg/kg then taper to 2–4 mg/kg q48h	Immunosuppressive
Triamcinolone (Aristocort®)	Dog, cat	PO	0.5–1 mg/kg q12–24 then taper to q48h	Anti-inflammatory
	Horse	IM	0.02–0.1 mg/kg	
		Intralesional	1–3 mg/site up to 1 mg total	
		Subconjunctival	1–2 mg	
Triamcinolone acetonide (Vetalog®)	Dog, cat	IM, SC	0.1–0.2 mg/kg repeat in 7–10d	
		Intralesional	1 mg for every centimeter of tumor q2wk	
Mineralocorticoids				
Desoxycorticosterone (Percorten-V®)	Dog, cat	IM, SC	2.2 mg/kg q25d	
Fludrocortisone (Florinef-Acetate®)	Dog	PO	0.015–0.02 mg/kg q24h	
	Cat	PO	0.05–0.1 mg/cat q12h	
Adrenal steroid inhibitors				
Ketoconazole (Nizoral®)	Dog	PO	10–15 mg/kg q12h	
	Cat	PO	5–10 mg/kg q12h	
	Horse	PO	30 mg/kg q12–24h	
Mitotane (Lysodren®)	Dog	PO	25 mg/kg/d for 10–14d, then 25–50 mg/kg/wk	Hyperadrenocorticism
		PO	50–75 mg/kg/d for 10d, then 75–100 mg/kg/wk	Adrenal tumor
	Cat	PO	25–50 mg q24h	
Selegiline (Anipryl®)	Dog	PO	1–2 mg/kg q24h	Might not work
Trilostane (Vetoryl®)	Dog	PO	2–10 mg/kg q24h	
	Horse	PO	0.4–1 mg/kg (total dose 120–240 mg) q24h	

(continued)

Name of drugs	Species	Route	Dose	Notes
Antidiabetic agents				
Insulin (regular)	Dog, cat	IM, SC	0.1–0.4 IU/kg q6–8h	Diabetic ketoacidosis, mild
		IV	0.5–1.0 IU/h or 0.025–0.05 U/kg	Diabetic ketoacidosis, severe
		IM	0.2 IU/kg once; then 0.1 IU/kg hourly until blood glucose is <250 mg/dL	Diabetic ketoacidosis, severe
	Horse	IM, SC	0.5 IU/kg	
Insulin (NPH)	Dog	SC	0.5–1 IU/kg q12–24h	
	Cat	SC	1–5 IU/cat q12h	
Insulin (PZI Vet®)	Dog	SC	0.5–1 IU/kg q12–24h	Long-acting
	Cat	SC	1–5 IU/cat q12–24h	
	Horse	IM, SC	0.15 IU/kg	
Insulin glargine (Lantus®)	Dog	SC	0.25 IU/kg q12h	
Lente insulin (Vetsulin®)	Dog	SC	0.5–1.0 IU/kg q12–24h	
	Cat	SC	0.5 IU/kg q12–24h	
Ultralente insulin	Dog	SC	0.5–1 IU/kg q12–24h (to effect)	
	Cat	SC	1–5 IU/kg q12–24h (to effect)	
	Cattle	SC	0.25 IU/kg q4–48h	
Metformin (Glucophage®, etc.)	Cat	PO	2–5 mg/kg q12	
Sulfonylureas				
Glimepiride (Amaryl®)	Cat	PO	1–2 mg/cat q24h	
Glipizide (Glucotrol®)	Cat	In food	2.5–5 mg/cat q8–12h	
Glyburide (Micronase®)	Cat	PO	0.2 mg/kg q24h	
Thyroid hormones				
Levothyroxine (Levotabs®, Soloxine®, etc.)	Dog	PO	20 mcg/kg q24h	
	Cat	PO	50–100 mcg/cat q24h	
	Horse	PO	10 mg in 70 mL syrup q24h	
Liothyronine (Cytomel®)	Dog	PO	4–6 mcg/kg q8h	
	Cat	PO	4.4 mcg/kg q8–12h	
Antithyroid agents				
Methimazole (Tapazole®, etc.)	Dog	PO	2.2 mg/kg q8–12h	
	Cat	PO	2.5–10 mg/cat q8–12h	
$Na^{131}I$	Cat	SC	1–5 mCi	
Anti-hypocalcemia agents				
Calcium gluconate	Dog, cat	IV slowly	94–140 mg/kg	
		PO	25–50 mg/kg q24h	
	All other species	IV slowly	150–250 mg/kg	
Calcitriol (Rocaltrol®)	Dog, cat	PO	1–3 ng/kg q12–24h	
Dihydrotachysterol (DHT®, Hytakerol®)	Dog, cat	PO	0.02–0.03 mg/kg q24h, maintenance: 0.01–0.02 mg/kg q24–48h	

(Continued)

Name of drugs	Species	Route	Dose	Notes
Human recombinant erythropoietin				
EPO (erythropoietin)	Dog, cat	SC	50–100 IU/kg 3 times/wk	

Chapter 15: Antimicrobial Drugs

Name of drugs	Species	Route	Dose	Notes
Sulfonamides				
Sulfachlorpyridazine (Vetisulid®)	Calves	IV	66–99 mg/kg for 1–5d	
Sulfadimethoxine (Albon®, etc.)	Dog, cat	PO, IV, SC	55 mg/kg initially, then 27.5 mg/kg q24h	
	Horse	IV, PO	55 mg/kg initially, then 27.5 mg/kg q24h	
	Cattle	IV, PO	55 mg/kg initially, then 27.5 mg/kg q24h for 5d	
Sulfamethazine (Sulmet®)	Dog, cat	PO	100 mg/kg once; then 50 mg/kg q12h	
Sulfamethoxazole (Gantanol®)	Dog, cat	PO	100 mg/kg once; then 50 mg/kg q12h	
Sulfaquinoxaline	Chicken	idw	0.04% for 2–3d, then 0.025% for 2d more	
	Turkey	idw	0.025% for 2–3d	
	Cattle	idw	0.015% for 3–5d	
Sulfasalazine (Azulfidine®)	Dog	PO	10–30 mg/kg q8–12h	
	Cat	PO	10–20 mg/kg q12–24h	
Sulfadiazine-trimethoprim (Tribrissen®)	Dog	PO, IV	15–30 mg/kg q12h	
	Cat	PO, SC	15–30 mg/kg q12h–24h	
	Horse	PO, IV	15–30 mg/kg q12h	
	Cattle	IM, IV	25–48 mg/kg q24h	
	Swine	IM	48 mg/kg q24h	
Sulfamethoxazone-trimethoprim (Bactrim®)	Dog	PO, IV	15–30 mg/kg q12h	
	Cat	PO, SC	15–30 mg/kg q12h–24h	
	Horse	PO, IV	15–30 mg/kg q12h	
	Cattle	IM, IV	25–48 mg/kg q24h	
	Swine	IM	48 mg/kg q24h	
Sulfadimethoxine-ormetoprim (Primor®)	Dog	PO	55 mg/kg (combined drug) 1st day of therapy, then 27.5 mg/kg	
Fluoroquinolones				
Ciprofloxacin (Cipro®)	Dog, cat	Po, IV	10-20 mg/kg q24h	
Danofloxacin (A180®)	Cattle	SC	6 mg/kg	
Difloxacin (Dicural®)	Dog	PO	5–10 mg/kg q24h	
Enrofloxacin (Baytril®)	Dog	IM, IV, PO	2.5–20 mg/kg	
	Cat	PO, IM	2.5–5 mg/kg	
	Horse		2.5–7.5 mg/kg q12h	
	Cattle	SC	2.5–5 mg/kg q24h for 3–5d	
		SC	7.5–12.5 mg/kg once	

(continued)

Name of drugs	Species	Route	Dose	Notes
Marbofloxacin (Zeniquin®)	Dog, cat	PO	2.75–5.5 mg/kg q24	
Orbifloxacin (Orbax®)	Dog, cat	PO	2.5–7.5 mg/kg q12–24h	
	Horse	PO	2.5–7.5 mg/kg q24h	
Penicillins				
Natural penicillins				
Penicillin G benzathine	Dog, cat	IM	50,000 IU/kg q5d	
	Cattle	IM, SC	44,000–66,000 IU/kg q2d	
Penicillin G potassium	Dog, cat	IV, IM	20,000–40,000 IU/kg q6–8h	
	Horse	IV, IM	10,000–50,000 IU/kg q6h	
		PO	20,000 IU/kg q6h	
		Intrauterine	5,000,000 UI	
Penicillin G procaine	Dog	IM	20,000–40,000 IU/kg q12–24h	
	Cat	IM, SC	20,000 IU/kg q12–24h	
	Horse	IM	20,000–50,000 IU/kg q8–12h	
	Cattle	IM, SC	44,000–66,000 IU/kg q24h	
	Swine	IM	40,000 IU/kg q24h	
Penicillin G sodium	Dog, cat	IV, IM, SC	20,000–40,000 IU/kg q6–8h	
	Horse	IV, IM	10,000–50,000 IU/kg q6	
Penicillin V	Dog, cat	PO	5.5–11 mg/kg q6–8h	
	Horse	PO	66,000–110,000 IU/kg q8h	
Penicillinase-resistant penicillins				
Cloxacillin (Orbenin®, Dry-Clox®)	Dog, cat	PO	20–40 mg/kg q8h	
Methicillin (Staphcillin®)	Dog, cat	IV, IM	20 mg/kg q6h	
	Horse	IM	25 mg/kg q4–6h	
		Subconjunctival	100 mg	
Nafcillin (Nafcillin®)	Dog, cat	IM	10 mg/kg q6h	
Oxacillin (Oxacillin®)	Dog, cat	PO, IM, IV	22–40 mg/kg q8h	
	Horse	IM, IV	25–50 mg/kg	
Broad-spectrum penicillins				
Aminopenicillins				
Amoxicillin (Amoxi-Tab®, Biomax®)	Dog, cat	PO	10–22 mg/kg q12h	
	Horse	PO	10–30 mg/kg q8h	
	Cattle	SC, IM	10–15 mg/kg q24h	
Amoxicillin + Clavulanic acid (Clavamox®)	Dog	PO	10–25 mg/kg	
	Cat	PO	10–20 mg/kg q8h	
	Horse	IV	15–25 mg/kg q6–8h	
Ampicillin (Polyflex®, etc.)	Dog, cat	IV, IM, SC	10–30 mg/kg q6–8h	
		PO	20–40 mg/kg q8h	
	Horse	IV, IM	10–50 mg/kg	

(Continued)

Name of drugs	Species	Route	Dose	Notes
	Cattle	IM, PO	4–10 mg/kg q24h	
	Swine	SC, IM	6–8 mg/kg q8h	
Ampicillin + Sulbactam (Unasyn®)	Dog, cat	IV	50 mg/kg (combined) q8h	
Carboxypenicillins				
Carbenicillin disodium (Geocillin®)	Dog, cat	IV, IM, SC	40–50 mg/kg q6–8h	
Carbenicillin indanyl sodium (Geopen®)	Dog, cat	PO	10–33 mg/kg q8h	
	Horse	IV, IM	50–80 mg/kg q8h	
		Subconjunc-tival	200 mg	
		Intrauterine	6 g	
Ticarcillin (Ticar®)	Dog, cat	IM, IV	33–50 mg/kg q4–6h	
	Horse	IV, IM	40–80 mg/kg q8h	
		Intrauterine	6 g	
Ticarcillin + Clavulanic acid (Timentin®)	Dog	IV, IM	40–110 mg/kg q6h	
	Cat	IV	40–50 mg/kg q6–8h	
	Horse	IV	50 mg/kg q6–8h	
		Intrauterine	6 g	
Ureidopenicillins				
Piperacillin (Pipercil®)	Dog, cat	IV, IM, SC	25–50 mg/kg q8–12h	
Cephalosporins				
Cefaclor (Ceclor®)	Dog, cat	PO	10–20 mg/kg q8h	
Cefadroxil (Cefa-Drops®)	Dog	PO	22–35 mg/kg q12h	
	Cat	PO	22–35 mg/kg q24h	
	Horse	PO	22 mg/kg q12h	
	Foal	IV	25 mg/kg q4–6h	
Cefazolin (Ancef®, Kefzol®)	Dog, cat	IV, IM, SC	10–30 mg/kg q4–8h	
Cefepime (Maxipime®)	Dog, cat	IV, IM	40–50 mg/kg q6–8h	
	Horse	IV	6 mg/kg q8h	
	Foal	IV	11 mg/kg q8h	
Cefixime (Supran®, Suprax®)	Dog	PO	5–12.5 mg/kg q12–24h	
	Cat	PO	5–12.5 mg/kg q12h	
Cefoperazone (Cefobid®)	Dog	IV, IM	22 mg/kg q12h for 7–14d	
	Horse	IV, IM	30–50 mg/kg q8–12h	
Cefpodoxime (Vantin®)	Dog, cat	PO	5–10 mg/kg q12h	
Cefotaxime (Claforan®)	Dog, cat	IV, IM	20–80 mg/kg q6h	
	Horse	IV, IM	15–30 mg/kg q6–12h	
Cefoxitin (Mefoxin®)	Dog, cat	IV, IM, SC	15–30 mg/kg q6–8h	
	Horse	IM	30–40 mg/kg q6–8h	
		IV	20 mg/kg q6h	
Ceftiofur (Naxcel®)	Dog, cat	SC	2.2–4.4 mg/kg q12–24h	
	Horse	IV, IM	1–5 mg/kg q12–24h	
		Intrauterine	1 g	
	Cattle	IM, SC	1.1–2.2 mg/kg q24h	
	Sheep, goat		1.1–2.2 mg/kg q24h for 3–5d	

(continued)

(*Continued*)

Name of drugs	Species	Route	Dose	Notes
Cephalexin (Keflex®, etc.)	Dog	PO	10–30 mg/kg q6–12h	
	Cat	PO	20–50 mg/kg q12h	
	Horse	PO	22–33 mg/kg q6h	
Cephalothin (Keflin®)	Dog, cat	IV, IM, SC	20–40 mg/kg q4–6h	
	Horse	IV, IM	20–40 mg/kg q6–8h	
		Subconjunc-tival	100 mg	
Cephapirin (Cefadyl®)	Dog, cat	IV, IM	10–30 mg/kg q4–8h	
	Horse	IV, IM	20–30 mg/kg q4–6h	
Carbapenems				
Imipenem (Primaxin®)	Dog, cat	IV, IM, SC	2.2–10 mg/kg q6–8h	
	Horse	IV slowly	15 mg/kg over 20 min q4–6h	
Meropenem (Merrem®)	Dog	SC	12 mg/kg q8h	
		IV	24–40 mg/kg q24h	
	Cat	SC	12 mg/kg q8h	
		IV	24–40 mg/kg q24h	
Monobactams				
Aztreonam (Azactam®)	Dog	IV, IM	12–25 mg/kg q8–12h	
Aminoglycosides				
Amikacin (Amiglyde-V®)	Dog	IV, IM, SC	15–30 mg/kg q24h	
	Cat	IV, IM, SC	10–20 mg/kg q24h	
	Horse	IM, SC	15–20 mg/kg q24h	
		Intrauterine	2 g	
	Foal	IV, IM	1–10 mg/kg q12h	
	Cattle	IM	10–25 mg/kg q8–12h	
Dihydrostreptomycin	Dog, cat	IM	10–20 mg/kg q12h	
	Horse	IM, SC	11 mg/kg q12h	
Gentamicin (Gentavet®, Gentocin®)	Dog	IV, IM, SC	2–4 mg/kg q8–12h or 6 mg/kg q24h	
	Cat	IV, IM, SC	3 mg/kg q8h	
	Horse	IV, IM, SC	2–4 mg/kg q12h–6h	
		IV, IM, SC	6.6–8.8 mg/kg q24h	
	Cattle	IM	4.4–6.6 mg/kg/d	
	Swine	idw	1.1–2.2 mg/kg/d	
Kanamycin (Kantrim®, Amforal®)	Dog, cat	IV, IM, SC	10 mg/kg q12h or 20 mg/kg q24h	
	Horse	IV, IM	7.5 mg/kg q8h	
		Intrauterine	1–2 g	
Neomycin (Neomix®, Biosol®)	Dog, cat	PO	10–20 mg/kg q6–12h	
	Horse	PO	1 g/horse q6h	
		PO	2 g/horse q12h	
		PO	0.5 g/foal q6h	
		PO	1.5 g/horse q12h	
	Cattle	PO	10–20 mg/kg q12h	
		IM	6.6–19.8 mg/kg q24h	
	Swine	PO	7–12 mg/kg q12h	
	Sheep, goat	PO	0.75–1 g/d q8–12h	
		In feed	70–140 g/ton	
Streptomycin	Dog, cat	IM	10–20 mg/kg q12h	
	Horse	IM, SC	11 mg/kg q12h	

Name of drugs	Species	Route	Dose	Notes
Tetracyclines				
Chlortetracycline (Aureomycin®)	Dog, cat	PO	25 mg/kg q6–8h	
	Cattle	IV, IM	6–10 mg/kg	
		PO	10–20 mg/kg	
	Swine	IV, IM	6–10 mg/kg	
		PO	10–20 mg/kg	
Doxycycline (Doxyrobe®)	Dog	IV, PO	5–10 mg/kg q12–24h	
	Cat	IV, PO	5 mg/kg q12–24h	
	Horse	PO	3–10 mg/kg q12h	
Minocycline (Minocin®)	Dog	PO	12.5–25 mg/kg q12h	
		IV	12.5 mg/kg q12h	
	Cat	PO	5–15 mg/kg q12h	
	Horse	PO	3 mg/kg q12h	
Oxytetracycline (Terramycin®)	Dog, cat	PO	20 mg/kg q8h	
		IV	7.5–10 mg/kg q8h	
	Horse	IV	5–20 mg/kg q24h	
	Cattle	IM	5–10 mg/kg q24h	
		IV	2.5–5 mg/kg q24h	
		PO	10–20 mg/kg q12h	
	Swine, sheep, goat	IV, IM	6–11 mg/kg	
		PO	10–20 mg/kg q6h	
Tetracycline (Panmycin®, etc.)	Dog, cat	PO	15–22 mg/kg q6–8h	
		IV, IM	4.4–11 mg/kg q8–12h	
	Horse	IV	6.6–11 mg/kg q12h	
	Cattle, sheep	PO	11 mg/kg	
	Swine	PO	22 mg/kg	
Chloramphenicol group (Amphenicols)				
Chloramphenicol (Chloromycetin®)	Dog	IV, IM, PO	30–50 mg/kg q6–8h	
	Cat	IV, IM, PO	30–50 mg/cat q12h	
	Horse	PO	25–50 mg/kg q6–8h	
	Foal	PO	4–10 mg/kg q6–8h	
	Horse	IV, IM	25 mg/kg q6–8h	
		Subconjunctival	50–100 mg	
Florfenicol (Nuflor®)	Dog	IM, SC	25–50 mg/kg q8h	
	Cat	IM, SC	25–50 mg/kg q12h	
	Cattle	IM	20 mg/kg q48h	
	Sheep, goat	IM	20 mg/kg/d for 2d	
Macrolides				
Azithromycin (Zithromax®)	Dog, cat	PO	5–10 mg/kg q24h for 3–5d	
	Horse	PO	10 mg/kg q24h for 5d followed by q48h	
Clarithromycin (Biaxin®, Adel®)	Dog, cat	PO	5–10 mg/kg q12h	
	Horse	PO	7.5 mg/kg q12h	

(continued)

Name of drugs	Species	Route	Dose	Notes
Erythromycin (Galimycin®, Ery-Tab®)	Dog	PO	10–20 mg/kg q8h	
		PO	0.5–1 mg/kg q8h	GI Prokinetic
	Cat	PO	10–20 mg/kg q8h	
	Horse	PO	25 mg/kg q12h	
		IV	0.1 mg/kg/ h	GI Prokinetic
	Cattle	IM	4–8 mg/kg q12–24h	
	Swine	IM	2.2–6.6 mg/kg q24h	
	Sheep	IM	2.2 mg/kg q24h	
Tilmicosin (Micotil®)	Cattle	SC	10 mg/kg q72h	
	Sheep	SC	10 mg/kg q72h	Not in lambs <15 kg
Tulathromycin (Draxxin®)	Cattle	SC	2.5 mg/kg	
	Swine	IM	2.5 mg/kg	
Tylosin (Tylan®, etc.)	Dog, cat	PO	10–40 mg/kg q12h	
	Horse	IM	10 mg/kg q12h	
	Cattle	IM, IV	5–10 mg/kg q24h	Not to exceed 5d
	Swine	IM	8.8–12.5 mg/kg q12h	Not to exceed 3d
	Sheep, goat	IM	10 mg/kg	Not to exceed 5d
Clindamycin (Antirobe®, Clinsol®)	Dog, cat	IM, IV, SC, PO	5–11 mg/kg q12h	
Lincomycin (Lincosin®)	Dog, cat	IV, IM, PO	15–25 mg/kg q12h	
	Swine	IM	11 mg/kg q24h for 3–7d	

Miscellaneous antibacterial drugs
Aminocyclitols

Name of drugs	Species	Route	Dose	Notes
Apramycin (Apralan®)	Swine	idw	20–40 mg/kg q24h	
	Cattle	idw	20–40 mg/kg q24h	
Spectinomycin (Adspec®)	Dog, cat	IM	5–12 mg/kg q12h	
		PO	22 mg/kg q12h	
	Horse	IM	20 mg/kg q8h	
	Cattle	IM, SC	15–39.6 mg/kg/d	
	Swine	IM, PO	10 mg/kg q12h	
Metronidazole (Flagyl®)	Dog, cat	PO	10–15 mg/kg q8–12h	
	Horse	PO, IV	10–25 mg/kg q6h	
Rifampin (RiFadin®)	Dog	IV, IM, PO	10–20 mg/kg q8–12h	
	Cat	IV, IM, PO	10–20 mg/kg q24h	
	Horse	PO	10–20 mg/kg q24h 3–5 mg/kg q12h with erythromycin	
Tiamulin (Denagard®)	Swine	idw	7.7 mg/kg q24h for 5d	
		idw	23.1 mg/kg q24h for 5d	*Haemophilus* pneumonia
Vancomycin (Vancocin®)	Dog, cat	IV slowly	15 mg/kg over 30–60 min q6	
	Dog	PO	10–20 mg/kg q6h for 5–7d	
	Horse	IV, PO	20–40 mg/kg q12h–6h	

Name of drugs	Species	Route	Dose	Notes
Polymixins				
Polymyxin B (Aerosporin®)	Dog, cat	IM	2 mg/kg q24h	
	Horse	PO	5,000–10,000 IU/kg q6h	
Polymixin E (Colistin®)	Horse	PO	5,000–10,000 IU/kg q6h	
Nintrofurans				
Furazolidone (Topazone®)	Dog, cat	PO	2.2–4 mg/kg q12h for 7–10d	
	Horse	PO	4 mg/kg q8h	
Nitrofurantoin (Furadantin®)	Dog, cat	PO	4 mg/kg q8h	
	Horse	PO	10 mg/kg q24h	
		IM	3 mg/kg q12h	
Nitrofurazone (NFZ Puffer®)	Dog	PO	4 mg/kg q8–12h × 5–7d	*Coccidia*
Novobiocins				
Novobiocin + Tetracycline (Albaplex®)	Dog	PO	22 mg/kg of each antibiotic q12h	
Antifungal agents				
Amphotericin B (Amphocin®, Fungizone®)	Dog	IV slowly	0.1–0.25 mg/kg q48h, 3 times/wk	Cumulative dose: 8–12 mg/kg
	Cat	IV slowly	0.25–0.5 mg/kg q48h, 3 times/wk	Cumulative dose: 4–8 mg/kg
	Horse	IV	0.05 mg/kg q48h for 1 month	
Azoles				
Clotrimazole (1%) (Lotrimin®, Mycelex®)	Dog, cat	Intranasal	50–60 mL per side over 1h via indwelling catheter	
	Horse	Intrauterine	500 mg q24h for 1 wk	
Fluconazole (Diflucan®)	Dog	PO	2.5–15 mg/kg q12–24h	
	Cat	PO	50–100 mg/cat q12–24h	
	Horse	PO	4 mg/kg q24h	
Itraconazole (Sporanox®)	Dog	PO	5–10 mg/kg q12–24h	
	Cat	PO	5–10 mg/kg q12 or 20 mg/kg q24h	
	Horse	PO	3 mg/kg q12h for up to 2 months	
Ketoconazole (Nizoral®)	Dog	PO	10–15 mg/kg q12h	
	Cat	PO	5–10 mg/kg q8–12h	
	Horse	PO	30 mg/kg q12–24h	
Flucytosine (5-FC®, Ancoban®)	Dog, cat	PO	50 mg/kg q8h or 75 mg/kg q12h combined with Amphotericin B	

(continued)

Name of drugs	Species	Route	Dose	Notes
Griseofulvin (microsize) (Fulcin®)	Dog	PO	50 mg/kg q24h for 42–56d (maximum dose: 110–132 mg/kg/d in divided doses)	
	Cat	PO	50–120 mg/kg divided daily	
	Horse	PO	10 g/450 kg q24h for 2 wk, then 5 g q24h for 7 wk	
	Swine	PO	20 mg/kg q24h for 6 wk	
Griseofulvin (ultramicrosize)	Dog	PO	5–10 mg/kg q24h for 42d	
	Cat	PO	10–15 mg/kg q12h	
	Cattle	PO	10–20 mg/kg q24h for 1–2 wk	
Nystatin (Natacyn®)	Dog	PO	50,000–150,000 IU q8h	
	Cat	PO	100,000 IU q6h	
	Horse	Intrauterine	250,000–1,000,000 IU	
Terbinafine (Lamisil®)	Dog, cat	PO	30–40 mg/kg q24h	
		PO	3–10 mg/kg q12h for 28d	Dermatophytosis
		PO	3–10 mg/kg x 42–84d	Onychomycosis
Antiviral agents Acyclovir (Zovirax®, Cicloviral®)	Cat	SC	10–25 mg/kg q12h	
		PO	200 mg q6h	
Amantadine (Symmetrel®, etc.)	Dog	PO	1.25–4 mg/kg q12–24h	
	Cat	PO	3 mg/kg q24h	
	Horse	IV	5 mg/kg q4h	Equine-2 influenza
Zidovudine (AZT) (Retrovir®)	Cat	SC	10 mg/kg q12h for 21d	FIV infections
		PO	5–20 mg/kg q8h	FIV infections
		PO	10–20 mg/kg q12h for 42d	FeLV

Chapter 16: Antiparasitic Drugs

Name of drugs	Species	Route	Dose	Notes
Nematocides **Benzimidazoles (BZDs)** Albendazole (Valbazen®, Albenza®)	Dog, cat	PO	25–50 mg/kg q12h for 3–5d	
	Horse	PO	25–50 mg/kg for 2–5d	
		PO	4–8 mg/kg for 1 month	*Echinococcus*
	Cattle	PO	7.5–15 mg/kg	
	Swine	PO	5–10 mg/kg	
	Sheep, goat	PO	7.5–15 mg/kg	

(Continued)

Name of drugs	Species	Route	Dose	Notes
Febantel (Rintal®)	Dog, cat	PO	10 mg/kg q24 for 3d	
Fenbendazole	Dog, cat	PO	50 mg/kg/d for 3d	
(Panacur®, Safe-Guard®)	Horse	PO	5 mg/kg	
		PO	10 mg/kg	*Parascaris equorum*
		PO	50 mg/kg/d for 3–5d	Verminous arteritis
		PO	50 mg/kg	*Strongyloides westeri*
		PO	50 mg/kg/d for 5d	*Onchocerca*
	Cattle	PO	5–10 mg/kg	
	Swine	PO	5–10 mg/kg for 3d	
	Sheep, goat	PO	5 mg/kg for 3d	
Oxfendazole (Synanthic®)	Horse	PO	10 mg/kg	
	Cattle	PO	4.5 mg/kg	
		IR	4.5 mg/kg	
	Swine	PO	3–4.5 mg/kg	
	Sheep	PO	5 mg/kg	
	Goat	PO	7.5 mg/kg	
Oxibendazole (Anthelcide EQ®)	Horse	PO	10–15 mg/kg	
	Cattle	PO	10–20 mg/kg	
	Swine	PO	15 mg/kg	
	Sheep	PO	10–20 mg/kg	
Nicotine-like nematocides				
Levamisole (Levasole®, Tramisol®)	Cattle	PO	5.5–11 mg/kg	
		SC	3.3–8 mg/kg	
		Topical	9 mg/kg	
	Swine	PO	8 mg/kg	
	Sheep, goat	PO	8 mg/kg	
Pyrantel pamoate (Nemex®, etc.) (Strongid-T®)	Dog			
	<2.5 kg	PO	10 mg/kg	
	>2.5 kg	PO	5 mg/kg	
	Cat	PO	20 mg/kg	
	Horse	PO	6.6 mg/kg	
Pyrantel tartrate (Strongid-C®) (Banminth®)	Horse	In feed	2.6 mg/kg q24h	
	Swine	In feed	22 mg/kg	
	Sheep, goat	In feed	25 mg/kg	
Morantel (Rumatel®)	Cattle	In feed	8.8–9.7 mg/kg	
	Sheep, goat	In feed	10 mg/kg	
Macrocyclic lactones				
Doramectin (Dectomax®, Dectomax Pour-On®)	Dog	SC	600 mcg/kg q1wk	Demodicosis
	Cat	SC	200 mcg/kg	
	Cattle	SC, IM	200 mcg/kg	
		Topical	500 mcg/kg	
	Swine	IM	300 mcg/kg	

(continued)

Name of drugs	Species	Route	Dose	Notes
Eprinomectin (Eprinex®)	Cattle	Topical	1 mL (5 mg)/10 kg	
Ivermectin (Ivomec®)	Dog	SC, PO	0.2–0.4 mg/kg	May not be safe
	Cat	SC	0.4 mg/kg	*Aelurostrongylus abstrusus*
	Horse	PO	0.2 mg/kg	
	Cattle	SC	0.2 mg/kg	
	Swine	SC	0.3 mg/kg	
	Sheep, goat	SC	0.2 mg/kg	
Milbemycin (Interceptor®, Sentinel®)	Dog	PO	0.5–2 mg/kg q24h for ≥3 months	Demodicosis
		PO	2 mg/kg q7d for 3 doses	Cheyletiellosis, scabies
	Cat	PO	2 mg/kg q1month	
Moxidectin (Proheart®)	Dog	PO	0.2 mg/kg	
(Advantage Multi®)	Dog	Topical	2.5 mg/kg	+ Imidacloprid
	Cat	Topical	1 mg/kg	
(Quest®)	Horse	PO	0.4 mg/kg	
(Cydectin®)	Cattle	Topical	0.5 mg/kg	
Selamectin (Revolution®)	Dog, cat	Topical	6 mg/kg	
Miscellaneous nematocides				
Dichlorvos (Atgard® C)	Swine	In feed	11.2–21.6 mg/kg once	
Emodepside + Praziquantel (Profender®)	Cat			
0.5–2.5 kg		Topical	0.35 mL (7.5 mg/30 mg)	
2.5–5 kg		Topical	0.7 mL (15 mg/60 mg)	
5–8 kg		Topical	1.12 mL (24 mg/95.8 mg)	
Piperazine (Pipa-Tabs®, etc.)	Dog, cat	PO	44–100 mg/kg	
	Horse	PO	88–110 mg/kg	
	Swine	PO	110 mg/kg	
		In feed	0.2–0.4%	
Drugs for Heartworm control				
Ivermectin (Ivomec®) (Heartgard®)	Dog	PO, SC	50 mcg/kg	
		PO	6–12 mcg/kg, q1month	Microfilaricide
	Cat	PO	24 mcg/kg q30–45d	
Melarsomine (Immiticide®)	Dog	Lumbar muscle	2.5 mg/kg twice 24h apart	Adulticide
Milbemycin (Interceptor®)	Dog	PO	0.5 mg/kg q1month	
		PO	0.5 mg/kg for 2 wk	Microfilaricide
	Cat	PO	2 mg/kg q1month	
Moxidectin (Advantage Multi®)	Dog, cat	PO	3 mcg/kg q1month	
	Dog	Topical	2.5 mg/kg q1month	+ Imidacloprid
	Cat	Topical	1 mg/kg q1month	
Selamectin (Revolution®)	Dog, cat	Topical	6 mg/kg q1month	
Anticestodal drugs				
Albendazole (Valbazen®, Albenza®)	Dog, cat	PO	25–50 mg/kg q12h for 3–5d	
	Cattle	PO	7.5–15 mg/kg	
	Sheep, goat	PO	7.5–15 mg/kg	

(Continued)

Name of drugs	Species	Route	Dose	Notes
Fenbendazole (Panacur®, Safe-Guard®)	Dog	PO	50 mg/kg/d for 3d	
	Cat	PO	50 mg/kg/d for 5d	
	Cattle	PO	5–10 mg/kg	
	Sheep, goat	PO	5 mg/kg for 3d	
Oxfendazole (Synanthic®)	Cattle	PO	4.5 mg/kg	
	Sheep	PO	5 mg/kg	
	Goat	PO	7.5 mg/kg	
Dichlorophene	Dog, cat	PO	100 mg/kg	
Epsiprantel (Cestex®)	Dog	PO	5.5 mg/kg	
	Cat	PO	2.75 mg/kg	
Praziquantel (Droncit®, Drontal®)	Dog			
	<6.8 kg	PO	7.5 mg/kg	
	≥ 6.8kg	PO	5 mg/kg	
	≤ 2.3kg	IM, SC	7.5 mg/kg	
	2.7 – 4.5 kg	IM, SC	6.3 mg/kg	
	>5 kg	IM, SC	5 mg/kg	
	Cat			
	<1.8 kg	PO	6.3 mg/kg	
	≥ 1.8kg	PO	5 mg/kg	
		IM, SC	5 mg/kg	
			2.5 mg/kg 18h for 2d	Paragonimiasis
	Horse	PO	0.5–1 mg/kg	
	Sheep, goat		10–15 mg/kg	
Pyrantel pamoate (Strongid-T®, etc.)	Horse	PO	13.2 mg/kg	

Drugs for control of liver flukes

Name of drugs	Species	Route	Dose	Notes
Albendazole (Valbazen®, Albenza®)	Cattle	PO	10 mg/kg	
Clorsulon (Curatrem®, Ivomec Plus®)	Cattle, sheep	PO	7 mg/kg	
		SC	2 mg/kg	+ Ivermectin

Antiprotozoal drugs
Anticoccidial agents

Name of drugs	Species	Route	Dose	Notes
Amprolium (Corid®, Amprovine®)	Dog	PO	100 mg in gelatin capsule q24h for 7–12d	Prophylaxis
		idw	30 mL of 9.6% solution/gallon (3.8 L)	
		In food	1.25 g of 20% powder	
	Cat	PO	60–100 mg total dose q24h for 7d	Prophylaxis
	Cattle	PO	10 mg/kg for 5d 5 mg/kg for 21d	Prophylaxis
	Swine	PO	25–65 mg/kg q12–24h for 3–4d	Prophylaxis
	Sheep, goat	PO	55 mg/kg q24h for 19d	Prophylaxis

(continued)

(Continued)

Name of drugs	Species	Route	Dose	Notes
	Chicken	In feed	0.012–0.024% for 3–5d	Prophylaxis
Clopidol (Coyden®)	Chicken	In feed	0.0125–0.025%	Prophylaxis
	Turkey	In feed	0.0125–0.025%	
Decoquinate (Deccox®, etc.)	Dog	PO	50 mg/kg q24h	Prophylaxis
	Cattle	In feed	0.5 mg/kg/d for ≥ 28d	Prophylaxis
	Sheep, goat	In feed	0.5 mg/kg/d during periods of exposure	Prophylaxis
	Chicken	In feed	60 g/ton	Prophylaxis
Diclazuril (Clinacox®)	Chicken	In feed	1 ppm	Prophylaxis. Can also be used for treatment
	Mammals	PO	2.5 mg/kg towards the age of 4 wk, to be renewed 15d later, prn	Can be used for treatment
Ponazuril	Mammals	PO	40–50 mg/kg	Treatment
Nicarbazin + Narasin	Chicken	In feed	27–45 g/ton each of narasin and nicarbazin	Prophylaxis
Pyrimethamine (Daraprim®)	Dog	PO	1 mg/kg q24h for 14–28d	5d for *Neosporum*
	Cat	PO	0.5–1 mg/kg q24h for 14–28d	
	Horse	PO	0.25 mg/kg q12h for 3d then q24h for 27d	
Robenidine (Robenz®)	Chicken	In feed	30 g/ton (0.0033%)	Prophylaxis
Ionophores				
Lasalocid (Bovatec®)	Cattle	In feed	1 mg/kg/d	Prophylaxis
Avatec®	Chicken Turkeys Rabbits	In feed	0.0075–0.0125%	Prophylaxis
Monensin (Coban® 60)	Chicken	In feed	90–110 g/ton	Prophylaxis
Rumensin® 80	Cattle	In feed	0.30–0.92 mg/kg/d	Prophylaxis
	Goat	In feed	0.30–2.2 mg/kg/d	Prophylaxis
Narasin (Maxiban® 72)	Chicken	In feed	27–45 g/ton	Prophylaxis
Salinomycin (Sacox® 60)	Chicken	In feed	40–60 g/ton	Prophylaxis
Sulfonamides				
Sulfadimethoxine-ormetoprim	Chicken	In feed	0.0125% sulfadimethoxine + 0.0075% ormetoprim	Prophylaxis and treatment
(Rofenaid®)	Turkey	In feed	0.00625% sulfadimethoxine + 0.00375% ormetoprim	
(Primor®)	Mammals	PO	55 mg/kg (combined drug) on d1, then 27.5 mg/kg, q24h.	Treatment of coccidiosis. Kittens may need lower dosage
Sulfamethazine	Chicken	In feed	128–187 mg/kg/d	
	Turkey	In feed	110–273 mg/kg/d	

(Continued)

Name of drugs	Species	Route	Dose	Notes
	Cattle	In feed	237.6 mg/kg (d1), 118.8 mg/kg (d2, d3, d4)	
	Swine	In feed	237.6 mg/kg (d1), 118.8 mg/kg (d2, d3, d4)	
Sulfaquinoxaline	Chicken	idw	0.04% for 2–3d then 0.025% for 2d more	
	Turkey	idw	0.025% for 2d–skip 3d– give for 2d—skip 3d and give 2d more	
	Cattle	idw	0.015% for 3–5d	
Zoalene (Zoamix®)	Chicken	In feed	0.0083–0.0125%	
	Turkey	In feed	0.0083–0.0125%	
EPM control				
Diclazuril (Protazil®)	Horse	PO	2.5 mg/kg q12h ≥ of 21d	
Nitazoxanide (Navigator®)	Horse	PO (d 1–5) PO (d 6–28)	25 mg/kg q24h 50 mg/kg q24h	
Ponazuril (Marquis®)	Horse	PO	5 mg/kg q24h for 28d	
Giardiasis control				
Albendazole (Valbazen®, Albenza®)	Dog, cat	PO	25 mg/kg q12h for 2d	
Fenbendazole (Panacur®)	Dog, cat	PO	25 mg/kg q12h for 2d	
Metronidazole (Flagyl®)	Dog	PO	50–65 mg/kg q24h for 5–7d	
	Cat	PO	50 mg/kg q24h for 5d	
Toxoplasmosis control				
Clindamycin (Clincaps®)	Dog, cat	PO, IM	10–20 mg/kg q12h for 4 wk	
Pyrimethamine-sulfadiazine	Dog	PO	0.25–0.5 mg/kg of Pyrimethamine, 30 mg/kg of sulfadiazine for 28d	
Trimethoprim-sulfadiazine (Tribrissen®)	Dog	PO	15 mg/kg q12h for 28d	
Cryptosporidiosis control				
Azithromycin (Zithromax®)	Dog	PO	15 mg/kg q12h for ≥ 7d	
	Cat	PO	15 mg/kg q12h for ≥ 7d	
	Horse	PO	10 mg/kg q24h	
Nitazoxanide (Navigator®)	Horse	PO	5 mg/kg q24h for 28d	
Paromomycin (Humatin®)	Dog	PO	50 mg/kg q12h for 10d	
	Cat	PO	50 mg/kg q12h for 10d	

(continued)

Name of drugs	Species	Route	Dose	Notes
Babesiosis control				
Imidocarb (Imizol®)	Dog	IM, SC	5–6.6 mg/kg repeat in 2 wk	
		IM, SC	5 mg/kg repeat in 14–21d	Ehrlichiosis
	Cat	IM	5 mg/kg repeat in 14d	*Cytauxzoon felis*
	Horse	IM	2.2 mg/kg	
	Sheep	IM	1.2 mg/kg; repeat in 10–14d	
Ectoparasiticides				
Insect development inhibitors				
Diflubenzuron (Dimilin®, Equitrol® II)	Horse	In feed	0.15 mg/kg/d	
Lufenuron (Program®)	Dog	PO	10 mg/kg q1month	
	Cat	PO	30 mg/kg q1month	
Insect nicotinic receptor agonists				
Imidacloprid (Advantage®)	Dog, cat	Topical	5–10 mg/kg q1month	
Nitenpyram (Capstar®)	Dog, cat	PO	1 mg/kg	
Spinosad (Comfortis®)	Dog, cat	PO	30 mg/kg q1month	
Fipronil (Frontline®)	Dog, cat	Topical	6.5–13 mg/kg q1month	

Chapter 17: Antineoplastic Drugs

Name of drugs	Species	Route	Dose	Notes
Alkylating agents				
Nitrogen mustards				
Chlorambucil (Leukeran®)	Dog	PO	2–6 mg/m^2 q24–48h	
		PO	20 mg/m^2 q1–2 wk	
	Cat	PO	2–6 mg/m^2 q48h or 20 mg/m^2 q2–3 wk	
	Horse	PO	20 mg/m^2 q2wk	
Cyclophosphamide (Cytoxan®)	Dog	PO	50 mg/m^2 q48h	
		PO	50 mg/m^2 q24h, 4d/wk	
		IV	100–300 mg/m^2 repeat in 2d	
	Cat	PO	200 mg/m^2 q2–3 wk	
Mechlorethamine (Mustargen®)	Dog	IV, IC	5 mg/m^2, repeat prn	
	Cat	IV	3 mg/m^2	
Melphalan (Alkeran®)	Dog	PO	0.05–0.1 mg/kg q24h for 10d; then 2–4 mg/m^2 q48h	
	Cat	PO	2 mg/m^2 q48h	
Nitroureas				
Busulfan (Myleran®)	Dog, cat	PO	3–4 mg/m^2 q24h	
		PO	0.1–0.2 mg/kg q24h	
Carmustine (BiCNU®)	Dog, cat	IV	50 mg/m^2 q6wk	
Dacarbazine (DTIC-Dome®)	Dog	IV	200–250 mg/m^2 q24h for 5d; repeat cycle q3wk	
		IV slowly	800–1000 mg/m^2 over 4–6h q3wk	

Name of drugs	Species	Route	Dose	Notes
Hydroxyurea (Hydrea®)	Dog	PO	30–50 mg/kg q24–48h	
	Cat	PO	25 mg/kg q24–48h	
Ifosfamide (Ifex®)	Dog <10 kg	IV	350 mg/m²	
	Dog >10 kg	IV	375 mg/m²	
	Cat	IV	350–500 mg/m²	
Lomustine (CCNU, CeeNU®)	Dog	PO	60–90 mg/m² q3–4 wk	
	Cat	PO	60 mg/m² q6wk	
Procarbazine (Matulane®)	Dog	PO	25–50 mg/m² q24h	
	Cat	PO	50 mg/m² q24h	
Streptozocin (Zanosar®)	Dog	IV	500 mg/m²	
Platinating agents				
Carboplatin (Paraplatin®)	Dog	IV	250–300 mg/m² q3–4 wk	
	Cat	IV	150–250 mg/m² q4wk	
Cisplatin (Platinol-AQ®)	Dog	IV, IC	50–70 mg/m² q3–4 wk	
	Do not use in cat			
Antimetabolites				
Azathioprine (Imuran®)	Dog	PO	50 mg/m² q12–48h	
		PO	2 mg/kg q24h initially, then 0.5–1.0 mg/kg q48h	
	Cat	PO	0.3 – 0.5 mg/kg q48h	
	Horse	PO	2–5 mg/kg q24h loading dose, then q48h for maintenance	
Cytosine arabinoside (Cytarabine®, CytosarU®)	Dog	IV, SC	100 mg/m² q24h for 4d; repeat prn	
	Cat	IV, SC	100 mg/m² q24h for 2d; repeat prn	
	Horse	IM, SC	200–300 mg/m² q1–2 wk with chlorambucil or cyclophosphamide	
5-Fluorouracil (5-FU®, Adrucil®)	Dog	IV, IC	150–200 mg/m² q1wk	
	Contraindicated in cats in any form			
Gemcitabine (Gemzar®)	Dog	IV	300 mg/m² administered over 25–30 min q1wk for 3–4 wk, then 1 wk break	
	Cat	IV	200 mg/m² in maintenance saline over 20 min	
6-Mercaptopurine (Purinethol®)	Dog	PO	50 mg/m² q24h to effect; then q48h or prn	

(*continued*)

(Continued)

Name of drugs	Species	Route	Dose	Notes
Methotrexate (Rheumatrex Dose Pack®)	Dog	PO	2.5 mg/m^2 q24h or 2–3 times/wk	
		IV	15–20 mg/m^2 q3wk	
	Cat	PO	2.5 mg/m^2 2–3 times/wk	
6-Thioguanine (Thioguanine Tabloid®)	Dog	PO	40 mg/m^2 q24h for 4–5d; then 40 mg/m^2 q3d	
	Cat	PO	25 mg/m^2 q24h for 1–5d; then repeat cycle q30d prn	
Mitotic spindle inhibitors				
Antibiotics				
Actinomycin D (Dactinomycin®)	Dog, cat	IV	0.7–1 mg/m^2 q3wk	
Doxorubicin (Adriamycin RDF®, Doxil®)	Dog			
≤ 10kg		IV	20–25 mg/m^2 q3wk	
≥ 10kg		IV	30 mg/m^2 q3wk	
	Cat	IV	20–25 mg/m^2 q3wk	
Mitoxantrone (Novantrone®, Mitoxal®)	Dog	IV	5 mg/m^2 q3wk	
	Cat	IV	5–6.5 mg/m^2 q3wk	
Taxane				
Paclitaxel (Taxol®)	Dog, cat	IV	5 mg/kg	
Vinblastine (Velban®)	Dog	IV	1–3 mg/m^2 q1wk	
	Cat	IV	2 mg/m^2 q1–2 wk	
Vincristine (Vincasar PFS®)	Dog	IV	0.5–1.0 mg/m^2 q1–2 wk	
	Cat	IV	0.5–0.75 mg/m^2 q1wk	
	Horse	IV	0.01–0.025 mg/kg q1wk	
Enzymes				
L-Asparaginase (Elspar®)	Dog	IM, IP, SC	400 IU/kg q1wk, for 3 wk or 10,000 IU/m^2 q1wk for 3 wk	
	Cat	IM, IP, SC	400 IU/kg q1wk, in combination with other protocols	
Miscellaneous				
Piroxicam (Feldene®)	Dog	PO	0.3 mg/kg q24h	
	Cat	PO	0.3 mg/kg q48h	
Mitotane (O,P′-DDD) (Lysodren®)	Dog	PO	50–75 mg/kg q24h divided for 10d to effect; then 75–100 mg/kg q3–7d prn	Adrenal tumor
Bleomycin (Blenoxane®)	Dog, cat	IV, SC	10–15 IU/m^2 q24h for 3–4d; then 10–15 IU/m^2 q7d	

Abbreviations: CRI, constant rate infusion; d, day(s); g, gram(s); h, hour(s); idw, in drinking water; IM, intramuscular; IP, intraperitoneal; IR, intraruminal; IU, international unit; IV, intravenous; MAC, minimal alveolar concentration; mcg, microgram(s); mg, milligram(s); min, minute(s); ng, nanogram(s); PO, *per os* (orally); ppm, parts per million; prn, *pro re nata* (when required); q, *qua'que* (every); SC, subcutaneous; tsp, teaspoon(s); wk, week(s).

Index

Note: Page numbers followed by (a) denote appendices, those by (f) denote figures, those by (t) denote tables, those by (q) denote study questions, and those by (e) denote explanations